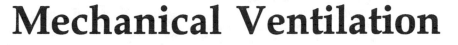

Mechanical Ventilation

Physiological and Clinical Applications

SUSAN P. PILBEAM, M.S., R.R.T.
Program Director, Respiratory Therapy Program
Greenville Technical College
Greenville, South Carolina

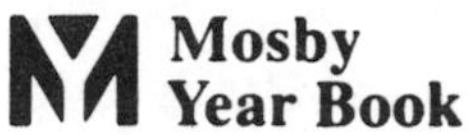
Mosby
Year Book

St. Louis Baltimore Boston Chicago London Philadelphia Sydney Toronto

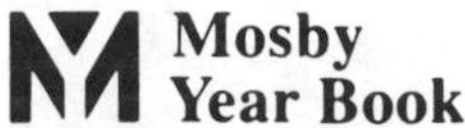

Dedicated to Publishing Excellence

Sponsoring Editor: David K. Marshall
Assistant Editor: Julie Tryboski
Assistant Managing Editor, Text and Reference: George Mary Gardner
Production Manager: Nancy C. Baker
Proofroom Manager: Barbara Kelly

Mosby–Year Book, Inc.
11830 Westline Industrial Drive
St. Louis, MO 63146

4 5 6 7 8 9 0 GW/PP 96

Library of Congress Cataloging-in-Publication Data
Pilbeam, Susan P., 1945–
Mechanical ventilation / Susan P. Pilbeam. —2nd ed.
p. cm.
Includes bibliographical references and index.
ISBN 0-8016-6360-1
1. Respiratory therapy. 2. Respirators. I. Title.
[DNLM: 1. Respiration, Artificial. WF 145 P637m]
RC735.I5P55 1992
617.5'40636–dc20
DNLM/DLC 92-18793
for Library of Congress CIP

MECHANICAL VENTILATION

Physiological and Clinical Applications

This book is dedicated to the pioneers—the respiratory therapists of the late 1960s and early 1970s—who "braved new frontiers." They were and are unique in their esprit de corps and unprecedented in their achievements.

Contributors

Thomas D. Baxter, B.S., R.R.T.
Director of Accelerated Programs
Respiratory Therapy
Greenville Technical College
Greenville, South Carolina

Robert L. Chatburn, R.R.T.
Director, Pediatric Respiratory Care
Rainbow Babies and Childrens Hospital
Cleveland, Ohio

Theresa Gramlich, M.S., R.R.T.
Respiratory Therapy Program
University of Arkansas for Medical Sciences
Little Rock, Arkansas

Cathleen Patterson, M.S.N., R.N.
Education Coordinator
Department of Professional Relations
Rainbow Babies and Childrens Hospital
Frances Payne Bolton School of Nursing
Case Western Reserve University
Cleveland, Ohio

Susan P. Pilbeam, M.S., R.R.T.
Program Director, Respiratory Therapy Program
Greenville Technical College
Greenville, South Carolina

David C. Shelledy, Ph.D., R.R.T.
Director of Respiratory Care
Athens Area Technical Institute
Athens, Georgia

Foreword

To someone new to respiratory care in the 1990s, whether in training for respiratory therapy, nursing, or medicine, this field presents a formidable array of electromechanical apparatuses, complex procedures, and unfamiliar technology. Its rapid evolution and ever-expanding list of acronyms can intimidate even the experienced clinician. And of the areas within respiratory care, none is more conceptually confusing, technically daunting, or rapidly changing than mechanical ventilation.

Here is a compact yet comprehensive guide to mechanical ventilation. Starting with a historical survey of the landmark developments in ventilatory support, it then defines mechanical ventilation's basic terms and concepts and reviews the principles of arterial blood gas interpretation by which mechanical ventilation is guided. After this introduction the book systematically covers the "nuts and bolts" of the topic: indications; basic physical aspects and concepts; modes; choice of tidal volumes, rates, and flows; and the potential effects, good and bad, of mechanical ventilation on the patient. Other chapters cover both invasive and noninvasive assessment and monitoring, available methods for augmenting oxygenation, and weaning from ventilatory support. The exclusive but important subjects of neonatal ventilatory support and home mechanical ventilation are addressed in separate chapters. Finally, a series of appendixes provides useful protocols, lists, formulas, and reference data on current ventilators. The book is written in a clear, direct style, and its chapters are organized to facilitate comprehension and the ready location of information.

Management of patients with mechanical ventilation can bring out two bedside phenomena that can render patient care suboptimal and also threaten the vital working relationship between respiratory care practitioner and physician. These 1990s phenomena are the *technology gap* and the *communication gap*. The technology gap can develop because ventilators and their modes have become so complex and changed so rapidly that physicians may not understand fully the implications of the therapy they order; the communication gap can result from reluctance on the part of some respiratory care practitioners to discuss suboptimal ventilator settings with ordering physicians. Both phenomena also can work in reverse, that is, with therapists being insufficiently familiar with the ventilators or modes they are using and physicians failing to explain to those at the bedside the rationale or intended effects of the therapy ordered. In most instances a common thread is an incomplete familiarity with the definitions, modes, procedures, physiologic effects, and complications described in this book. Mastery of the material contained herein can make ventilator management safer, less uncomfortable, and more clinically appropriate and can facilitate the teamwork that is so vital to effective respiratory care.

DAVID J. PIERSON, M.D.
Professor of Medicine
University of Washington School of Medicine
Medical Director
Respiratory Care
Harborview Medical Center
Seattle, Washington

Preface

Mechanical Ventilation: Physiologic and Clinical Applications, originally part of the Faculty Lecture Series in Respiratory Care, is a textbook on ventilatory management in the critically ill adult patient. As in the past, it is intended to be used as an educational tool by health care practitioners involved in caring for patients who require mechanical ventilatory support, that is, students in respiratory care programs, respiratory care practitioners, nurse clinicians, medical students, and pulmonary fellows. It is assumed that the reader already has a working knowledge of respiratory anatomy and physiology, pulmonary diseases, and arterial blood gas interpretation, although some of these areas are reviewed briefly in the text.

One of the most difficult tasks facing a respiratory care educator is teaching the concepts involved in mechanical ventilation. What in part makes this so difficult is the rapidly expanding knowledge base. In the early 1970s there were five ventilators commonly used by hospitals; that number has expanded to more than 50, and their function can change on an annual basis. When ventilators were introduced there were two basic methods of ventilation; now there are as many as 10, depending on how you count them.

The intent of this text is to make the basic concepts of ventilation as simple as possible and at the same time remain true to the current medical literature. I wanted to keep it simple without distorting the scientific truth through the simplicity. Every effort was made to make the reading level easier by using shorter sentences and simpler words whenever possible. I want to thank Mary Watson for her studies on reading levels, which made me more aware of this problem in respiratory care textbooks.

Although the basic format remains the same as in the original text, some additional information and chapters have been added. Greater emphasis has been placed on the use of graphic representations of volume, pressure, flow, and time curves, in keeping with the newer CRT monitoring capabilities of the newer microprocessor-controlled ventilators. The methods of pressure support, pressure control, and other recently developed ventilatory techniques are emphasized throughout the text. Chapter 5, which covers physical aspects of mechanical ventilation, now encompasses a more up-to-date method of ventilator classification that makes it easier to include the current generation of ventilators. This is in thanks to Rob Chatburn, who has been a major influence in respiratory care literature in this area.

There is now a separate chapter on noninvasive gas monitoring and calculation of shunt and dead space (Chapter 9). Methods for improving oxygenation are contained in Chapter 10; these include positive end-expiratory pressure (PEEP), continuous positive airway pressure (CPAP), and inverse ratio ventilation (IRV). IRV is a fairly new and still experimental form of ventilation in the adult patient; for this reason, it is covered here.

Chapter 11 is new in this edition and covers the basics of hemodynamic monitoring. A brief review of related terms (e.g., cardiac output, stroke volume, preload, afterload, contractility, and vascular resistance) is provided. The indications, use, and hazards of the pulmonary artery catheter are included. Pulmonary vascular pressure, both normal and abnormal, also is discussed. It was not intended that this chapter replace a textbook on hemodynamic monitoring but provide a basic understanding, particularly for students who do not have the luxury of taking a course in this content area.

In addition to traditional methods of weaning, Chapter 12 also describes use of intermittent mandatory ventilation (IMV), synchronous intermittent mandatory ventilation (SIMV), pressure support, and mandatory minute ventilation as methods of discontinuation and weaning from ventilator support.

Mechanical ventilation in adult patients is the primary focus of the text, but in this second edition the decision was made to add a chapter to cover some basic concepts in neonatal and pediatric assessment, resuscitation, and ventilation. The purpose is to provide the general respiratory care practitioner with enough information to be able to identify an infant in respiratory distress, provide resuscitation efforts, and initiate ventilatory support.

Finally, Chapter 14 on home mechanical ventilation was added to the text to cover this very rapidly growing and important area. It includes discussions of negative pressure ventilation, CPAP, and bilevel PEEP (inspiratory and expiratory positive airway pressure).

The original text ended with a chapter on high-frequency ventilation. This has been deleted, primarily because this mode of ventilation has not become widely used. Its use still is experimental and restricted primarily to infants. Future research may reveal its greatest application and promote greater use.

With the exception of Appendix M, there is little to no discussion of specific ventilators. I wanted to write only about "how to" and not "with what." It is difficult to impossible to write a text on the current ventilators in use and being added to use without being out of date by the time the text is printed. I'll leave this to those more courageous than I.

SUSAN P. PILBEAM, M.S., R.R.T.

Acknowledgments

This book would not have been possible without the support of many of my colleagues and friends. I would especially like to thank the following persons for reviewing my work: Tom Baxter, B.S., R.R.T.; Robin Chatburn, R.R.T.; Lisa Conry, M.S., R.R.T.; Deborah David, Vijay Deshpande, M.S., R.R.T.; Robert Kacmarek, Ph.D., R.R.T.; Wanda Perry, M.In.Ed., R.R.T.; Anthony Rogers, Deborah Turk, B.S., R.R.T.; and James Woody, B.S., R.R.T. Special thanks go to my editor, David Marshall, who has made this difficult task a pleasant experience.

I am grateful to Patricia Travis for both her help with word processing and her artwork. Thanks for artwork also to Deborah Reynolds.

Finally, special thanks go to all the students through all these years who have taught me so much. "All education is self-education. A teacher is only a guide to point out the way, and no school, no matter how excellent, can give you an education" (Louis L'Amour, *The Lonesome Gods*, Bantam Books, 1983).

SUSAN P. PILBEAM, M.S., R.R.T.

Acknowledgments

Contents

Chapter **1**

History of Mechanical Ventilation

On completion of this chapter the reader will be able to:

1. State the historical influence of Hippocrates, Aristotle, Galen, Paracelsus, and Hooke on the theory of respiration and breathing.
2. List chronologically seven events that influenced the development of resuscitation techniques from 1744 through the early 1900s.
3. Name the three persons responsible for the development of the first successful negative pressure iron lung–type ventilator.
4. Describe the methods used to provide an airway and ventilate the lungs in polio victims in the 1952 polio epidemic of Copenhagen.
5. State the influence of each of the following persons on the development of the artificial airway and techniques for its insertion: Smellie, Fothergill, Jackson, Macewen and Kirstein, Tuffier and Hallion, Fell and O'Dwyer, and Matas.
6. Explain the use of the negative pressure chamber developed by Sauerbruch and its later adaptation by Brauer.

7. Name the early positive pressure ventilators developed in the 1940s and 1950s.
8. Discuss the development of IPPB devices as designed by Bennett and Bird in the 1940s and 1950s.
9. Describe the early development of PEEP and CPAP from its early inception by Barach to its use in the early 1970s.
10. Explain the development of IMV and high-frequency ventilation.

HISTORY OF MECHANICAL VENTILATION

Before one begins a text on mechanical ventilation it seems appropriate to provide some background or history to the reader. The main reason for doing this is to give an insight into how historical discovery often preceded clinical adaptation of a technique—not by days but usually by decades.

Perhaps the best example of this is in cardiopulmonary resuscitation. Andreas Vesalius wrote a report of successful resuscitation in an animal in 1555. Because of human prejudice, lack of insight, and unadaptability, it took 400 years before this technique was put into practice. Dr. James M. Hurst put it aptly in his article in *Respiratory Care:*

> Quite simply, all new techniques, be they mechanical ventilatory support or other technological advances, are time-intensive until sufficient familiarity with these techniques allows routine application. Likewise, ridicule and lack of acceptance frequently precede the accepted application of any new technique.[16]

History not only informs us of where we have been, but often predicts the place to which we will return. The so-called modern techniques touted today as new ideas are often remnants of past innovations, forgotten or ignored at their inception either because they were ahead of their time or because their importance was not yet realized.

There is often in medicine, as in other aspects of human life, "nothing new under the sun." What are presented as new discoveries are most likely many years old. It is just the unfortunate human condition that often prevents us from adapting to genuinely new ideas for a very long time. Nowhere is this more true than in the arena of medical care.

EARLY HISTORY

Descriptions on the theory of respiration and air appear in the early writings of the Egyptian, Chinese, and Greek peoples. The act of artificially inducing pressure breathing into another person is documented as far back as the Old

Testament, written around 800 B.C.: "The prophet Elisha went up and lay upon the child, and put his mouth on his mouth, and his eyes on his eyes, and his hands upon his hands, and stretched himself upon him, and the flesh of the child became warm . . . the child sneezed seven times and opened his eyes" (II Kings 4:34–35). While this may be stretching the interpretation, it seems a reasonable speculation that resuscitation did occur.

Hippocrates (c. 460–375 B.C.) gave an early description of what he thought was the function of breathing in his "Treatise on Air." He describes the treatment for situations where suffocation was imminent: "One should introduce a cannula into the trachea along the jawbone so that the air can be drawn into the lungs."[8, 15] This is probably the first written instance of endotracheal intubation. Aristotle (384–322 B.C.) noticed that animals placed in airtight boxes died. He thought this was because they could not cool themselves. While his deduction was incorrect, his experiments did demonstrate that fresh air was essential for maintaining life.

Galen, a Greek physician of the second century A.D., was well known. His teachings were followed for centuries after his death. He had done extensive study of anatomy by dissecting dogs, pigs, apes, and oxen. His assumption was that human anatomy was similar. For example, the ape has a segmented sternum, and for centuries it was believed that humans did also.

For 1,300 years after Galen, religious and political influence forbade the dissection and scientific study of the human body. Punishment for such activity was death by burning at the stake. Galen's statements were accepted as they were, without question. No wonder they call it the Dark Ages. It took a few brave souls in the 16th century to finally start turning things around.

In experimenting with lung function, Paracelsus (1493–1541) used a fire bellows connected to a tube inserted in a patient's mouth as a device for assisting in ventilation. This 1530 study credits him with the first form of mechanical ventilation. Around the same time (c. 1541–1564), Vesalius tried introducing a reed into an animal's trachea, and through resuscitation managed to successfully restore a dying animal's heart beat. Vesalius' resuscitation efforts were simple intermittent positive pressure ventilation (IPPV).

Actually, Vesalius was quite a character. He was the first person we know of to brave the potential grave consequences and perform dissection on human cadavers. His report of illustrated human anatomy comprised seven volumes and was the first accurate description of the human body. However, his colleagues were not very accepting or appreciative of his efforts. Story has it that Vesalius had to make a pilgrimage to the Holy Land to avoid punishment for his "crimes" and that he died during the journey. Dr. E. Trier Mörch provides a wonderful early history of Vesalius for the interested reader.[17]

Another early explorer of ventilation was Robert Hooke (1635–1703). Hooke was interested in establishing the exact cause of death when the thorax was opened during surgery. He experimented with dogs and found that he was able to sustain an animal's life by using a fire bellows connected to an opening cut into the trachea below the epiglottis. He could maintain ventilation even when the animal's thorax was opened. It was thought previously that it was the movement of the thorax that prevented asphyxiation. He further examined his hypothesis by cutting a hole into the lung while the thorax was open and supplying a constant flow of air through the trachea and into the lung by using two bellows instead of one. The constant airflow kept the lung inflated adequately to sustain life and maintain a regular heart beat. Hooke concluded that it was not the motionlessness of the lungs or thorax that resulted in death; rather it was the cessation of fresh airflow into the lungs.

This case of an induced pneumothorax is similar to that of a patient treated in a Washington hospital in 1990 who had suffered severe trauma and had developed a pneumothorax. The staff was able to successfully ventilate the patient's lungs despite large air leaks through an open lung injury. Testing the gases that escaped from the chest tube, they found these gases high in carbon dioxide. It was like having another airway for the removal of carbon dioxide.

The patient lived, and eventually left the hospital. More than 300 years after Hooke we again see an example of exactly what he was talking about. While the presence of an open pneumothorax might have prevented adequate ventilation and even caused death, it was intuitively discovered to be another route for the flow of air through the lungs.[1]

RESUSCITATION

In spite of Hooke's presentation of his material to the Royal Society of England in 1667, nearly two centuries passed before his theory was applied to human surgery. It was another 100 years before John Fothergill of England (1744) reported a successful case of mouth-to-mouth resuscitation. Fothergill speculated that a bellows also could be used for the same purpose. Since the thought of touching the dead was not widely accepted at the time, no further attempts were made at mouth-to-mouth resuscitation until about 1750.

The Dutch were more aggressive about taking steps to try to save drowning victims.[13] Considering the number of waterways around Amsterdam and the countryside, this is not surprising. In 1767 the Dutch formed the Society for the Rescue of Drowned Persons, or the Humane Society. One of the more progressive findings was to keep the victim warm, give mouth-to-mouth breathing, and compress the chest and stomach to assist exhalation. Another technique was to blow tobacco smoke into the rectum and lower bowel of the victim. Saving effort also included "bleeding" by lancing the jugular vein, induced vomiting by giving ipecacuanha wines, and inducing sneezing by the use of "spirit of quicklime" in the nostrils.[17]

John Hunter of London in 1775 developed a double bellows system for resuscitation, one for blowing air in and the second for drawing the bad air out.

He also recommended the use of finger pressure over the larynx to help prevent gastric inflation with air. This technique was adapted for patient use by the Royal Humane Society in 1782 and started another trend in early ventilation.

E. Coleman of Scotland recommended a silver catheter for tracheal intubation that was much wider than those used before. Bellows were used for inspiration and a bleed-in for oxygen. He also recommended application of electrical current by electrodes placed over the apex and base of the heart.

Other scientists who explored the use of artificial respiration and published their works included Edmund Goodwyn of London (1786) and Lord Daniel Herholdt and Carl Gottlob Rafn (1796) of Copenhagen, who scientifically explored and reported methods of resuscitation that have application today. However, not many people read Danish, and it was another 150 years before the Danes' work, "Life-Saving Measures for Drowning Persons," received any real recognition.[17]

In 1911, Dräger designed an artificial breathing device that was used for resuscitation by fire and police units. The Dräger pulmotor held the head of the victim in the head-tilt position. Pressure by the operator on the cricoid cartilage helped prevent gastric inflation. A mask held on the face along with correct positioning of the head provided an airway. Inflation was accomplished with positive pressure. The device was powered by a compressed gas cylinder, and operation was essentially automatic[25] (Fig 1–1).

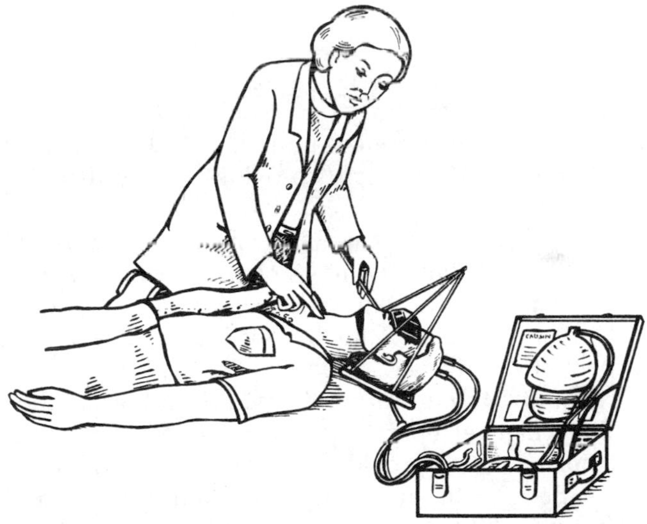

FIG 1–1.
The Dräger pulmotor (1911) used for resuscitation and powered by compressed air. (Redrawn from Mushin WL, Rendell-Baker L, Thompson PW, et al: *Automatic Ventilation of the Lungs*, ed 2, Oxford, England, Blackwell Scientific Publishers Ltd, 1969, p 197. Used by permission.)

NEGATIVE PRESSURE VENTILATORS

Iron Lung Style

From the mid 1800s to the early 1900s an incredible number of devices were invented that applied negative pressure (pressure below ambient) around the body. These devices became known as negative pressure ventilators, or "iron lungs." An interesting review, *The Evolution of the "Iron Lung"* was published by John H. Emerson of Cambridge, Massachusetts in 1978.[12]

The iron lung became successful in two designs. In one the body was enclosed in an iron box or cylinder and the patient's head protruded out one end; the other design was a box or shell that fitted over the thoracic area only. Both devices were designed to apply negative pressure around the body or thoracic cavity. This negative pressure was transmitted to the intrapleural space, and room air would enter through the patient's mouth.

Although physicians believed this was the normal physiologic mechanism of breathing, many of the early designs did not work. In 1864 Alfred F. Jones of Lexington, Kentucky, patented one of the early barorespirators, devices that alternately applied positive and negative ventilation. The patient sat inside a box resembling an old-fashioned steam bath with his or her head protruding through the top. Positive pressure helped expiration while alternating negative pressure around the body assisted inspiration (Fig 1–2).

In 1876 Dr. Woillez of Paris designed the first spirophore. This device operated like the iron lung (Fig 1–3). He had high hopes of using the device for resuscitating drowning victims along the Seine, but funds for the project never materialized. Over the next 80 years a profusion of similar barospirometers and iron lungs were developed. These were sometimes successful in treating respiratory arrest or respiratory insufficiency, but no single design really became popular until the 1920s. Dr. E. Trier Mörch, in "History of Mechanical Ventilation," provides an excellent review of many of these exotic devices.[17]

The first really successful negative pressure ventilator was designed in 1928 by engineer Philip Drinker, physiologist Louis Agassiz Shaw, and Dr. Charles F. McKhann. At the Department of Ventilation, Illumination, and Physiology of the Harvard Medical School, they built a chamber of sheet metal in which the patient's body was enclosed. The patient's head remained outside. A rubber collar fitted snugly around the neck and sealed the chamber from the outside air. This chamber operated off a rotary blower and an alternating valve. Though cumbersome, it provided one of the first widely used respirators.[10]

Because the iron lung made nursing care and physiotherapy difficult, Dr. James L. Wilson developed an entire room on the same principles of ventilation. This allowed for the simultaneous care of several patients, and was used successfully at Children's Hospital in Boston during a polio epidemic.

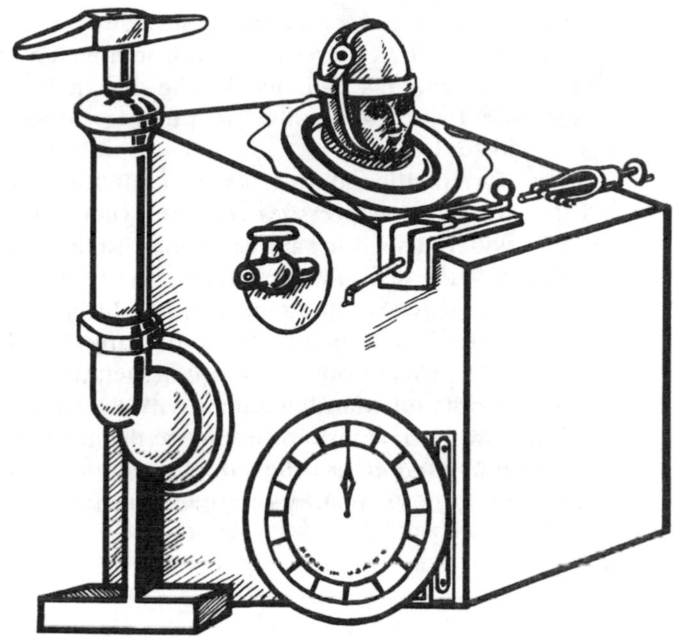

FIG 1–2.
An early negative pressure device designed by Alfred F. Jones in 1864. (Redrawn from Young JA, Crocker D: *Principles and Practices of Inhalation Therapy*. Mosby–Year Book Inc, 1970. Used by permission.)

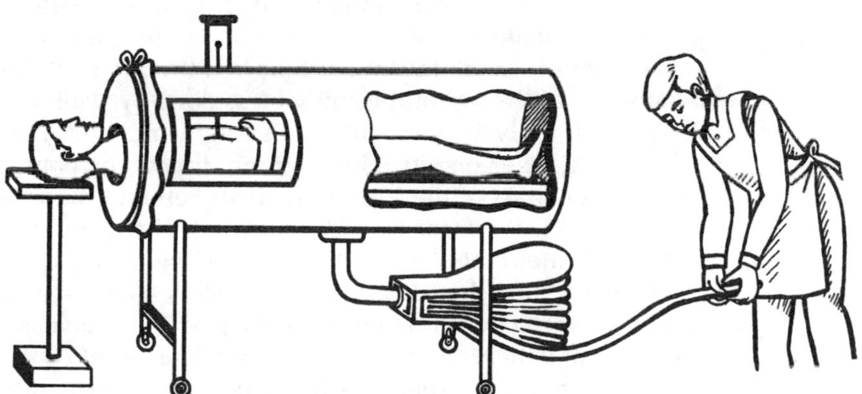

FIG 1–3.
A negative pressure device designed for resuscitation by Woillez in 1876. (Redrawn from Young JA, Crocker D: *Principles and Practices of Inhalation Therapy*, Mosby–Year Book Inc, 1970. Used by permission.)

Dr. August Krogh of Denmark saw the Drinker ventilator on a visit to the United States. When he returned to Copenhagen in 1931 he designed a similar unit for use with his patients. To the design he added a hood that could be placed over the patient's head to provide carbogen therapy (95% oxygen/5% carbon dioxide).

The aforementioned Emerson simplified the ideas of Drinker and Shaw and developed a negative pressure ventilator that was simpler and less expensive. It, too, was widely used for paralyzed polio victims and patients requiring artificial ventilation.[21] He also added a transparent airtight dome that fitted over the patient's head. It was designed to provide positive pressure breaths intermittently at the mouth. In this way the tank could be opened by nurses and physicians to provide care in an unhurried manner and the patient's lungs still could be ventilated. Many problems with the iron lung persist: bulk, difficulty in handling the patient, problems in sterilization, and the hazards of use with hypovolemic patients. It continues, however, to be a successful method of providing long-term ventilatory support, especially to patients with neuromuscular disorders.

Chest Cuirass

The word cuirass (Fr. *cuirasse,* breastplate) was used to describe a piece of armor for protecting the chest. It has also come to mean a type of negative pressure ventilator that covers the thorax and sometimes the abdomen as well. This particular type of ventilator was described first in the late 1800s. In Austria Ignez von Hauke (1974), in Hungary Rodolf Eisenmenger (1901), and in the United States Alexander Graham Bell (1882) made early chest cuirass–negative pressure ventilators.

A variety of other inventions followed the successful use of this device. One large study of the use of the cuirass was done by Wallace and his associates. Of 248 patients, only 16 were not successfully ventilated. These failures were associated with either obesity, chronic lung disease, or poor fit of the shell. Emerson's chest cuirass of the 1950s fit patients better because he used a wraparound piece of plastic ("raincoat") under the shell. The cuirass itself was powered by a vacuum cleaner motor (Fig 1–4).

Patients with chronic paralytic disorders have been successfully ventilated on cuirass ventilators at home for as long as 25 to 30 years. The cuirass is still in use today in patients on home ventilators. The use of plastic shells has also made it easier, if not less expensive, to mold shells to fit patients who are normally hard to fit. One of the practical drawbacks is that not only the thorax but the abdomen often is exposed to the negative pressure. Thus there is a tendency for air to enter the stomach. This produces some unseemly belching, but does not appear to interfere with ventilation in patients adapted to its use.

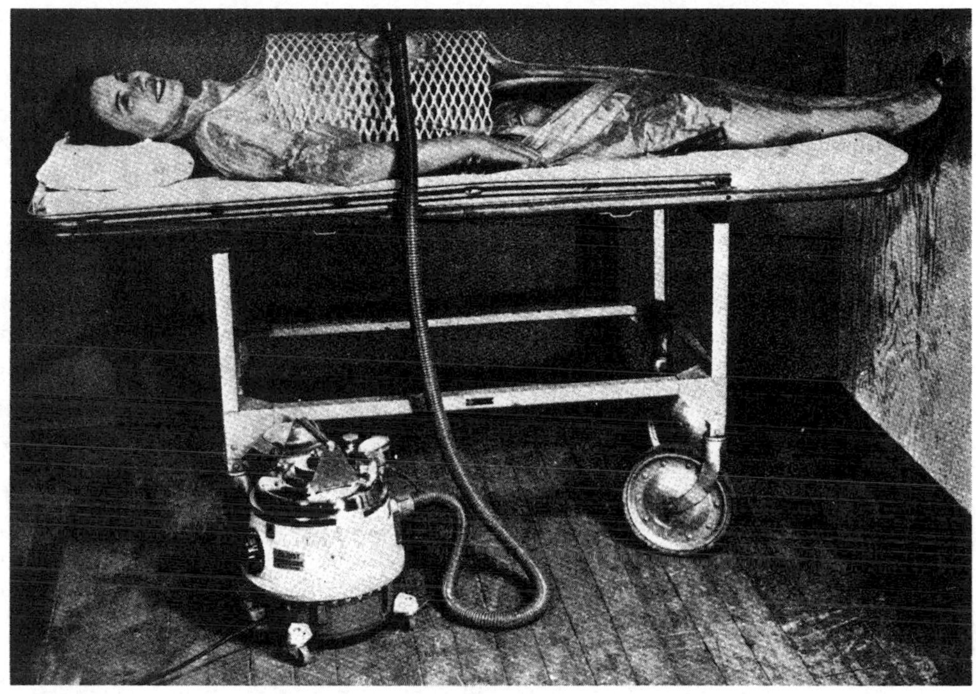

FIG 1–4.
The chest respirator developed by Emerson. (Courtesy of J.H. Emerson Co., Cambridge, Mass.)

POLIOMYELITIS EPIDEMIC IN SCANDINAVIA – 1952

Some episodes in our history are so dramatic that not only do they make great headlines, they have impact on the future of the world community. The polio epidemic that occurred in Copenhagen in 1952 was such an event. Polio had affected various countries prior to this, but none of these incidents were so widespread or dramatic.

From mid-July to early December of 1952, 2,722 patients with polio were treated in the Community Disease Hospital of Copenhagen.[23] Of these, 315 patients required ventilatory support. At the time, only uncuffed tracheostomy tubes were available for airway management. There were no humidifiers, and only one iron lung and six chest cuirasses for ventilation of all the patients.[17] One of the chief anesthesiologists in the hospital, Bjorn Ibsen, was consulted after 27 of the first 31 patients had died within 3 days. Dr. Ibsen employed ventilatory techniques used, at the time, only in the operating room: cuffed tracheostomy tubes and manual artificial ventilation. The survival of the first patient managed by this method prompted the rest of the house staff to adopt the technique.

The medical school in Copenhagen closed for nearly a year to allow the medical students to participate around-the-clock in the manual ventilation of paralyzed polio victims. Dr. Mörch, in a chapter on the history of mechanical ventilation, dramatically describes the herculean task it was.[17] Nearly 500 patients were already in the hospital, and nearly 50 more were admitted daily. Drs. Lassen and Ibsen organized teams of volunteer "ventilators" from the 260 auxillary nurses, 250 medical students, and 27 technicians. In addition, some noted anesthesiologists were in Copenhagen at the time: Dr. Henrik H. Bendixen (Columbia University, New York), Henning Pontoppidan (Massachusetts General Hospital, Boston), and Christian C. Rattenborg (University of Chicago). The names of these three men are an integral part of the development of respiratory care in the United States and are remembered by all respiratory therapists who have been in practice since the 1960s.

Many of the principles of positive pressure ventilation were started during the Danish epidemic, including the use of cuffed tubes, the periodic "sigh" breath, and weaning by reduction of assisted breaths. Toward the end of the epidemic a few positive pressure ventilators became available – the Engström, the Lundi and the Bäng – which became popularly known as the "mechanical students."

The polio epidemic in the United States in the early 1950s was attended by similar experiences. Some regions used iron lung ventilators; others used those and the two available positive pressure ventilators – the Jefferson and the Mörch. The successful management and survival of victims of this terrible and highly infectious disease gave the biggest possible promotion to the use of mechanical ventilation of patients. Now victims of paralytic diseases did not have to die from respiratory failure. The successful development of the Salk and Sabin vaccines brought an end to the polio epidemic of the 1950s. Polio centers began to close, and by the 1960s those permanently paralyzed surviving patients were able to go home with the iron lung and chest cuirass or to stay in general hospital wards.

In spite of the experience gleaned from these events, many problems related to ventilatory care still remained. They included trauma from intubation, airway problems from lack of humidification, and nonsterile suctioning techniques leading to frequent respiratory infections. I can remember caring for patients in a unit where a red rubber suction catheter was used a full 24 hours before replacement. It was kept in a long metal tube hung from the bed, where it soaked in a quaternary ammonium (Zephiran) solution. *Pseudomonas* organisms now are known to be resistant to this quaternary ammonium compound. We were no doubt reinfecting patients with a gram-negative organism known to be associated with secondary pneumonias. Eventually the increasing number and variety of patients who needed ventilatory support helped establish the special units we call intensive care units that are so prevalent in hospitals today.

EARLY ENDOTRACHEAL TUBES, ANESTHESIA, AND THORACIC SURGERY

One of the early problems of artificial ventilation was establishing and maintaining an airway. Some of the early investigators used tubes or reeds, but not without the drawbacks of gastric inflation, infection, and trauma. In 1763 Smellie successfully inserted a flexible metal tube through the mouth and into the trachea. He observed that blowing into the tube not only allowed positive pressure to ventilate the lungs, but it also was useful for suctioning.[29,30] In 1797 Fothergill applied the use of a nasal tube to the principle of ventilation with the fire bellows and created a successfully functioning artificial ventilation device.[12]

Between the late 1700s and the late 1800s most of the research in respiratory care was done in the physiology laboratory and concerned gas exchange, the transport of respired gases, and regulation of respiration. The mid-1800s, however, saw several new developments. It was during this time that anesthetic agents began to be used. The popularity of surgery increased, and the problems of ventilating patients were studied with a greater intensity. Efforts at resuscitation or assisting nonsurgical patients also received a boost. From this point on, artificial ventilation took two paths: surgeons and anesthesiologists looked for methods for ventilating patients during surgery, while other physicians and inventors designed methods for treating patients with apnea and other breathing difficulties.

Between 1880 and 1910 thoracic surgery was investigated widely in hopes of establishing safe techniques for maintaining survival after this procedure. The application of anesthetic agents provided surgeons with the opportunity to explore the chest, but to do so without causing death still remained a problem. Whenever the chest was entered the lungs collapsed. Early surgeons and anesthesiologists began devising ways to keep the lungs functioning during thoracic surgery. Some thought that simply preventing the lung from collapsing would keep the patient alive, since it had worked this way with animal experiments; others, however, were convinced that the movement of fresh air into and out of the lungs was essential, just as Hooke had shown nearly 200 years earlier.

One important development was the endotracheal tube invented in 1880 by Macewen,[8] as well as the simultaneous development of the direct vision "autoscope" by Kirstein in Berlin in 1895[25] and the laryngoscope by Jackson in Pittsburgh in 1895. Two surgeons, Tuffier and Hallion, working in France in the mid-1890s, successfully operated on a patient and performed a partial lung resection. Their technique involved introducing a cuffed endotracheal tube into the patient's trachea and using a nonrebreathing valve device to artificially ventilate the lungs rhythmically.[8,25] These ideas did not spread further, primarily because of lack of physician skill in this technique and a general reluctance to learn it.

The combined experimental results of Fell and O'Dwyer in Buffalo resulted in an apparatus that used a laryngeal cannula to provide an open airway. The airway was attached through a flexible tube to a foot-operated bellows. The external end of the endotracheal tube had two branches, one connected to the bellows and one to the operator's thumb. During inspiration the operator covered one branch with his thumb, forcing the air from the bellows into the lungs. During expiration the thumb was removed and the accumulated air from the lungs was allowed to pass into the room.[8] O'Dwyer was aware at this time that expiration could proceed passively (Fig 1–5).

In 1898 the surgeon Rudolph Matas used the Fell-O'Dwyer apparatus and successfully performed a chest wall resection. In 1902 he had modified the device enough to operate it from a compressed air source[20] (Fig 1–6). Despite the

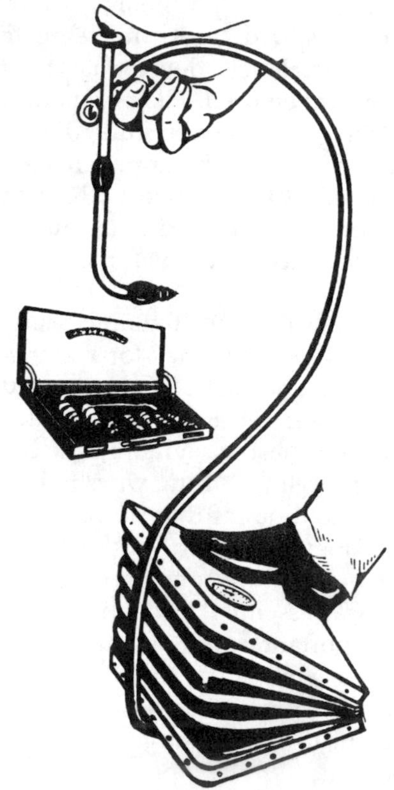

FIG 1–5.
A ventilating device with attached artificial airway operated by a foot bellows. It was similar to the original Fell apparatus and incorporated O'Dwyer's laryngeal tube (1888). (Redrawn from Mushin WL, Rendell-Baker L, Thompson PW, et al: *Automatic Ventilation of the Lungs*, ed 2, Oxford, England, Blackwell Scientific Publishers Ltd, 1969, p 186. Used by permission.)

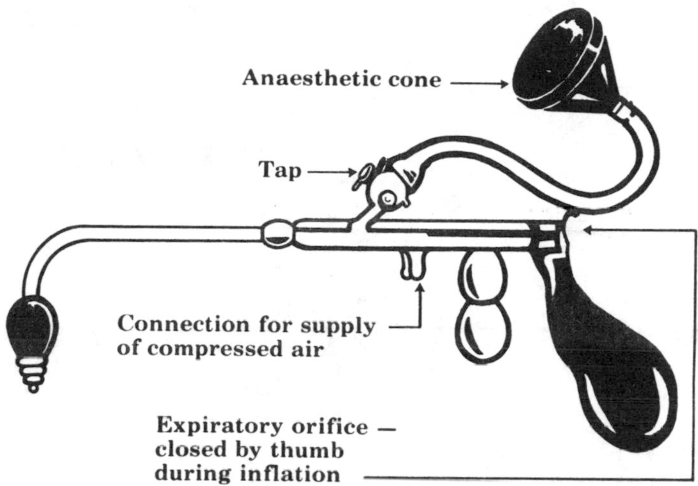

FIG 1–6.
Matas' adaptation of the Fell-O'Dwyer apparatus which used compressed air for power rather than the foot (1902). (Redrawn from Mushin WL, Rendell-Baker L, Thompson PW, et al: *Automatic Ventilation of the Lungs*, ed 2, Oxford, England, Blackwell Scientific Publishers Ltd, 1969, p 186. Used by permission.)

success of these devices, they were largely ignored by the medical community, in part because of lack of skill in using the equipment.

In Germany in 1904 the surgeon Ferdinand Sauerbruch was working on a device for thoracic surgery. Sauerbruch concluded that if the lungs could be kept inflated during surgery, as they are in the intact chest, the patient's respiratory needs could be provided for. He designed an operating chamber large enough to house both the surgeon and the patient, although the patient's head protruded (Fig 1–7). A mechanical pump maintained the pressure in the chamber at a constant -10 cm H_2O. In animal experiments this procedure was successful and the animals survived surgery. Sauerbruch concluded that by maintaining lung inflation successful thoracic surgery could be performed, but he said nothing about ventilation or providing an inspiratory and expiratory phase. The device necessitated that the surgeon remain inside the chamber to operate, and Sauerbruch did perform a lobectomy under these conditions in 1908.[8, 25]

In 1905 Brauer reversed the principles of Sauerbruch and enclosed only the patient's head inside of a much smaller chamber (Fig 1–8). His device applied a constant positive pressure of about $+10$ cm H_2O to the upper airway and thus maintained a constant inflation of the lung when the chest wall was open. This device was less cumbersome, and some surgeons used it instead of Sauerbruch's pressure chamber. Both chambers were widely used in Europe until around 1940.

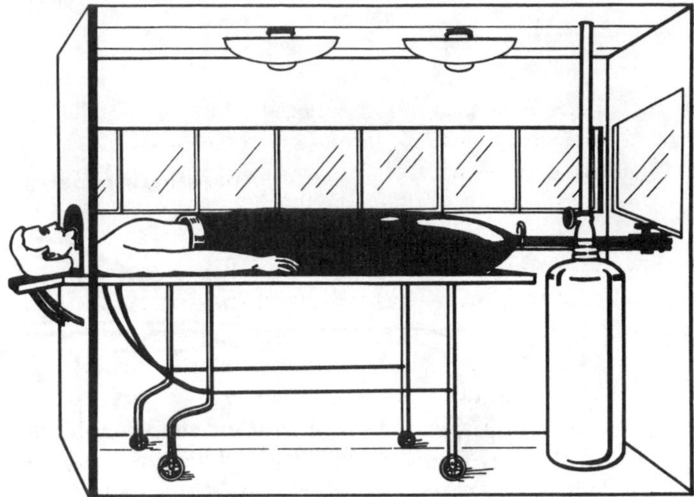

FIG 1–7.
A negative pressure chamber designed by Sauerbruch in 1904 for use in thoracic surgery procedures. (Redrawn from Mushin WL, Rendell-Baker L, Thompson PW, et al: *Automatic Ventilation of the Lungs,* ed 2, Oxford, England, Blackwell Scientific Publishers Ltd, 1969, p 188. Used by permission.)

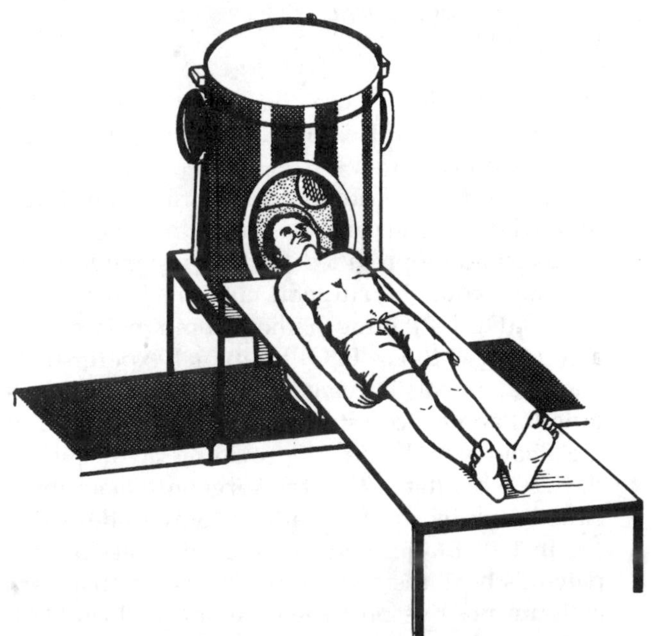

FIG 1–8.
Brauer's continuous positive pressure head chamber for supporting ventilation during thoracic surgery (1905). (Redrawn from Mushin WL, Rendell-Baker L, Thompson PW, et al: *Automatic Ventilation of the Lungs,* ed 2, Oxford, England, Blackwell Scientific Publishers Ltd, 1969, p 189. Used by permission.)

The American laryngologist Chevalier Jackson advocated the skill of intubation as early as 1913. Janeway, in the same year, successfully used an automatic positive pressure assistor applied to an endotracheal tube and performed surgery on a patient. Despite these developments, the value of controlled ventilation was still being debated as late as 1950.

Thus between the 1890s and 1930s many advances were made in experimental surgery and in techniques of intubation and ventilation during surgery. For American surgeons the pressure chambers of Sauerbruch and Bauer never became very popular. The greatest interest in the United States was in the area of intubation and artificial ventilation.

Although surgeons and medical physicians were anxious to find some safe way into the airway, use of the early narrow tubes and techniques of intubation practiced by Jackson and Janeway never were followed. The difficulty of trying to make the right-angle turn between the oral and nasal cavities and the larynx made a lot of people nervous. Tracheal intubation was considered very dangerous, and the technique of direct endotracheal intubation fell by the wayside for many years. Nevertheless, during World War I Ivan Whiteside Magill and E. S. Rowbotham, of London, changed, simplified, and published their techniques on tracheal intubation. The technique of endotracheal intubation as we know it today evolved from their investigations. Once it was learned how to straighten out the right angle between the oral cavity and the larynx things became a lot easier. By lifting and extending the patient's head, the curve turned into a straight line.

EVOLUTION OF POSITIVE PRESSURE VENTILATORS

The development of ventilators as we know them began with the combined history of cardiopulmonary physiology, resuscitation, anesthesia, intubation, and differential (negative or positive) pressure chambers. It evolved around disease problems and epidemics such as the polio epidemic. This historical development is probably best described in Mushin's classic text *Automatic Ventilation of the Lungs.* This text had a profound influence on my early education.

By the time World War II began, British Army physicians were using controlled ventilation with cyclopropane during surgery. Prolonged ventilatory support outside the operating room for medical or surgical patients was still not generally employed. In German-occupied Denmark the Danish anesthesiologist E. Trier Mörch designed his own device.

Unable to obtain one of the spiropulsators designed in Sweden by Giertz and Anderson in the early part of the century, he began to build the Mörch respirator, which provided intermittent inflation by a motor-driven piston pump. This first design was used during thoracic surgery by a number of surgeons in Denmark between 1940 and 1949. Mörch eventually moved to the United States in the early 1950s, and there began successful use of the Mörch ventilator. During the same time John Gibbon and Chris Andreason developed another widely available ventilator for the American market, the Jefferson ventilator (1950). Competitors soon evolved, and included the Stephenson CRU (1956), the Bennett ventilator (1957), the Bird Mark 4 ventilator (1959), and the Emerson postoperative ventilator, a piston-operated device designed to provide prolonged continuous ventilatory support to patients. Numerous ventilators were designed and used. Some were successful commercially; others were successful in patient management but never became well known.

INTERMITTENT POSITIVE PRESSURE BREATHING

The therapeutic use of positive pressure gas blowing into the lungs was certainly understood as a method to keep an apneic patient alive. But additional uses for this positive pressure breath were described as early as 1937 by Barach, Eckman, and Ginsburg, and again in 1945 by Motley and his associates.[24] Barach found intermittent positive pressure breathing (IPPB) beneficial in the treatment of pulmonary edema and other edemas. Discovery of effective cardiac drugs soon surpassed any transient benefits from edema that IPPB provided. However, their study of the use of IPPB for oxygen delivery during high-altitude flying had an important impact on flying in World War II.

Motley, Cournand, and Werk used IPPB for barbiturate-related respiratory failure, asthma attacks, and carbon monoxide poisoning, among other maladies. They used the Burns pneumatic balance resuscitator, as developed by the US Air Force, for their studies. It turned out that the military machine and its associated geniuses in the United States and Europe had a significant input into the medical development of positive pressure devices. In attempting to find a way to maintain oxygenation in pilots flying at high altitudes, the government hired V. Ray Bennett in 1942 to develop a method for accomplishing this task. The valve he designed for this purpose later became incorporated into an IPPB device. In 1956 the Puritan Compressed Gas Association purchased Bennett's company, and the results of their endeavors produced the Puritan Bennett PR-1 and PR-2 IPPB machines, which are still in use for IPPB aerosol treatments and positive pressure ventilation.

In World War II Forrest Bird was commissioned in the Army Air Corps as a pilot. His war-related flying experiences led him to develop a device to ease the problems of breathing at high altitudes. Later modifications of his device proved valuable and effective to a friend who had emphysema. This pilot, designer, and entrepreneur was strongly influenced by Dr. Barach and by Dr. Andre Cournand, who helped him incorporate some of his ideas along with theirs. "In fact, the conception and medical testing of the Bird Mark 7 came about under the medical supervision of Dr. Cournand at Bellevue Hospital in New York."[7] The original device had been used as a pressure suit regulator in aviation. Forrest Bird modified the device, and it became the first Bird Mark 7, well known to this day to all respiratory care practitioners (Fig 1–9). In the 1960s the Bird Mark 7 sold for the astonishing price of $375, a bargain even then. Bird eventually founded a school of "inhalation therapy" in Palm Springs, California, which probably was the first of its kind.

The IPPB devices developed by Bennett and Bird, among other similar but less widely used instruments, became popular as "breathing treatment" machines. These devices aerosolized a medication in a cup and delivered the aerosol to the patient during a positive pressure inspiration. The popularity of IPPB treatments began in the 1960s and hit an all-time high in the 1970s. It was not so much the scientifically proved benefit of the device, but a blind acceptance that it *might* be good that provided for its unquestioning success. Couple this with the amount of money a hospital could make through its "inhalation therapy department" by the staggering number of these treatments given to

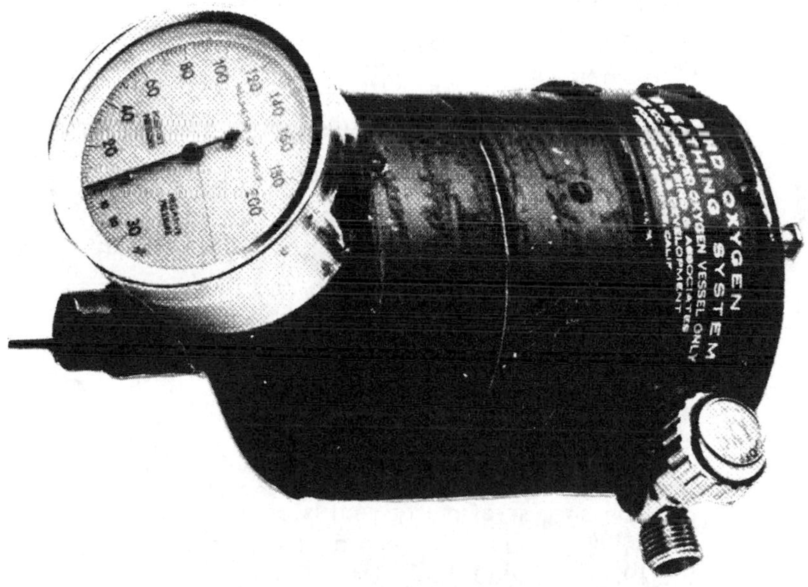

FIG 1–9.
The original Bird Mark 7, built inside a coffee can. This was the first Bird breathing device to use magnets for the control of gas movement (1951). (From Branson RD: *AARC Times*, 1990; 14(Dec):53. Used by permission.)

patients with all types of admitting diagnoses and it is no wonder it was widely used.

Studies during the mid to late 1970s finally disproved the benefit of IPPB over less expensive methods of medication delivery in all but a few applications, and IPPB became all but nonexistent. But the other and often overlooked use of the Bird and Bennett machines was for mechanical ventilation of the apneic patient or the patient in respiratory failure. These machines never became as popular as devices that could deliver a fixed volume through the use of piston or bellows. However, they could—and still do—provide an alternative method of ventilation during transport of a patient, for short-term ventilation such as in the radiology department during a procedure and in the recovery room as a "wake-up" ventilator.

DISEASE PROCESSES AND MECHANICAL VENTILATION

The historical development of mechanical ventilation has taken several parallel courses. First there was the effort by scientists to investigate how the process of breathing keeps us alive. Then there were attempts to resuscitate the dying and the various resuscitation techniques used. Finally extended mechanical ventilatory support was attempted in victims of diseases such as polio. Patients had a chance for recovery if they did not die first of respiratory failure. Some of these attempts extended from the surgical suites, where anesthesiologists had developed various methods of maintaining the airway and supporting ventilation.

From the very early history of Paracelsus and Vesalius to the mid 1900s mechanical ventilation has plodded a long slow path. But the world in the 1950s and 1960s took on a new pace and a new approach. The early ventilators such as the Mörch, the Emerson Post-Op, and the Jefferson had been designed for use in the paralyzed and apneic patient, such as the polio victim. It was these early designs that basically governed the way we would ventilate patients' lungs for the next 40 years. A huge variety of ventilators were made and marketed from the late 1960s to the present. They included those such as the Arp (designed for neonatal patients but never extensively marketed) to Puritan Bennett's MA-1, which became as common as the light bulb.

The success of many ventilators depended on their simplicity of use, dependability, and service records. To name just a few, ventilators that appeared in the 1970s included the Gill, the Ohio 560 and 550, the Monaghan 225, the IMV (intermittent mandatory ventilation) Emerson and Baby Bird, the BEAR 1, the Bourns LS-104, the Engström, the Foregger, and the Siemens Servo. Some survived because of their successful designs and service records. Others buried themselves with their flaws. Still others were bought out by the competition and never seen again.

The most notable result of this profusion of inventions was development of a competitive market. Manufacturers discovered that money could be made with a successfully designed ventilator, and technology had advanced enough to provide a variety of new ventilating and monitoring techniques.

POSITIVE END-EXPIRATORY PRESSURE AND CONTINUOUS POSITIVE AIRWAY PRESSURE

In 1967 Ashbaugh, Petty, and colleagues[2] revived the idea of continuous positive pressure breathing (CPPB), which has become more popularly known as positive end-expiratory pressure (PEEP). This technique was introduced by Poulton and Barach[15] in the 1930s for treatment of acute pulmonary edema due to cardiac failure. With the development of diuretic therapy and cardiac drugs, the treatment for congestive heart failure had become drug therapy rather than pressure breathing.

In the early 1940s the military, in its efforts to provide adequate oxygen to high-altitude-flight pilots, adapted PEEP to increase the partial pressure of alveolar oxygen.[4] This technique, however, had adverse effects on the cardiovascular system. Its use resulted in reduction of cardiac output and impeded venous return to the heart. It was replaced with the IPPB devices.[3] Thus PEEP as a technique in the treatment of certain types of respiratory failure did not become useful in medicine until the late 1960s. In 1971 Gregory and his colleagues[17] reported the use of continuous positive airway pressure (CPAP) in the treatment of idiopathic respiratory distress syndrome (IRDS) in newborns. Positive pressure breathing became useful in the care of infants as well as adults.

PEEP and CPAP remain popular modes of assisting with ventilation in patients with adult respiratory distress syndrome (ARDS). This disorder has been known since World War I, and began to receive a lot of attention beginning with the Vietnam War, when it was called Da Nang lung and shock lung syndrome. War trauma victims can develop very stiff lungs, which are difficult to oxygenate. Chest films show a pattern of whiteout that appears to be a pulmonary edema. Although ARDS is attributed to a variety of causes, its exact nature remains a mystery. Mortality from ARDS is between 40% and 60%. Despite a great many studies, the statistics predicting patient death from ARDS have not changed since the Vietnam era. PEEP and CPAP remain two of the few methods of oxygenating patient lungs that have shown some success.

This fact also makes us aware of one of our failures. The peculiar nature of ARDS seems to point out one design flaw in mechanical ventilation as we know it. The ventilators we use, mostly volume ventilators, never were designed for use in this type of lung condition. PEEP and CPAP offer some respite, but they also remain unsuccessful. Still, mechanical ventilation with PEEP remains one of the best ways we have to maintain ventilation and oxygenation in patients with

ARDS. It will be interesting to see what the future will provide as a method to successfully manage ARDS patients.

INTERMITTENT MANDATORY VENTILATION

In the early 1970s Kirby and his associates developed a technique of ventilating infants with IRDS called intermittent mandatory ventilation (IMV).[18] With IMV the patient can breathe spontaneously from a reservoir system while the ventilator provides a positive pressure breath at intermittent intervals. Shortly thereafter, Downs and co-workers adapted the IMV system for adult ventilation. It was proposed not only as a method for ventilation in adults but also as a method by which to discontinue mechanical ventilation. This technique was so successful that it rapidly became popular. Some respiratory therapy departments adapted IMV systems to all the ventilators they were using. New ventilators now have built-in IMV systems and an added feature called SIMV, or synchronized IMV. This design makes the ventilator sensitive to the patient's inspiratory effort and waits to provide the mandatory machine breath until the patient starts breathing in. IMV and SIMV have never been proved to be physiologically different, yet patients report being "more comfortable" with the SIMV system. It also raised the price of ventilators by about $2,500 when it first became available. So much for the price of new technology!

HIGH-FREQUENCY VENTILATION

The year 1971 also saw the introduction of high-frequency positive pressure ventilation (HFPPV) by Oberg and Sjöstrand of Sweden. The concept of ventilating at rates higher than normal is unusual but supports the idea that it is not the rhythmic inflation of the lungs that successfully keeps us alive but the fresh supply of air.

In 1667 Hooke reported in a paper presented to the Royal Society of London that he had kept a dog alive with an open thorax by providing a continuous flow of air through a hole cut in the visceral pleura (outer coat of the lungs). Hooke had shown more than 300 years ago that the lungs do not have to keep inflating and deflating to maintain life.

In 1955 J. H. Emerson, who had designed the iron lung and the Emerson Post-Op ventilator, patented a ventilator for "vibrating portions of a patient's airway." Emerson can probably be credited with inventing the first modern high-frequency ventilator. His ventilator could provide between 100 and 1,500 "vibrations" per minute. But unfortunately, the use of his device as a ventilator was about 20 years too early.

Newer methods of providing high-frequency ventilation were extensively explored in the late 1970s and early 1980s.[9] HFPPV provides a way of ventilating patients without a wide fluctuation in intrapleural pressures. While an incredible amount of research is still being done with this technique, it remains only an alternative method of ventilation. Most of its use is restricted to infants, and it still has not been demonstrated to be better than more traditional modes of ventilation.

VENTILATION IN THE COMPUTER AGE

Table 1–1 briefly lists some of the historical events that have marked the evolution of mechanical ventilation. One item not noted on this list is the computer. Although its development has spanned many decades, its impact on mechanical ventilation has become important only since the 1980s. In the mid-1980s ventilator designs began not only to incorporate computers for monitoring but also to use microprocessors for actual ventilator operation. The Puritan Bennett 7200 ventilator was one of the first—but it certainly will not be the last.

More and more sophistication is seen in the modernization of ventilator techniques and patient monitoring. It has become a source of frustration for respiratory therapists who have been practicing respiratory care since the 1960s. The frustration stems from their historical training. Early designs such as the Emerson, the MA-1, and the Bird Mark 7 used to be studied until the typical therapist could disassemble, repair, and reassemble all six ventilators then available on the market.

Now, however, there probably is closer to sixty than six ventilators.

Almost all of the newer designs are run by microprocessors—circuit boards and microswitches—rather than pistons and bellows. Now respiratory care school graduates can turn the knobs or press the touch pad, but the internal workings remain a mystery. This has pushed us into an era where the extensive understanding of a ventilator's operation is limited to trying to understand why the blasted alarm is going off and won't be silenced. But manufacturers are taking care of even that. Now microprocessor ventilators have screens that give you a message telling why the alarm is jangling and what you can do to correct the problem.

This advancement makes me a bit uneasy. Is my unease just a reluctance to adapt to a rapidly changing technology? Or is it my concern that not fully understanding all of a ventilator's intricacies and peculiarities of operation may leave me with the feeling that I might be jeopardizing a patient's well-being? I think Mörch put it aptly when he wrote: "Often we have to decide whether to sacrifice reliability and simplicity for the sometimes dubious advantages that a highly sophisticated piece of apparatus may provide."[17] And James M. Hurst commented: ". . . the blind enthusiasm for special forms of ventilatory support

TABLE 1–1.
History of Mechanical Ventilation

Date	Event
800 BC	Biblical quotation of resuscitation
460 BC to 370 BC	Hippocrates described the function of breathing in "Treatise on Air" and treatment for suffocation by cannulation of the trachea
384 BC to 322 BC	Aristotle noted that air is essential for life
1493 AD to 1541 AD	Paracelsus used a fire bellows to assist ventilation in a patient
1541 to 1564	Vesalius used a reed in an animal's trachea and restored a dying animal's heart beat
1635 to 1703	Hooke noted that it was fresh air and not the movement of the thorax that was essential to life
1763	Smellie used a flexible metal tube in the trachea to blow air into the lungs
1775	Hunter used an expiratory and an inspiratory bellows for ventilation in animals
1786	Kite had a volume-limiting mechanism that he used in a bellows device, for the first volume was considered important
1790	Courtois used a piston and cylinder in place of a bellows for ventilation
1796	Fothergill used a nasal tube and a fire bellows for artificial ventilation
1864	Jones patented one of the earliest negative pressure ventilators which resembled a steam bath
1876	Woillez designed the spirophore which was similar in operation to the iron lung
1860 to 1950	A profusion of negative pressure devices were invented
1880	Macewen developed the endotracheal tube
1895	Kirstein developed the direct vision autoscope
	Jackson invented the laryngoscope
1886	Tuffier and Hallion successfully performed a partial lung resection by using a cuffed endotracheal tube and a nonrebreathing valve
1893	Fell and O'Dwyer used a laryngeal cannula connected to a foot-operated bellows for ventilation during surgery
1896, 1902	Matas used compressed air to power the Fell-O'Dwyer apparatus during surgery
1904	Sauerbruch used continuous negative ventilation around the body to sustain ventilatory requirements during surgery
1905	Brauer used constant positive pressure at the upper airway to sustain ventilation during surgery
1909	Janeway and Green developed an intermittent positive pressure ventilator (IPPV) for surgical use
1909	Meltzer and Auer designed an apparatus using tracheal cannulation and a compressed air source
1911	Dräger designed the pulmotor for resuscitation
1928	Drinker and Shaw designed a negative pressure ventilator known as the iron lung that was intended for long-term ventilatory support
1931	Emerson developed an iron lung similar to Drinker and Shaw's that became widely used commercially
1940	Crafoord, Frenckner, and Andreason designed the spiropulsator, an IPPV ventilator
1941 to 1945	Mörch designed an IPPV ventilator
1952	The polio epidemic began in Copenhagen
1967	Positive end-expiratory pressure (PEEP) with mechanical ventilation was introduced
1971	Continuous positive airway pressure (CPAP) was introduced in the treatment of idiopathic respiratory distress syndrome (IRDS) of newborns
1971	Oberg and Sjöstrand introduced the use of high-frequency positive pressure ventilation (HFPPV)
1973	Intermittent mandatory ventilation (IMV) as a technique for weaning patients from ventilatory support was introduced
1980	High-frequency positive pressure ventilation (HFPPV) gains the literature as an experimental approach to mechanical ventilation

must be bridled by carefully controlled clinical investigations."[16] And I can't help but imagine that in another 20 years we will look back at all of these new advances—but with the retrospect of history. Hindsight is, after all, 20/20.

Tom Baxter, a co-worker of mine, summarized it neatly when he said:

> The function of the ventilator, no matter how many bells and whistles the manufacturer has added to it, is still only to blow air into the patient's lungs. The function of the respiratory care practitioner is to make sure this is done in a manner that is most beneficial to the patient.

REFERENCES

1. American Association for Respiratory Care Teleconference: *Respiratory Problems Following Trauma,* September 14, 1990.
2. Ashbaugh DG, Bigelow DB, Petty TL, et al: Acute respiratory distress in adults. *Lancet* 1967; 2:319–323.
3. Barach AL, Eckman M, Eckman I, et al: Studies on positive pressure respiration III. Effect on continuous positive pressure breathing on arterial blood gases at high altitude. *J Aviat Med* 1947; 18:139.
4. Barach AL, Fenn WO, Ferris EB, et al: The physiology of pressure breathing. *J Aviat Med* 1947; 18:73.
5. Barach AL, Hylan AB, Petty TL: Perspectives in pressure breathing. *Respir Care* 1975; 20:627–642.
6. Bird Corporation: *Specifications and Instructions for the Bird Pneumioband.* Palm Springs, Calif, Bird Space Technology, 1966.
7. Branson RD: Pioneers in respiratory care: Forrest M. Bird, Ph.D. *AARC Times* 1990; 14:51–57.
8. Comroe JH: *Retrospectroscope: Insights Into Medical Discovery.* Menlo Park, Calif, Von Gehr Press, 1977.
9. DeHaven CB: Newer techniques: High frequency positive pressure ventilation. *Curr Rev Respir Ther* 1988; 2:171–176.
10. Drinker P, McKhann CF: The use of a new apparatus for the prolonged administration of artificial respiration: I, A fatal case of poliomyelitis. *JAMA* 1929; 92:1658–1660.
11. Elliot LS. A pictorial history of mechanical respiration devices. *Respir Ther,* Jan/Feb, 1979; pp 52-54.
12. Emerson JH: *The Evolution of the "Iron Lung."* Cambridge, Mass, JH Emerson Co, 1978.
13. Fothergill DA: Apparatus for the recovery of drowned persons in 1797. *Resp Care* 1974; 19:1020.
14. Gandevia B: The breath of life: An essay on the earliest history of respiration. *Respir Care* 1972; 17:2–6.
15. Heironimus TW: *Mechanical Artificial Ventilation.* Springfield, Ill, Charles C Thomas, Publisher, 1971.

16. Hurst JM: What's the Gas About Specialized Ventilatory Support? *Respir Care* 1987; 32:781–784.
17. Kirby RR, Banner MJ, Downs JB: *Clinical Applications of Ventilatory Support.* New York, Churchill Livingstone, Inc, 1990.
18. Kirby R, Robinson E, Shultz J, et al: Continuous flow ventilation as an alternative to assisted or controlled ventilation in infants. *Anesth Analg* 1971; 51:871–875.
19. Kirby RR, Smith RA, Desautels DA: *Mechanical Ventilation.* New York, Churchill Livingstone Inc, 1985.
20. Matas R: Artificial respiration by direct intralaryngeal intubation with a new graduated air-pump, in its application to medical and surgical practice. *Am Med* 1902; 3:97–103.
21. McPherson SP: *Respiratory Therapy Equipment.* St Louis, Mosby–Year Book, Inc, 1981.
22. Meltzer ST, Auer J: Continuous respiration without respiratory movements. *J Exp Med* 1909; 2:622.
23. Meyers RA: Mechanical support of respiration. *Surg Clin North Am* 1974; 54:1115–1123.
24. Motley HL, Lang LP, Gordon B: Use of intermittent positive pressure breathing combined with nebulization in pulmonary disease. *Am J Med* 1948; 5:853–857.
25. Mushin WL, Rendell-Baker L, Thompson PW, et al: *Automatic Ventilation of the Lungs,* ed 2. Oxford, England, Blackwell Scientific Publishers Ltd, 1969.
26. Rarey KP, Youtsey JW: *Respiratory Patient Care.* Englewood Cliffs, NJ, Prentice-Hall, Inc, 1981.
27. Rau JL: Continuous mechanical ventilation—Part I. *Crit Care Update* October 1981, p 11.
28. Scott F: Arp ventilator gets another look. *The Advance for Respiratory Care Practitioners,* July 16, 1990, p 12.
29. Young JA, Crocker D: *Principles and Practices of Inhalation Therapy,* ed 1. St Louis, Mosby–Year Book, Inc, 1970.
30. Young JA, Crocker D: *Principles and Practices of Respiratory Therapy,* ed 2. St Louis, Mosby–Year Book, Inc, 1976.

Chapter **2**

Basic Terms and Concepts of Mechanical Ventilation

On completion of this chapter the reader will be able to:

1. Define the following terms: ventilation, internal and external respiration, transairway pressure, transpulmonary pressure, transrespiratory pressure, transthoracic pressure, pressure at the body surface, mouth pressure, airway

opening pressure, airway pressure, alveolar pressure, and intraalveolar pressure.
2. Explain the concept of normal ventilation.
3. Define compliance and resistance in relation to ventilation.
4. Describe negative pressure ventilation and compare its function to normal lung ventilation.
5. Graph a positive pressure curve for a mechanical breath, and label plateau pressure, peak pressure, and baseline pressure.
6. Graph changes in flow, volume, alveolar pressure, upper airway pressure, and transairway pressures against time with a constant flow ventilator.
7. Give an equation for calculating time constants and discuss their importance in determining inspiratory and expiratory time.

REVIEW OF NORMAL MECHANICS IN SPONTANEOUS VENTILATION

The purpose of this chapter is to review the basic concepts of ventilation. With an understanding of how air moves into and out of the lungs, it is easier to see how mechanical ventilation is accomplished. In addition, terms commonly applied to airway pressure measurements and lung characteristics are defined. This section is followed by an introduction to the basic terms frequently used in mechanical ventilation.

Ventilation and Respiration

Spontaneous breathing or spontaneous ventilation is simply the movement of air into and out of the lungs. The main purpose of ventilation is to bring in fresh air for gas exchange in the lung and to allow the exhalation of air that is high in carbon dioxide. The exchange of gas is accomplished inside the lung between the alveoli and the pulmonary capillaries, which are adjacent to the alveoli.

Respiration is defined as the movement of gases across a membrane. Oxygen moves from the lung into the bloodstream and carbon dioxide moves from the bloodstream into the alveoli. This is called *external respiration.* At the cellular level carbon dioxide moves out of cells and into the blood and oxygen moves from the blood into the cells. This is termed *internal respiration.*

Normal ventilation, the drawing of air into the lungs, is accomplished by the expansion of the thorax or chest cavity. It occurs when the muscles of inspiration, the diaphragm and external intercostals, contract. During contraction, the diaphragm descends and enlarges the vertical dimension of the thoracic cavity. The external intercostals contract and raise the ribs slightly, increasing the circumference of the thorax.

During exhalation, when air leaves the lungs, the muscles relax. The diaphragm moves upward to its resting position and the ribs return to their normal position. The volume of the thoracic cavity decreases and air is forced out of the alveoli. Exhalation is normally a passive maneuver.

Gas Flow and Pressure Gradients During Ventilation

An important point involved in ventilation is the basic concept of why gases flow. Whenever you have a tube or airway, in order for air to flow from one end of the tube to the other end, you must have a pressure difference, or *pressure gradient.* The pressure at one end of the tube must be higher than the pressure at the other end. Air or fluid will always flow from the point where the pressure is highest to the point where the pressure is lowest.

Thus, changes in lung volumes occur as a result of gas flows that are caused by pressure changes. We commonly measure pressures in centimeters of water pressure (cm H_2O). These pressures are given a baseline value of zero. The zero reference is equal to atmospheric pressure; for example, 760 mm Hg (1,034 cm H_2O) is the pressure at sea level. Remember that 1 mm Hg equals 1.36 cm H_2O.

During spontaneous ventilation the conductive airways begin at the mouth and nose and end at the alveolar level. Whenever the pressures at the mouth and at the alveoli are equal, no gas flows. At the end of inspiration there is no gas movement. Nor is there gas movement at the end of exhalation. So the pressures across the conductive tube are equal. There is no pressure gradient.

Mouth pressure (PM) is often called pressure at the airway opening (Pawo) or airway pressure (Paw). It can also be called upper airway or proximal airway pressure. Unless positive pressure is applied to the upper airway, Pawo is usually zero. A similar measurement is pressure at the body surface (Pbs). This is equal to zero (atmospheric) unless the person is exposed to a pressurized chamber such as a hyperbaric chamber or a negative pressure ventilator such as an iron lung. A third commonly measured pressure is pressure in the alveoli (PA), which is also called intrapulmonary pressure. Alveolar pressure changes as the intrapleural pressure changes. Intrapleural pressure (Ppl) is a measurement of pressure in the potential space between the parietal and visceral pleura. Normal intrapleural pressure is about -5 cm H_2O at the end of exhalation before inspiration begins. It is about -10 cm H_2O at the end of inspiration.

There are four basic pressure gradients used to describe normal ventilation (Table 2–1). These are described below and pictured in Figure 2–1.[3]

Transthoracic Pressure (Pw).—Pw is the pressure difference between the alveolar space (PA) and the body's surface (Pbs). Pw = PA − Pbs. It represents the pressure needed to expand or contract both the lungs and the chest wall simultaneously.

TABLE 2–1.

Terms and Pressure Gradients in the Respiratory System

Terms	
C	Compliance
R	Resistance
Raw	Airway resistance
P_M	Pressure at the mouth (same as Pawo)
$\bar{P}_{AW}$	Airway pressure (any place in the airway)
Pawo	Pressure at the airway opening; mouth pressure; mask pressure
Pbs	Pressure at the body surface
P_A	Alveolar pressure
Ppl	Intrapleural pressure
Pmus	Pressure due to respiratory muscle contraction
Pressure gradients	
Transrespiratory pressure (P_{TR}) = Pawo − Pbs	
Transthoracic pressure (Pw) = P_A − Pbs	
Transairway pressure (P_{TA}) = Paw − P_A	
Transpulmonary pressure (P_L) = P_A − Ppl	

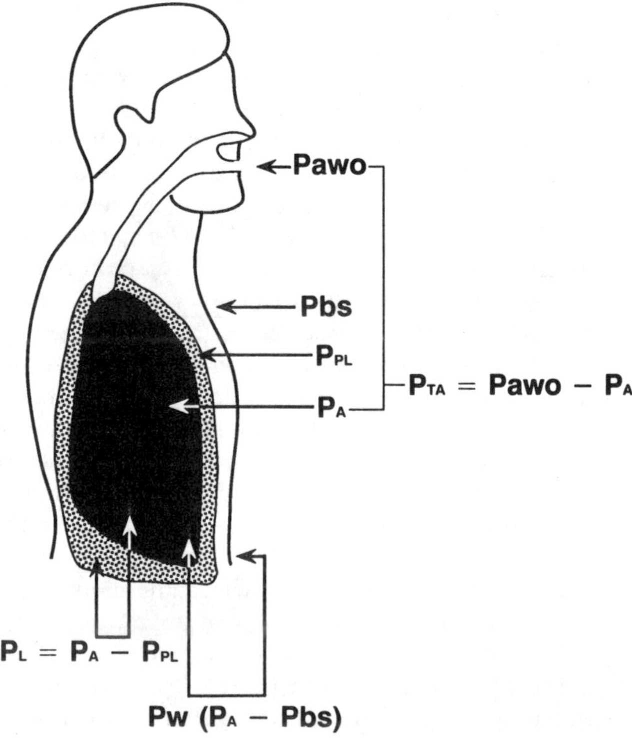

FIG 2–1.
The various pressure gradients in the respiratory system: transairway pressure, transpulmonary pressure, and transthoracic pressure. See Table 2–1 for abbreviations.

Transairway Pressure (PTA).—PTA is the pressure gradient between the airway (Paw) and the alveolus. Airway pressure is usually measured at the airway opening, Pawo. PTA = Paw − PA. It is responsible for airway movement in the conductive airways. It represents the pressure due to airway flow resistance.

Transrespiratory Pressure (PTR).—PTR is the pressure gradient between the airway opening and the body surface (Pawo − Pbs). This is the pressure required for inflation during positive pressure ventilation. The Pbs in this situation is atmospheric and is usually given the value zero. In this case Paw becomes the pressure read on a ventilator gauge.

Transrespiratory pressure is represented by two components: Pw (pressure required to overcome elastance) and PTA, or pressure required to overcome airway flow resistance. PTR = Pw + PTA. Thus, (Pawo − Pbs) = (PA − Pbs) + (Paw − PA).

Transpulmonary Pressure (PL).—PL is the pressure difference between the inside of the lung and the outside of the lung, in other words between the alveolus (PA) and the pleural space (Ppl). It is sometimes abbreviated PTP. PL = PA − Ppl.[13, 22]

PL is responsible for maintaining alveolar inflation and is sometimes referred to as alveolar distending pressure. All modes of ventilation try to increase PL by either decreasing Ppl (negative pressure ventilators) or increasing PA by increasing Pawo.

With negative pressure ventilation Pbs becomes negative and this negative pressure is transmitted to the pleural space. PL increases. With positive pressure ventilation Pbs remains atmospheric but the pressures at the upper airways (Pawo) and in the conductive airways (Paw) become positive. Therefore, PA becomes positive and PL increases.

Some authors refer to PL as the pressure between the airway (Paw) and the pleural surface (Ppl)[13]: Paw − Ppl. They state that the lung volume is directly related to PL. There is really not much difference between Paw and PA during positive pressure ventilation. For this reason, both abbreviations are used.

During normal, spontaneous inspiration (Fig 2–2), as the volume of the thoracic space increases, the pressure in the pleural space, intrapleural pressure (Ppl), becomes more negative in relation to atmospheric pressures. This is as you would expect according to Boyle's law. For a constant temperature, as the volume increases the pressure decreases. This negative *intrapleural pressure* goes from about −5 cm H_2O at end-expiration to about −10 cm H_2O at end-inspiration. This is transmitted to the alveolar space. The *intrapulmonary* or intraalveolar (PA) pressure becomes more negative relative to atmospheric pressure. The transpulmonary pressure, PL, or the pressure gradient across the lung, widens (Table 2–2). As a result, the alveoli have a negative pressure.

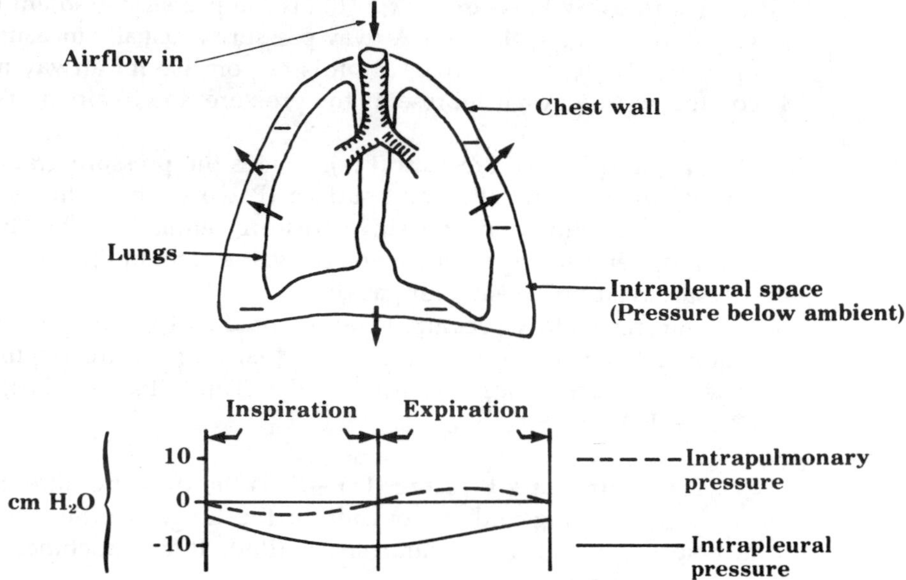

FIG 2–2.
The mechanics of spontaneous ventilation and the resulting pressure waves.

TABLE 2–2.
Changes in Transpulmonary Pressure at End-Expiration and End-Inspiration

	Pressure		
	Intraalveolar	Intrapleural	Transpulmonary
End-expiration	0 cm H_2O	-5 cm H_2O	$P_L = 0 - (-5) = +5$ cm H_2O
End-inspiration	0 cm H_2O	-10 cm H_2O	$P_L = 0 - (-10) = +10$ cm H_2O

Pressure at the mouth or body surface is still atmospheric. This creates a pressure gradient between the mouth (zero) and the alveolus of -10 cm H_2O. The transairway pressure gradient (P_{TA}) is approximately $[0 - (-10)]$ or 10 cm H_2O. Air flows from the mouth into the alveoli and the alveoli expand. When the volume of gas builds up in the alveoli and the pressure returns to zero, the airflow stops. This marks end-inspiration. There is no more movement of gas into the lungs. Pressure at the mouth and in the alveoli is equal to zero or atmospheric pressure (see Fig 2–2).

During exhalation, the muscles relax. The thoracic volume decreases to normal and Ppl is back to a normal resting level of about -5 cm H_2O. Pressure inside the alveolus now increases and becomes slightly positive. This is a result of the elastic lung tissue recoiling and the ribs and diaphragm rebounding to their normal positions. This puts pressure on the alveoli. Pressure at the mouth is now lower than inside the alveoli. The transairway pressure gradient causes air to move out of the lungs. When the pressure in the alveoli and the mouth finally equalize at zero (ambient), exhalation ends.

This process describes the normal movement of air into and out of the lungs. Understanding this gives a basic knowledge of what inventors are trying to accomplish when they build mechanical ventilators.

Compliance

There normally exist two types of forces that oppose the inflation of the lungs—elastic forces and frictional forces. The elastic forces are due to the elastic properties of the lungs and thorax. The frictional forces are due to two factors: first, the resistance of the tissues and organs as they move and become displaced during breathing; second, the resistance to gas flow through the airways.

The compliance of any structure is the relative ease with which the structure distends. A balloon that is easy to inflate is very compliant. One that is hard to inflate is noncompliant. Compliance (C) is the opposite or inverse of the property called elastance (e): $C = 1/e$ or $e = 1/C$. Elastance is the tendency of a structure to return to its original form after being stretched. For example, which is more elastic, a golf ball or a tennis ball? The answer is, a golf ball. It tends to retain its original form. Which is more compliant? The tennis ball.

Pulmonary physiology uses the term compliance to describe and measure the elastic forces opposing lung inflation. Compliance is defined as the change of volume which corresponds to the change in pressure: $C = \Delta V/\Delta P$. Normally, volume is measured in liters or milliliters and pressure in centimeters of water pressure.

Normal compliance of the lungs is actually the sum of the compliance of both the lung tissue and the surrounding thoracic structures. In the spontaneously breathing individual, the total compliance is about 0.1 L/cm H_2O. The value for compliance varies a great deal depending on the posture, position, and level of consciousness of the subject. It can range anywhere from 0.02 L/cm H_2O to 0.17 L/cm H_2O, i.e., 20 to 170 mL/cm H_2O.

Suppose we calculate the amount of pressure that would be needed to attain a tidal volume (V_T) of 0.5 L (500 mL). Remember that $C = \Delta V/\Delta P$. ΔP will be $\Delta V/C$. If the compliance is 0.1 L/cm H_2O and volume is 0.5 L, pressure will be 0.5 L/0.1 cm H_2O, or 5 cm H_2O. An alveolar pressure change of 5 cm H_2O would be needed to achieve a V_T of 0.5 L in a person with normal lung compliance.

In intubated and mechanically ventilated patients with normal lungs, the compliance value will vary from 40 to 50 mL/cm H_2O in males and from 35 to 45 mL/cm H_2O in females to as high as 100 mL/cm H_2O in either sex. With changes in the conditions of the lungs or thoracic wall, the compliance value will also change. Monitoring changes in compliance is a valuable method for looking at changes in the patient's condition during mechanical ventilatory support. This is usually done under conditions of no gas flow and is referred to as a static compliance (Cs) or effective compliance (see Chapter 8). Diseases which reduce compliance will tend to increase the pressure needed to deliver the same volume.

Resistance

Resistance or frictional forces associated with ventilation are due to the anatomic structures of the conductive airways, and the tissue viscous resistance of the lungs and adjacent tissues and organs. As the lungs and thorax move during ventilation, the movement and displacement of structures create resistance to breathing. These structures include the lungs, abdominal organs, rib cage, and diaphragm. The tissue resistance stays constant under most circumstances. For example, an obese patient or one with fibrosis has an increased tissue resistance, but it usually does not change significantly when the patient is being mechanically ventilated. On the other hand, if a patient develops ascites or fluid build-up in the peritoneal cavity, then the tissue resistance will change.

What is most often evaluated during mechanical ventilation is resistance of the airways. The ability of air to flow through the conductive airways depends on the gas viscosity, gas density, the length and diameter of the tube, and the flow rate of the gas through the tube. In clinical situations, viscosity, density, and the tube or airway length remain fairly constant. Careful attention is given to the airway lumen and the flow rate of the gas. This is true since the airway diameter might change with changes in the patient's condition. The diameter might decrease with bronchospasm, increased secretions, with mucosal edema, and with the use of endotracheal tubes of different diameters. The flow rate of the gas into the lungs can generally be controlled on most mechanical ventilators.

At the end of the expiratory cycle, before the ventilator cycles into inspiration, there is no flow of gas. Alveolar and mouth pressure are equal. Since there is no flow, there is no resistance to flow. When the ventilator cycles on and creates a positive pressure at the upper airway, the gas attempts to move into the lower pressure zones in the alveoli. However, its movement is impeded or blocked by having to pass through the endotracheal tube and the upper conductive airways. Some of the molecules are slowed down as they collide with the tube and the bronchial walls. In doing this they are exerting energy or pressure against the passages. In reality, this causes the airways to expand. The cost of doing this results in a loss of some of the pressure or gas molecules that were intended for the alveoli. In addition, as the gas molecules flow through the airway, the layers of gas flow over each other. This, too, causes resistance to flow which is called viscous resistance.

The relationship of gas flow, pressure, and resistance in the airways is described by the equation for airway resistance: Raw = P_{TA}/flow, where Raw is airway resistance, PTA is the pressure difference between the mouth and the alveolus, or the transairway pressure, and flow is the gas flow. Resistance is usually expressed in centimeters of water per liter per second. In normal conscious individuals with a gas flow of 0.5 L/sec, the resistance is about 0.6 to 2.4 cm H_2O/L/sec. The actual amount varies over the entire respiratory cycle. The variation occurs because the flow during spontaneous ventilation is usually slower at the beginning and the end of the cycle, and fast in the middle. With artificial airways in place, normal airway resistance is increased. The smaller the internal diameter of the tube, the greater the resistance to flow. Resistance is in the range of about 6 cm H_2O/L/sec, or greater than normal.

Diseases of the airway also increase resistance. In conscious nonintubated subjects with emphysema and asthma, the resistance may range from 13 to 18 cm H_2O/L/sec. Still higher values will occur with other severe types of obstructive disorders. The disadvantage of higher airway resistance to breathing is obvious. With higher resistance, more of the pressure for breathing is lost to the airway resistance and never reaches the alveoli. With less pressure in the alveolus, less volume of gas is available for gas exchange.

Another disadvantage of high resistance is that more force must be exerted to try and get the gas to flow through the obstructed airways. To achieve this force, spontaneously breathing patients use their accessory muscles to try and breathe. This generates higher intrapleural pressures and a greater pressure gradient in order to achieve a flow of gas. The same occurs during mechanical ventilation. More pressure is exerted to try and "blow" the air into the patient's lungs through airways that are obstructed or through a small endotracheal tube.

MECHANICAL VENTILATION

In developing ways to mimic or replace the normal mechanisms of breathing, three methods have been developed. These are negative pressure ventilation, positive pressure ventilation, and high-frequency ventilation.

Negative Pressure Ventilation

Negative pressure ventilation attempts to mimic the actual function of the respiratory muscles to allow breathing through normal physiologic mechanisms. A good example of a negative pressure ventilator is the tank ventilator, or the "iron lung." In this method, the patient's head is exposed to ambient pressure. Either the thoracic area or the entire body is encased in an airtight container that is subjected to negative pressure, i.e., pressure less than atmospheric. When negative pressure is generated around the thoracic area, this negative pressure is transmitted across the chest wall, into the intrapleural space, and finally into the

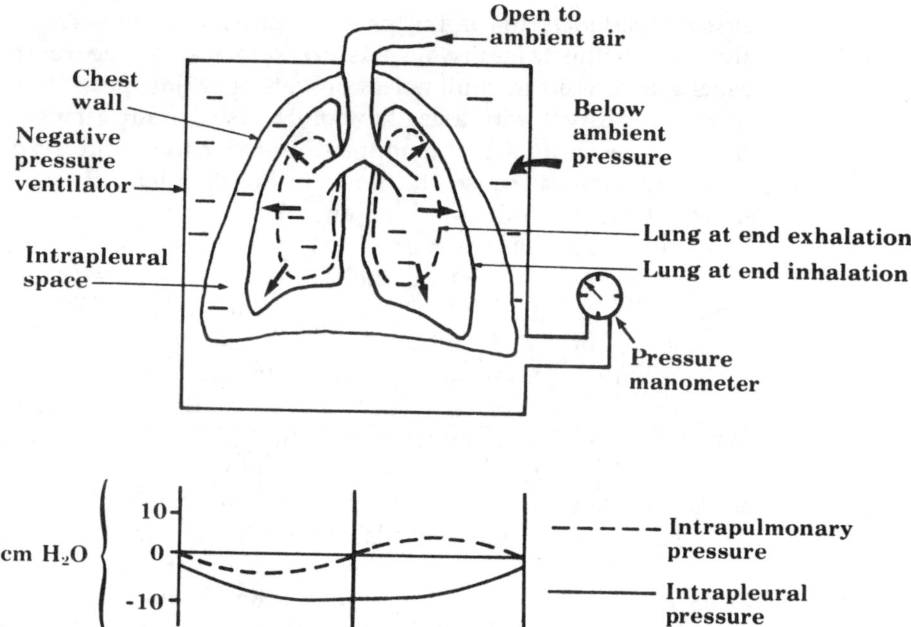

FIG 2–3.
Negative pressure ventilation and the resulting lung mechanics and pressures.

intraalveolar space. The intrapulmonary or intraalveolar space becomes increasingly negative in relation to the pressure at the mouth. A pressure gradient exists. Air moves into the lungs. In this way, the negative pressure ventilator resembles normal lung mechanics. Expiration occurs when the negative pressure around the chest wall is removed. The normal elastic recoil allows air to flow out of the lungs passively (Fig 2–3).

These ventilators have significant advantages. The upper airway can be kept open without the use of an endotracheal tube or tracheotomy. Patients are able to talk and eat. Negative pressure ventilation also has fewer physiologic disadvantages.[23] This is mostly because negative pressure ventilation is like normal lung-thorax mechanics. With hypovolemic patients, however, the negative pressure on the abdomen is not fully compensated for by normal cardiovascular responses. Patients can have significant pooling of blood in the abdomen and reduced venous return to the heart.

While the negative pressure ventilator declined in popularity through the 1970s and early 1980s, it is now showing a bit of a revival. Newer methods of creating negative pressure breathing suits and better ways to fit the chest cuirass have resulted in a resurrection of these once very popular ventilators. Their current use is mostly for care of patients in the home setting. They are used with patients who require some ventilatory support, such as at night for sleeping. But these patients are not usually ventilator-dependent. Negative pressure ventilators are often used in patients who have chronic respiratory failure of neurologic origin such as polio and amyotrophic lateral sclerosis.[10] Further discussion of negative pressure ventilation is provided in Chapter 14.

Positive Pressure Ventilation

Positive pressure ventilation occurs when a mechanical ventilator literally blows air into the patient's lungs by way of the endotracheal tube. Pressure is positive at the mouth and zero in the alveoli so air moves into the lungs owing to this gradient. For example, if the pressure at the mouth or upper airway is +15 cm H_2O and the pressure in the alveolus is zero, the gradient is: $P_{TA} = Pawo - P_A$, or 15 − (0) = 15 cm H_2O.

At any point during inspiration the inflating pressure at the upper (proximal) airway will equal the sum of the pressures required to overcome the elastic resistance of the lung and chest wall and the resistance of the airways. The pressure in the alveolus builds progressively and becomes more positive. Positive P_A is transmitted across the visceral pleura. The intrapleural space may become positive at the end of inspiration (Fig 2–4).

At the end of inspiration the ventilator stops delivering positive pressure. Mouth pressure returns to ambient (zero). Alveolar pressure is still positive. This creates a gradient between the mouth and the alveolus and air flows out. Exhalation is passive. The muscles do not have to actively contract. Alveolar pressure returns to zero or ambient and exhalation ends.

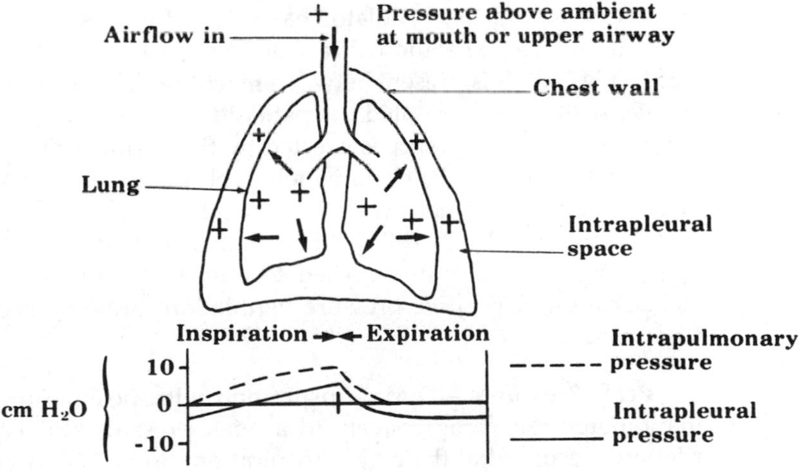

FIG 2–4.
The mechanics and pressures associated with positive pressure ventilation. Intrapleural pressures are above ambient during end-inspiration.

High-Frequency Ventilation

High-frequency positive pressure ventilation is the use of high ventilating rates that are above normal with low ventilating volumes that are below normal. There are three basic modes of high-frequency ventilation: (1) high-frequency positive pressure ventilation (HFPPV), which uses respiratory rates between about 60 and 100 breaths/min; (2) high-frequency jet ventilation (HFJV), which uses rates between about 100 and 400 to 600/min; and (3) high-frequency oscillation, which uses rates in the thousands up to about 4,000/min. These are more correctly defined by the type of ventilator used rather than the specific rates of each. Ventilation with high frequency has been used primarily in infants with respiratory distress and in adults or infants with open air leaks such as bronchopleural fistulas.

Measuring Pressures During Positive Pressure Ventilation

At any point in a respiratory cycle, you can look at the manometer or pressure gauge of a ventilator and take a reading. This reading is measured either very close to the mouth (proximal airway pressure) or on the inside of the ventilator where it closely estimates pressure at the mouth or airway opening.

Baseline Pressures.—Pressures are read from a baseline value (Fig 2–5). Normally, baseline is zero on the manometer and indicates that during expiration and before inspiration, there is no additional pressure at the airway. Pressure is atmospheric.

Sometimes baseline takes on a higher value than zero. This occurs only if the person operating the ventilator has selected a pressure higher than zero to be present during exhalation. We call this positive end-expiratory pressure, or PEEP (Fig 2–6). It is present between machine-delivered breaths. This means that the ventilator has prevented the patient from exhaling to zero or atmospheric. A certain resistance pressure is exerted by the ventilator's expiratory valve so that the patient cannot exhale completely. This increases the volume left in the lungs at the end of a normal exhalation. In other words there is an increased functional residual capacity (FRC). PEEP that is applied by the operator is sometimes called extrinsic PEEP as opposed to auto-PEEP, or intrinsic PEEP, which is a complication of positive pressure ventilation. More is discussed about PEEP in Chapter 11.

Peak Pressures.—During inspiration with positive pressure ventilation the manometer rises progressively to a peak pressure (P_{Peak}). This is the highest pressure recorded at the end of inspiration. P_{Peak} is also called peak inspiratory pressure (PIP) or peak airway pressure (see Fig 2–5).

The pressures measured *during* inspiration are actually the sum of two pressures: first, the pressure required to force the gas through the resistance of

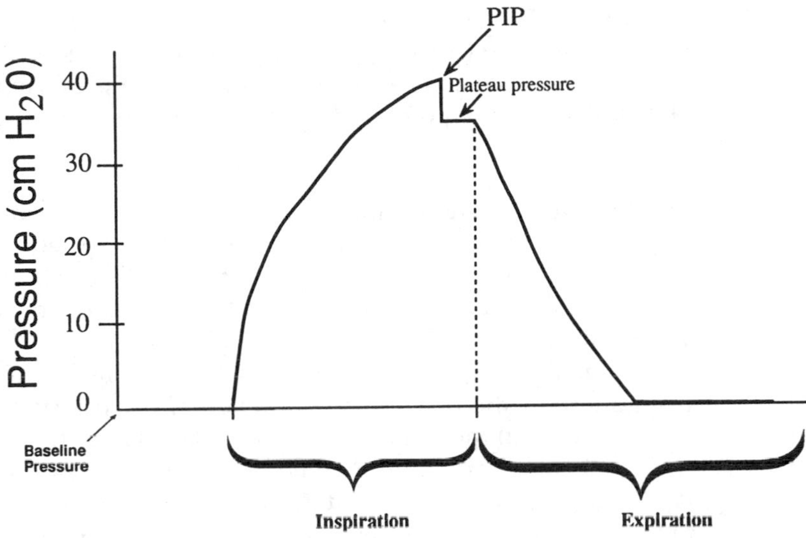

FIG 2–5.
The upper airway pressures during a positive pressure breath. Pressure rises during inspiration to peak inspiratory pressure *(PIP)*. With a breath hold, the plateau pressure can be measured. Pressures fall back to baseline during expiration.

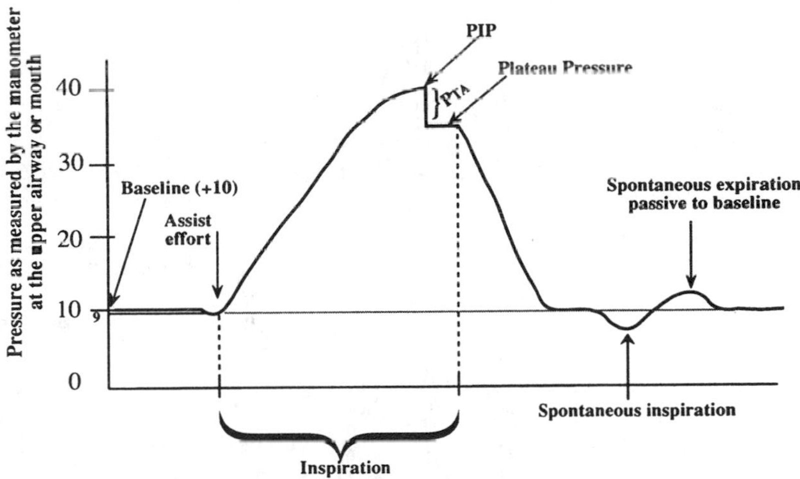

FIG 2–6.
The airway pressures during both a mechanical, positive pressure breath and a spontaneous breath. Both of these are at an elevated baseline. Positive end-expiratory pressure (PEEP) = +10 cm H_2O. To assist a breath the pressure drops below baseline by 1 cm H_2O. Assist effort is at +9 cm H_2O. *PIP* = peak inspiratory pressure; *PTA* = transairway pressure.

the airways, P_{TA}; second, it reflects the gas volume as it fills the alveoli. Pressure on the manometer or gauge is the sum of the pressure lost in the conductive airways due to airway resistance (P_{TA}), and the pressure required to inflate the alveoli (P_A). At any point during inspiration, the pressure on the gauge equals $P_{TA} + P_A$.

Plateau Pressure.—Another valuable pressure measurement is plateau pressure. Plateau pressure is actually a pressure measurement that is taken after a breath has been delivered to the patient and before exhalation has begun. In this instance, exhalation is prevented by the ventilator for a fraction of a second when this maneuver is selected.

Plateau pressure measurement is like holding your breath at the end of inspiration. At the point of breath holding, the pressure inside the alveoli and mouth are equal (no gas flow). But the relaxation of the respiratory muscles and the elastic recoil of the lung tissues is exerting force on the inflated lungs. This creates a positive pressure and is read on the manometer as a positive pressure. Since it is during a breath hold, or pause, the reading is stable. It "plateaus" at a certain pressure (Figs 2–5 to 2–7).

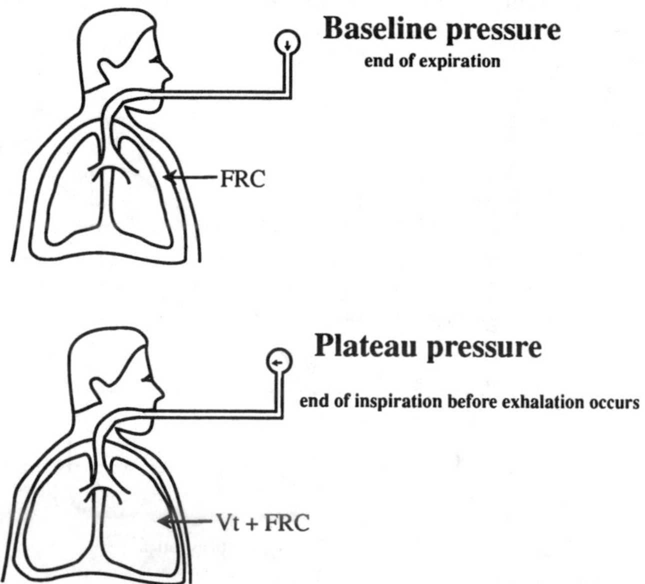

FIG 2–7.
At baseline pressure and the end of expiration, the volume remaining in the lungs is the functional residual capacity *(FRC)*. At the end of inspiration before exhalation starts, the volume in the lungs is the tidal volume (V_T) plus the FRC. The pressure measured at this time with no flow of air is called *plateau pressure.*

Plateau pressure is sometimes used interchangeably with the term alveolar pressure (P_A) or intrapulmonary pressure. The two are close in value, but not always equal. Plateau pressure reflects the effect of the elastic recoil of the lungs and chest on the gas volume inside the alveoli *and* any pressure exerted by the volume in the ventilator circuit. A true, stable plateau will allow pressure equalization so that P_A = Pawo = pressure on manometer.

Pressure at the End of Exhalation.—Air can be trapped in the lungs during mechanical ventilation if not enough time is allowed for exhalation. In order to avoid this, one should measure the pressure in the ventilator at the end of exhalation before inhalation begins. The reading normally equals the desired baseline pressure, be it zero or PEEP. If it is greater than the normal baseline, air trapping is present. This is called auto-PEEP or intrinsic PEEP (see Chapter 7).

Measuring Airway Resistance

We can take measurements for PIP and P_A. We cannot easily measure airway resistance pressure or P_{TA}; however, we can calculate its value. PIP − P_A = P_{TA}. This allows us to determine how much pressure is going to the airways and how much to alveoli where it is functional in gas exchange. For example, if the PIP is 25 cm H_2O and the plateau pressure is 20 cm H_2O, how much pressure is lost to the airways due to airway resistance? 25 cm H_2O − 20 cm H_2O = 5 cm H_2O. Actually, 5 cm H_2O is about a normal amount of pressure to lose to airway resistance (Raw) when a patient has an endotracheal tube of the proper size in place. If the PIP is 40 cm H_2O and the plateau pressure is 25 cm H_2O, how much pressure is going to Raw? This value is high and indicates an increase in Raw: 40 cm H_2O − 25 cm H_2O = 15 cm H_2O.

Mechanical ventilators often have dials which give specific flow rate settings. Some ventilators also have monitors which read the actual gas flow rate value. With this additional information, one can calculate an estimate of Raw on a ventilated patient. This calculation assumes that flow is constant. If the flow rate is constant at 60 L/min, and we use the pressure reading above for P_{TA}, we can estimate Raw. First, since Raw is usually measured in centimeters of water per liter per second, we must convert the flow to liters per second rather than using liters per minute: 60 L/min = 60 L/60 sec, or 1 L/sec. We can now substitute our values into the equation for Raw.

$$\text{Raw} = (\text{PIP} - \text{Plateau pressure})/\text{flow}$$

$$\text{Raw} = 15 \text{ cm } H_2O/(1 \text{ L/sec})$$

$$\text{Raw} = 15 \text{ cm } H_2O/(\text{L/sec})$$

For an intubated patient, this is a high value for Raw and may be due to secretions or bronchospasm. A respiratory care practitioner should be careful about listening to breath sounds and determining the possible cause of the increased resistance. Some of the newer microprocessor ventilators have the capability of calculating resistance. This calculation is determined on the basis of where the pressure and flow is being measured. If the measurements are internal to the ventilator, they are less accurate than those measured at the airway opening. For example, some ventilators measure flow at the exhalation valve and pressure on the inspiratory side of the ventilator. These values will pick up the resistance to flow through the patient circuit and not just patient airway resistance. They are less accurate than those calculations which use measurements taken at the airway opening.

Measuring Lung or Chest Wall Compliance

Recall that compliance is a volume measured per unit of pressure. In mechanically ventilated patients compliance calculations use the plateau pressure measured at static or no flow conditions. One also uses the pressure at end-exhalation. You then measure the volume that is actually exhaled from the patient's lungs. This is most easily done by measuring the volume at the patient wye-connector (Fig 2–8). The equation for calculating static compliance (Cs) in the ventilated patient is:

$$C_{\text{LUNG}} = (\text{exhaled } V_T)/(\text{Plateau pressure} - \text{EEP})$$

where EEP = end-expiratory pressure or baseline pressure. By measuring the baseline pressure and subtracting this from our plateau pressure reading we can determine the pressure change that was required to achieve our exhaled V_T (see Fig 2–8). Using only these two pressures eliminates any Raw pressure from our reading. Dividing this pressure change into the actual exhaled V_T will give us our patient's lung compliance, or static compliance.

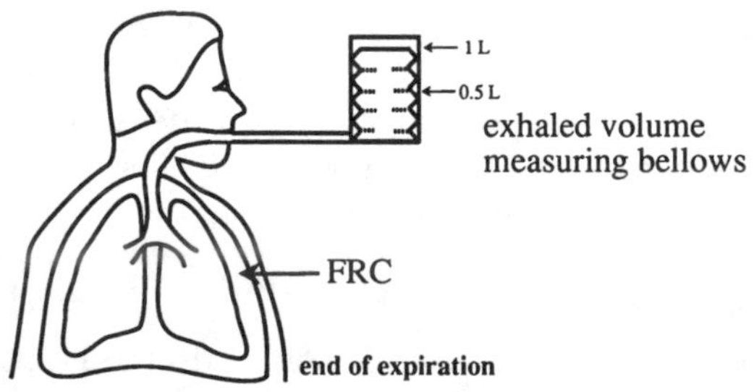

FIG 2–8.
A bellows device measuring the volume of gas as it is exhaled from the patient. Many ventilators now use a flow transducer to measure the exhaled tidal volume. *FRC* = functional residual capacity.

GRAPHICS OF BASIC POSITIVE PRESSURE BREATHS

Later in the book the physical aspects of ventilation are covered along with monitoring techniques. Basic to learning these concepts is an understanding of the interrelation of pressure, time, flow, and volume during mechanical ventilation. Part of the explanation of these incorporates the use of the graphs. In this section exercises in graphing will provide an introduction to these concepts. Newer microprocessor ventilators now provide graphic reading of these curves as well as graphs of compliance and airway resistance. For this reason, it is very important for the student of mechanical ventilation to understand how to read these graphs.

Fundamentals of Pressure, Time, Flow, and Volume

How much volume or air will fill a patient's lungs during mechanical ventilation depends on two basic factors – the patient's lung characteristics (compliance and resistance) and the force or power causing gas flow into the lungs. Imagine, for example, that you have two people trying to blow up two new balloons. One person is very strong and muscular. The other is very weak and feeble. The weak person will only generate a small amount of pressure to inflate the balloon. Less flow will go into the balloon and less volume. The strong person will generate a lot of pressure to inflate the balloon. The flow will be high so the balloon will fill faster and with a greater volume. This is comparable to a ventilator with a strong source of power vs. one with a very weak source of power. The following four principles explain the basic interrelation of pressure, volume, time, and flow:

1. The volume delivered depends on the amount of flow and how much time is given in which the flow is to occur.
2. The flow rate of gas into the lungs depends on the difference in pressure between the power source, the ventilator, and the pressure inside the lungs. The greater this pressure gradient, the greater the flow rate.
3. The pressure in the lung depends on the stiffness of the lung and the volume delivered. If the lung is easy to inflate (very compliant), it does not take much pressure to inflate it. If the lung is very stiff (low compliance value), it requires more pressure to inflate it.
4. The pressure measured at the mouth (Pawo) depends on the resistance of the conductive tube and the compliance of the lungs. Looking just at the tube, the larger the size (diameter) of the tube, the easier and greater the potential flow. Whereas, the smaller the diameter, the lower the flow and the greater the resistance in trying to achieve a specific flow.

High Energy Source Ventilator

Let us use an example of a ventilator which has a high-power source. One such ventilator would be one that uses a cylinder of compressed gas connected to a 50-psig (pounds per square inch gauge) regulator. The 50-psig pressure is equal to about 3,500 cm H_2O above atmospheric (1 psig = ~70 cm H_2O of pressure). Recall that PA is very low, nearly zero.

Connecting a 50-psig gas source to a lung is, of course, dangerous. But if a clamp were placed in line between the gas source and the lungs, it could regulate the amount of flow allowed to pass (Fig 2–9). The clamp, in technical terms, is called high internal resistance. With this type of ventilator, no matter how stiff the lung, any desired gas flow or volume could be achieved. No amount of back pressure on the system would slow the flow down coming from the cylinder because of the high pressure source. It could produce a constant

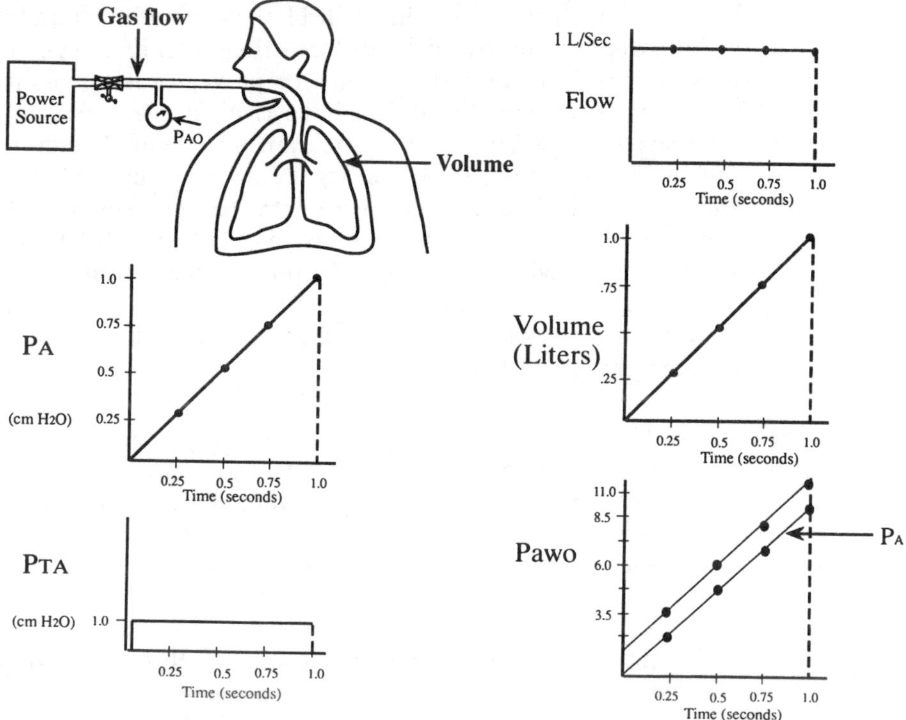

FIG 2–9.
A high-energy source ventilator with high internal resistance. Flow is constant. Volume rises as an ascending ramp during inspiration. Alveolar pressure *(PA)* also rises as an ascending ramp. Transairway pressure *(PTA)* is a rectangular waveform, just like the flow curve. Monitored gauge pressures *(Pawo)* are the sum of PTA and PA.

flow of gas. Also, no matter how much airway resistance is present between the ventilator and the lung, it will not affect the high energy source pressure. The source will stay at 50 psig.

Graphic Examples

Using the ventilator described above, let us imagine we have a patient with normal lung compliance of 0.1 L/cm H_2O, a normal Raw of 1.0 cm H_2O/L/sec, an average gas flow of 60 Ls/min (1 L/sec), and an inspiratory time of 1 second. What type of curves would this generate after 0.25, 0.5, 0.75, and 1.0 second?

The specific curves we are generating are (1) flow, (2) volume delivery, (3) alveolar pressure, and (4) transairway pressure, and (5) pressure at the airway opening (Pawo = PA + PTA). For each time interval on the horizontal axis we need to calculate the value for each of the variables (flow, volume, and pressure) on the vertical axis since they will change (vary) over time.

In drawing the curves we use a constant flow ventilator. Always draw the flow curve first. Second, calculate the volume delivered at every 0.25-second interval. Third, use the volume calculated for each 0.25 second to calculate PA (PA = $\Delta V/C$). Fourth, calculate PTA using flow and resistance values. Flows must be in liters per second. Finally, add the values of PTA and PA for each 0.25-second interval. This will be Pawo. Remember Pawo = PTA + PA.

The values calculated below are all graphed on Figure 2–9.

Flow.—Flow is volume per unit time and for this ventilator it is constant at 60 L/min or 1 L/sec (60 L/min × 60 sec/min = 1 L/sec)

Time	Variable: FLOW
0.25 sec	1 L/sec
0.5 sec	1 L/sec
0.75 sec	1 L/sec
1.00 sec	1 L/sec

Volume.—Volume is the product of inspiratory time and flow.

Time	Variable: VOLUME
0.25 sec	0.25 sec × 1 L/sec = 0.25 L
0.5 sec	0.5 sec × 1 L/sec = 0.50 L
0.75 sec	0.75 sec × 1 L/sec = 0.75 L
1.00 sec	1.00 sec × 1 L/sec = 1.00 L

Pressures

Alveolar pressure (PA) = volume/compliance

Time	Variable: ALVEOLAR PRESSURE
0.25 sec	0.25 L/(0.1 L/cm H_2O) = 2.5 cm H_2O
0.5 sec	0.5 L/(0.1 L/cm H_2O) = 5.0 cm H_2O
0.75 sec	0.75 L/(0.1 L/cm H_2O) = 7.5 cm H_2O
1.00 sec	1.00 L/(0.1 L/cm H_2O) = 10.0 cm H_2O

Transairway pressure (PTA) = flow × Raw

Time	Variable: TRANSAIRWAY PRESSURE
0.25 sec	1 L/sec × 1.0 cm H_2O/(L/sec) = 1.0 cm H_2O
0.5 sec	1 L/sec × 1.0 cm H_2O/(L/sec) = 1.0 cm H_2O
0.75 sec	1 L/sec × 1.0 cm H_2O/(L/sec) = 1.0 cm H_2O
1.00 sec	1 L/sec × 1.0 cm H_2O/(L/sec) = 1.0 cm H_2O

Pressure at Airway Opening (Pawo) = PA + PTA

The total pressure at the airway opening or mouth is the sum of pressure due to airway resistance plus alveolar pressure.

Time	Variable: AIRWAY OPENING PRESSURE
0.25 sec	2.5 cm H_2O + 1.0 cm H_2O = 3.5 cm H_2O
0.5 sec	5.0 cm H_2O + 1.0 cm H_2O = 6.0 cm H_2O
0.75 sec	7.5 cm H_2O + 1.0 cm H_2O = 8.5 cm H_2O
1.00 sec	10.0 cm H_2O + 1.0 cm H_2O = 11.0 cm H_2O*

*Peak inspiratory pressure (PIP).

Note that with a constant flow the pressure lost to Raw is constant. The curve representing PTA always parallels flow. Also note that with a constant flow, the rise in volume is at a constant rate. And it is important that the PA curve resemble the volume delivery curve.

Compliance Curves

Another graph that is available with newer computer monitoring is the graph of volume and pressure. Recall that these two variables describe compliance ($C = \Delta V/\Delta P$). During the monitoring of these curves gas flow is still occurring. As a result, they also provide some information about Raw.

Note that in Figure 2–10 line *AB* represents the volume-pressure relationship of the normal lung. This is under *no flow* conditions. Since compliance represents the elastic component of the lungs, the shaded area marked triangle *ABE* represents the amount of mechanical work required to overcome the elastic resistance properties of the lungs.

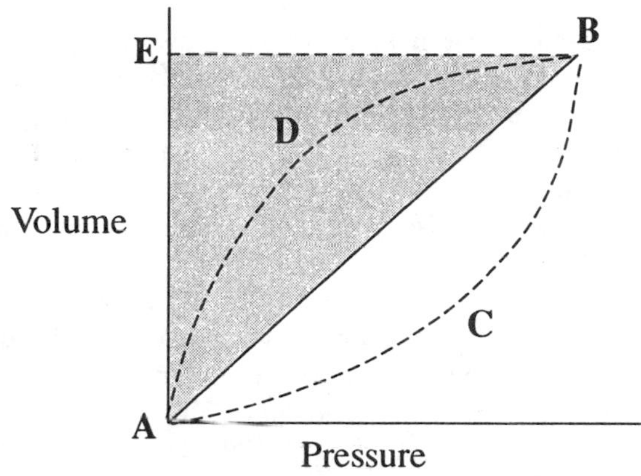

FIG 2–10.
A volume pressure curve in the normal lung. *Shaded area* represents the amount of mechanical work required to overcome the elastic resistance properties of the lung. See text.

With less compliant (stiffer) lungs, greater pressure is needed for a given volume. The line *AB* rotates to the right. With more compliant lungs, less pressure is needed to achieve the same volume. The line *AB* rotates to the left. Examples of stiff lung conditions include fibrotic diseases of the lung; conditions that flood the alveoli with fluids, such as pulmonary edema and pneumonia; and conditions that deflate alveoli, i.e., atelectasis. Conditions that are more compliant (left shift) are diseases such as emphysema or aging.

With flow present, the straight-line relationship no longer exists. Instead, the line is curved during inspiration and expiration. A certain amount of extra pressure is needed during inhalation (curve *ACB*) and exhalation (curve *BDA*) to overcome the resistance of the airways and the tissues or nonelastic (frictional) forces opposing ventilation.

The total mechanical work of breathing is the sum of the shaded triangle *ABE* and the curved area *ACB*. The inspiratory work due to tissue resistance, especially Raw, is the curve *ACB*. The expiratory work is represented by the curve *ADB*.

When lung compliance is normal but there is more Raw present, such as an obstructed airway, the amount of pressure needed to overcome airway resistance increases. The ellipse *ACBD* gets fatter or tends to bulge.

TIME CONSTANTS AND UNEVEN VENTILATION

The changes in compliance and resistance that occur in the lungs do not occur evenly throughout the lung parenchyma. Small parts may be affected by increased resistance, others by low compliance, and others will be entirely normal. Because of this, different areas of the lung will fill faster than others.

Imagine that each small unit of the lung is like a small inflatable balloon attached to a short soda straw. The amount of volume that each balloon receives in relation to other small units will depend on its compliance and resistance—assuming other factors are equal such as ventilating pressure and location in the lung zones.

As the normal lung unit fills, it fills within a fairly reasonable period of time and with a large volume (Fig 2–11,A). On the other hand, if the balloon is very stiff (low compliance/high elastance), it fills rapidly but with a much smaller volume for the same amount of filling pressure (Fig 2–11,B). By further contrast,

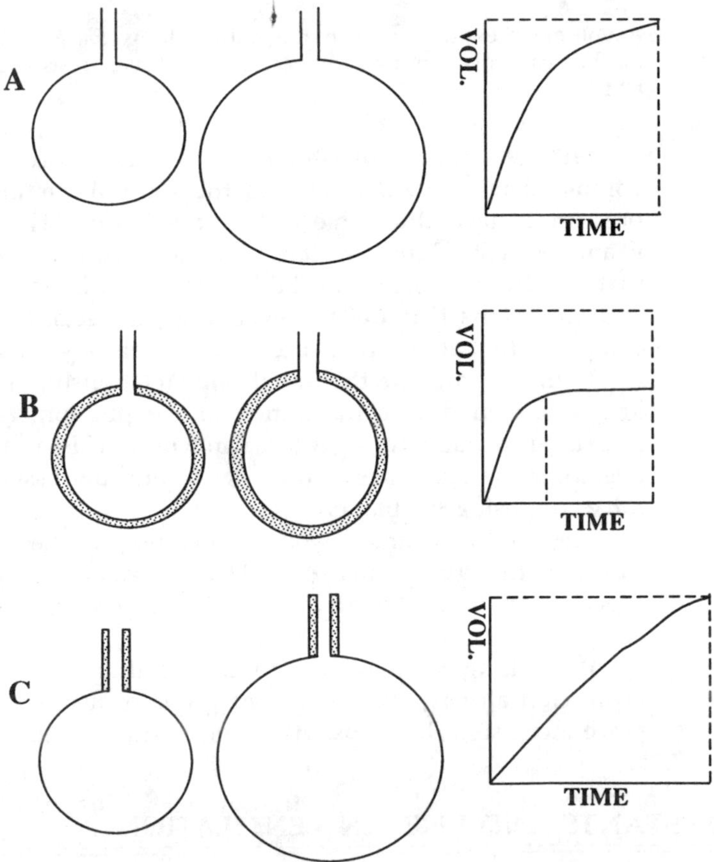

FIG 2–11.
A, filling of a normal lung unit. **B,** low compliance unit that fills quickly but to a lesser amount. **C,** increase in resistance. The unit fills slowly. If time were to end at the same time as in **A,** the volume in **C** would be lower.

if the balloon is normal, but our straw very narrow (high resistance), the lung unit fills very slowly and with a smaller volume than would normal units were inspiration short. The shorter the time for inhalation, as occurs with a high respiratory rate or fast inspiratory flow rates, the lower the lung volume for units that are not normal and that fill slowly (Fig 2–11,C).

In normal lung units (see Fig 2–11,A) filling can be nearly complete before exhalation begins. Stiff lung units (see Fig 2–11,B) fill and empty quickly, but never receive as much volume as normal lung units. High-resistance units (see Fig 2–11,C) fill slowly. The rest of the lung could very well begin exhalation before high-resistance units have received their entire volume.

The amount and rate of filling of each lung unit depends on the compliance and resistance of that unit. The rate at which individual units fill is called the *time constant.* The time constant is a mathematical expression that has been derived in other texts.[4,12] This derivation will not be done here. But a basic understanding of the time constant is important to understand lung ventilation. A time constant is the product of compliance and resistance ($C \times R$). For example, if the compliance is 0.1 L/cm H_2O and the resistance is 1 cm H_2O/L/sec, the time constant will be:

$$0.1 \text{ L/cm } H_2O \times 1 \text{ cm } H_2O/(\text{L/sec}) = 0.1 \text{ second}$$

One time constant allows 63% of either the inspiratory phase or the expiratory phase to occur. Two time constants allow about 86% of either phase to occur. Three time constants allow about 95% of either phase, and four time constants allow 99.3% of inspiration or expiration to occur. Five time constants theoretically allow nearly all of inspiration or expiration to occur. In our example, five time constants would equal 5×0.1 second or 0.5 second.

Calculation of time constants becomes important in setting up a ventilator's inspiratory time and expiratory time. An inspiratory time of less than four to five time constants may cause incomplete delivery of the V_T. Prolonging inspiratory time allows an even distribution of ventilation and adequate V_T delivery. However, if it is too long, it may slow the respiratory rate to a level at which enough minute ventilation ($\dot{V}_E$) in 1 minute is not possible.

An expiratory time of less than four to five time constants may lead to incomplete emptying of the lungs. This can increase FRC and cause inadvertent PEEP or auto-PEEP, also known as air trapping. Some authors believe that using the 95% time point of three time constants is adequate.[12] Exact time settings would really require careful observation of the patient and measurement of end-expiratory pressure to determine which better is tolerated. There are fast-filling lung units with short time constants and slow-filling lung units with long time constants. Long time constants are a product of units with increased resistance or increased compliance, or both. These take more time to fill and empty. Short time constants are a product of reduced airway resistance or low compliance, or both. These take less time to fill and empty.

The most difficult thing to remember is that the lung is rarely an even mixture of ventilating units. Some units will empty and fill faster than others. The best thing a clinician can do is determine how the majority of the lung is functioning and base treatment of the patient according to this and the patient's response to therapy.

STUDY QUESTIONS

Exercise 1

This exercise helps to understand the graphs that are produced by some microprocessor ventilators. Doing the graphing exercise and calculations also helps the reader gain a better understanding of the relation between flow, volume, and pressures in the ventilated patient.

Assume you have a patient being ventilated by a volume-controlled ventilator. It is set to deliver a constant flow of gas during inspiration until it reaches the volume ordered by the physician. You are given the following information about the patient's lung characteristics and the ventilator parameters: (1) C = 20 mL/cm H_2O; (2) Raw = 15 cm H_2O/L/sec; (3) flow rate is constant at 40 L/min; (4) the ordered V_T is 1,000 mL; and (5) the end-expiratory pressure is zero (no PEEP). Calculate and graph the following from the known information.

1. Calculate the flow rate in liters per second.
2. Record under variable the flow at each 0.25 second of time that is present during inspiration. Graph the flow below (Fig 2–12,A) at 0.25-second intervals.
3. Calculate and graph the volume delivered at each 0.25-second interval during inspiration: Volume = time × flow (Fig 2–12,B).
   Note that the ordered V_T of 1,000 mL was delivered in about 1.5 seconds. A volume-controlled ventilator would stop the inspiratory phase at this point. For all graphs from this point on, we need only calculate for times up to 1.5 seconds.
4. Using the volume, calculate and graph the alveolar pressure. Recall that $C = \Delta V/\Delta P$. $P_A - EEP = \Delta P$ and $EEP = 0$. $P_A = V/C$. The volume is taken from the calculations of volume in Exercise 3 for each 0.25-second interval (see Fig 2–16,C).
5. Calculate and graph the transairway pressure (P_{TA}). Recall Raw = P_{TA}/flow. Therefore, P_{TA} = Raw × flow. Both Raw and flow have constant values. P_{TA} will have the same value for each 0.25-second interval (Fig 2–12,D).
6. Add the values of P_A and P_{TA} to determine the Pawo at each 0.25-second interval. Graph these values. Note that at the zero point on the *xy* = axis the Pawo will not go to zero. The pressure rises vary rapidly as the flow be-

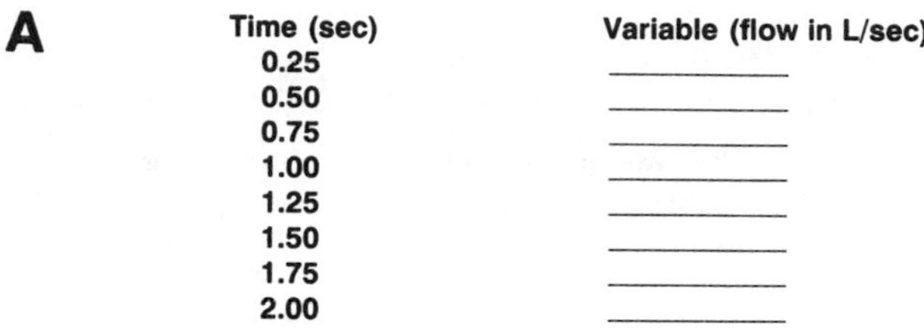

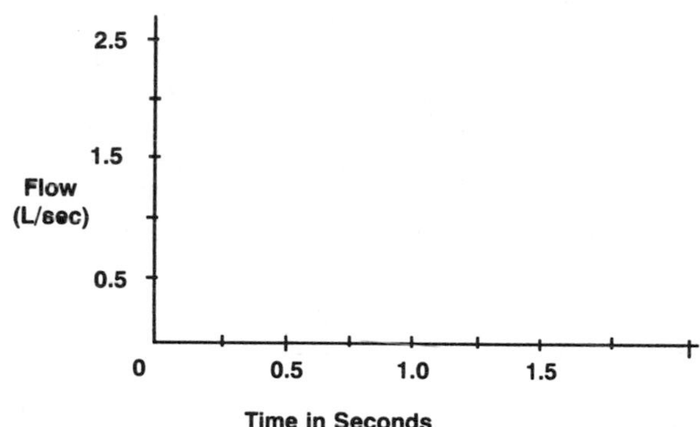

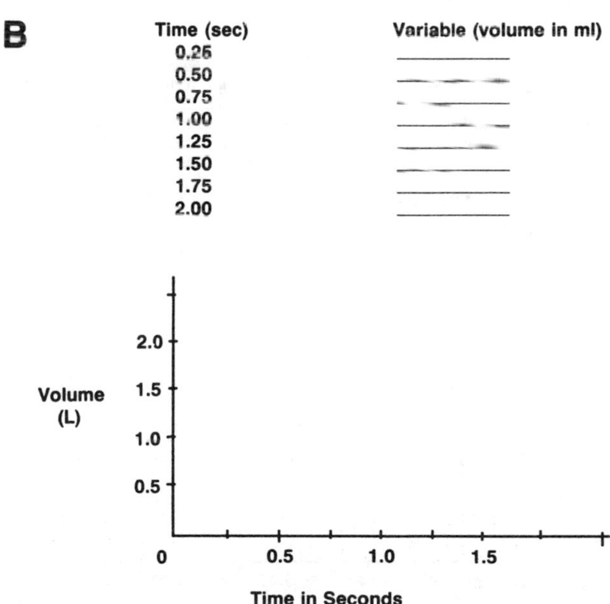

FIG 2–12.
A–B, graphic exercises. See text for explanation.

(Continued.)

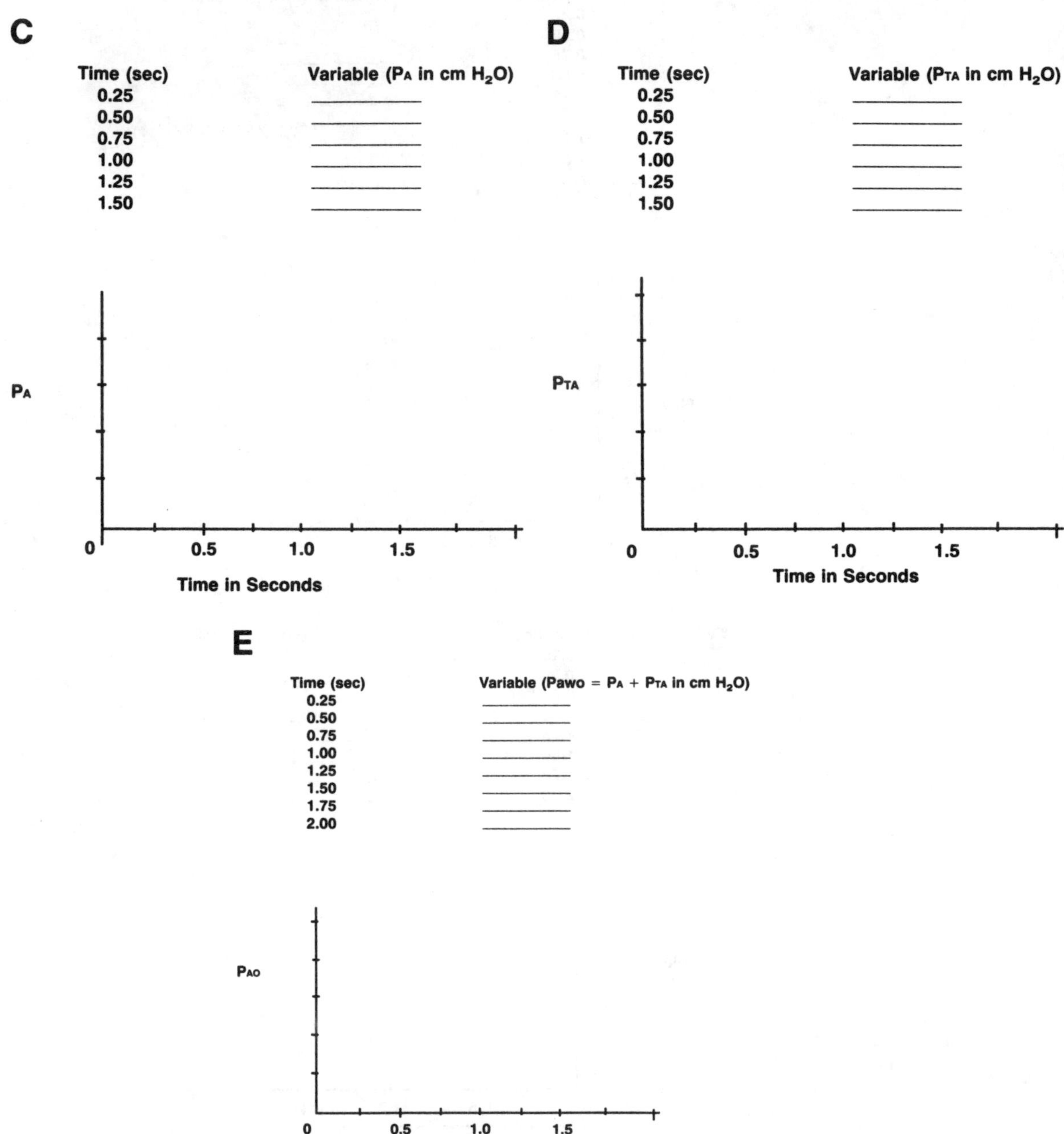

FIG 2–12 (cont.).
C–E, graphic exercises. See text for explanation.

A

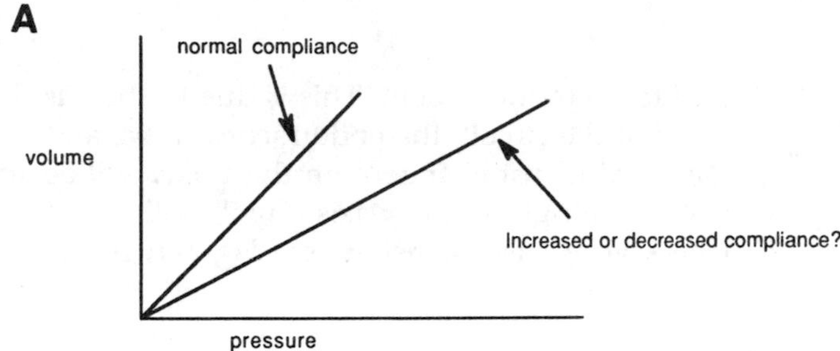

B

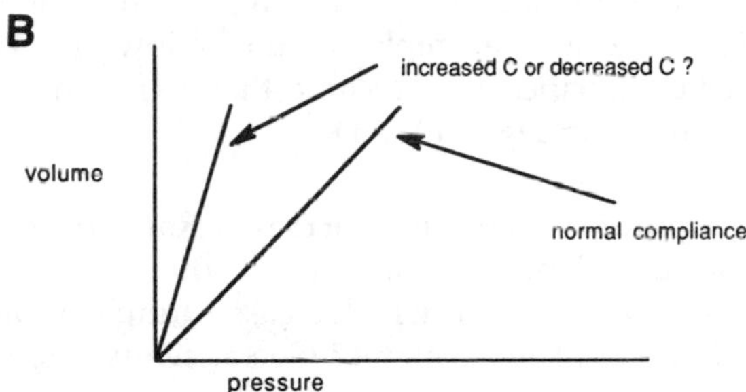

C

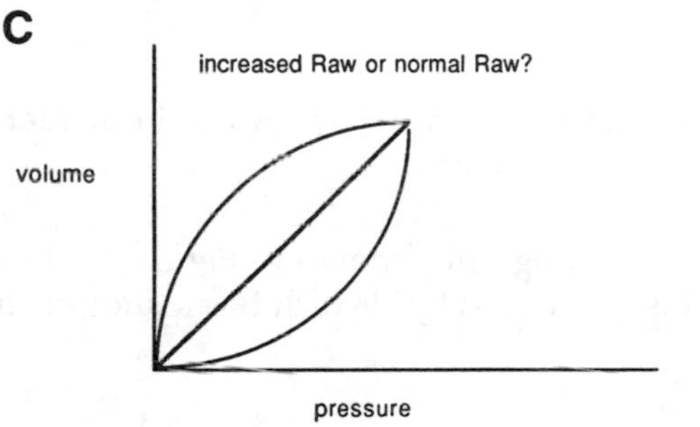

D

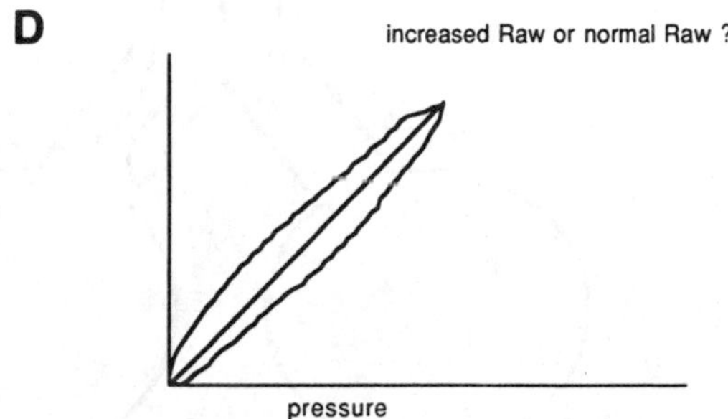

FIG 2–13.
A and **B,** exercises for evaluating compliance *(C)*. **C** and **D,** exercises for evaluating airway resistance. See text.

gins to go to the patient. This is due to the gas flow encountering the resistance of the circuit, the endotracheal tube, and the patient's airways. The Pawo value just near zero on the x-axis will be approximately equal to P_{TA} just to the right of the y-axis (Fig 2–12,E).

7. Check your answers below (see Fig 2–16,A–E).

Exercise 2

The curves in Figures 2–13,A–D represent compliance curves of volume and pressure. These give examples of the following: (1) increased compliance, (2) decreased compliance, (3) increased Raw, (4) normal Raw. Match the above (1–4) with the curves in Fig 2–13,A–D.

1. What conditions can cause increased Raw? How can this be detected on ventilated patients? (See answers below.)
2. What conditions can cause decreased lung compliance? How can this be detected on ventilated patients? (See answers below.)

Exercise 3

This exercise is intended to provide the reader with a little greater understanding of time constants.

1. Which of the lung units shown in Figure 2–14 will receive more volume during inspiration? Why? Which has a shorter time constant?

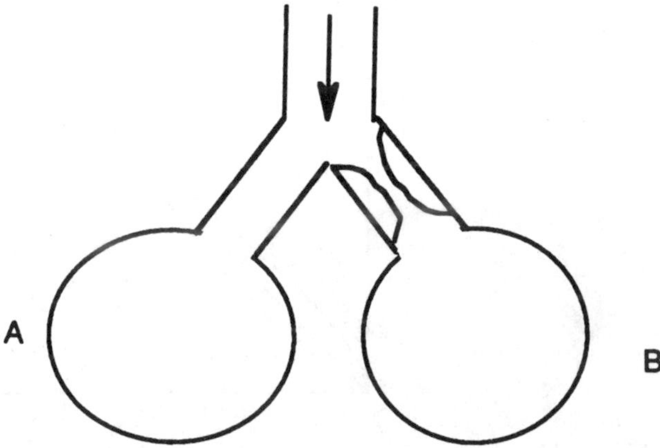

FIG 2–14.
Unit *A* is normal. Unit *B* shows an obstruction in the airway. See text.

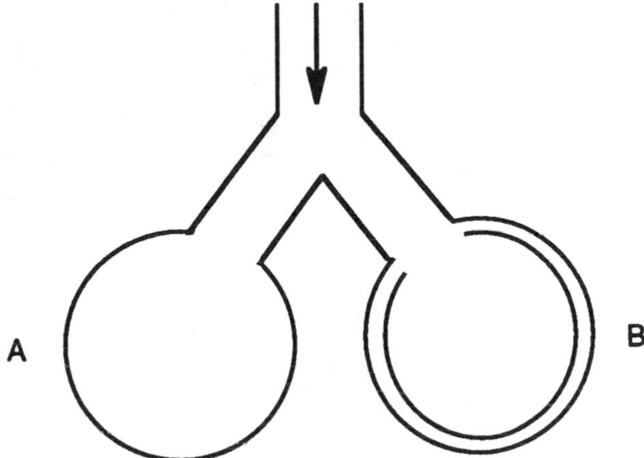

FIG 2–15.
Unit *A* is normal. Unit *B* shows decreased compliance. See text.

2. Which of the lung units shown in Figure 2–15 will fill more quickly? Which has the shortest time constant? Which will receive the greatest volume? Why?

ANSWERS TO STUDY QUESTIONS

Exercise 1

1. 40 L/min = 40 L/60 sec = ⅔ L in 1 second = 0.667 L/sec.
2. Figure 2–16,A.
3. The volume delivered at each 0.25-second interval during inspiration. Volume = time/flow (Fig 2–16,B). For all graphs from this point on, we only calculate for 1.5 seconds, since this marks the point where inspiration ends.
4. C = ΔV/ΔP. P_A − EEP = ΔP change and EEP = 0. P_A = V/C. The volume is taken from the calculations of volume in 3 for each 0.25-second interval. The curve for P_A will look like the curve for volume (Fig 2–16,C).
5. The transairway pressure (P_{TA}). Raw = P_{TA}/flow and P_{TA} = Raw × flow. Raw and flow are constant. The P_{TA} will look like the curve for flow (Fig 2–16,D).
6. The Pawo variable (Pawo = P_A + P_{TA} in cm H_2O) (Fig 2–16,E). The Pawo is the same pressure you would see on the ventilator's pressure gauge during inspiration. The Pawo value at 1.5 seconds (end-inspiration) is the peak pressure reading. If you did a plateau measurement at this point, the pressure would be minus P_{TA} (no flow, no resistance) and would be the plateau pressure which approximately equals the P_A.

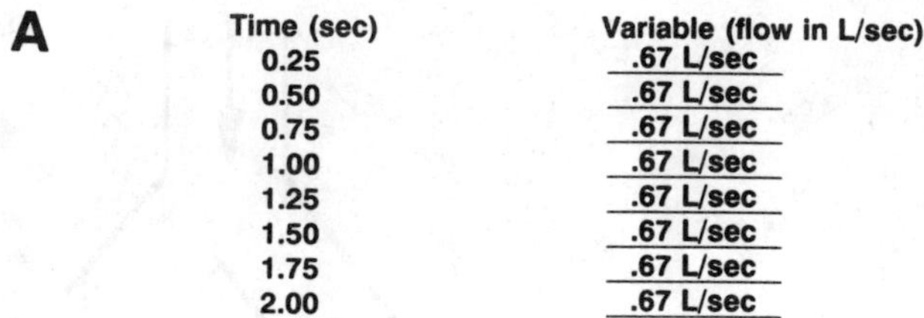

A

Time (sec)	Variable (flow in L/sec)
0.25	.67 L/sec
0.50	.67 L/sec
0.75	.67 L/sec
1.00	.67 L/sec
1.25	.67 L/sec
1.50	.67 L/sec
1.75	.67 L/sec
2.00	.67 L/sec

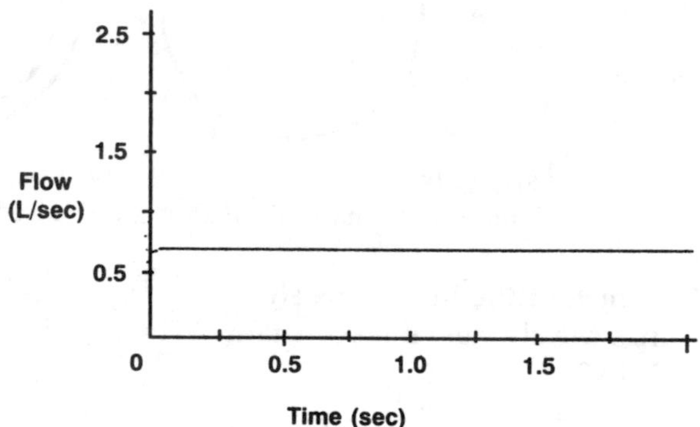

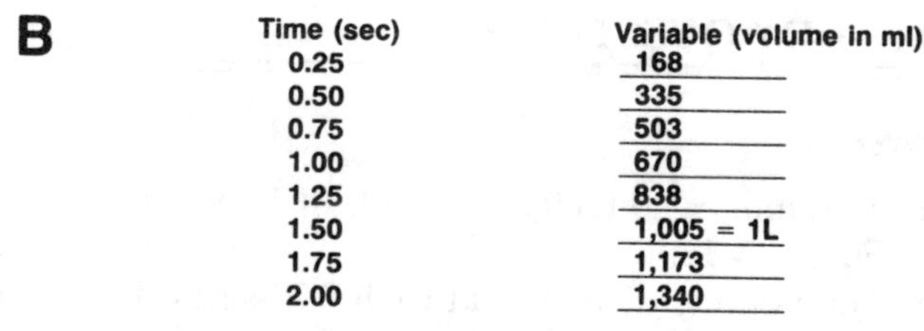

B

Time (sec)	Variable (volume in ml)
0.25	168
0.50	335
0.75	503
1.00	670
1.25	838
1.50	1,005 = 1L
1.75	1,173
2.00	1,340

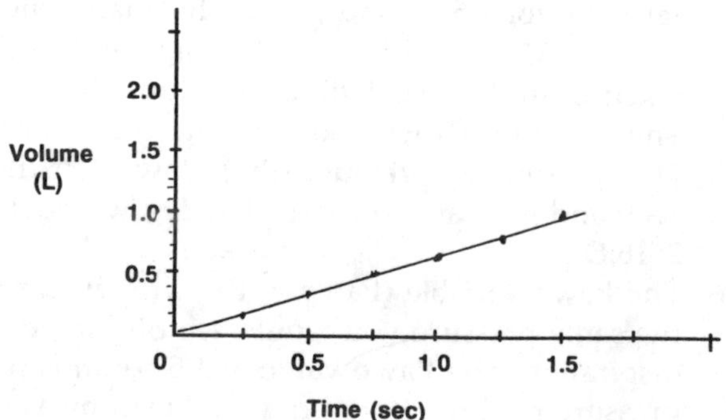

FIG 2–16.
A–B, Answers to exercise 1.

C

Time (sec)	Variable (P_A in cm H_2O)
0.25	8.4
0.50	16.8
0.75	25.1
1.00	33.5
1.25	41.9
1.50	50.3

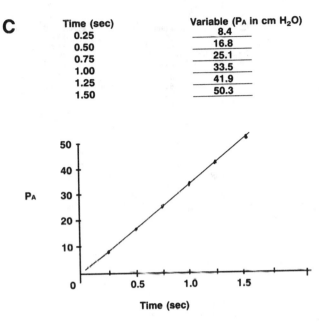

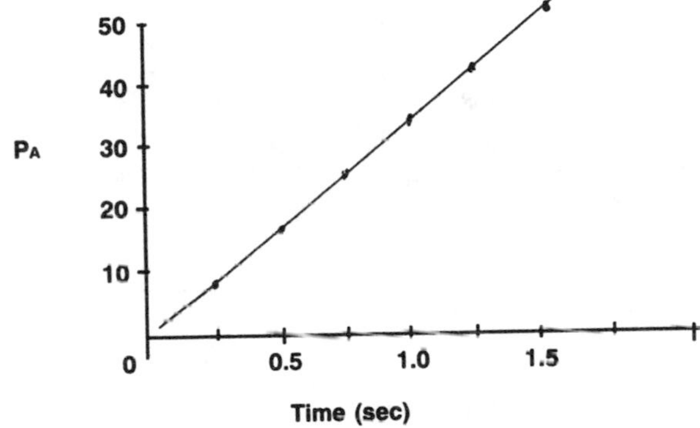

D

Time (sec)	Variable (P_{TA} in cm H_2O)
0.25	10
0.50	10
0.75	10
1.00	10
1.25	10
1.50	10

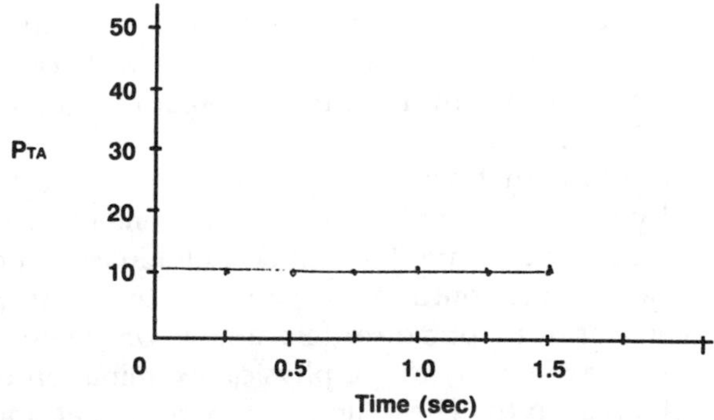

FIG 2–16 (cont.).
C–D.

(Continued.)

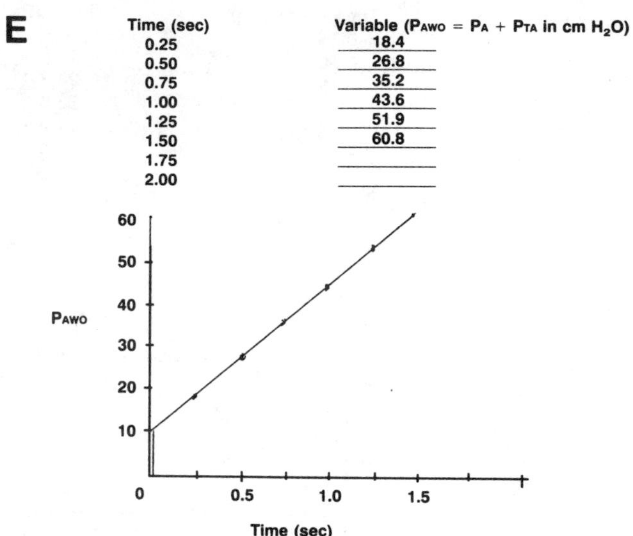

E

Time (sec)	Variable ($P_{AWO} = P_A + P_{TA}$ in cm H_2O)
0.25	18.4
0.50	26.8
0.75	35.2
1.00	43.6
1.25	51.9
1.50	60.8
1.75	
2.00	

FIG 2–16 (cont.).
E, Answers to exercise 1.

Exercise 2

Figure 2–13,A shows decreased compliance. More pressure is required for the same volume.

Figure 2–13,B shows increased compliance. Less pressure is required for the same volume.

Figure 2–13,C shows increased Raw.

Figure 2–13,D shows normal Raw.

1. Increased secretions, mucosal edema, or anything that narrows the airway can cause increased Raw. This can be detected on ventilated patients by listening to breath sounds and noting increased PIP and P_{TA}.
2. Anything that occupies space normally occupied by pulmonary parenchyma or that inhibits alveolar movement can cause decreased lung compliance. Examples include pulmonary edema, pneumonia, consolidation, lung contusion, aspiration, atelectasis, pleural effusion, pneumothorax, fibrotic disorders, and so on. These can be detected on ventilated patients by doing physical examination of the chest, observing changes in the chest film, and by noting an increase in PIP and plateau (alveolar) pressure.

Exercise 3

1. Unit *A* will receive more volume. There is less resistance to gas flow. Unit *A* has a shorter time constant. Time constant = Raw × C. Since unit *B* has a higher Raw, its time constant will be greater. It will take longer to fill than unit *A*.
2. Unit *B* will fill more quickly. It has the shortest time constant. Since compliance on unit B is *low,* then its time constant (Raw × C) will have a smaller value. Stiff alveoli with poor compliance fill quickly, but they do not fill with the same volume for a given positive pressure. If pressure delivery to both units is the same, then A will have a greater volume. Recall, C = V/P and V = C × P.

REFERENCES

1. Banner MJ, Gallagher TJ, Bluth LJ: A new microprocessor device for mean airway pressure measurement. *Crit Care Med* 1981; 9:51–53.
2. Chatburn RL: *Classification of Mechanical Ventilators.* Dallas, American Association for Respiratory Care, 1988.
3. Chatburn RL: A new system for understanding mechanical ventilators. *Respir Care* 1991; 36:1123–1155.
4. Chatburn RL, Craig KC: *Fundamentals of Respiratory Care Research.* East Norwalk, Conn., Appleton-Lange, 1988.
5. Chatburn RL, Lough MD: *Handbook of Respiratory Care,* ed 2. St Louis, Mosby–Year Book, Inc, 1990.
6. Cherniak V, Vidyasager D: Continuous negative wall pressure in hyaline membrane disease: One year experience. *Pediatrics* 1972; 49:753–760.
7. Deshpande VM, Pilbeam SP, Dixon RJ: *A Comprehensive Review in Respiratory Care.* East Norwalk, Conn, Appleton-Lange, 1988.
8. Egan DF: *Fundamentals of Respiratory Therapy.* St Louis, Mosby–Year Book, Inc, 1973.
9. Gherini S, Peters RM, Virgilio RW: Mechanical work in the lungs and work of breathing with positive end expiratory pressure and continuous positive airway pressure. *Chest* 1979; 76:251–256.
10. Holtackers TR, Loosbrook LM, Gracey DR: The use of the chest cuirass in respiratory failure of neurologic origin. *Respir Care* 1982; 27:271–275.
11. Hubmayr RD, Abel MD, Rehder D: Physiologic approach to mechanical ventilation. *Crit Care Med* 1990; 18:103–113.
12. Kacmarek RM, Stoller JK: *Current Respiratory Care.* Philadelphia, BC Decker, Inc, 1988.
13. Kirby RR, Banner MJ, Downs JB: *Clinical Applications of Ventilatory Support,* ed 2. New York, Churchill Livingstone, Inc, 1990.
14. Kirby RR, Graybar GB: Intermittent mandatory ventilation. *Int Anesthesiol Clin* 1980; 18:1–189.

15. Kirby R, Robinson E, Schultz J: Continuous-flow ventilation as an alternative to assisted or controlled ventilation in infants. *Anesth Analg* 1972; 51:871–875.
16. Lough MD, Chatburn RL, Schrock WA: *Handbook of Respiratory Care.* St Louis, Mosby–Year Book, Inc, 1983.
17. Marks A, Asher J, Bocles L, et al: A new ventilator assistor for patients with respiratory acidosis. *N Engl J Med* 1963; 268:61–68.
18. Mushin WW, Rendell-Baker L, Thompson PW, et al: *Automatic Ventilation of the Lungs.* Philadelphia, FA Davis Co, 1980.
19. Nunn JF: *Applied Respiratory Physiology.* Boston, Butterworths & Co, 1977.
20. Primiano FT, Chatburn RL, Lough MD: Mean airway pressure: Theoretical considerations. *Crit Care Med* 1982; 10:378–383.
21. Pulmonary terms and symbols: A report of the ACCP-ATS Joint Committee on Pulmonary Nomenclature. *Chest* 1975; 67:583–593.
22. Scanlan CL, Spearman CB, Sheldon RL: *Egan's Fundamentals of Respiratory Care,* ed 5. St Louis, Mosby–Year Book, Inc, 1990.
23. Shapiro BA, Harrison RF, Trout CA: *Clinical Application of Respiratory Care.* St Louis, Mosby–Year Book, Inc, 1979.
24. Shapiro BA, Harrison RA, Walton JR, et al: Intermittent demand ventilation (IDV): A new technique for supporting ventilation in critically ill patients. *Respir Care* 1976; 21:521–525.
25. Spearman CB, Sheldon RL, Egan DF: *Fundamentals of Respiratory Therapy.* St Louis, Mosby–Year Book, Inc, 1982.
26. *Volume Ventilator Adult Operating Manual.* Emeryville, Calif, Searle Cardiopulmonary Group, 1974.
27. West JB: *Respiratory Physiology—the Essentials,* ed 3. Baltimore, Williams & Wilkins Co, 1985.

Chapter 3

Arterial Blood Gas Review

On completion of this chapter the reader will be able to:

1. List the normal values for venous and arterial blood gas data.
2. Calculate a change in pH due to changes in the ventilatory status ($Paco_2$).
3. Determine the bicarbonate from the pH (hydrogen ion content) and $Paco_2$.
4. Estimate the bicarbonate based on ventilatory changes in $Paco_2$.
5. Calculate changes in bicarbonate based on changes in pH.

ARTERIAL BLOOD GAS REVIEW

REVIEW OF ARTERIAL BLOOD GASES

This chapter assumes that the reader has a good understanding of arterial blood gas (ABG) interpretation and acid-base balance. There are several references listed at the end of this chapter which provide good review material. Also at the end of this chapter is an exercise on ABG interpretation. Exercise 1 gives the reader an opportunity to test his or her knowledge of this concept. Table 3–1 reviews normal values and Table 3–2 gives the causes of some common blood gas abnormalities.

When caring for patients who are receiving mechanical ventilatory support, it is essential to be able to quickly evaluate changes in blood gas results and determine how they relate to changes in alveolar ventilation, dead space, oxygenation, ventilation-perfusion ($\dot{V}/\dot{Q}$) imbalance, and metabolism. It is appropriate at this point to expand on the basic foundation of ABG interpretation. There are four methods for evaluating ABG results which are useful in the clinical setting. These are:

1. Alveolar ventilation and its relation to changes in partial pressure of oxygen (P_{AO_2}) and carbon dioxide (P_{ACO_2}) in the alveoli.
2. Relation of alveolar ventilation to arterial carbon dioxide tension (Pa_{CO_2}) and carbon dioxide production ($\dot{V}_{CO_2}$).
3. Changes in Pa_{CO_2} affecting arterial oxygen tension (Pa_{O_2}).
4. pH changes associated with changes in Pa_{CO_2} and bicarbonate (HCO_3^-).

During ventilation, air flow and gas exchange between the lungs and the environment are accomplished when pressure changes between these two areas allow for gas movement. As ambient air is brought in, it provides the needed oxygen for the cells. As the air from the alveoli leaves the lungs, it carries with it the excessive carbon dioxide from the metabolism in cells. While the act of ventilation can perform these functions, it cannot guarantee the exchange of gas at the alveolar-capillary level. External respiration depends on the integrity of the alveolar-capillary membrane and the cardiovascular system.

TABLE 3–1.
Normal Arterial Blood Gas Values*

	Arterial	Venous
Dissolved CO_2	1.2	1.5
Combined CO_2	24.0	27.1
Total CO_2	25.2	28.6
P_{CO_2} (mm Hg)	40	46
Dissolved O_2 (vol%)	.3	.12
Combined O_2 (vol%)	19.5	14.7
Total O_2 (vol%)	19.8	14.82
P_{O_2} (mm Hg)	90	40
pH	7.40	7.37

*Sea level, ambient air conditions. Values are in millimoles per liter unless noted otherwise.

TABLE 3–2.
Examples of Common Arterial Blood Gas Abnormalities

Conditions	pH	$Paco_2$	HCO_3^-	PaO_2*	Causes
Normal	7.35–7.45	35–45	24–28	80–100	Normal ventilation without pulmonary pathologic condition
Respiratory					
Acute acidosis	7.00–7.34	>45	24–28	80	Hypoventilation, sedation, drug overdose, cardiopulmonary arrest, chest trauma, pneumothorax, CNS trauma, etc
Chronic acidosis (compensated)	7.35–7.45	>45	30–48	<80	Hypoventilation, COPD, chronic neuromuscular disease, muscle wasting, late CNS injury, etc
Acute alkalosis	7.42–7.70	<35	24–28	>80	Increased alveolar ventilation, hypoxemia (if Pao_2 is low), pain, anxiety, mechanical ventilation, cirrhosis of the liver, pulmonary emboli (if Pao_2 is low), severe infection, fever, salicylate intoxication, etc
Chronic alkalosis (compensated)	7.35–7.45	<35	12–24	80–100	Long-term mechanical ventilatory support with increased alveolar ventilation, etc
Metabolic					
Acute acidosis	7.00–7.34	35–46	12–22	80–100	Ketoacidosis, uremic acidosis, loss of HCO_3 (diarrhea), etc.
Compensated acidosis	7.35–7.45	<35	12–22	>80	Respiratory compensation for metabolic acidosis as with diabetic acidosis and lactic acidosis, etc
Acute alkalosis	7.42–7.70	35–46	30–48	80–100	HCO_3^- ingestion, HCl loss, vomiting, GI suction, diuretic-induced K+ or Cl^- loss, steroids, etc
Compensated alkalosis	7.35–7.45	>45	30–48	<80	Primary hypokalemic metabolic alkalosis, with dehydration/azotemia (rare)

*Assuming no pulmonary pathologic condition other than respiratory hypoventilation, and no therapeutic oxygen.

CHANGES IN ALVEOLAR VENTILATION ASSOCIATED WITH CHANGES IN P_{AO_2} AND P_{ACO_2}

Under normal circumstances, alveolar ventilation provides air to the alveoli at a rate of about 4 to 5 L/min (see Appendix A). At this level, enough gas exchange can occur in the lung to keep ABG values within a normal range. The relationship of alveolar ventilation to P_{AO_2} and P_{ACO_2} is described by the graph in Figure 3–1. Values are normal with an alveolar ventilation of about 4.5 L/min. As

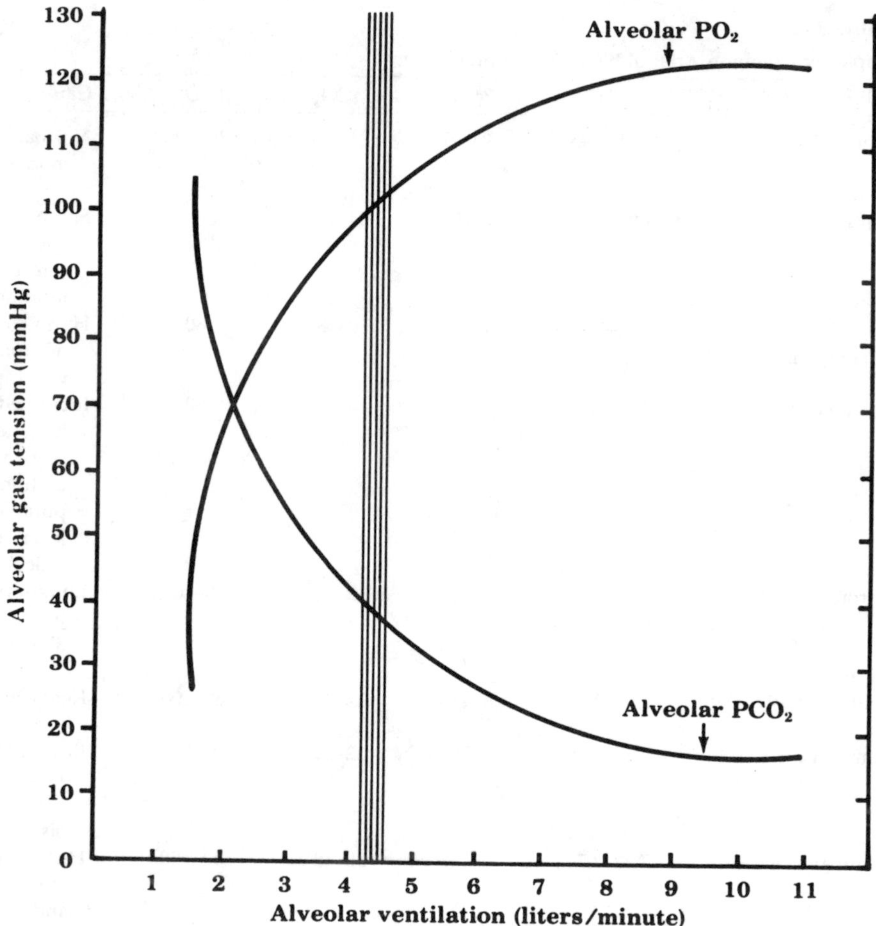

FIG 3–1.
Effect of alveolar ventilation on alveolar gases.

alveolar ventilation increases, the P_{ACO_2} decreases until it plateaus at about 20 to 25 mm Hg. Hyperventilation also increases the P_{AO_2} above normal. The P_{AO_2} will plateau at approximately 120 mm Hg. With hypoventilation there is a reduction in alveolar ventilation resulting in a rise in P_{ACO_2} and a fall in P_{AO_2}.

ALVEOLAR VENTILATION, Pa_{CO_2} AND $\dot{V}_{CO_2}$

There is another way of describing the relationship of alveolar ventilation ($\dot{V}_A$) to the physiologic measurement of $\dot{V}_{CO_2}$. Cellular metabolism is responsible for producing CO_2 with the lungs being the primary organ for removing the CO_2. How much is being produced and how well it is being removed by the lungs is expressed in the following formula, where $Paco_2$ describes the balance between CO_2 production and alveolar ventilation:

$$Paco_2 = \frac{\dot{V}co_2}{\dot{V}A}$$

Using $\dot{V}co_2$ in milliliters per minute and $\dot{V}A$ in liters per minute, this equation can be rewritten as:

$$Paco_2 = \frac{0.863 \times \dot{V}co_2}{\dot{V}A}$$

where 0.863 corrects for $\dot{V}A$ being reported in liters per minute at body conditions (BTPS) and $\dot{V}co_2$ being reported in milliliters per minute at standard conditions (STPD).

For example, when the $\dot{V}A$ is 4.5 L/min and the $\dot{V}co_2$ is 200 mL/min, the $Paco_2$ will be 38 mm Hg. If the $\dot{V}A$ were half normal (2.25 L/min) and the $\dot{V}co_2$ were normal, the $Paco_2$ would be:

$$Paco_2 = \frac{0.863 \times 200 \text{ mL/min}}{2.25 \text{ L/min}}$$

$$Paco_2 = 76.7 \text{ mm Hg}$$

CHANGES IN $Paco_2$ AFFECTING Pao_2

Changes in $Paco_2$ will also affect the Pao_2. This relationship is best described by the alveolar air equation which is presented in detail in Appendix B. This equation assumes that the $Paco_2$ is equal to the $PAco_2$. A simplified form of the alveolar air equation is as follows: $PAo_2 = PIo_2 - (Paco_2/0.8)$, where PIo_2 is the partial pressure of inspired oxygen. The factor 0.8 will change slightly with changes in fractional concentration of oxygen in inspired gas (FIo_2). Note that the amount of oxygen in the alveoli will depend, in part, on the amount of CO_2 present (Dalton's law of partial pressures). This is an easy formula to use in situations where quick clinical evaluation of ABGs is needed and a calculator is not readily available.

At sea level (760 mm Hg) and at a normal FIo_2 of 0.21 with a water vapor pressure of 47 mm Hg (saturated at 37°C), the PIo_2 will equal 149 mm Hg based on the equation $PIo_2 = FIo_2 (PB - 47) = 0.21 \times (760 - 47)$, where PB is barometric pressure. Using the simplified version of the alveolar air equation, $P_{AO_2} = P_{IO_2} - (P_{ACO_2}/0.8)$, when the Pa_{CO_2} is 40 mm Hg, the P_{AO_2} will be equal to 149 − (40/0.8), or 99 mm Hg. As the Pa_{CO_2} rises owing to hypoventilation, the P_{AO_2} will fall. For example, if the Pa_{CO_2} = 80 mm Hg, the P_{AO_2} will be 149 − 80/0.8) or 49 mm Hg. When this occurs, less oxygen is present in the alveoli. As a result, less oxygen is available to the blood and tissues.

Under normal physiologic conditions, the alveolar oxygen is always greater than the arterial oxygen. This is called the alveolar-arterial oxygen difference $[P(A - a)O_2]$. Normal values for the difference are approximately 5 mm Hg in a 20-year-old, as a result of normal anatomic shunts. This value increases by approximately 4 mm Hg per decade after 20 years of age.[4]

During hyperventilation, the P_{AO_2} will increase due to the drop in Pa_{CO_2}. For example, if the Pa_{CO_2} were 20 mm Hg and the P_{IO_2} were 149 mm Hg, the P_{AO_2} would be 149 − (20/0.8), or 124 mm Hg. Since more oxygen is now available in the alveoli, more oxygen can be delivered to the arterial blood. This assumes that the levels of shunting and diffusion are normal and that there are no other pathologic conditions causing hypoxemia.

In general, as the Pa_{CO_2} increases by 1 mm Hg, the Pa_{O_2} will decrease by 1.25 mm Hg.[7] For example, if the Pa_{CO_2} increases from 40 to 50 mm Hg, a Pa_{O_2} at 100 mm Hg will decrease to about 88 mm Hg.

CHANGES IN pH, Pa_{CO_2}, AND BICARBONATE

As the Pa_{CO_2} increases, the level of acid available in the blood also increases. The pH becomes more acidotic and has a lower numeric value. The advantage of knowing the value of pH and Pa_{CO_2} is that it allows one to evaluate a patient's condition and determine the cause of the instability in these variables. The relationship between the pH (H^+ concentration), the Pa_{CO_2} (mm Hg), and the HCO_3^- level (mEq/L) can be described by the Henderson equation[12]:

$$[H^+] = \frac{24 \times Pa_{CO_2}\ (\text{mm Hg})}{HCO_3^-\ (\text{mEq/L})}$$

where $[H^+]$ is the hydrogen ion concentration is nanomoles per liter (nmol/L) and the number 24 is derived from the dissociation constant for carbonic acid (Table 3–3). For example, if the Pa_{CO_2} is 62 mm Hg and the HCO_3^- is 26 mm Hg, the $[H^+]$ is calculated as follows:

$$[H^+] = \frac{24 \times 62}{26} = 57\ \text{nmol/L}$$

TABLE 3–3.
Relationship Between pH and Hydrogen Ion $[H^+]$ Concentration

	pH	Approximate $[H^+]$ nanomoles Concentration (nmol/L)
Alkalosis	8.0	10
	7.8	15
	7.7	20
	7.6	25
	7.5	30
Normal	7.4	40
Acidosis	7.3	50
	7.2	65
	7.1	80
	7.0	100

For a $[H^+]$ concentration of 57 nmol/L, the pH will be close to 7.20, or approximately 7.23.

When the pH is 7.40 and the $Paco_2$ is 50 mm Hg, the HCO_3^- will be 30 mEq/L:

$$[H^+] = \frac{24 \times Paco_2}{HCO_3^-}$$

$$HCO_3^- = \frac{24 \times Paco_2}{[H^+]}$$

$$HCO_3^- = \frac{24 \times 50 \text{ mm Hg}}{40} = 30 \text{ mEq/L}$$

Remember that these determinations are estimations of the actual value. They can be useful in clinical situations for a quick determination of a patient's HCO_3^-, pH, or $Paco_2$ value when two of the factors are known.

DETERMINING ACUTE VS. CHRONIC HYPERCAPNIA

Calculation and evaluation of the ratio between the change in H^+ concentration and the change in $Paco_2$ can be used to determine acute, chronic, or acute-on-chronic hypercapnia in a patient.[4] In acute hypercapnia, $\Delta[H^+]/\Delta\ Paco_2$ will be about 0.7. In chronic hypercapnia, the ratio is about 0.3 or less. In acute-on-chronic hypercapnia, the ratio is between 0.3 and 0.7. Consider the following: the $Paco_2$ is 80 mm Hg and the HCO_3^- is 28 mEq/L; the pH is 7.19.

$$[H^+] = \frac{24 \times 80}{28} = 68 \text{ nM/L}$$

This represents a net change in $[H^+]$ of 28 nmol/L from normal ($\Delta[H^+] = 68 - 40 = 28$). The change in $Paco_2$ is: $\Delta Paco_2 = 80 - 40 = 40$ mm Hg. The ratio is: $\Delta[H^+]/\Delta Paco_2 = 28/40 = 0.7$. This represents an acute hypercapnia.

Acute-on-chronic hypercapnia is similar to the following:

$$pH = 7.25,\ Paco_2 = 92 \text{ mm Hg},\ HCO_3^- = 38 \text{ mEq/L}$$

$$[H^+] = \frac{24 \times 92}{38} = 58 \text{ nmol/L}$$

$$[H^+] = 58 - 40 = 18 \text{ nmol/L}$$

$$Paco_2 = 92 - 40 = 52 \text{ mm Hg}$$

$$\Delta[H^+]/\Delta Paco_2 = 18/52 = 0.35$$

The above method of evaluating hypercapnia and the relationship between pH, $Paco_2$, and HCO_3^- is valuable in distinguishing the types of hypercapnia. Since different types require different treatments, it is important clinically to understand this concept.

PH CHANGES DUE TO $Paco_2$

There is another similar equation that can help to evaluate the relationship between the $Paco_2$ level and the pH as shown in Table 3–4.[13] By using this method one can determine if changes in pH are reflections of changes in $Paco_2$ or are due to metabolic changes. For example, if the $Paco_2$ is 80 mm Hg, this is 40 mm Hg above the normal of 40 mm Hg. The pH would decrease by about 0.2 and would be equal to about 7.20 if the change were due to hypoventilation. During hyperventilation, if the $Paco_2$ were 20 mm Hg, this is 20 mm Hg less than

TABLE 3–4.

Relationship Between Changes in $Paco_2$ and pH

When starting at a $Paco_2$ of 40 mm Hg, for every 20 mm Hg increase in $Paco_2$, the pH decreases by 0.10 units. For example:

$Paco_2$ = 40 mm Hg	pH = 7.40	HCO_3^- = 24 mEq/L
$Paco_2$ = 60 mm Hg	pH = 7.30	HCO_3^- = 26 mEq/L
$Paco_2$ = 80 mm Hg	pH = 7.20	HCO_3^- = 28 mEq/L

This is true in persons with normal blood buffers (remember that this is an approximation).

When the $Paco_2$ decreases 10 mm Hg, the pH increases by 0.10 units.

$Paco_2$ = 30 mm Hg	pH = 7.50	HCO_3^- = 22 mEq/L
$Paco_2$ = 20 mm Hg	pH = 7.60	HCO_3^- = 20 mEq/L

As $Paco_2$ increases, Pao_2 decreases.

normal and one would expect the pH to be 7.60. If it were not close to 7.60 but was actually 7.50, then one would conclude that the pH was not entirely due to ventilatory changes. This would suggest metabolic acidosis with respiratory alkalosis. Again, this relationship is an estimation intended to aid in rapid clinical assessment of the patient.

CHANGES IN PLASMA BICARBONATE DUE TO CHANGES IN $Paco_2$

The association of increased HCO_3^- with increased $Paco_2$ is also shown in Table 3–4. As CO_2 is added to the blood it raises the HCO_3^- level and vice versa. Recall the equilibrium equation for CO_2 in water:

$$CO_2 + H_2O \longleftrightarrow H_2CO_3 \longleftrightarrow H^+ + HCO_3^-$$

If you add CO_2 on the left, it produces more HCO_3^- on the right, as well as acid. During hypoventilation CO_2 is increased. For each 10 mm Hg increase in $Paco_2$, the HCO_3^- increases 1 mEq/L. As $Paco_2$ decreases by 10 mm Hg with hyperventilation, HCO_3^- decreases about 1.5 mEq/L.[9, 11]

For example, if $Paco_2$ is 40 mm Hg and the HCO_3^- is 24 mEq/L and the $Paco_2$ increases to 50 mm Hg, the HCO_3^- will increase to 25 mEq/L owing to the rise in CO_2. Looking in the other direction, if $Paco_2$ is 40 mm Hg and the HCO_3^- is 24 mEq/L and the $Paco_2$ decreases to 20 mm Hg, the HCO_3^- will decrease to 21 mEq/L.

If hypoventilation or hyperventilation continues for 2 to 3 days, normal kidney function will help correct the pH and compensate by retaining or excreting HCO_3^-. Remember the above example where $Paco_2$ = 50 mm Hg and HCO_3^- = 25 mEq/L. As hypoventilation produces a respiratory acidosis, the kidneys compensate by retaining about 2 mEq/L of HCO_3^- for every 10 mm Hg increase in $Paco_2$. The HCO_3^- will rise to about 27 mEq/L.

On the other hand, during hyperventilation the plasma becomes more alkalotic. This is compensated in the kidneys by the excretion of HCO_3^- causing a 3 mEq/L decrease for every 10 mm Hg decrease in $Paco_2$. Recalling the above example, with $Paco_2$ = 20 mm Hg, HCO_3^- is 21 mEq/L. The HCO_3^- will fall to about 15 mEq/L (3 mEq/L/10 mm Hg) after a few days of renal compensation.[8]

METABOLIC CHANGES IN BICARBONATE AND pH

There is another rule of thumb that can help to describe the relationship between the pH and the HCO_3^-. Changes in pH that are due to metabolic and not respiratory changes can be estimated by the equation which states that a pH change of 0.15 is approximately equal to a change in base of 10 mEq/L. Suppose there is an increase of pH from 7.40 to 7.55 (an increase of 0.15). The base will change by 10 mEq/L. If the base were normal (HCO_3^- = 24 mEq/L) at the outset, one would expect it to increase by 10 mEq/L, or HCO_3^- = 34 mEq/L with a pH rise from 7.40 to 7.55 due to metabolic causes. Imagine a decrease in pH from 7.40 to 7.25 (a decrease of 0.15). One would expect the HCO_3^- to decrease by 10 mEq/L, from a normal of 24 mEq/L to 14 mEq/L. This is true as long as the change in pH was due to purely metabolic causes.

SUMMARY

Consideration of ABG evaluation and the interrelation between $\dot{V}_A$ and pH, $Paco_2$, and Pao_2 are important concepts when monitoring and evaluating patients in the clinical setting, particularly those in need of mechanical ventilatory support. The interpretation should always be done with care.

STUDY QUESTIONS

Exercise 1

Interpret the following blood gas values:

1. pH 7.39
$Paco_2$ 44 mm Hg
Pao_2 89 mm Hg
HCO_3^- 25 mEq/L
2. pH 7.12
$Paco_2$ 42 mm Hg
Pao_2 155 mm Hg
HCO_3^- 13 mEq/L
3. pH 7.25
$Paco_2$ 65 mm Hg
Pao_2 55 mm Hg
HCO_3^- 28 mEq/L
4. pH 7.52
$Paco_2$ 32 mm Hg
Pao_2 105 mm Hg
HCO_3^- 26 mEq/L
5. pH 7.42
$Paco_2$ 33 mm Hg
Pao_2 102 mm Hg
HCO_3^- 21 mEq/L
6. pH 7.55
$Paco_2$ 38 mm Hg
Pao_2 98 mm Hg
HCO_3^- 32 mEq/L
7. pH 7.37
$Paco_2$ 66 mm Hg
Pao_2 68 mm Hg
HCO_3^- 36 mEq/L
8. pH 7.29
$Paco_2$ 73 mm Hg
Pao_2 69 mm Hg
HCO_3^- 31 mEq/L
9. pH 7.33
$Paco_2$ 65 mm Hg
Pao_2 78 mm Hg
HCO_3^- 33 mEq/L
10. pH 7.52
$Paco_2$ 25 mm Hg
Pao_2 99 mm Hg
HCO_3^- 20 mEq/L

11. pH 7.10
    $Paco_2$ 99 mm Hg
    Pao_2 22 mm Hg
    HCO_3^- 30 mEq/L
12. pH 7.32
    $Paco_2$ 60 mm Hg
    Pao_2 78 mm Hg
    HCO_3^- 29 mEq/L
13. pH 7.25
    $Paco_2$ 24 mm Hg
    Pao_2 110 mm Hg
    HCO_3^- 9 mEq/L
14. pH 7.55
    $Paco_2$ 50 mm Hg
    Pao_2 83 mm Hg
    HCO_3^- 41 mEq/L
15. pH 7.51
    $Paco_2$ 20 mm Hg
    Pao_2 112 mm Hg
    HCO_3^- 15 mEq/L
16. pH 7.21
    $Paco_2$ 90 mm Hg
    Pao_2 45 mm Hg
    HCO_3^- 35 mEq/L
17. pH 7.35
    $Paco_2$ 46 mm Hg
    Pao_2 44 mm Hg
    HCO_3^- 25 mEq/L
18. pH 7.49
    $Paco_2$ 21 mm Hg
    Pao_2 98 mm Hg
    HCO_3^- 16 mEq/L
19. pH 7.38
    $Paco_2$ 60 mm Hg
    Pao_2 61 mm Hg
    HCO_3^- 36 mEq/L
20. pH 7.20
    $Paco_2$ 60 mm Hg
    Pao_2 55 mm Hg
    HCO_3^- 23 mEq/L
21. pH 7.49
    $Paco_2$ 43 mm Hg
    Pao_2 98 mm Hg
    HCO_3^- 33 mEq/L
22. pH 7.10
    $Paco_2$ 13 mm Hg
    Pao_2 75 mm Hg
    HCO_3^- 4 mEq/L
23. pH 7.58
    $Paco_2$ 59 mm Hg
    Pao_2 77 mm Hg
    HCO_3^- 55 mEq/L
24. pH 7.54
    $Paco_2$ 29 mm Hg
    Pao_2 56 mm Hg
    HCO_3^- 23 mEq/L
25. pH 7.31
    $Paco_2$ 60 mm Hg
    Pao_2 75 mm Hg
    HCO_3^- 30 mEq/L
26. pH 7.43
    $Paco_2$ 24 mm Hg
    Pao_2 119 mm Hg
    HCO_3^- 15 mEq/L
27. pH 7.43
    $Paco_2$ 41 mm Hg
    Pao_2 94 mm Hg
    HCO_3^- 26 mEq/L
    BE* +2
    Sao_2* 95%
28. pH 7.52
    $Paco_2$ 30 mm Hg
    Pao_2 45 mm Hg
    HCO_3^- 24 mEq/L
    BE +2
    Sao_2 86%

* BE = base excess; Sao_2 = oxygen saturation.

29. pH 7.15
    $Paco_2$ 80 mm Hg
    Pao_2 80 mm Hg
    HCO_3^- 27 mEq/L
    BE 0
    Sao_2 90%
30. pH 7.20
    $Paco_2$ 55 mm Hg
    Pao_2 55 mm Hg
    HCO_3^- 21 mEq/L
    BE −8
    Sao_2 79%
31. pH 7.60
    $Paco_2$ 40 mm Hg
    Pao_2 85 mm Hg
    HCO_3^- 39 mEq/L
    BE +10
    Sao_2 97%
32. pH 7.54
    $Paco_2$ 25 mm Hg
    Pao_2 52 mm Hg
    HCO_3^- 21 mEq/L
    BE +8
    Sao_2 90%
33. pH 7.25
    $Paco_2$ 65 mm Hg
    Pao_2 39 mm Hg
    HCO_3^- 28 mEq/L
    BE +15
    Sao_2 65%
34. pH 7.39
    $Paco_2$ 38 mm Hg
    Pao_2 65 mm Hg
    HCO_3^- 24 mEq/L
    BE 0
    Sao_2 92%

Exercise 2

1. List the normal arterial values for the following: pH, total CO_2, $Paco_2$, Cao_2, Pao_2, Sao_2.
2. Give the normal venous values for the following: pH, $Pvco_2$, Cvo_2, Pvo_2, Svo_2.
3. An excitable patient is admitted to the outpatient clinic following an emotional trauma. ABGs on room air are: $Paco_2$ = 20 mm Hg, Pao_2 = 110 mm Hg, Sao_2 = 99%. What would you expect the pH to be if the blood gas changes were due to respiratory changes only? How would you interpret these gases? What treatment would you recommend for the patient?
4. A patient in the emergency room is being treated for severe congestive heart failure. ABGs on room air are: $Paco_2$ = 78 mm Hg, Pao_2 = 65 mm Hg, Sao_2 = 85%. What would the pH be if these results were due to hypoventilation alone? How would you interpret the acid-base status? What respiratory treatment would you recommend?
5. An ABG has a pH of 7.30, and a $Paco_2$ of 25 mm Hg. What is the estimated HCO_3^- based on these two values?
6. An ABG has a pH of 7.39, and a $Paco_2$ of 61 mm Hg. What is the estimated HCO_3^- based on these two values?
7. How much effect will an increase in $Paco_2$ from 40 to 50 mm Hg have on an HCO_3^- level of 25 mEq/L?
8. A patient hyperventilates from a $Paco_2$ of 40 to 30 mm Hg. The HCO_3^- is 24 mEq/L initially. What will the HCO_3^- be after the $Paco_2$ change?

9. A patient with chronic obstructive pulmonary disease (COPD) has normal blood gases: $Paco_2$ = 52 mm Hg, Pao_2 = 55 mm Hg, and pH = 7.39 with an HCO_3^- of 33 mEq/L. The patient begins to vomit and the pH rises to 7.53. How will the pH change possibly change the HCO_3^-?
10. A patient has the following ABG values: $Paco_2$ = 38 mm Hg, pH = 7.30, HCO_3^- = 18 mEq/L. The patient's HCO_3^- increases to 28 mEq/L after intravenous (IV) administration of HCO_3^-. What would you expect the pH to change to?
    a. 7.40.
    b. 7.45.
    c. 7.15.
    d. 7.55.
    e. It will not change.

ANSWERS TO STUDY QUESTIONS

Exercise 1

1. Normal.
2. Uncompensated metabolic acidosis with hyperoxemia.
3. Uncompensated respiratory acidosis with moderate hypoxemia.
4. Uncompensated respiratory alkalosis with hyperoxemia.
5. Compensated respiratory alkalosis with hyperoxemia.
6. Uncompensated metabolic alkalosis.
7. Compensated respiratory acidosis with mild hypoxemia.
8. Partially compensated respiratory acidosis with mild hypoxemia.
9. Partially compensated respiratory acidosis with mild hypoxemia.
10. Partially compensated respiratory alkalosis.
11. Partially compensated respiratory acidosis with severe hypoxemia.
12. Partially compensated respiratory acidosis with mild hypoxemia.
13. Partially compensated metabolic acidosis with hyperoxemia.
14. Partially compensated metabolic alkalosis.
15. Partially compensated respiratory alkalosis with hyperoxemia.
16. Partially compensated respiratory acidosis with moderate hypoxemia.
17. Normal acid-base status with moderate hypoxemia; probable venous sample.
18. Partially compensated respiratory alkalosis.
19. Compensated respiratory acidosis with mild hypoxemia.
20. Uncompensated respiratory acidosis with moderate hypoxemia.
21. Uncompensated metabolic alkalosis.
22. Partially compensated metabolic acidosis with mild hypoxemia.
23. Partially compensated metabolic alkalosis with mild hypoxemia.

24. Uncompensated respiratory alkalosis with moderate hypoxemia; probable hyperventilation due to hypoxia.
25. Partially compensated respiratory acidosis with mild hypoxemia.
26. Compensated respiratory alkalosis with hyperoxemia.
27. Normal ABGs.
28. Uncompensated respiratory alkalosis with moderate hypoxemia.
29. Uncompensated respiratory acidosis.
30. Combined metabolic and respiratory acidosis with moderate hypoxemia.
31. Uncompensated metabolic alkalosis.
32. Combined respiratory and metabolic alkalosis with moderate hypoxemia.
33. Partially compensated respiratory acidosis with severe hypoxemia; this can occur with COPD in acute respiratory failure.
34. Normal acid-base status with mild hypoxemia.

Exercise 2

1. pH = 7.40, total CO_2 = 25.2 (mmol/L), $Paco_2$ = 40 mm Hg, Cao_2 = 19.8 vol%, Pao_2 = 80–100 mm Hg, Sao_2 = 97%.
2. pH = 7.37, $Pvco_2$ = 46 mm Hg, Cvo_2 = 14.8 vol%, Pvo_2 = 40 mm Hg, Svo_2 = 75%.
3. With a decrease in $Paco_2$ of 20 mm Hg, the pH should increase by 0.2. The pH value would be about 7.60. This is an example of respiratory alkalosis. The patient needs to rebreath CO_2, perhaps by breathing into a plastic bag, and the patient should be calmed down.
4. The increased $Paco_2$ of 78 mm Hg is about 40 mm Hg above the normal $Paco_2$. The pH would be about 7.20, a decrease from normal of 0.2. This is a respiratory acidosis. The patient needs ventilatory support.
5. HCO_3^- = (24 × $Paco_2$)/[H^+]; HCO_3^- = 24 × 25/50; HCO_3^- = 12 mEq/L.
6. HCO_3^- = (24 × $Paco_2$)/[H^+]; HCO_3^- = 24 × 61/40; HCO_3^- = 36.6 mEq/L.
7. An increase in $Paco_2$ from 40 to 50 mm Hg (10 mm Hg) will increase the HCO_3^- level from 25 to 26 mEq/L.
8. $Paco_2$ drops by 10 mm Hg; HCO_3^- will decrease by 0.15 to 22.5 mEq/L.
9. An increase in pH of 0.15 will increase the HCO_3^- by 10 mEq/L. The expected HCO_3^- will be about 43 mEq/L.
10. b.

REFERENCES

1. Barnes TA, Lisbon A: *Respiratory Care Practice.* St Louis, Mosby–Year Book, Inc, 1988.
2. Burton GG, Hodgkin JE: *Respiratory Care: A Guide to Clinical Practice,* ed 2. Philadelphia, JB Lippincott Co, 1984.

3. Burton GG, Hodgkin JE, Ward JJ: *Respiratory Care: A Guide to Clinical Practice,* ed 3. Philadelphia, JB Lippincott Co, 1991.
4. Demers RR, Irwin RS: Management of hypercapneic respiratory failure: A systemic approach. *Respir Care* 1979; 24:328–335.
5. Eubanks DH, Bone RC: *Comprehensive Respiratory Care—A Learning System,* ed 2. St Louis, Mosby–Year Book, Inc, 1990.
6. Kacmarek RM, Mack CW, Dimas S: *The Essentials of Respiratory Care,* ed 3. St Louis, Mosby–Year Book, Inc, 1990.
7. Light RW: Conservative treatment of hypercapneic acute respiratory failure. *Respir Care* 1983; 28:561–569.
8. Murray JF: Pathophysiology of acute respiratory failure. *Respir Care* 1983; 28:531–541.
9. Otis AB: Quantitative relationships in steady-state gas exchange, in *Handbook of Physiology.* Section 3; *Respiration.* Fenn WO, Rahn H (section eds). Washington, DC, American Physiological Society, 1964.
10. Scanlan CL, Spearman CB, Sheldon RL: *Egan's Fundamentals of Respiratory Care,* St Louis, Mosby–Year Book, Inc, 1990.
11. Shapiro BA: Fundamentals of acid-base balance and blood gas analysis, in *Annual Refresher Course Lectures.* Chicago, American Society of Anesthesiology, 1983; 126:1–7.
12. Shapiro BA, Harrison RA, Walton JR: *Clinical Application of Blood Gases.* St Louis, Mosby–Year Book, Inc, 1977.
13. Shapiro BA, Harrison RA, Trout C: *Clinical Application of Respiratory Care.* St Louis, Mosby–Year Book, Inc, 1979.
14. Sorbini CA, Grassi V, Solinas E, et al: Arterial oxygen tension in relation to age in healthy subjects. *Respiration* 1968; 25:3–13.

Chapter 4

Establishing the Need for Mechanical Ventilation

On completion of this chapter the reader will be able to:

1. Define acute respiratory failure and respiratory insufficiency.
2. List respiratory, cardiovascular, and neurologic findings in mild to moderate hypoxia and severe hypoxia.
3. List respiratory, cardiovascular, and neurologic findings in mild to moderate hypercarbia and severe hypercarbia.
4. Name three categories of disorders that may lead to respiratory insufficiency or acute respiratory failure.
5. Give normal values for vital capacity, maximum inspiratory pressure, peak expiratory pressure, FEV_1, peak expiratory flow rate, V_D/V_T ratio. $P(A - a)O_2$, and arterial:alveolar P_{O_2} ratio.

6. List critical values that indicate the need for ventilatory support for the following: vital capacity, maximum inspiratory pressure, peak expiratory pressure, FEV_1, peak expiratory flow rate, VD/VT ratio, $P(A - a)O_2$, and arterial-alveolar PO_2 ratio.
7. Name the five standard criteria for the institution of mechanical ventilatory support.
8. Give the four goals of therapy for the mechanically ventilated patient.
9. From a case study, identify the findings that indicate the need for ventilatory support.

ACUTE RESPIRATORY FAILURE AND RESPIRATORY INSUFFICIENCY

The purpose of ventilation, be it spontaneous or artificial, is to assist in the maintenance of homeostasis. This is particularly true where it relates to the acid-base status of the blood and the levels of oxygen and carbon dioxide being exchanged.

Any condition in which respiratory activity is completely absent or is inadequate to maintain oxygen uptake and carbon dioxide clearance is referred to as *acute respiratory failure.*[32] If adequate gas exchange is being maintained, but at a great expense to the breathing mechanism of the subject, this is referred to as *respiratory insufficiency.*[44] This condition can eventually lead to acute respiratory failure.

Clinically, acute respiratory failure may be defined as the inability of the patient to maintain the arterial partial pressure of oxygen (PaO_2), carbon dioxide ($PaCO_2$), and pH at acceptable levels. This is generally considered to be (1) a PaO_2 below the predicted normal range for the patient's age under ambient air conditions, (2) $PaCO_2$ levels above 50 mm Hg and rising, and (3) a falling pH of 7.25 or less.[29, 35]

Since the conditions of respiratory insufficiency and acute respiratory failure can lead to coma and death, it is important to be able to recognize these conditions quickly in the clinical setting. They identify the need for mechanical ventilatory support.

ACUTE CARBON DIOXIDE RETENTION AND HYPOXEMIA

The presence of hypercarbia and hypoxemia are sure signs of respiratory problems. These two usually occur together. For this reason, it is hard to distinguish between their clinical features. The importance of doing so is academic in any case since the presence of either is detrimental to the patient's well-being and requires respiratory care.

TABLE 4-1.
Features of Hypoxia and Hypercarbia

	Mild to Moderate	Severe
Hypoxia		
Respiratory findings	Tachypnea Dyspnea Paleness	Tachypnea Dyspnea Cyanosis
Cardiovascular findings	Tachycardia Mild hypertension Peripheral vasoconstriction	Tachycardia, eventual bradycardia, arrhythmias Hypertension and eventual hypotension
Neurological findings	Restlessness Disorientation Headaches Lassitude	Somnolence Confusion Blurred vision Tunnel vision Loss of coordination Impaired judgment Slow reaction time Manic-depressive activity Coma
Hypercarbia		
Respiratory findings	Tachypnea Dyspnea	Tachypnea and eventual bradypnea
Cardiovascular findings	Tachycardia Hypertension Vasodilation	Tachycardia Hypertension and eventual hypotension
Neurological findings	Headaches Drowsiness	Hallucinations Hypomania Convulsions Coma
Signs	Sweating Redness of the skin	

The basic features found in patients with conditions of hypoxia and hypercarbia are shown in Table 4–1. Initial evaluation of the patient should include several observations. First, one must evaluate the patient's level of consciousness. Is the patient awake or asleep? If asleep or unconscious, is the patient arousable, and if so, to what extent? Second, look at skin color and appearance and texture. Is there evidence of cyanosis in the nail beds or lips? Is the patient pale and diaphoretic? Third, determine the respiratory rate, the heart rate (HR), and the blood pressure (BP). Is the body temperature elevated? These signs and measurements will provide rapid and useful information about the patient's condition.

Tachycardia and tachypnea are early indicators of hypoxia. If the HR decreases by 10 beats/min after several minutes on oxygen, then the probable cause of the tachycardia is hypoxia. If it does not decrease, then hypoxia may or may not be present. Some conditions of hypoxia, such as severe shunting, are refractory to oxygen therapy and as a result oxygen therapy would not significantly reduce the tachycardia.

In patients with respiratory insufficiency or failure, elevated $Paco_2$ levels always occur with hypoxia unless the patient is on oxygen therapy. Elevation of arterial CO_2 leads to an increased cerebral blood flow and is often accompanied by headaches. Severe hypercarbia will eventually lead to CO_2 narcosis, cerebral depression, coma, and death.

The combined effect of hypoxia, hypercarbia, and acidosis can lead to ventricular arrest or fibrillation.[3] These findings emphasize the importance of being able to identify the patient in acute or impending respiratory failure and to begin prompt therapy. Use of supplemental oxygen therapy, maintenance of a patent airway, physical examination of the chest, and an arterial blood gas evaluation are the next steps in attending to the patient.

PATIENT HISTORY AND DIAGNOSIS

There are certain types of disorders and situations that make individuals more likely to develop respiratory failure. These generally fall into three categories: (1) disorders of the central nervous system (CNS), (2) problems with neuromuscular function, and (3) increased work of breathing.

Central Nervous System Disorders

Disorders associated with the CNS are listed in Table 4–2. They include such conditions as depression of the respiratory centers induced by drugs or trauma. As the respiratory centers are affected, the minute ventilation ($\dot{V}_E$) is decreased. Since the anatomic dead space does not change, the alveolar ventilation ($\dot{V}_A$) also decreases. This leads to an increase in the ratio of dead space volume to tidal volume (V_D/V_T). As $\dot{V}_A$ decreases, the $Paco_2$ increases and the Pao_2 decreases. The resulting onset of hypoventilation and later respiratory failure becomes clinically apparent.

Disorders of the brain, such as tumors or trauma, can alter the general pattern of clinically observed respiration. For example, a head injury might result in cerebral hemorrhage and increased pressure on the brain tissue. If significant, this can alter cerebral function; such patients might be seen with Cheyne-Stokes patterns of respiration or Biot's breathing. Another significant observation is that as the $Paco_2$ rises above 70 mm Hg it can act as a CNS depressant, and respirations can be further reduced. Hypoxia, which accompanies this process, might act as a respiratory stimulant to the peripheral receptors. If the CNS were already compromised, its ability to respond would be reduced.

TABLE 4–2.
Disorders Associated With Hypoventilation and Possible Respiratory Failure

Disorders of the CNS associated with reduced drive to breath
Depressant drugs (barbiturates, tranquilizers, narcotics, general anesthetic agents)
Brain or brainstem lesions (stroke, trauma to head or neck, cerebral hemorrhage, tumors, spinal cord injury)
Pickwickian syndrome or sleep apnea syndrome due to central problems
Inappropriate oxygen therapy
Disorders associated with neuromuscular function
Myasthenia gravis
Tetanus
Botulism
Guillain-Barré syndrome
Polio
Muscular dystrophy
Drugs (curare, nerve gas, succinylcholine, insecticide poisoning)
Disorders resulting in increased work of breathing
Pleural effusions, hemothorax
Pneumothorax, flail chest, rib fracture
Kyphoscoliosis, chest wall deformity, obesity
Interstitial pulmonary fibrotic diseases
Increased airway resistance (asthma, emphysema, chronic bronchitis, croup, epiglottitis, acute bronchitis)
Aspiration, adult respiratory distress syndrome (ARDS), cardiogenic pulmonary edema, drug-induced pulmonary edema
Pulmonary emboli
Increased metabolic rate with accompanying pulmonary problems
Airway emergencies
Postoperative pulmonary complications

In addition to compromising normal ventilation, cerebral abnormalities can affect normal reflex responses such as swallowing. If the glottic response is affected, it becomes important to protect the airway from obstruction by the tongue or aspiration caused by poor epiglottic reflex.

In patients with closed head injury, controlled hyperventilation is indicated. Lowering of the $Paco_2$ and increasing the pH through mechanical ventilation results in reduced cerebral perfusion and a reduction in intracranial pressures.

Problems With Neuromuscular Function

Some of the more common neuromuscular disorders and dysfunctions that can lead to respiratory failure are listed in Table 4–2. These are usually a result of either motor nerve damage, problems with transmission of nerve impulses at the neuromuscular junction, or muscle dysfunction. These problems can be caused by drugs, viruses, bacteria and their toxins, or autoimmune disorders. In some cases, such as Guillian-Barré syndrome, the cause is unknown.

Drug-induced neuromuscular failure usually has a rapid onset. Substances such as curare, nerve gas, and succinylcholine all alter the neuromuscular transmission of impulses. In diseases such as myasthenia gravis, days to years may elapse before respiratory failure results. The maximum inspiratory pressure, expiratory force, and vital capacity of these patients should be monitored every 2 hours to identify changes in the respiratory status. These measurements are inexpensive, noninvasive, and provide important information.

Baseline blood gas evaluations and repeat testing for significant changes in the patient's condition provide further data. Evaluation of the patient's clinical condition, along with the history and diagnosis, may show the need for mechanical ventilatory support. Once problems such as tetanus, botulism, and Guillian-Barré syndrome begin to affect the respiratory system, there is nothing to stop their progress. If the patient is worsening, the practitioner should not wait until the patient is in an acute situation before intervening.

Increased Work of Breathing

An increase in the work of breathing can lead to respiratory failure secondary to respiratory muscle fatigue.[18] Normally, the work of breathing accounts for 1% to 4% of the total oxygen consumption at rest.[34] An increased work of breathing usually registers as a greater rate and depth of respiration. Oxygen consumption by the respiratory muscles increases[27] and may be as high as 35% to 40% in some patients.[24] More work is required to move the same tidal volumes owing to an airway obstruction or restrictive disorder or both. Tolerance to increased ventilatory work is probably limited by fatigue of the respiratory muscles in response to the increased demands of ventilation.[18, 35] Table 4–2 lists some of the causes of increased work of breathing which can induce hypoventilation, respiratory insufficiency, and eventual respiratory failure.

For example, in patients with severe chest injury, the occurrence of flail chest, pneumothorax, or hemothorax can impair the mechanics of breathing and affect the ability to oxygenate. The reduction of $\dot{V}_A$ leads to increased dead space, increased V_D/V_T ratio, hypoxemia, hypercarbia, and acidosis. In addition, ventilation-perfusion ($\dot{V}/\dot{Q}$) mismatching aggravates the ability to maintain gas exchange. While respiratory centers may be intact and able to respond to hypercarbia and hypoxemia, the increased respiratory efforts result in little benefit to the patient. Regardless of the effort of increased respiratory rate, the Pa_{O_2} may continue to fall, the Pa_{CO_2} to rise, and the pH to decrease.

Eventually, the increased work of breathing may, in some patients, result in rapid shallow breathing and paradoxical abdominal movement.[18] With asynchronous movement the abdomen moves out on exhalation and in on inhalation. This is the reverse of normal where the chest wall and abdomen move outward together on inspiration and inward on exhalation. The dyssynchronous motion of the chest and abdomen indicates fatigue of the diaphragm.[9]

PHYSIOLOGIC MEASUREMENTS IN ACUTE RESPIRATORY FAILURE

There are specific physiologic measurements which indicate the need for mechanical ventilation, regardless of the cause. The advantage of these measurements is that they can be done quickly and with minimal cost and risk to the patient. These measurements and their values are generally grouped into three categories: (1) ventilatory mechanics, (2) ventilation, and (3) oxygenation (Table 4–3).

Ventilatory Mechanics

Ventilatory mechanics include measurements of inspiratory and expiratory force. These include the maximum inspiratory pressure (MIP, or PImax), also called inspiratory force (IF), negative inspiratory force (NIF), and negative inspiratory pressure. MIP is now the most widely used term for this measurement. Other ventilatory mechanics measurements are the maximum peak expiratory pressure (PEP), vital capacity (VC), respiratory frequency or rate (f), tidal volume (VT), and occasionally the one-second forced expiratory volume (FEV_1). These parameters are reliable indicators of the mechanical ability of the subject to move air into and out of the lungs and to produce a strong cough. Measurement of

TABLE 4–3.
Indications of Acute Respiratory Failure and Need for Mechanical Ventilatory Support

Criteria	Normal Range	Critical Value*
Ventilatory mechanics		
Maximum inspiratory pressure (MIP) (cm H_2O)	−50–−100	<−20
Peak expiratory pressure (PEP) (cm H_2O)	+100	<+40
Vital capacity (VC) (mL/kg)	65–75	<15
Tidal volume (VT) (mL/kg)	5–8	<5
Respiratory frequency (f) (breaths/min)	12–20	>35
Forced expired volume at 1 sec (FEV_1) (mL/kg)	50–60	<10
Ventilation		
pH	7.35–7.45	<7.25
$Paco_2$ (mm Hg)	35–45	>55 and rising
VD/VT	0.3–0.4	>0.6
Oxygenation†		
Pao_2 (mm Hg)	80–100	<70 (on O_2)
$P(A\text{-}a)o_2$ (mm Hg)	25–65	>450 (on O_2)
Arterial/alveolar Po_2	0.75	<0.15

*Indicates need for mechanical ventilatory support.
†Indicates need for oxygen therapy or PEEP or CPAP.

MIP, PEP, VC, and FEV_1 require a maximum effort on the part of the patient to be accurate.

MIP and PEP are usually measured with a Bourdon gauge pressure manometer (Fig 4–1). The device is connected to the patient's airway by means of a mask, mouthpiece, or endotracheal tube adaptor. By instructing the patient to inhale and exhale in a closed system, these values can be determined.

MIP measurements have been found to be most consistent and accurate when measured with a one-way valve in the system to allow exhalation into the room but to prevent inspiration.[28] This may improve the function of the diaphragm at lower lung volumes.[5, 28] A total of eight to ten consecutive breaths are monitored. The measurement is stopped when MIP reaches its most negative value. This may take about 20 seconds.[20] The patient is monitored during this time to make sure there is no worsening of his or her conditon. MIP is normally −50 to −100 cm H_2O. Values between 0 and −20 cm H_2O are considered inadequate for producing a V_T large enough to produce a good cough.

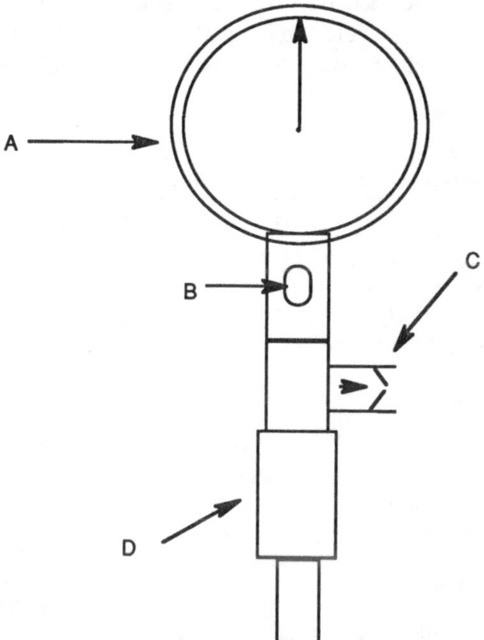

FIG 4–1.
Maximum inspiratory pressure measuring device. *A* is the pressure measuring device. *B* is the port that is occluded with the thumb during the procedure. *C* is a one-way valve connection that allows exhalation to the room, but does not allow inhalation of air. *D* is the connection to the patient's mouth or endotracheal tube.

A PEP of +40 cm H_2O is required for an adequate cough. A value of 100 cm H_2O is considered normal. Values less than +40 cm H_2O are considered inadequate.[33] This measurement is not as commonly used in clinical practice as the MIP determination.

A volume of twice the normal VT is considered necessary to produce an adequate cough for clearing the airway. For this reason, measurement of VC is important to be sure of how high a volume a patient can attain. Vital capacity is the volume measured from maximum inspiration to maximum expiration. The normal VC is 65 to 75 mL/kg and may go as high as 100 mL/kg. Values less than 15 mL/kg are considered inadequate to maintain normal ventilation and cough mechanisms.[35] Volumes can be easily measured at the bedside using such simple devices as a respirometer.[31] This measurement requires the patient's cooperation and good instruction on the part of the clinician. If the patient is unable to cooperate, measurement of exhaled VC immediately after a 20-second MIP determination can be done. This gives a VC equivalent to VC measured by standard techniques.[21]

The respiratory rate is normally about 12 to 20 breaths/min.[34] When adult rates exceed 35 breaths/min for extended periods of time, this signals problems of inadequate $\dot{V}_E$ or hypoxemia, or both. Elevated respiratory rates increase the work of breathing and can lead to fatigue and probably respiratory collapse.

Tidal volume is the most direct bedside measure of lung expansion[36] and can be evaluated using a respirometer fitted to a face mask. Tidal volumes of 5 to 8 mL/kg are considered normal while those less than 5 mL/kg may indicate the need for mechanical ventilation.

Minute ventilation is the product of tidal volume and respiratory rate ($V_T \times f$). The normal value is about 5 to 6 L/min and is directly related to a patient's metabolic rate. When the $\dot{V}_E$ exceeds 10 L/min, acute respiratory failure is probable. The $\dot{V}_E$ necessary to maintain a stable Pa_{CO_2} may become so high that the work of breathing cannot be sustained by the patient.[18, 26]

Another important ventilatory maneuver is the FEV_1. Normally the FEV_1 is approximately 83% of the VC or 50 to 60 mL/kg of ideal body weight.[35] An FEV_1 of less than 10 mL/kg is considered critical. The measurement of FEV_1 requires the use of a bedside spirometer and requires patient cooperation and coaching from the clinician.[31] Sometimes this is *not* an appropriate measurement to perform on a patient who is severely short of breath and in acute respiratory failure.

The peak expiratory flow rate is not usually included with ventilatory mechanics, but it is an excellent method for determining whether or not the patient is maintaining adequate airway patency. A peak flowmeter is used to evaluate the maximum expiratory flow rate. Acceptable values range from 500 to 600 L/min. When values begin to decrease, this is an indication of increased airway resistance. Values less than 75 to 100 L/min are cause for alarm and indicate severe airflow obstruction. Low exhaled flow rates are often seen in patients during an asthma attack.

Ventilation

The second major indicator of acute respiratory failure is ventilation. The best single indicator of adequate ventilation is the $PaCO_2$. The $PaCO_2$, along with the pH, helps to determine if the patient's condition is acute or chronic. Normal $PaCO_2$ is about 35 to 45 mm Hg. A $PaCO_2$ of more than 55 mm Hg associated with a falling pH (<7.25) is indicative of acute hypoventilation or acute respiratory acidosis.[35]

The patient history, diagnosis, and clinical evaluation will confirm this conclusion. An elevated $PaCO_2$ also suggests that the V_D is increased in relation to the V_T. The normal V_D/V_T range is between 0.3 and 0.4 at normal V_T values. Values greater than 0.6 indicate a critical increase in dead space. For example, if a patient had a 1,000-mL V_T and a V_D/V_T of 0.6, then for each breath taken, only 40% is contributing to alveolar gas exchange; 60% is going to areas of the pulmonary system that are not in contact with the pulmonary capillary bed. That is, only 400 mL of the 1,000 mL is in contact with pulmonary blood flow. Under these conditions, the patient must increase the rate and depth of breathing in attempting to achieve an adequate gas exchange. This represents a condition of respiratory insufficiency or respiratory failure. Increased V_D/V_T ratios manifest as rising $PaCO_2$ values with accompanying falls in PaO_2 or as unchanging $PaCO_2$ values with a rising $\dot{V}_E$. This $\dot{V}/\dot{Q}$ mismatching may also be due to pulmonary thromboemboli, or pulmonary vascular injury or destruction.

The measurement of the V_D/V_T ratio requires the collection of expired gases and the simultaneous evaluation of $PaCO_2$ (see Chapter 9). This is a time-consuming procedure and for patients in severe respiratory insufficiency it is not well tolerated. For this reason, the V_D/V_T evaluation is not generally used in the assessment of a patient who might need mechanical ventilatory support. The best indicator is to watch for a rising $\dot{V}_E$ with no change or a slight increase in $PaCO_2$. This may mean an increase in V_D/V_T or an increase in CO_2 production.

Oxygenation

The third, and last, category of physiologic measurements used to indicate the condition of respiratory distress is that of oxygenation. The PaO_2 is one index of tissue oxygenation. Normal PaO_2 is 80 to 100 mm Hg but varies with age and body position. A PaO_2 of less than 70 mm Hg on an oxygen mask indicates inadequate oxygenation.[35] A decrease in PaO_2 can be attributed to aging, hypoventilation, diffusion defects, $\dot{V}/\dot{Q}$ mismatching, or shunting.[45] To further evaluate oxygenation, the alveolar-arterial oxygen difference [$P(A - a)O_2$] can be calculated (see Appendix B). The normal range is about 2 to 30 mm Hg on room air. Values greater than 450 mm Hg on supplemental oxygen are considered critical. When the PaO_2 is low and the $P(A - a)O_2$ is high, then hypoxemia is due to one of the other three general causes: shunt, diffusion, or $\dot{V}/\dot{Q}$ mismatching. In such situations the $Paco_2$ might even be lower than normal, indicating hyperventilation to compensate for hypoxemia.

The ratio between the arterial and alveolar oxygen pressure (Pao_2/PAO_2) is another way to evaluate oxygenation. It is easier to understand than the $P(A - a)O_2$. The Pao_2/PAO_2 ratio is normally about 0.75. If you divide a Pao_2 of 100 mm Hg by a PAO_2 of 105 mm Hg, also normal values, the ratio is 0.95. So normal can range from 0.75 to 0.95. Normal values show that of the oxygen available in the alveolus, 75% to 95% is getting into the artery. A value of 0.15 or less is critical. Basically this shows that of the amount available in the alveolus, only 15% (0.15) is getting into the artery.

Some clinicians go one step further and divide the Pao_2 by the FIO_2. This saves having to calculate the PAO_2. Normal values can be calculated as follows: 100 mm Hg/0.21 = 476. A severe abnormality might be a Pao_2 of 40 mm Hg on an FIO_2 of 1.0: 40 mm Hg/1.0 = 40. Normal values would be close to 475 and decline as they become worse.

By themselves situations of severe hypoxemia are treated with oxygen therapy. Refractory hypoxemia, under some conditions, can be treated with positive end-expiratory pressure (PEEP) or continuous positive airway pressure (CPAP) (see Chapter 10). However, when hypoxemia is accompanied by increased work of breathing, rising $Paco_2$ values, and a falling pH, then mechanical ventilatory support is needed.

SUMMARY

The standard criteria for the institution of mechanical ventilatory support are as follows:

1. Apnea or absence of breathing when reversible disease is present.
2. Acute respiratory failure.
3. Impending respiratory failure.
4. Severe hypoxemia attributed to increased work of breathing or an ineffective breathing pattern.

It should be kept in mind that no single parameter should determine the decision for treatment. History, physical assessment, arterial blood gas evaluation, lung mechanics, prognosis—all should be considered. The goals of therapy for the mechanically ventilated patient should always be remembered while caring for the patient.[13] They are:

1. To provide the pulmonary system with the support needed to maintain an adequate level of alveolar ventilation.

2. To reduce the work of breathing until the cause of respiratory failure can be removed.
3. To restore normal acid-base balance to the arterial and systemic areas.
4. To increase oxygen transfer and oxygenation to the body organs and tissues.

CASE HISTORIES

Case 1

A 23-year-old woman is admitted to the hospital following ingestion of an unknown quantity of drugs and alcohol. She was found unconscious in her apartment by friends. She is unconscious and nonresponsive to verbal command. Her pulse is 124 beats/min. Blood pressure is 85/50 mm Hg. Her respiratory rate is 15 breaths/min. Exhaled V_T is 300 mL, or about half of predicted value. Arterial blood gases on room air are: Pa_{O_2} = 60 mm Hg; Pa_{CO_2} = 69 mm Hg; and pH = 7.24. Breath sounds reveal bilateral coarse crackles, especially in the bases.

Drugs and alcohol are known to depress the respiratory centers of the brain and also to weaken the normal glottic response, and these are most likely the cause of the patient's low respiratory rate and V_T. The bilateral crackles may be due to aspiration. Weakening of the normal glottic response causes failure of the glottis to protect the airway during vomiting. It is not uncommon for drugs and alcohol to cause nausea and vomiting.

The arterial blood gases indicate acute respiratory failure. The most important action here for the respiratory care practitioner is to protect the airway, i.e., to intubate and provide ventilation. In drug overdose, it is sometimes possible to treat the patient pharmacologically. This depends on the types of drugs ingested. For example, narcotic overdoses can be treated with naloxone (Narcan). The physician would try to establish the type and quantity of drugs ingested and treat the patient appropriately.

Case 2

A 30-year-old man is admitted to the hospital emergency room complaining of weakness of the limbs, tingling of the hands and feet, and increasing lack of coordination. Two weeks previously he had been treated for a flulike illness. The diagnosis of Guillian-Barré syndrome is made based on the history and physical findings. The respiratory care practitioner obtains a baseline blood gas which is within normal limits. MIP is −70 cm H_2O and VC is 4.3 L (predicted = 4.8 L). Over a 36-hour-period the patient is monitored every 2 hours for VC, MIP, V_T, and respiratory rate. Values progressively decrease to a VC of 2.1 L (44% of predicted; 23 mL/kg). MIP is −32 cm H_2O. A repeat arterial blood gas evaluation on room air shows: Pa_{O_2} = 70 mm Hg, Pa_{CO_2} = 48 mm Hg, and pH = 7.34.

Knowing the patient's diagnosis and clinical findings, the physician decides to intubate and begin respiratory support. Guillian-Barré syndrome is a rapidly progressing, ascending, bilateral, flaccid muscle paralysis. Once it begins, it can go on to affect all the respiratory muscles, as well as other skeletal muscles. There are no current drug treatments which will stop its progress. For this reason, it is important in this case for the physician to intervene before the patient goes into complete respiratory failure.

Case 3

A patient with status asthmaticus has been treated in the emergency room for several hours. Administration of intravenous and aerosolized bronchodilators is not effective in reducing airway obstruction and the work of breathing. The patient has a respiratory rate of 37 breaths/min. Scattered wheezes are present in both lungs. Breath sounds are distant. Exhaled V_T is 500 mL. Peak expiratory flow rate is 70 L/min. Arterial blood gases on 50% oxygen show: Pa_{O_2} = 73 mm Hg, Pa_{CO_2} = 28 mm Hg, and pH = 7.46. The Pa_{O_2}/PA_{O_2} ratio is 0.23. Only 23% of the alveolar oxygen is getting into the arteries.

Hyperventilation in moderate or severe attacks of asthma is probably localized to areas of the lung where resistance to flow is lowest. Other areas of the lung are underventilated, resulting in shunting and low oxygenation. In patients with status asthmaticus this pattern may go on for hours. How long the patient is able to tolerate this amount of work and hypoxemia varies among patients. If the persistent bronchospasm and mucous plugging cannot be stopped, this will lead to a situation where the Pa_{CO_2} will start to rise despite high $\dot{V}_E$ values.

After 2 more hours of treatment, the patient develops a Pa_{O_2} of 75 mm Hg on 80% oxygen. Pa_{CO_2} = 56 mm Hg, pH = 7.31, $\dot{V}_E$ = 18 L/min.

Serious consideration must be given to intubation under mild sedation and mechanical ventilatory support. This is often a difficult decision to make in a fully conscious and distressed patient.[20] Unfortunately, it may be the only alternative. The scenario that follows will sometimes result in a reduction in the previously strong respiratory efforts. Rates and V_T may start to fall. The patient may become stuporous or uncontrollably agitated.[36] These are often signs of fatigue. This is another example of impending respiratory failure where aggressive care was needed before the patient went into failure or arrest.

Case 4

An 83-year-old woman with severe kyphoscoliosis is admitted to the hospital from a nursing home. She is diagnosed with pneumonia. Evaluation of the patient shows a very weak, pale woman with decreased skin turgor. Blood pressure is 110/72 mm Hg. The pulse rate is 110 beats/min. The respiratory rate is 28 breaths/min and shallow. Breath sounds reveal bilateral crackles scattered throughout both lungs. After 3 days of hospitalization and antibiotic therapy the patient worsens. Arterial blood gases on a 2-L/min nasal cannula show: Pao_2 = 58 mm Hg, $Paco_2$ = 68 mm Hg, and pH = 7.24. The decision is made to intubate the patient and begin ventilatory support. The combination of her severe, chronic, restrictive disorder plus the unresolved pneumonia resulted in blood gases that indicated acute respiratory failure.

Case 5

A man with chronic obstructive pulmonary disease (COPD) is brought in by ambulance to the emergency room. He was placed on a partial rebreathing mask at 12 L/min during transport. His respiratory rate is only 6 breaths/min. The patient appears to be sleeping. Normal blood gases on room air are: Pao_2 = 41 mm Hg, $Paco_2$ = 68 mm Hg, and pH = 7.38. Current blood gases on an estimated FIO_2 of 0.5 are: Pao_2 = 65 mm Hg, $Paco_2$ = 94 mm Hg, and pH = 7.18.

In this situation a patient with chronic CO_2 retention was placed on an oxygen concentration that was too high. His hypoxic drive was reduced. As a result his respiratory rate was low and his level of consciousness depressed. Oxygen-induced hypoventilation will most often happen in patients with CO_2 retention in the presence of severe hypoxemia and acidosis.[2, 39] As long as the pH stays above 7.2, and the patient stays alert and cooperative, there is little danger. But with an increasing level of CO_2, severe acidosis and unconsciousness will result.

The Pao_2 fell as the $Paco_2$ increased ($PAO_2 = PIO_2 - Paco_2/0.8$). If the oxygen is removed from the patient at this point, the PIO_2 will decrease, but the $Paco_2$ will stay where it is unless ventilation is increased. This will further aggravate the condition. For example, suppose this patient is removed from oxygen therapy. His PAO_2 will drop significantly:

$$\text{Initial } PAO_2 \text{ est} = (760 - 47) \times 0.5 - 94/0.8 = 356.5 - 117.5 = 239 \text{ mm Hg } PAO_2$$
$$\text{if } O_2 \text{ mask is removed} = (760 - 47) \times 0.21 - 94/0.8 = 32 \text{ mm Hg}$$

With the PAO_2 at 32 mm Hg, the Pao_2 would be even lower. This will result in severe hypoxemia which may produce cerebral anoxia. Some method of increasing $\dot{V}A$ must be instituted before oxygen therapy is removed.

It is premature to place such a patient on ventilatory support. Several measures can be taken. If the patient is arousable, he should be encouraged to take several deep breaths while the oxygen mask is switched to a low-concentration Venturi mask. Keeping the patient in the upright or semi-Fowler's position may be helpful. Respiratory stimulants might also be used, but their use is controversial in this setting.

Finally, a resuscitation bag and mask can be used and the concentration of oxygen gradually reduced if the patient is difficult to arouse. This must be done with caution to avoid hyperventilation while allowing blood gases to improve. If the patient is still not conscious and ventilation does not improve, intubation and mechanical ventilation may be required.

STUDY QUESTIONS

1. Define acute respiratory failure.
2. Name two respiratory findings in mild hypoxia.
3. Name two cardiovascular findings in mild hypoxia.
4. Name one cardiovascular finding in severe hypercarbia.
5. List two CNS problems associated with a reduced drive to breathe.
6. Name two neuromuscular disorders associated with reduced respiratory drive.
7. Name two disorders which increase the work of breathing and may require mechanical ventilatory support.
8. Give the normal values for the following and the values that would indicate a patient needs mechanical ventilation: $Paco_2$, pH, MIP, VC, f.
9. Which of the following items indicate the presence of respiratory problems that might require ventilatory support?
    I. MIP of −17 cm H_2O.
    II. VC of 2.1 in a 70-kg man.
    III. V_D/V_T of 0.65.
    IV. $Paco_2$ of 81 mm Hg and pH of 7.19.
    V. Pao_2 of 65 mm Hg on room air.
    a. I and III.
    b. II and V.
    c. I, III, and IV.
    d. I, II, III, and IV.
    e. I, II, III, IV, and V.
10. An unconscious patient is brought to the emergency room and arterial blood gas analysis on room air shows the following: pH = 7.23, $Paco_2$ = 81 mm Hg, Pao_2 = 43 mm Hg. In the absence of additional data, which of the following forms of therapy are indicated?
    a. Oxygen with a nonrebreathing mask.
    b. CPAP mask.
    c. Intermittent positive pressure breathing (IPPB) treatment with albuterol.
    d. Oxygen with a nasal cannula at 4 L/min.
    e. Intubation and mechanical ventilatory support.
11. A patient is seen in the emergency room. She exhibits paralysis of the lower extremities that is getting progressively worse. Vital capacity is 12

mL/kg; the MIP measurement is less than 30 cm H_2O. Blood gas analysis has been requested but is not yet available. What type of therapy do you think this patient is most likely going to need?
   a. Aerosol treatment with a bronchodilator with a metered dose inhaler.
   b. Oxygen therapy.
   c. Mechanical ventilatory support.
   d. Incentive spirometry to improve muscle strength.
   e. A narcotic blocking agent.
12. A patient with botulism is beginning to develop progressive muscle paralysis. The respiratory care practitioner has been monitoring MIP and VC every 2 hours. The most recent results show that the patient continues to deteriorate. MIP is -27 cm H_2O and VC is 32 mL/kg. Which of the following would you recommend?
   a. Gastric lavage.
   b. Oxygen therapy.
   c. Medication to reverse the paralysis.
   d. Mechanical ventilatory support.
   e. Incentive spirometry to improve muscle strength.
13. A patient in the emergency room arrives from the scene of a motor vehicle accident. He is unconscious and nonresponsive. Arterial blood gases on a nonrebreathing mask show a Pa_{O_2} of 47 mm Hg, Pa_{CO_2} of 93, and pH of 7.09. Which of the following would you recommend?
   a. Recheck vital signs.
   b. Intubate and ventilate.
   c. Change to a Venturi mask and coach the patient to breathe.
   d. Recommend the administration of bicarbonate.
   e. Begin cardiopulmonary resuscitation (CPR).
14. A patient with a history of COPD and CO_2 retention is admitted to the emergency room. He was brought in by ambulance and is receiving oxygen by partial rebreathing mask. He appears to be sleeping, but arouses when talked to. HR = 100 beats/min, BP = 128/78 mm Hg, f = 5 breaths/min. Breath sounds reveal bilateral crackles and wheezes. Which of the following would you recommend *immediately?*
   a. Change to a Venturi mask and coach the patient to breathe.
   b. Intubate and ventilate.
   c. Recheck vital signs.
   d. Recommend aerosol treatment with a bronchodilator on compressed air.
   e. Begin CPR.
15. A patient with myasthenia gravis is beginning to develop progressive muscle paralysis. The respiratory care practitioner has been monitoring MIP and VC every 2 hours. The most recent result shows that the patient continues to deteriorate despite treatment with anticholinesterase drugs.

MIP = −25 cm H_2O and VC = 23 mL/kg. Which of the following would you recommend?
   a. Gastric lavage.
   b. Oxygen therapy.
   c. Medication to reverse the paralysis.
   d. Mechanical ventilatory support.
   e. Incentive spirometry to improve muscle strength.

ANSWERS TO STUDY QUESTIONS

1. Definition of acute respiratory failure: any condition in which respiratory activity is completely absent or is inadequate to maintain oxygen uptake and carbon dioxide clearance: a $Paco_2$ of 50 to 55 mm Hg and rising, a pH of 7.25 and falling, and a Pao_2 below normal predicted.
2. See Table 4–1.
3. See Table 4–1.
4. See Table 4–1.
5. See Table 4–2.
6. See Table 4–2.
7. See Table 4–2.
8. See Table 4–3.
9. c.
10. e.
11. c.
12. d.
13. b.
14. a.
15. d.

REFERENCES

1. Aldrich TK, Prezant DJ, Karpel JP, et al: Maximal inspiratory pressure is not a reliable test of inspiratory muscle strength in respiratory failure. *Chest* 1989; 96(suppl):175S.
2. Aubier M, Murciano D, Milic-Emili J, et al: Effects of administration of O_2 on ventilation and blood gases in patients with chronic obstructive pulmonary disease during acute respiratory failure. *Am Rev Respir Dis* 1980; 122:747–754.
3. Ayres SM, Mueller H: Hypoxia and hypercarbia and cardiac arrhythmias: The importance of regional abnormalities of vascular distensibility. *Chest* 1973; 63:981–985.
4. Branson RD, Hurst JM, Davis K: Measurement of maximum inspiratory pressure (MIP): Comparison of two techniques. *Respir Care* 1988; 33:950.

5. Branson RD, Hurst JM, Davis K, et al: Comparison of maximum inspiratory pressure (MIP) measurements: Manual versus the P-B 7200a. *Respir Care* 1988; 33:951.
6. Branson RD, Hurst JM, Davis K Jr, et al: Measurement of maximal inspiratory pressure: A comparison of three methods. *Respir Care* 1989; 34:789–794.
7. Bone RC: Treatment of respiratory failure due to advanced obstructive lung disease. *Arch Intern Med* 1980; 140:1018.
8. Burke JF, Wolfe RR, Mullany CJ, et al: Glucose requirements following burn injury. *Ann Surg* 1979; 190:274–285.
9. Burrow B, Knudson RJ, Kettel LJ: *Respiratory Insufficiency.* St Louis, Mosby–Year Book, Inc, 1975.
10. Carlotto D, Sinclair S, Kemper M, et al: Serial maximal inspiratory pressure measurement during weaning. *Respir Care* 1988; 33:949.
11. Cherniak RM: The management of acute respiratory failure. *Chest* 1970; 58:427–452.
12. Cherniak RM: *Pulmonary Function Testing.* Philadelphia, WB Saunders Co, 1977.
13. Didier E: Principles in the management of assisted ventilation. *Chest* 1970; 58:423–428.
14. Gordon E: Critical care of the patient with head trauma, in *33rd Annual Refresher Course Lectures.* Chicago, American Society of Anesthesiology, 1982; 142:1–7.
15. Gietzen JW: Blood gas corner #29—A case of oxygen induced hypoventilation. *Respir Care* 1991; 36:431–433.
16. Hieronimus TW: *Mechanical Artificial Ventilation: A Manual for Students and Practitioners. American Lecture Series.* Springfield, Ill, Charles C Thomas, Publishers, 1970.
17. Huch A, Huch AB, Rooth B: Continuous transcutaneous oxygen tension measured with a heated electrode. *Scand J Clin Lab Invest* 1973; 31:269–275.
18. Hudson LD: Evaluation of the patient with acute respiratory failure. *Resp Care* 1983; 28:542–552.
19. Hudson LD: Respiratory failure: Etiology and mortality. *Respir Care* 1987; 32:584–593.
20. Kacmarek RM, Chapman MC, Young-Palazza PJ, et al: Comparison of two methods to determine inspiratory force. *Respir Care* 1988; 33:950.
21. Kacmarek RM, Cheever P, Foley K, et al: Determination of vital capacity in mechanically ventilated patients: A comparison of techniques (abstract). *Respir Care* 1990; 35:129.
22. Kacmarek R, Cycyk-Chapman MC, Young-Palazzo PJ, et al: Determination of maximal inspiratory pressure: A clinical study and literature review. *Respir Care* 1989; 34:868–878.
23. Kacmarek R, Stoller JK: *Current Respiratory Care.* Philadelphia, BC Decker, Inc, 1988.
24. Levison H, Cherniack RM: Ventilatory cost of exercise in chronic obstructive pulmonary disease. *J Appl Physiol* 1968; 25:21.
25. Lifschitz MD, Brasch R, Cuomo AJ, et al: Marked hypercarbia secondary to severe metabolic alkalosis. *Ann Intern Med* 1972; 77:405–409.
26. Long CL, Schaffel N, Geiger JW, et al: Metabolic response to injury and illness: Estimation of energy and protein needs from indirect calorimetry and nitrogen balance. *JPEN* 1979; 3:452–456.
27. Marini JJ: The role of the inspiratory circuit in the work of breathing during mechanical ventilation. *Respir Care* 1987; 32:419.

28. Marini JJ, Smith TC, Lamb V: Estimation of inspiratory muscle strength in mechanically ventilated patients: The measurement of maximal inspiratory pressure. *J Crit Care* 1986; 1:31–38.
29. Martz KV, Joiner J, Shepherd RM: *Management of the Patient-Ventilator System: A Team Approach.* St Louis, Mosby–Year Book, Inc, 1979.
30. McPherson SP: *Respiratory Therapy Equipment.* St Louis, Mosby–Year Book, Inc, 1981.
31. Mushin WW, Rendell-Baker L, Thompson PW, et al: *Automatic Ventilation of the Lungs.* Philadelphia, FA Davis Co, 1980.
32. O'Donohue WJ, Baker JP, Bell GM, et al: Respiratory failure in neuromuscular disease: Management in a respiratory intensive care unit. *JAMA* 1976; 235:733–735.
33. Otis AB: The work of breathing. *Physiol Rev* 1954; 34:449.
34. Pierson DJ: Indications for mechanical ventilation in acute respiratory failure. *Respir Care* 1981; 28:570–578.
35. Pontoppidan H: Treatment of respiratory failure in non-thoracic trauma. *Trauma* 1968; 8:938–944.
36. Pontoppidan H, Geffin B, Lowenstein E: Acute respiratory failure in the adult [first of three parts]. *N Engl J Med* 1972; 287:690–698.
37. Pontoppidan H, Geffin B, Lowenstein E: Acute respiratory failure in the adult [second of three parts]. *N Engl J Med* 1972; 287:743–752.
38. Rattenborg C, Via-Reque E: *Clinical Use of Mechanical Ventilation.* St Louis, Mosby–Year Book, Inc, 1981.
39. Rau JL: Continuous mechanical ventilation—Part II. *Crit Care Update* 1981 (Nov); 5–20.
40. Rogers RM, Juers JA: Physiological considerations in the treatment of acute respiratory failure. *Basics Respir Disease* 1975; 3:1–6.
41. Ruppell G: *Manual of Pulmonary Function Testing.* St Louis, Mosby–Year Book, Inc, 1975.
42. Shapiro BA: Fundamentals of acid-base balance and blood gas analysis, in *Annual Refresher Course Lectures.* Chicago, American Society of Anesthesiology, 1983; 126:1–7.
43. Shapiro BA, Harrison RF, Trout CA: *Clinical Application of Respiratory Care.* St Louis, Mosby–Year Book, Inc, 1979.
44. Sorbini CA, Grassi V, Solinas E, et al: Arterial oxygen tension in relation to age in healthy subjects. *Respiration* 1968; 25:3–13.
45. Swinburne AJ, Fedullo AJ, Wahl GW, et al: Acute respiratory failure in patients with chronic obstructive pulmonary disease and acute bronchitis: Factors associated with survival after mechanical ventilation. *Chest* 1989; 96(suppl):175S.
46. Tuller MA, Mehdi F: Compensatory hypoventilation and hypercapnea in primary metabolic alkalosis. *Am J Med* 1971; 50:281–290.

Chapter 5

Physical Aspects of Mechanical Ventilation

On completion of this chapter the reader will be able to:

1. Name the five components of the internal control system of ventilators.
2. Describe the eight mechanical drive mechanisms available on mechanical ventilators.
3. Explain the function of each of the four output control valves discussed in the text.
4. Define internal and external circuit.
5. Give the functional parts of an external circuit and added optional components.
6. List and explain the three most frequent methods of triggering inspiration.
7. Describe the following: IMV, SIMV, PS, PC, MMV, HFV, APRV, and inflation hold.
8. Explain the function of volume controllers, flow controllers, and pressure controllers.
9. Discuss how changes in patient lung characteristics affect P_A, P_{TA}, and PIP with a constant flow controller.
10. Describe the effects of changing lung characteristics on the flow pattern of a ventilator with low to moderate pressure drive.
11. Explain how pressure, volume, and flow are limited during inspiration and how they can alter volume or pressure delivery.
12. List the four cycling mechanisms and describe their function.
13. Define the following: NEEP, PEEP, CPAP, IPAP, EPAP, expiratory retard, and expiratory hold.

14. Classify a ventilator based on power source, triggering mechanism(s), inspiratory phase delivery, cycling mechanism(s), and expiratory phase variables.

PHYSICAL ASPECTS OF MECHANICAL VENTILATION

In order to properly care for a critically ill patient on ventilatory support, it is essential to know the various functions of the ventilator being used. One needs to understand how the ventilator interacts with the patient and how changes in the patient's lung condition can alter the ventilator function. The basic purpose of this chapter is to look at the physical characteristics of mechanical ventilators to see how they provide ventilation and how they interact with the patient.

Ventilators have certain properties in common. Because of these properties they tend to be grouped or classified together by common traits. Methods of classifying ventilators have varied considerably over time. This chapter reviews a classification that correlates with most texts in respiratory care and includes a new way of incorporating the function of the newer, microprocessor-controlled ventilators.[6, 7] It is not my intention in this chapter to review all of the ventilators that are currently available on the market. This may be found elsewhere[10, 13, 15] and in the literature provided by the manufacturer. Rather, this chapter purposes to provide a basic understanding of how ventilators physically operate.

FUNDAMENTAL CHARACTERISTICS OF VENTILATORS

Probably the simplest way to look at a ventilator is as if it were a "black box." You plug it into an electrical outlet or a high pressure gas source and gas comes out the other end. The person that operates the ventilator sets certain knobs or controls to determine the pattern of gas flow coming out of the machine. Inside the black box is a control system that interprets what the operator sets. It then provides the desired output. These basic characteristics can be given specific names (Table 5–1):

1. The electrical or gas source is called the ventilator's power source or its "input" power.
2. The internal control system monitors and controls the following:
   a. Control systems are open and closed loop systems that control ventilator function.

TABLE 5–1.
Basic Characteristics of Mechanical Ventilators

1. Power source or input power
2. Internal control system
   a. Control systems
   b. Mechanical drive mechanism
   c. Control panel
   d. Output control valve
   e. Pneumatic circuit

b. A mechanical drive mechanism causes gas to flow to the patient. The power source gives the energy to this piece of equipment to function. One example of this is a piston driven by an electrical motor.
c. The control panel is the outside panel that is monitored and set by a ventilator operator or respiratory care practitioner. The internal control system reads and uses this information to control the function of the mechanical drive mechanism.
d. The output control valve interacts with the mechanical drive mechanism to control the gas waveforms being delivered to the patient. Older ventilators like the Puritan Bennett MA-1 and the Emerson do not have a valve such as this. The newer microprocessor ventilators do.
e. The pneumatic (patient) circuit is the plastic tubing that connects the patient to the ventilator.

Each of these components is reviewed individually below.

POWER SOURCE OR INPUT POWER

The power used by the ventilator to achieve either positive or negative pressure is provided by electrical power, pneumatic (gas) power, or a combination of the two. You connect the ventilator to this power source. The control system or decision-making system can use either electronics, pneumatics, or fluidics, or a combination of the three for controlling the function of the ventilator internally.

Electrically Powered Ventilators

Electrically powered ventilators are fairly common and rely entirely on electricity to function. The electrical source can be either a wall outlet or battery. Battery power is usually only used for the short term, such as transporting a ventilated patient or in the home for a back-up power source should wall electricity fail.

The electrical energy is controlled by an on/off switch. It can then control motors, electromagnets, potentiometers, or rheostats. These, in turn, control the timing mechanisms for inspiration and expiration, the flow of gas, and the alarm systems. The electrical power may operate such things as fans, bellows, solenoids, and transducers. All these operations help achieve a controlled gas flow to the patient.

Examples of electrically controlled and powered ventilators are the MA-1 and the Emerson 3-PV. The Emerson uses an electrically powered motor to drive a rotary piston which provides gas flow. The MA-1's electrical power drives a compressor which provides compressed air to power a bellows. The bellows provides the gas to the patient.

Internal electrically powered circuits can also control *electronic* devices such as resistors, capacitors, diodes, and transistors. Combinations of these can form integrated circuits. These, along with circuit boards, may form complicated electronic devices such as microprocessors. More on this later.

Pneumatically Powered Ventilators

Ventilators which depend entirely on a compressed gas source for power are also available. Ventilators that operate using 50-psig (pounds per square gauge) gas sources have built-in internal reducing valves so that the operating pressure is lower than the source pressure.

There are two types of pneumatically powered ventilators: (1) pneumatic and (2) fluidic. Pneumatic types may use needle valves, Venturi entrainers (injectors), flexible diaphragms, and spring-loaded valves to control the flow, volume delivery, and inspiratory-expiratory function. An example of a pneumatically powered and operated ventilator is the Bird Mark 7. Fluidic ventilators use the principles of fluidics such as the Coanda effect for control of operation. An example of a fluidic ventilator is the Monaghan 225/SIMV. It is pneumatically powered from a 50-psig gas source and fluidically controlled internally.

Combined Power Ventilators

Some ventilators use both an electrical power source and one or two 50-psig gas sources. The gas sources, mixtures of air and oxygen, provide for a variable fractional concentration of oxygen in inspired gas (FIO_2) and they may also provide the power for inspiration. The electrical power may be used to control capacitors, solenoids, and electrical switches that govern the phasing of inspiration and expiration and the monitoring of gas flow. These are considered both pneumatically and electrically powered. They may also be pneumatically or electronically controlled.

For example, the Siemens Servo 900 series of ventilators use gas power to provide the driving force or flow to the patient. They use electricity to control special stepper motors that regulate the opening and closing of scissors-like valves for inspiration and expiration. Electronic logic controls the function of the scissor valves. These ventilators are considered pneumatically powered and electronically controlled.

Positive and Negative Pressure Ventilators

How air flow into the lungs is achieved by the ventilator is based on two different ways of changing the transrespiratory pressure—the pressure at the airway opening less pressure at the body surface (Pawo − Pbs).[7] The ventilator controls pressure at either the airway opening or at the body's surface. If the ventilator provides negative pressure around the body, it is a negative pressure ventilator. The physiologic effect of these two techniques is described in Chapter 2.

Basically, the negative pressure ventilator causes a negative pleural pressure greater than normal which is transmitted to the alveoli. As a result a pressure gradient develops between the airway opening and the alveoli and air flows in. The volume delivered will depend on the pressure difference between the alveolus (P_A) and the pleural space (Ppl)—transpulmonary pressure (P_L) = P_A − Ppl—and the compliance of the lung.

The positive pressure ventilator makes the pressure at the airway opening positive and air flows into the alveoli. Positive pressure at the end of inspiration is transmitted to the pleural space so that it becomes slightly positive. Again, volume delivery will depend on the pressure distending the alveoli (P_L) and the compliance of the lung.

INTERNAL CONTROL SYSTEM

Control Systems

The development of the computer has had a great impact on new medical devices. The microprocessor ventilators are discussed throughout this chapter. At this point we will simply look at one aspect of computer or microprocessor control—the loop system. Most ventilators that are not microprocessor-controlled are called *open loop* systems. This is an "unintelligent" system. The operator sets a control or knob, e.g., to set a tidal volume (V_T). The ventilator delivers that volume to the patient circuit. It is called "unintelligent" because it cannot change its operation. If the volume were to leak out of the patient circuit and never get to the patient, this ventilator would not make any changes in its function to correct for this leak. It simply puts out or "outputs" the volume and does *not* care where it goes. This is an open loop system (Fig 5–1,A).

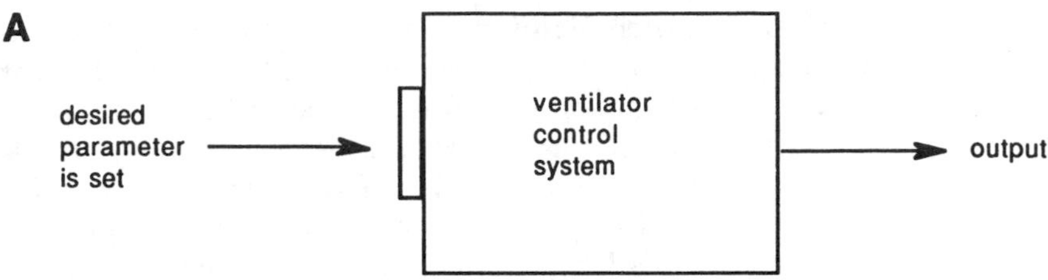

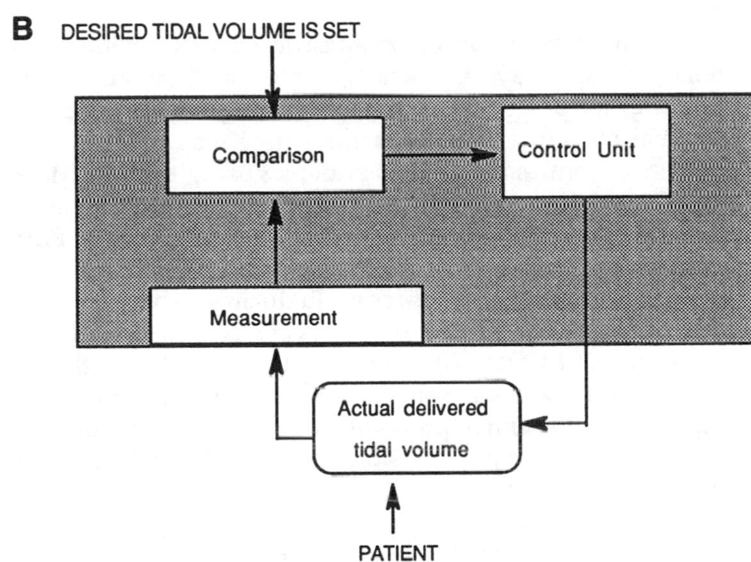

FIG 5–1.
A, Open loop system. B, Closed loop system using a tidal volume as the measured parameter.[6]

Closed loop systems are more intelligent. A closed loop system compares the set control variable to the measured control variable. For example, it might compare the volume setting to the measured volume exhaled by the patient. If the two differ, the programming tells the ventilator to either alarm or alter the volume delivery (Fig 5–1,B).

Mechanical Drive Mechanisms

The various types of devices involved in inspiratory flow delivery include the drive mechanisms which generate the force for inspiratory gas flow. A few of the more common drive mechanisms are described here.[9, 10, 15, 17]

Spring-Loaded Bellows.—The Servo 900 ventilator uses a spring-loaded bellows to act as the force behind the breath. In this ventilator a preblended mixture of oxygen and air at the desired F_{IO_2} flows into a bellows. This bellows has a spring on the top that applies a force. This provides a force per unit area, or a pressure (P = force/area). On the Servo 900 this is called the working pressure. When the scissors-like inspiratory valve opens, the pressure forces gas into the patient's lungs. The tighter the spring, the greater the force and the greater the pressure. This system generates a pressure of up to 120 cm H_2O. As the bellows empties, the spring relaxes and the pressure decreases. The pressure source is not constant, but decreases at the end of inspiration (Fig 5–2).

High Pressure Gas or Pneumatic Drive.—Cylinders or compressed gas or bulk gas supply systems which employ wall outlets provide high pressure gas (50 psig) for power. These are used along with needle valves (Fig 5–3) or high internal resistance flow regulators. They may use fluidic devices or pneumatic devices to control the system, examples being the Bird Mark 7 and 8, the Puritan Bennett PR-1 and -2, and the Monaghan 225/SIMV (fluidic). They also may use electronic or microprocessor control as is found in the Puritan Bennett 7200.

Pressure-Reducing Valves.—Reducing valves take high pressure sources and reduce them to lower pressures (50–200 cm H_2O). In mechanical ventilators, these pressures would have to be at levels safe for the human lung (<80 cm H_2O). The PR-2 is an example of a ventilator that has a built-in reducing valve that lowers the source pressure (50 psig) to what is desired (0–50 cm H_2O) (Fig 5–4). The pressure chosen is displayed on the front manometer marked control pressure.

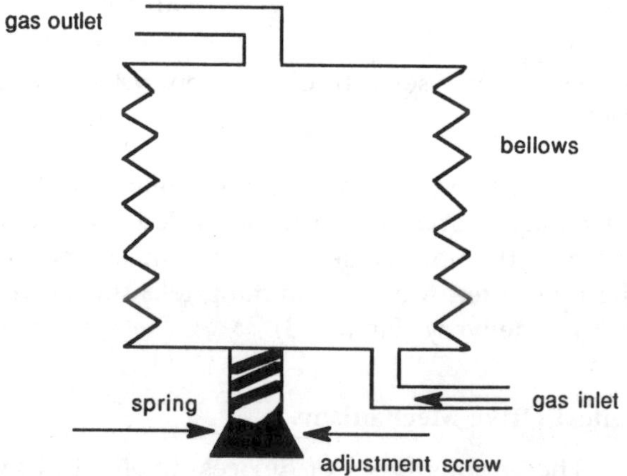

FIG 5–2.
Spring-loaded bellows as in the Siemens Servo 900 series.

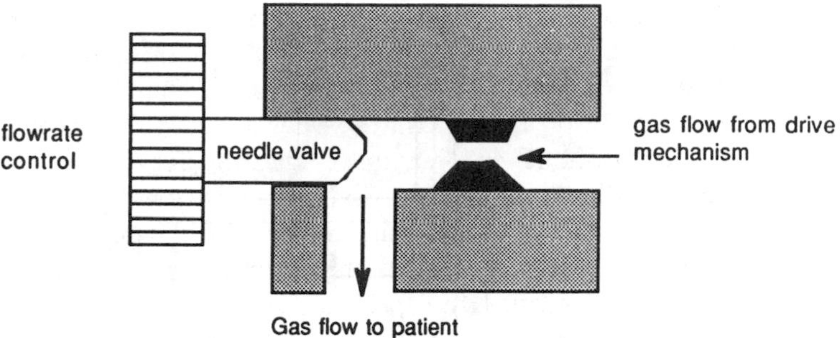

FIG 5–3.
Needle valve for controlling gas flow to the patient.

Linear Drive Piston.—In a direct drive or linear drive piston, an electrical motor is connected by special gearing to a piston rod or arm (Fig 5–5). The rod moves a piston forward inside a cylinder housing in a linear fashion at a constant rate. This creates a constant or rectangular wave flow of gas to the patient. The direct drive piston is an example of what is called a constant flow generator. An example of a linear drive piston is the Bourns LS104-150 ventilator.

Rotary Drive Piston.—The Emerson 3-MV and the Emerson Post-Op (3-PV) ventilators use this type of drive mechanism. It is called either a rotary drive, nonlinear drive, or an eccentric drive piston. An electric motor rotates a drive wheel. As the wheel rotates forward, the piston arm moves forward. The head of the piston creates a positive pressure "breath" inside the piston housing. As the wheel continues to turn, the piston arm moves away from the piston housing. Exhalation occurs during this phase (Fig 5–6). The unusual property of this mechanism is that the rate at which the gas is compressed in the housing changes. The fastest rate of gas delivery is when the piston arm is at the top of the wheel during its forward motion. At the beginning and end of inspiration, the forward movement of the piston is less rapid. The resulting flow pattern is slow at the beginning of inspiration, is at its greatest speed at midinspiration, and then tapers off at end-inspiration. This pattern is called a sine wave and is discussed later in this chapter.

Venturi Injectors or Entrainers.—The Bird Mark 7 uses a Venturi entrainer when it is operated on the air/mix mode. In this instance, a high pressure gas source coming from the center body passes through a Venturi device. This entrains room air from the ambient chamber side of the machine. The gas then flows through the pressure chamber and to the patient (Fig 5–7). The end result is a higher gas flow to the patient. This is one example of the use of Venturi injectors. Other ventilators use this type of device to operate other internal parts of the ventilator besides the drive mechanism. One example is the peak flow

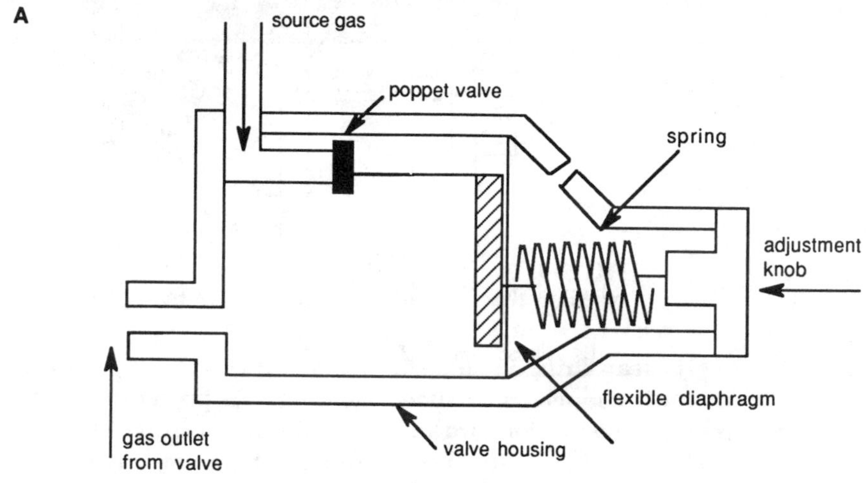

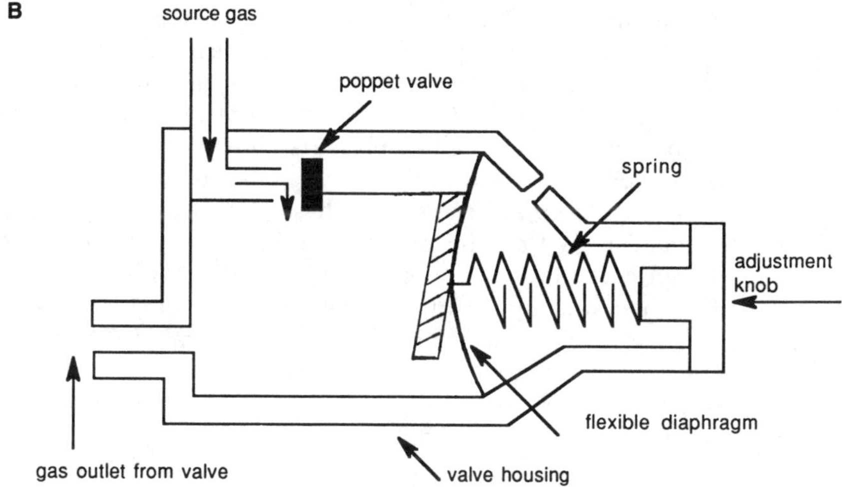

FIG 5–4.
A, Puritan Bennett PR series spring-loaded reducing valve.[10] The valve is off. Pressure inside the valve equals spring tension. **B,** pressure inside the valve is lower than the spring tension. This opens the poppet valve and allows inflow of gas from the gas source into the valve and out toward the patient.

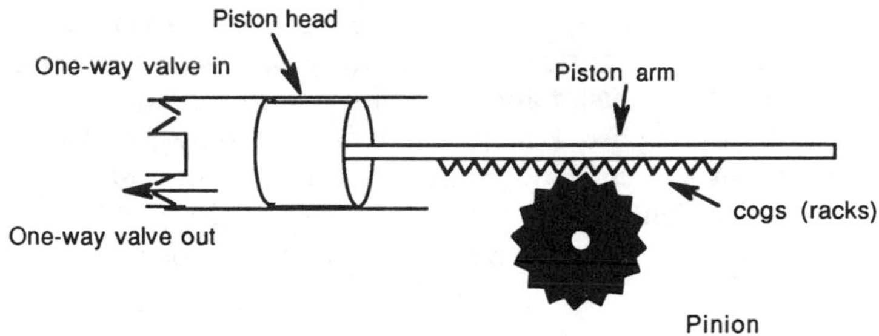

FIG 5–5.
Linear drive piston. The gears engage the cogs and move the piston arm forward in a linear motion.

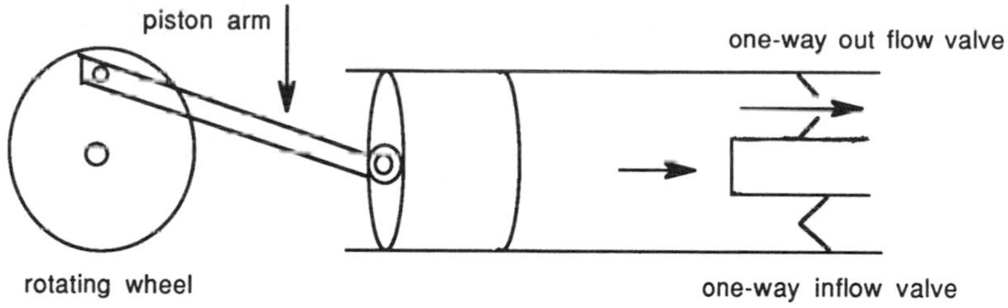

FIG 5–6.
Rotary (eccentric) wheel-driven piston. The forward motion of the piston is most rapid when the piston arm is at the top of the rotating wheel. Inspiratory flow is greatest at this time.

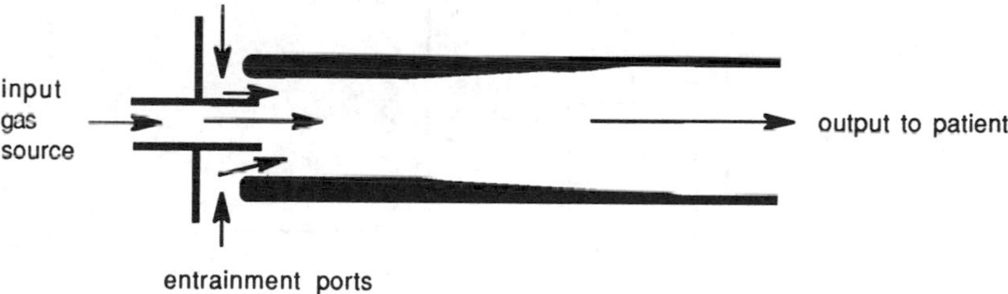

FIG 5–7.
Venturi injector or entrainer.

control on the MA-1 which operates on a Venturi. Some positive end-expiratory pressure (PEEP) valves also function in this manner.

Blower.—In this drive mechanism, an electric motor powers a blower. This is a series of blades like a fan that rotates at a high constant speed. The pressure generated by the blower is the source pressure or generating pressure of the ventilator. An example is the MA-1. A built-in compressor (blower) causes gas to flow to a cannister that contains a bellows. When the blower is on it forces air into the cannister and the bellows empties. The gas from the bellows goes to the patient (Fig 5–8). The pressure generated by the MA-1 compressor is about 7 psig (about 490 cm H_2O). It is reduced to about 1.8 psig after it passes through a Venturi entrainer. Under most conditions this is enough working pressure to provide a constant pressure source and a constant gas flow to the patient. Other

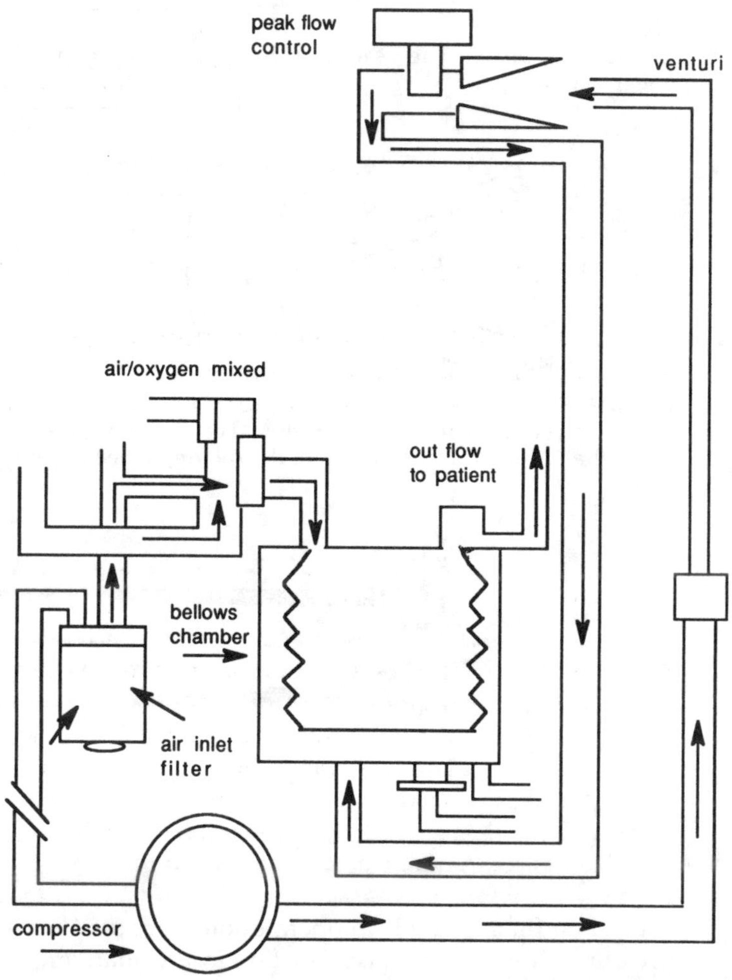

FIG 5–8.
Puritan Bennett MA-1 compressor with bellows and Venturi at peak flow knob. The MA-1 compressor acts as the drive mechanism. Driving pressure is decreased as it passes through the Venturi at the peak flow control.

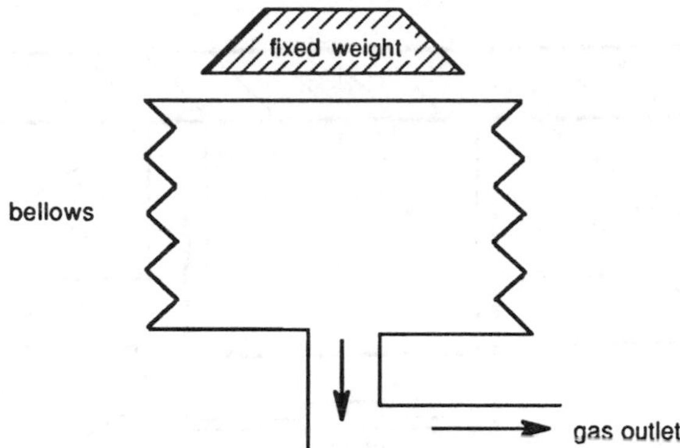

FIG 5–9.
Weighted bellows. This provides a constant force or pressure during inspiration.

ventilators with a blower or compressor include the MA-2, BEAR 1 and 2, (compressors), Air-Shields (blower), and Ohio CCV 2/SIMV (rotary blower).

Weighted Bellows or Weighted Drive Mechanism.—Flow is the result of gravity acting on a weight over the top of a bellows or piston. (Fig 5–9). An example is the Chemstron Gill-1 (no longer manufactured).

Control Panel

The control panel has a variety of available knobs or settings: V_T and rate, inspiratory time, F_{IO_2}, etc. These controls are set by the operator. Basically they control four parameters: flow, volume, pressure, and time. These values can be varied over a wide range. For each ventilator the manufacturer provides a list of ranges for these variables. For example, volume, V_T, ranges from 200 to 2,000 mL on most adult ventilators.

In Chapter 2 it was pointed out that volume, flow, and pressure vary or change during inspiratory time when a breath is given to a patient. They are called "control" variables because the ventilator has control over how they change. Part of this control is based on what the operator selects when the ventilator is set. A major part of understanding ventilator classification is knowing how the control variables work in a specific ventilator.

Output Control Valves

This section describes some of the different output control valves which may interact with the drive mechanism in determining the pattern of flow delivery in a ventilator.

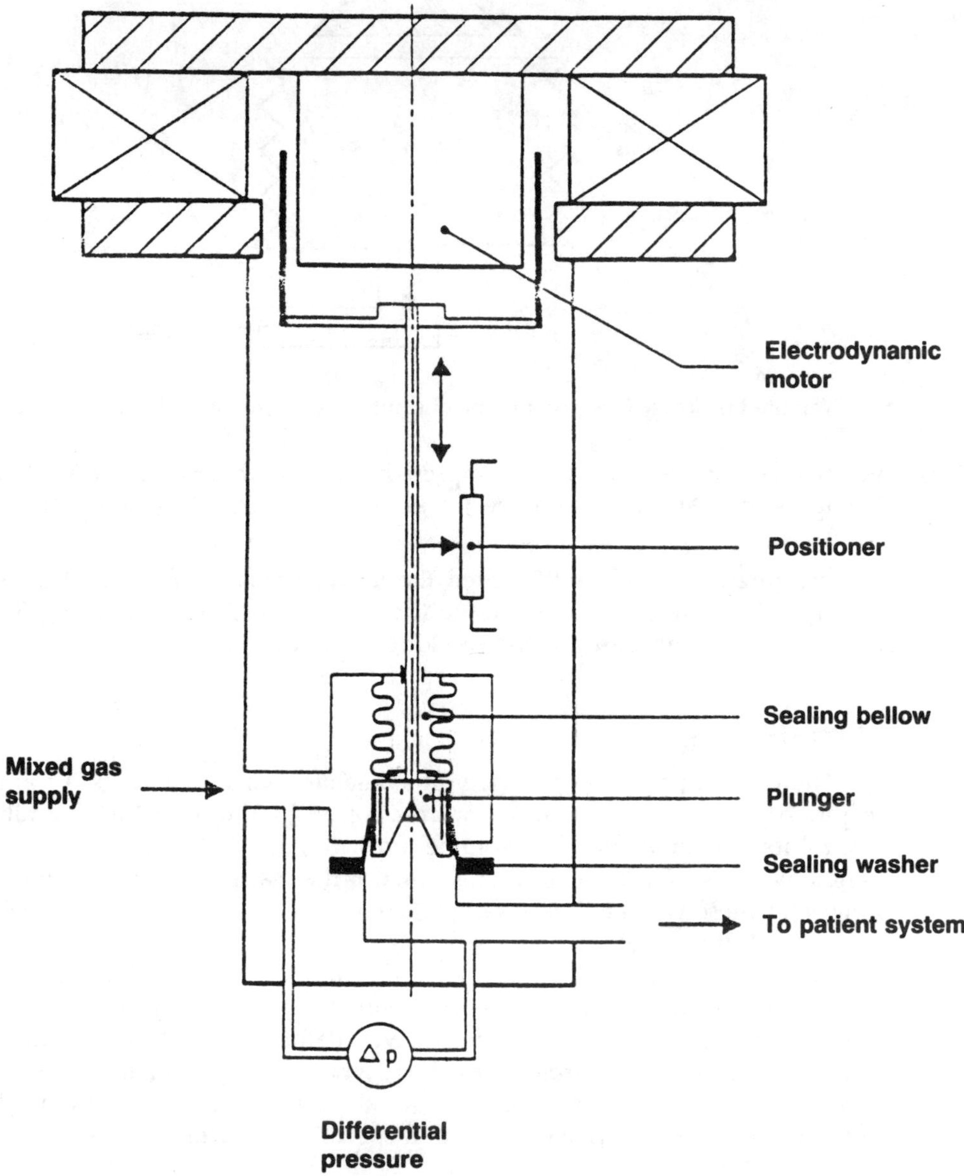

FIG 5–10.
Hamilton Veolar servo-controlled flow valve. The electrodynamic motor controls the movement of the plunger allowing controlled amounts of the mixed gas supply to pass to the patient. (Courtesy of Hamilton Medical, Inc., Reno, Nev.)

Resistance-Type or High-Resistance Valve.—This valve is designed for ventilators which operate off high pressure gas sources. The valve reduces the pressure source to deliver a safe level of pressure to the patient. One example is a clamp between the high pressure source and the patient. Another example is the needle valve on the flow control knob of the Mark 7 (see Fig 5–3).

Proportional Valve.—The proportional solenoid valve is a small valve which is a microprocessor-controlled solenoid. It regulates the flow of the air or oxygen source. The precise and rapid valve movement allows control of the gas flow pattern. An example of a ventilator which has this type of valve setup is the Bennett 7200. Another example is the Hamilton Veolar (Fig 5–10). A high speed proportional servo valve controlled by a microprocessor uses an electrodynamic motor (like a music speaker) to move a piston up and down. The piston is connected to a potentiometer and a small plunger or cylinder. A current is sent to the electrodynamic motor which raises and lowers the plunger, allowing flow to the patient.

Stepper Motor with Valve.—A motor controls a lever arm on a hinged clamp device like a scissor valve. The stepper motor moves in rapid discrete steps to open or close the valve. It is electronically operated. This valve controls the flow of gas to the patient. Examples of ventilators with this type of valve are the Servo 900, the Bird 6400, and the BEAR 5 (Fig 5–11).

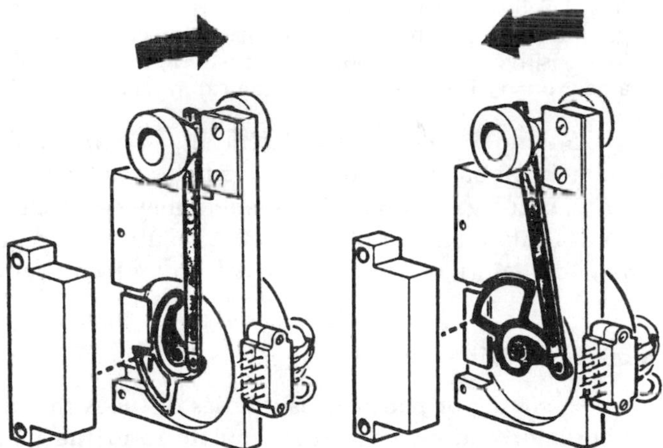

FIG 5–11.
Stepper motor and scissor valve on the Siemens Servo 900C. On the motor is a cam that controls the moving arm. On the left the valve is shown in the closed position. On the right the valve is completely open. (Courtesy of Siemens Life Support Systems, Schaumburg, Ill.)

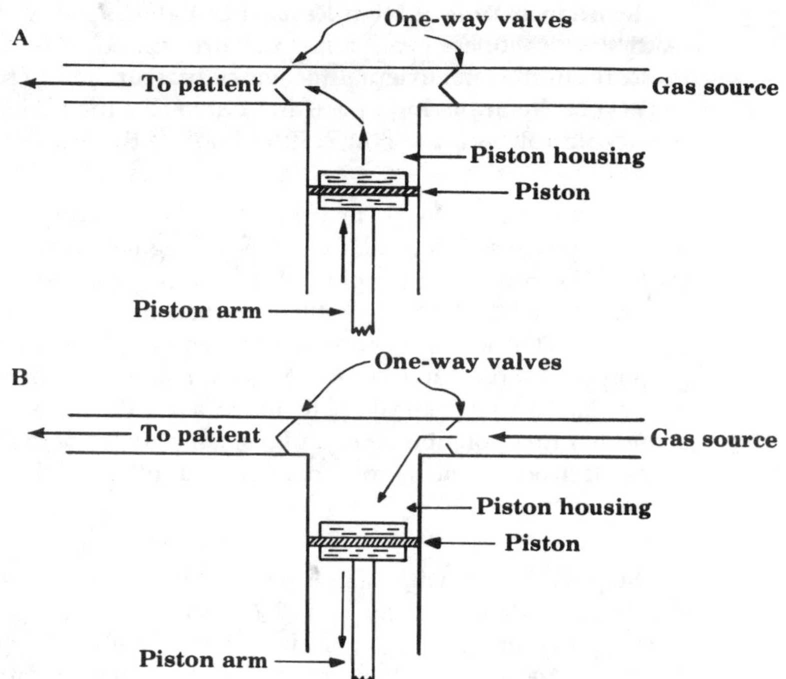

FIG 5–12.
Single-circuit ventilator. Gas goes directly from the power source to the patient, as seen in this simplified version of the IMV Emerson. **A,** the piston moves up and compresses the gas inside the piston housing. This gas is forced under pressure to the patient. This results in a positive pressure inspiratory breath. **B,** the piston moves down and draws gas from a gas source. This occurs during the expiratory phase.

Solenoid Valve.—An electrically generated magnetic force controls this valve in an on/off manner and regulates the amount of flow from a blended and pressurized gas source. The solenoid may be an electronic interface valve (Infrasonics Infant Star), a plunger (BEAR Cub), or a pinch valve (Bunnell Life Pulse Jet Ventilator), or the Ohmeda Advent, which uses an electrovalve.

Pneumatic Circuit

A circuit, or pathway, is a series of tubes that allows gas to flow inside the ventilator and between the ventilator and the patient. The pressure gradient achieved by the ventilator through its power source generates the airflow that passes through the circuits en route through the machine and to the patient. The gas is first directed from the generating source inside the ventilator through the internal circuits or tubes to its outside surface. Gas then flows through an external circuit or patient circuit to the patient. It then exits from the patient and passes through an exhalation limb, and thence through the exhalation valve.

Internal Circuit.—If the internal circuit allows the gas to go directly from its power source into the patient, it is called a *single-circuit* ventilator. The source of the gas can either be externally compressed gas, as in the Bird Mark 7, or the internal pressurizing source such as a piston (Emerson 3-MV). With the Emerson ventilator, room air or oxygen is drawn into a piston cylinder during its downstroke and is then pushed into the patient's airway or the upstroke (Fig 5–12).

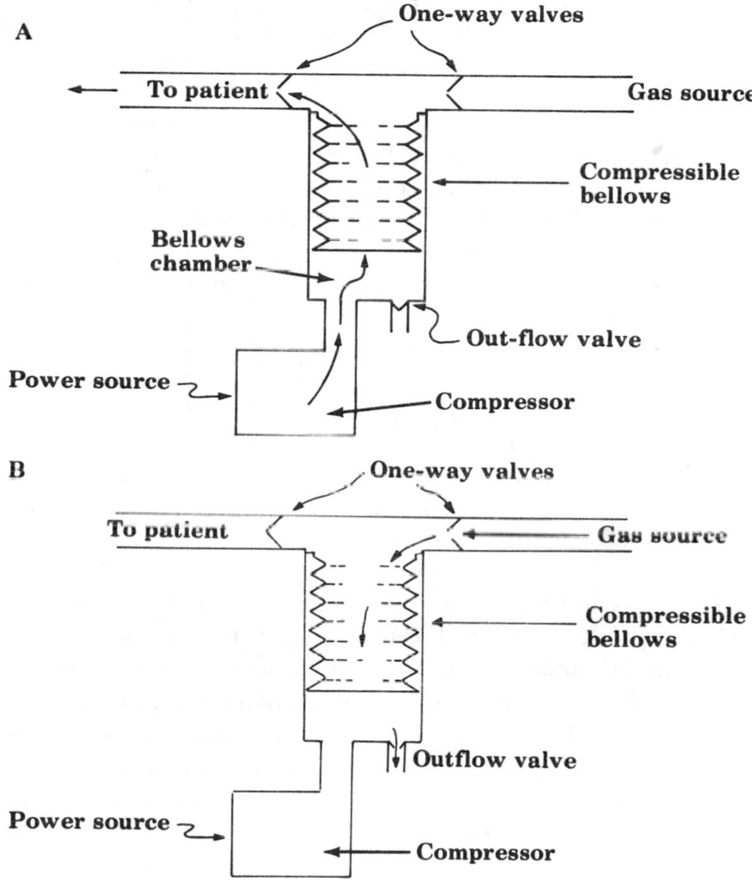

FIG 5–13.
In this double-circuit ventilator, gas that goes to the patient is not in direct contact with the power source, as seen in this schematic representation of the Puritan Bennett MA-1 in its simplest form. **A,** the compressor produces a high pressure gas source which is directed to a chamber. The chamber holds a collapsible bellows and the bellows contains the desired gas mixture which will go to the patient. The pressure in the chamber forces the bellows upward resulting in a positive pressure breath. **B,** After the inspiratory breath is delivered, the compressor no longer sends pressure to the chamber and exhalation occurs. The bellows drops to its original position and fills with the desired delivery gas in preparation for the next breath.

A second type of internal circuit is the *double circuit*. The primary power source generates a gas flow that compresses another mechanism. This creates a second gas flow that goes to the patient. An example is the MA-1. In this unit, ventilator gas is compressed into a chamber containing a bellows. This then compresses the bellows. The air that was in the bellows then flows to the patient (Fig 5–13).

External Circuit.—The external circuit or patient circuit concerns the positive pressure ventilator to the patient's artificial airway. The patient circuit requires several basic elements in order to provide a positive pressure breath. (Fig 5–14,A):

a. A main inspiratory line connecting the ventilator output to the patient's airway adaptor or connector.
b. An adaptor to fit this tube to the patient's airway. This is also called a patient connector or wye adaptor because of its shape.
c. An expiratory line to carry expired gas away from the patient and to the exhalation valve.
d. An expiratory valve to conduct the patient's exhaled gas from the expiratory line to the room. During inspiration this valve closes so that gas can only go to the patient's lungs. Sometimes this valve is mounted directly on the ventilator and at other times it is part of a manifold.
e. An expiratory valve line to power the expiratory valve. Sometimes this is mounted internally in the ventilator below or behind the exhalation valve and cannot be seen.

When a ventilator begins the inspiratory phase, gas flows through the main inspiratory tube to the patient. Gas also flows into the expiratory valve line to the exhalation valve. This closes the exhalation valve during inspiration (see Fig 5–14,A). In newer-generation ventilators the exhalation valve may be controlled by a mechanical device rather than a positive pressure flow of gas. This device is then mounted internally and its function is not normally visible (Fig 5–14,B). During exhalation the flow from the ventilator stops. The exhalation valve opens. Air no longer enters the patient's lungs. The patient is able to passively exhale through the expiratory port. In addition to these essential parts, additional items are added to the circuit when a patient is being mechanically ventilated to optimize gas delivery and ventilator function (Fig 5–14,C). Minimally, these include:

1. Device to warm and humidify inspired air.
2. Thermometer to measure inspired air temperatures.
3. Apnea or low pressure alarm to indicate when a leak is present or that the patient is not ventilating adequately.

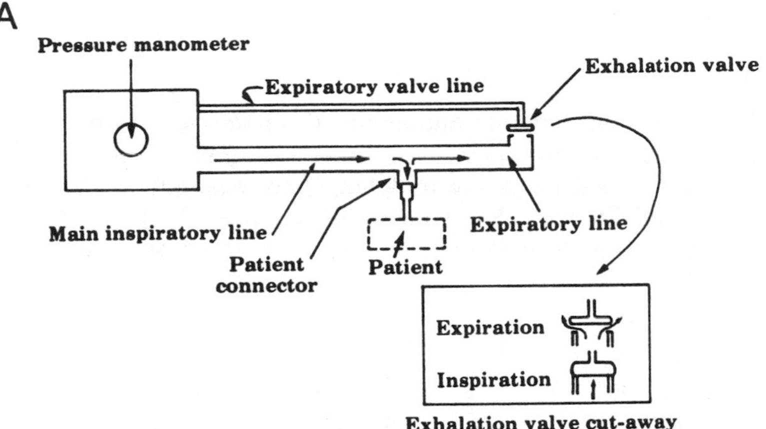

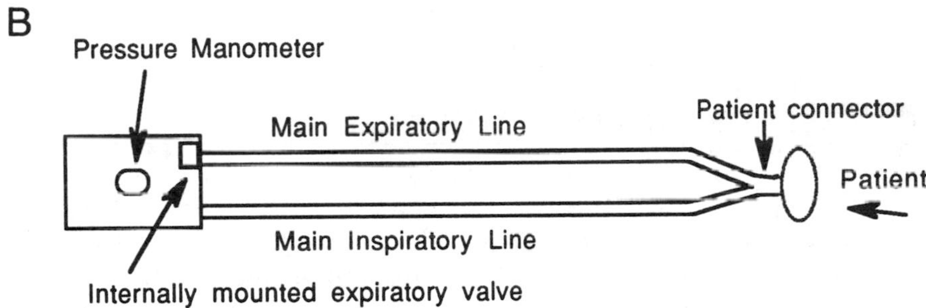

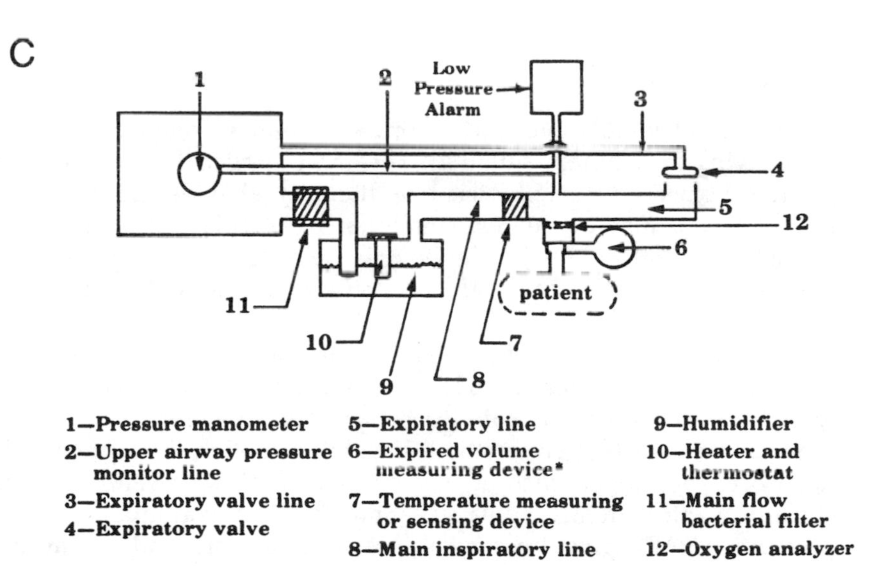

FIG 5–14.
Basics of a patient circuit. **A**, the basic components of a patient circuit required to provide a positive pressure breath. The exhalation valve is mounted externally. **B**, an internally mounted exhalation valve. The expiratory valve line is not visible. It is inside the ventilator. **C**, a patient circuit containing additional components which are required for optimal functioning during continuous mechanical ventilation.

4. Nebulizer line to power a micronebulizer for delivery of aerosolized medications.
5. Volume-measuring device to determine the patient's exhaled volume.
6. Bacterial filters to filter gas going to the patient.
7. Pressure gauge to measure pressures at the upper airway. This is usually built into the ventilator.

Additional monitoring devices might include: oxygen analyzers, pulse oximeters, capnographs (end-tidal CO_2 monitors), and flow and pressure sensors to monitor patient lung compliance and airway resistance and display the information graphically.

THE FOUR PHASES OF THE RESPIRATORY CYCLE

The physical and mechanical operation of any ventilator relies on its ability to accomplish all of the parts of the normal cycle of ventilation. These include the mechanisms which (1) begin inspiration (end-expiration), (2) control the inspiratory phase, (3) begin exhalation (end-inspiration), and (4) control the expiratory phase.

Modes of Ventilation

Modes of ventilation are a shorthand used to describe how a ventilator is behaving in a certain situation. The term applied to a mode of ventilation is often coined by the physician or therapist that developed that particular mode. A *mode* may be defined simply as a particular set of control and phase variables.[7] In other words, we describe a mode by the pressure, flow, and volume patterns that occur over time when that method of ventilation is used on a patient.

Historically, methods of initiating inspiration were often referred to as modes. The most common modes that triggered the ventilator into inspiration were time triggering (the *control mode*), pressure triggering (the *assist mode*), and time or pressure triggering (the *assist-control* mode). Since then, other modes have been developed such as intermittent mandatory ventilation (IMV), synchronized intermittent ventilation (SIMV), PEEP, continuous positive airway pressure (CPAP), pressure control, pressure support, and airway pressure release ventilation.

In this section the different and most common methods (modes) of ventilation and their general uses are described. We begin with the four mechanisms that make up a total breath.

BEGINNING OF INSPIRATION: THE TRIGGERING MECHANISM

The mechanism which begins inspiration and marks the end of expiration is the triggering mechanism. The ventilator may be triggered by pressure, flow, time, and volume, although in reality the volume variable is seldom used.

Controlled Ventilation (Time Triggering)

One of the first triggering mechanisms used on mechanical ventilators was time-triggered, or controlled ventilation. This refers to ventilation provided either by machine or resuscitator bag. The rate of breathing is controlled by the ventilator operator. In this mode of ventilation a patient cannot obtain fresh air or get a breath from the machine by making an inspiratory effort. Thus, the term *control mode.* Controlled ventilation is *time*-triggered. After a certain time interval has passed the ventilator cycles into inspiration. The control knob for this is commonly a rate control knob. For example, if the rate is set at 12 breaths/min, a breath will occur every 5 seconds (60 sec/min divided by 12 breaths/min = 5 seconds). The internal timing device on the ventilator triggers inspiration after 5 seconds has elapsed.

Early ventilators, such as the first Emerson Post-Op had only the control mode and made no provision for the patient's own efforts to breathe. The machine automatically controlled breathing (Fig 5–15). Controlled ventilation is recommended for patients with apnea or who are paralyzed.

Assisted Ventilation (Pressure Triggering)

Recognizing that some patients might attempt spontaneous breathing during mechanical ventilation, machines were developed that could sense changes in pressure at the upper airway when the patient attempted to inspire. When the negative pressure is detected, the machine is then triggered and it delivers a

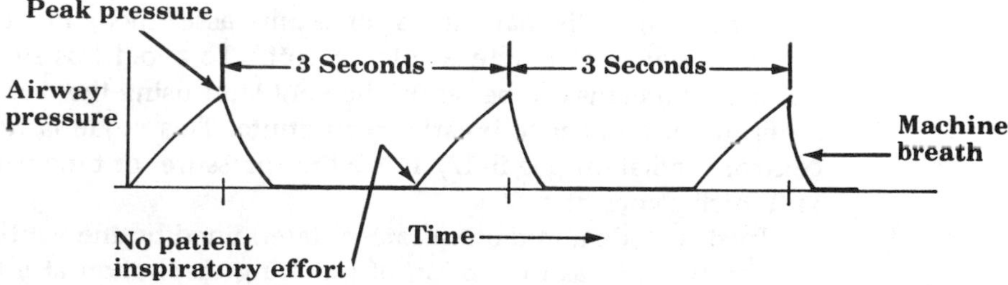

FIG 5–15.
Controlled ventilation pressure curve. Patient effort will not trigger a mechanical breath. Inspiration occurs at equal timed intervals.

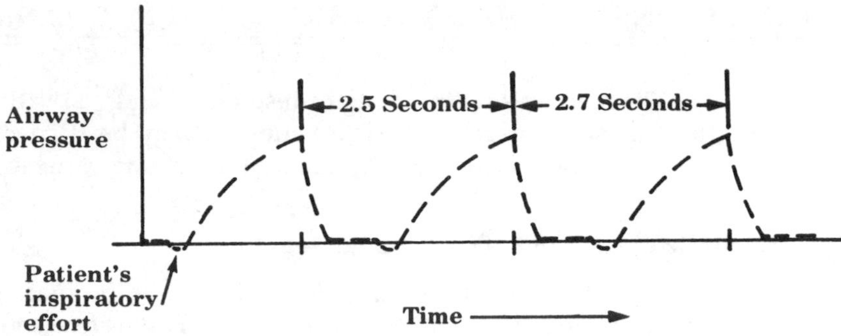

FIG 5–16.
Assist pressure curve. Patient effort (negative pressure deflection from baseline) occurs before each positive pressure machine breath. Breaths may not occur at equal timed intervals.

positive pressure breath known as an assisted breath. Thus the machine is *pressure*-triggered. This type of ventilator pattern is called *assisted ventilation* (Fig 5–16). The operator must set the sensitivity setting, which is also called the "patient effort" or "patient triggering" device. This sensitivity determines how much of a pressure change must be detected before the ventilator is triggered. Less pressure means the machine is more sensitive. The assist and SIMV (see below) modes of ventilation are pressure-triggered into inspiration.

The same type of ventilation can be done by someone manually ventilating a patient with a resuscitation bag. When you sense the patient breathing in, you can give a positive pressure breath. In assist ventilation, the patient initiates the breath and establishes the respiratory rate.

Assist-Control Ventilation

Clinicians have learned that even though some patients begin to breathe spontaneously and the assist mode can be used, occasionally the patient will stop breathing. If the patient was on a pure assist mode he or she would receive no breaths at all. The rate would be "off." To avoid this situation, a minimum number of breaths can be set on the ventilator using the rate knob to guarantee a minimum number of breaths per minute. This mode is referred to as assist-control ventilation (Fig 5–17). It is either pressure- or time-triggered, depending on which comes first.

In this mode a minimum rate is determined by the ventilator control knob, but the patient has the option of initiating inspiration at a faster rate. For the mode to work correctly, the ventilator operator must always be sure that the ventilator is "sensitive" to the patient's efforts.

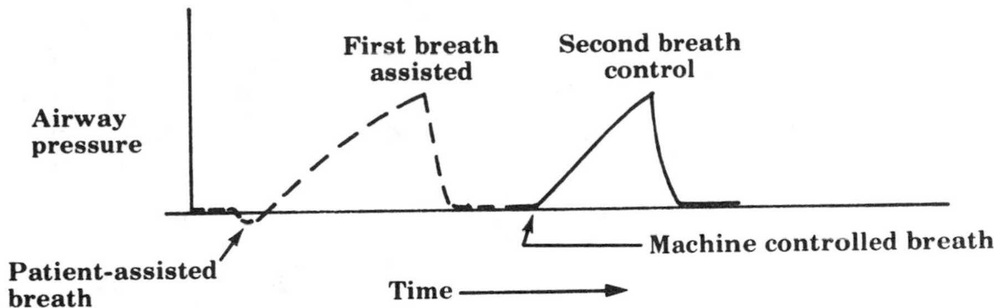

FIG 5–17.
Assist-control pressure curve. An assisted breath shows negative deflection of pressure before inspiration while a controlled breath does not.

Flow Triggering

If a ventilator is capable of measuring the inspiratory flow effort from a patient and of then triggering flow delivery, it is said to be *flow-triggered*. At the present time only a few ventilators use flow triggering—the Puritan Bennett 7200a, originally in the flow-by mode only, and the Servo 300 when set for flow sensitivity. The Puritan Bennett 7200ae is currently being programmed and may offer flow triggering in other modes in the near future.

When the ventilator detects a certain drop in the gas flow due to patient inspiration, it will increase the gas flow through the circuit. Whether it augments flow or actually provides a pressure-limited or volume-limited breath depends on the ventilator and the mode in use.

Intermittent Positive Pressure Breathing (IPPB)

During controlled ventilation, since a positive pressure breath is delivered intermittently, this type of ventilation is referred to as intermittent positive pressure breathing (IPPB) or ventilation (IPPV). The early development of mechanical ventilation in the 1950s was accompanied by the adaptation of small, portable IPPB devices that were used to deliver aerosolized medications. As a result, the term IPPB in modern usage implies an aerosol treatment. IPPV implies the mechanical support of breathing in the nonbreathing patient on a continuous basis.

Alternative Methods (Modes) of Ventilation

Intermittent Mandatory Ventilation (IMV).—In IMV periodic flow- or volume-limited mechanical breaths occur at preset time intervals. The operator sets the IMV rate and V_T and flow for the machine breath. The ventilator is time-triggered. Flow and volume are limited to the amount for which they are

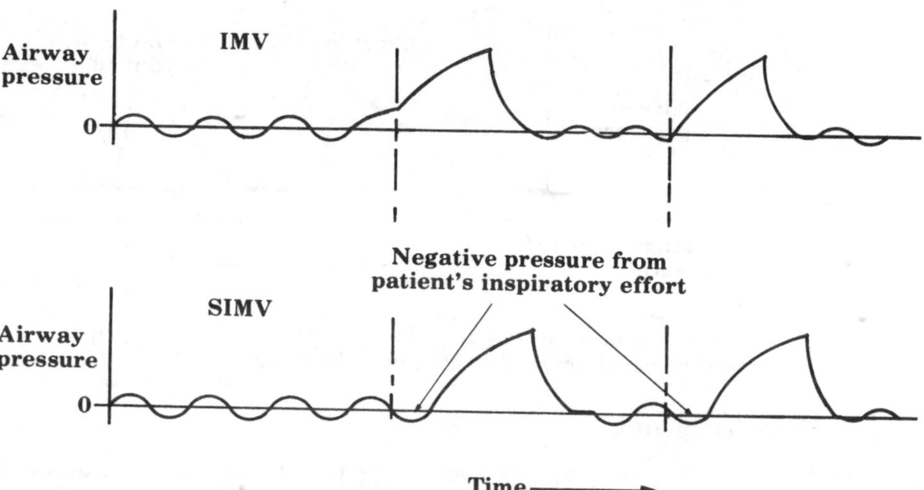

FIG 5–18.
Difference between intermittent *(IMV)* and synchronized intermittent ventilation *(SIMV)*. Spontaneous breathing in both modes is usually at ambient pressures. Machine breaths in the IMV mode are an equal distance apart. During SIMV, machine breaths are not necessarily an equal distance apart. An inspiratory effort (negative deflection) usually occurs before each SIMV breath.

set. Between the machine breaths, patients breathe spontaneously at any desired volume level. The spontaneous baseline is usually at ambient pressures (zero gauge pressure) (Fig 5–18). Gas flow through the circuit can be continuous so that spontaneous breaths are unassisted. If the ventilator has a demand valve, then spontaneous breaths are actively supported.[7]

This mode of ventilation was initially used for ventilation of infants to help alleviate the problems associated with trying to synchronize mechanical breaths in the assist-control mode with the rapid respiratory rates of infants. IMV helps reduce the effects of positive pressure ventilation by reducing the amount of time that positive pressure is applied to the pulmonary system. It also allows the patient to maintain a reasonable spontaneous breathing pattern and can be used as a method of weaning patients from mechanical ventilation.

IMV can also be adjusted so that when the patient breathes spontaneously, the pressures at the mouth are above zero, i.e., the baseline is positive. The mode is then called IMV with PEEP or CPAP. IMV is also available on some ventilators with pressure support for spontaneous breaths. The ventilator then performs as a time-triggered, flow- or volume-limited ventilator for machine breaths and a pressure-triggered, pressure-limited machine for spontaneous breaths. More about these methods of ventilation later in this chapter.

Newer microprocessor ventilators are able to provide IMV breaths that are pressure-limited rather than flow- or volume-limited. The machine breaths will be what are called "pressure-control" breaths.

Synchronized Intermittent Mandatory Ventilation (SIMV).—Successful use of IMV resulted in the development of SIMV. In this mode the patient is allowed to breath spontaneously through the ventilator circuit. At a predetermined timed interval set by the operator, the ventilator waits for the next inspiratory effort from the patient. Sensing the effort the ventilator assists the breath by synchronously delivering a positive pressure machine breath (see Fig 5–18). The operator usually sets the rate, V_T, flow, and sensitivity for the SIMV breath. The mode is pressure-triggered and flow- or volume-limited. Machine breaths are set up on a timing mechanism. Once the positive machine breath is delivered, the ventilator is once again insensitive to patient airway pressure changes until the next preset timed interval comes about and the patient again triggers a machine breath. If the patient fails to initiate ventilation in the set time frame, the ventilator will usually give a breath.

SIMV was originally designed to eliminate the problem which could occur with IMV. With IMV, if a machine-timed positive pressure breath accidently occurred at the time the patient spontaneously inhaled, the lungs received huge volumes of air. This was referred to as "breath stacking" and was a concern as it could cause barotrauma or rupture of lung tissue. However, this problem can be avoided with IMV simply by setting a peak pressure limit to prevent excessive build-up of pressure at the airway. Thus, large volumes, once they reach the pressure limit, are vented into the air, or the machine simply ends inspiration.

With SIMV, if the patient fails to make an inspiratory effort during the timed interval in which the ventilator is sensitive to the patient's inspiratory effort, the ventilator cycles. When and how this occurs depends on the particular ventilator being used. This can prevent the problem of lack of ventilation if the patient becomes totally apneic. SIMV is occasionally referred to as intermittent demand ventilation (IDV) or intermittent assisted ventilation (IAV) or augmented ventilation.

As with IMV, SIMV can be used with a positive baseline pressure or with pressure support for spontaneous breaths (Fig 5–19). Microprocessor ventilators like the Servo 300 can also provide SIMV breaths using a preset pressure (pressure control breath; see below). Here a preset pressure is given to the patient for the SIMV breath rather than a preselected V_T. This is an SIMV breath which is pressure-triggered and pressure-limited.

Pressure Support.—Pressure support is a special form of assisted (pressure-triggered), pressure-limited ventilation. The ventilator provides a constant pressure of air once it senses that the patient has made an inspiratory effort (see Fig 5–19). The pressure reached during inspiration is set by the operator. Inspiration usually stops when a predetermined flow level is achieved. How much volume the patient receives for the preset pressure is entirely dependent on lung characteristics (airway resistance and lung compliance) and the inspiratory effort of the patient. The more actively the patient inspires, the more of a pressure

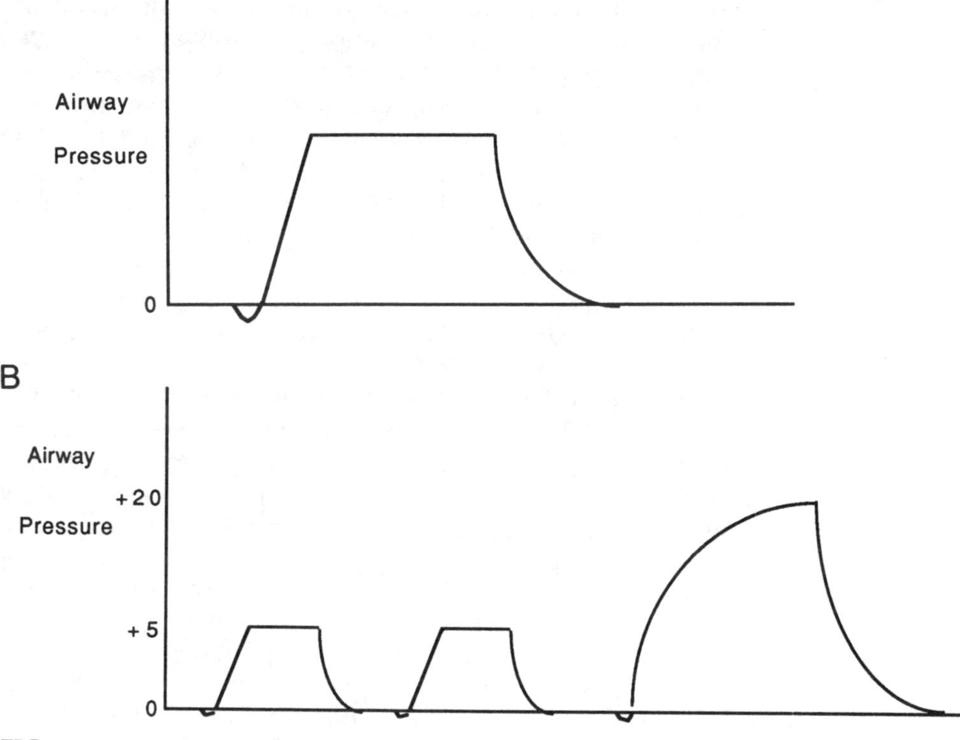

FIG 5–19.
A, pressure support breath--pressure triggered, pressure limited. **B,** SIMV with pressure support.

gradient is created between the mouth, alveolar level, and the intrapleural space. Greater patient effort will result in greater volume delivery.

This mode of ventilation is often used with another form of ventilation, such as IMV, to provide assistance to spontaneous breaths. This helps reduce the work of breathing that results from trying to breathe through the ventilator circuit, demand valve, and endotracheal tube.

Pressure Control.—Pressure control is a mode of ventilation that began to gain popularity in the late 1980s. In this type of ventilation the patient may be paralyzed and sedated and the ventilator is time-triggered and pressure-limited. The patient may also be breathing spontaneously on some ventilators and these breaths are pressure-triggered. Tidal volume is based on the compliance and resistance of the patient's lungs and the spontaneous breathing effort if the patient is breathing spontaneously.

The ventilator provides a constant pressure of air to the patient during inspiration (Fig 5–20,A). The length of inspiration and the pressure level are set by the operator, as is the rate of ventilation. During the early use of this mode the inspiratory time was often increased to longer than the expiratory time, which is not physiologically normal. However, under some conditions the longer inspiratory time provided better oxygenation. Because of the longer inspiratory time, this mode is sometimes called pressure control inverse ratio ventilation (PCIRV). The patient is often unable to fully exhale and this results in gas trapping or auto-PEEP. Its early use was restricted to patients with very stiff lungs who were not successfully ventilated by conventional methods.

Other uses of pressure control will become available as clinical studies prove the usefulness of this ventilator mode. For example, it can be used as an alternative mode of ventilation. Volume-limited or controlled ventilation has been used for many years to ventilate patients. However, in some types of patients it may not be the best choice. Further clinical trials are needed to ascertain other uses of pressure control. One option is SIMV with pressure control. The mandatory breath provides a constant pressure at the upper airway (Fig 5–20,B).

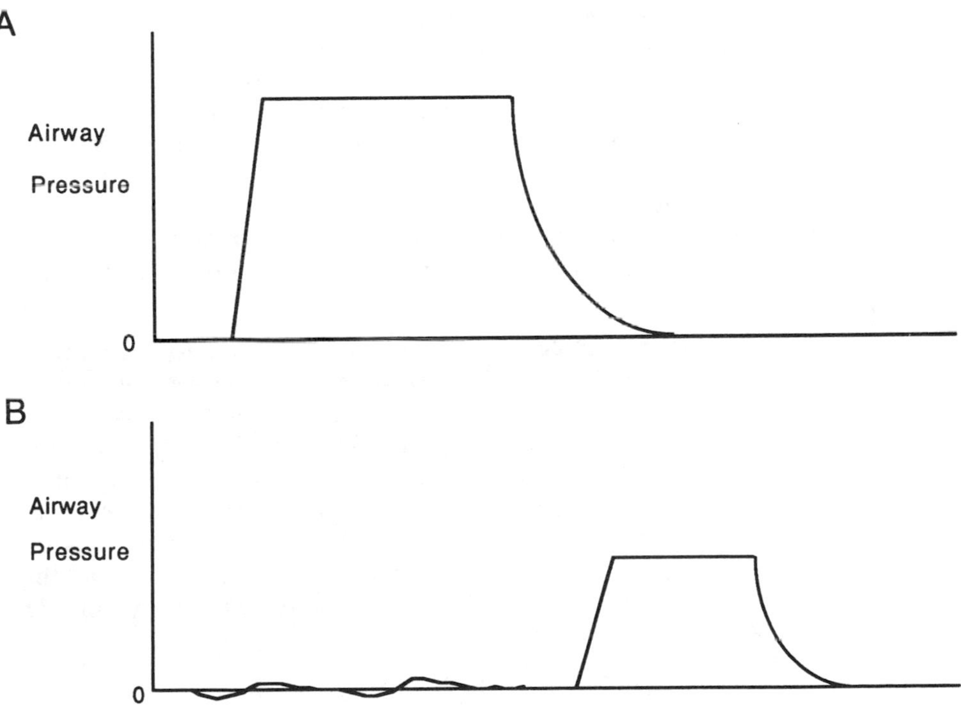

FIG 5–20.
A, pressure-control or pressure-limited breath that provides a constant pressure at the upper airway during inspiration. Flow is a descending ramp. **B,** pressure control with SIMV where the machine breaths are pressure-limited and the spontaneous breaths are unassisted.

Mandatory Minute Ventilation (MMV).—During the 1970s a method of ventilation was designed for weaning or discontinuing of ventilation. It was called *minimum* or *mandatory minute ventilation* (MMV). An operator set a minimum minute ventilation ($\dot{V}_E$). The ventilator monitored the patient's breathing. If the desired $\dot{V}_E$ was not delivered, the ventilator would provide positive pressure machine breaths with preset volumes. However, if the patient began to do a lot of breathing without ventilator assistance, the ventilator reduced the amount of support it provided. If the patient met the preset $\dot{V}_E$ setting, the ventilator would remain passive.

Unfortunately, sometimes patients would begin to breathe at a rapid rate with very shallow breaths. This pattern increases dead space ventilation without effectively increasing alveolar ventilation. However, the ventilator only reads the total volume in 1 minute regardless of how the patient accomplishes it. The result is a worn-out patient. The upshot: the method did not sell.

Since that time, however, newer monitoring techniques, alarms, and a more sophisticated computer ventilation control have eliminated that problem. Operators can now set high and low respiratory rate alarms and high and low V_T alarms. The mode is again being used.

MMV is also called extended mandatory minute ventilation, minimum minute ventilation, or augmented minute ventilation. It is similar to SIMV except that the mandatory breaths are not delivered if the patient is able to maintain the $\dot{V}_E$ spontaneously. MMV is used as a method of weaning patients from ventilatory support. The way it operates depends on the type or brand of ventilator being used. Some ventilators operate by delivering additional V_T volumes. Others increase the pressure support level on the spontaneous breaths.

Inflation Hold.—Inflation hold is designed to maintain air in the lungs at the end of inspiration. This helps to increase the peripheral distribution of gas and improve oxygenation. Inflation hold allows a positive pressure inspiratory breath to be delivered by the ventilator. Then, at the end of inspiration, the expiratory valve is blocked and the air stays in the patient's lungs for a fraction of a second (pause time). The pressure on the manometer will be seen to build to a peak during inspiration. Then it levels. The pressure reading during this phase is called plateau pressure. This technique of breath-holding is referred to as inspiratory pause, end-inspiratory pause, inspiratory hold, or inflation hold (Fig 5–21).

High-Frequency Ventilation.—A unique mode of providing mechanical ventilation to patients is high-frequency ventilation (HFV). This technique was reported in the late 1960s and has been given a significant amount of attention since. Workers in Scandinavia, Europe, and Canada have used it to maintain ventilation during surgical procedures, for infants, and in special adult cases. Its use in the United States has been largely restricted to infants with respiratory distress in whom standard modes of ventilation are not successful.

High-frequency ventilation is defined as the delivery of small VT values at high ventilation rates. HFV actually has about three categories. High-frequency positive pressure ventilation describes ventilating rates up to approximately 100 breaths /min. High-frequency jet ventilation (HFJV) is mainly distinguished by the fact that it is delivered by a small-bore catheter or injector. Tidal volumes are smaller than normal. Respiratory rates range from 100 to 500 to 600 breaths/min.

High-frequency oscillation has rates up to 4,000 breaths/min. These rapid oscillations are often superimposed on the patient's spontaneous breathing pattern. If the respiratory muscles are paralyzed, the ventilator forces gas both in and out of the lungs. This creates a positive gas flow on inspiration and a negative gas flow on expiration. Some research has been done to see if this can be used not only as a mode of ventilation but as a way to internally percuss the chest and improve removal of secretions.

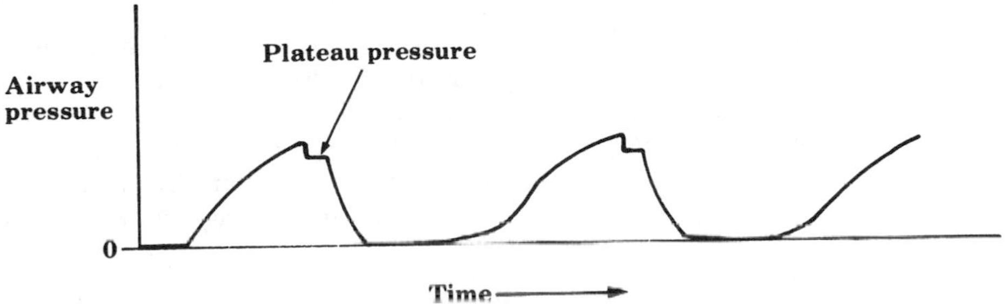

FIG 5–21.
Intermittent positive pressure ventilation *(IPPV)* with inflation hold or end-inspiratory pause leading to a pressure plateau, i.e., plateau pressure.

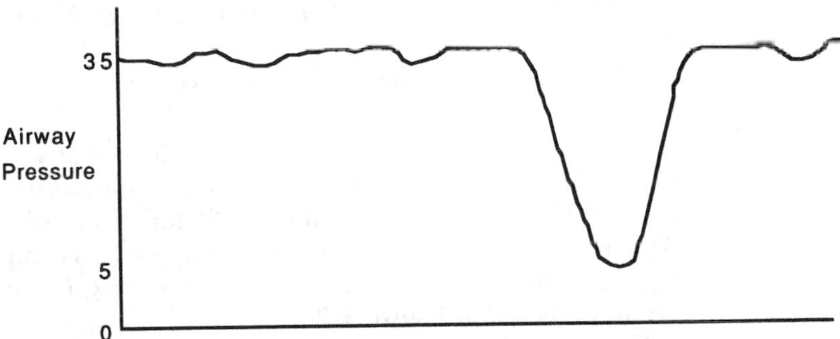

FIG 5–22.
Airway pressure release ventilation allows a patient to breathe spontaneously at a positive baseline pressure. Intermittently, at time-triggered intervals, the baseline drops to another preselected value. After a brief timed interval the original baseline is resumed.

Airway Pressure Release Ventilation.—Airway pressure release ventilation (APRV) was designed by Drs. Christine Stock and John B. Downs in 1987. It is basically a form of spontaneous breathing at a positive baseline pressure (CPAP). Periodically this baseline pressure is released to a lower pressure level (Fig 5–22). At this point the lungs are allowed to deflate passively. The length of the release time is generally no longer than 1 to 2 seconds at most. This mode is similar to pressure-controlled ventilation with an inverse inspiratory-expiratory (I/E) ratio. The primary difference is that pressure-controlled inverse ratio ventilation in its early trials was primarily used as a controlled mode of ventilation. APRV may be an alternative mode to help improve oxygenation with lower mean airway pressures.

THE INSPIRATORY PHASE

Model of Ventilation in the Lung During Inspiration

During either spontaneous breathing or mechanical ventilation, two forces (pressures) act on the respiratory system. The forces, due either to muscle action or ventilator action, are called *muscle pressure* and *ventilator pressure.* These forces result in motion, described as flow, to give an end product, volume delivery. The resulting volume delivery depends on the compliance of the lungs (elastic recoil pressure) and the resistance to gas flow during volume delivery (flow resistance pressure). The forces and resulting motion are described below:

Muscle pressure + ventilator pressure =
elastic recoil pressure + flow resistance pressure

This simplified equation, known as the "equation of motion of the respiratory system," has been derived by Chatburn[5, 6] and can be expressed as follows:

$$\text{Pmus} + \text{P}_{\text{TR}} = \text{V/C} + \text{R} \times \text{flow}$$

Pmus is the pressure generated by the muscles of ventilation. If they are not active, this is equal to zero. P_{TR} is the transrespiratory pressure (Pawo − Pbs), basically the pressure read on the ventilator gauge during inspiration during IPPV. V is volume-delivered. C is respiratory system compliance, R is respiratory system resistance, and flow is the gas flow during inspiration. A model of this equation is shown in Figure 5–23.

The reason for showing this equation is to show how really simple the concept of ventilation is. Only two forces can provide ventilation: the patient's muscles or the ventilator. If the patient is apneic or paralyzed, the ventilator provides all the work of breathing. The result of the work is represented by the

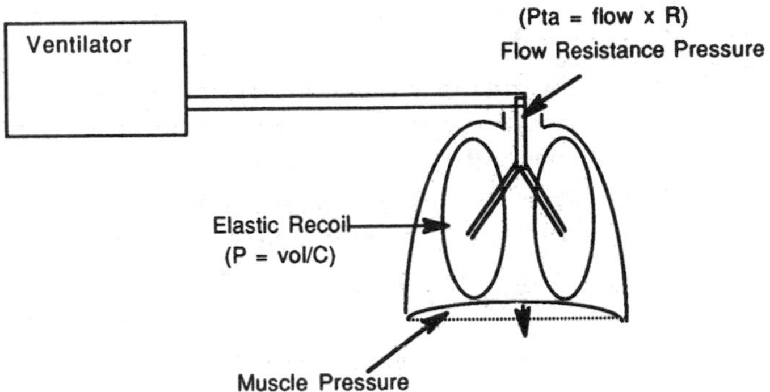

FIG 5–23.
Equation of motion model.

right side of the equation. These are pressure in the airway (P_{TA}) and alveolar pressure (P_A). Airway pressure results from the resistance to flow of gases through the conductive airways: Resistance = P_{TA}/flow. Alveolar pressures result from the elastic recoil of the lung tissues: C = volume delivered/P_A. During inspiration compliance and resistance stay fairly constant for any one breath. What changes during inspiration are pressure, volume, and flow. These three parameters, or variables, *can* change. They are controlled by the ventilator during inspiration. Only one of these three variables plus time can be controlled by the ventilator for any single breath. Knowing this makes it easy to classify how a ventilator functions during inspiration.

The Ventilator Output

The inspiratory delivery of gas is perhaps the most important single characteristic of a ventilator. In positive pressure ventilation, the function of the ventilator during inspiration is to force air into the patient's lungs. Inspiration is generated by the drive mechanism of the ventilator. How it is delivered and how flow, volume, and pressure are controlled are determined by the drive mechanism and the output control valve. The ability of a ventilator to maintain a flow, volume, or pressure pattern during inspiration depends on one or both of these mechanical devices.

One of the things that has complicated how ventilators are classified during inspiration has been the use of such terms as high pressure generators and low pressure generators. Another problem that has arisen is that the function of a ventilator can change if pressures at the mouth change dramatically. In addition, the development of the newer microprocessor-controlled ventilators has made it possible for the person using the ventilator to precisely control how the ventilator operates. To keep classification simple, some basic points can be kept in mind:

1. Ventilator operation during inspiration is divided into four types: pressure controllers (pressure generators), flow controllers (flow generators), volume controllers, and time controllers.
2. A pressure controller keeps the same pattern of pressure at the mouth regardless of changes in patient lung conditions. This pattern can be constant or nonconstant. The pressure source (driving pressure) is usually less than five times the pressures reached at the airway opening (about 100–300 cm H_2O).

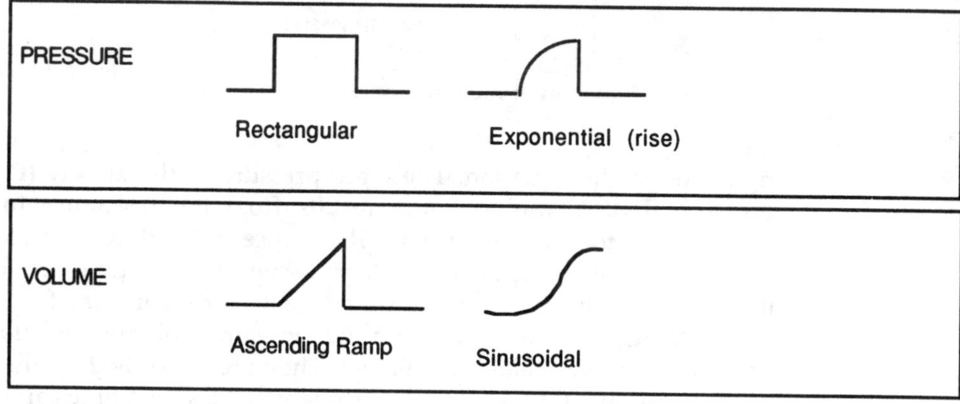

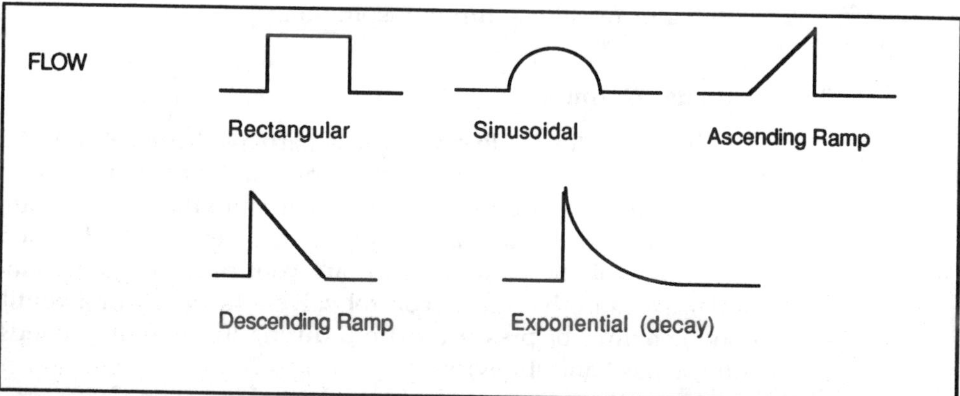

FIG 5–24.
Examples of curves for pressure, volume, and flow. Pressure curves are usually rectangular or rising exponential. Volume curves are usually ramp or sinusoidal. Flow ramps can take on any variety of forms. The most common are rectangular, ramp, sinusoidal, and decaying exponential.

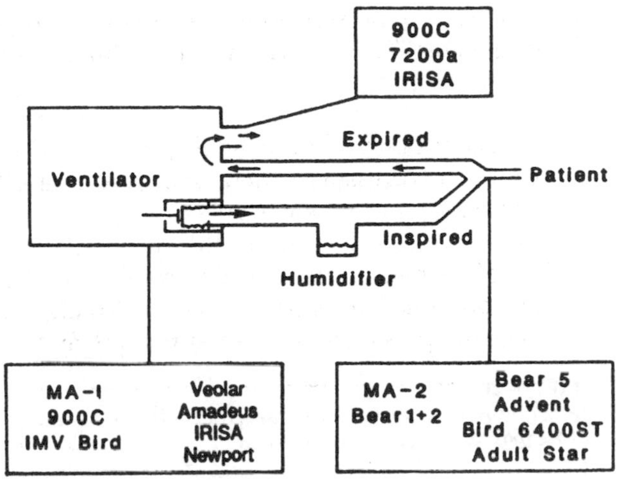

FIG 5–25.
Pressure monitoring sites of old and new ventilators. The Irisa ventilator uses measurements of pressure from inspired and expired sides in an effort to calculate proximal airway pressure. (From Branson RD: *Respir Care* 1991;36:365. Used by permission.)

3. A flow controller keeps the same pattern of flow at the mouth regardless of changes in patient lung conditions. This pattern can be constant or nonconstant. The pressure source (driving pressure) is usually more than five times the pressures reached at the airway opening (about 300–3,500 cm H_2O).
4. The flow, volume, or pressure waveform produced at the mouth is usually one of four shapes[7] (Fig 5–24).
   a. Rectangular, also called square or constants.
   b. Exponential, also called accelerating or increasing.
   c. Sinusoidal, also called sine wave.
   d. Ramp, available as accelerating or descending ramp.

The airway pressure patterns or graphs such as those included in this section actually describe what a person would see if he or she watched the ventilator pressure manometer as it was delivering air to the patient. The manometer measures pressure at either the upper or proximal airway where the patient is connected to the ventilator, or internally. Figure 5–25 shows where pressure sensors are usually located. The pressure is the sum of the elastic and resistance properties of the lungs and thorax.

The flow pattern measured at the mouth or exhalation valve can be seen on some ventilators (Fig 5–26). Newer microprocessor-controlled ventilators have the ability to display the parameters they monitor on a screen. Some, like the BEAR 5, come with a built-in screen. Others, like the Hamilton Veolar, can

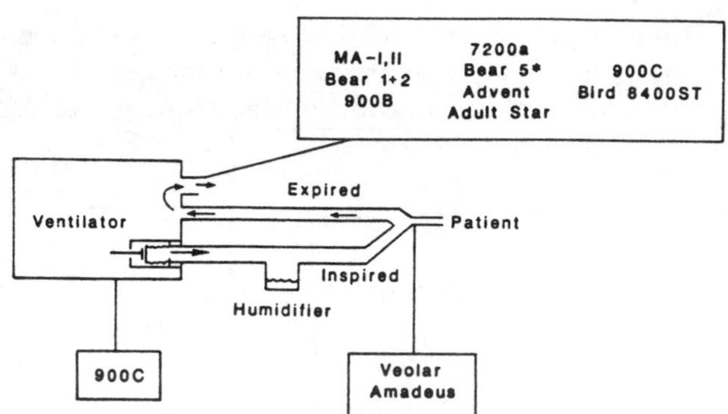

FIG 5–26.
Placement of flow-volume transducers in old and new ventilators. (From Branson RD: *Respir Care* 1991;36:367. Used by permission.)

be connected to a monitor. These give not only flow patterns but pressure and volume as well. This information can help with the classification of the ventilator.

Ventilator Classification During Inspiration

This section deals with the classification of ventilations during inspiration. It includes volume controllers, flow controllers, and pressure controllers. Volume controllers or limiters are few in number and only a few are covered here. Other ventilators are classified as flow controllers or pressure controllers. These are subdivided into two groups: constant and nonconstant.

Volume Controllers.—Remember that flow is actually volume per unit of time (flow = V_T/inspiratory time). If changes in compliance and resistance do not change volume, they will not change the flow pattern. The distinctive feature of a volume controller is that it measures the volume it delivers. Volume change can be measured by the displacement of a piston or bellows. Ventilators that (1) keep a constant volume change in the face of changing lung mechanics and (2) use a piston or bellows or similar device for volume delivery, and (3) measure the displacement of that device are volume controllers. An examle is the MA-1. Ventilators that measure flow and display volume are *not* volume controllers. Examples are the Servo 900C, Servo 300, Puritan Bennett 7200a, BEAR 5, Ohmeda Advent, and Hamilton Veolar.

Flow Controllers.—With the flow controller, the ventilator controls the flow of gas going to the patient. The flow pattern that it produces does not vary and is not affected by changes in the patient's lung characteristics. The *pressure* pattern *will* vary with changes in compliance and resistance. Volume is not measured. The two categories of flow generators or flow controllers are constant flow generators and nonconstant flow generators. The characteristics of a constant flow controller are:

1. It delivers a constant gas flow, also called a square wave or rectangular wave.
2. Regardless of changes in the patient's lung conditions, the flow stays constant.
3. The pressure measured during gas delivery varies with lung conditions.
4. The pressure due to airway resistance (flow resistance) is constant.
5. Pressures at the manometer and in the alveoli rise in a linear fashion throughout inspiration.
6. Volume is not measured although flow may be measured and displayed as volume.

This is one of the most common types of ventilation pattern used. Most ventilators in use today are capable of producing a rectangular flow pattern. In order to produce a constant gas flow that does not vary in the face of changing lung conditions, it must have a lot of power behind its gas delivery. Ventilators that have high internal or working pressure sources have this capability.

A ventilator that can generate pressures far in excess of what will be reached at the upper airway is what is needed for a rectangular flow delivery. For example, a ventilator that uses a 50-psig gas source offers far higher pressures than are needed to ventilate the human lung. A pressure of 50 psig is about 3,500 cm H_2O. Pressures generated at the mouth are in the range of 10 to 100 cm H_2O. So the gradient which generates flow is very high [3,500 cm H_2O – (10–100) cm H_2O]. Changes in lung compliance and airway resistance will not affect the flow rate because they cannot significantly affect the pressure gradient that causes the flow. If a ventilator can produce five times or more the amount of pressure seen at peak inspiration it is considered a constant flow ventilator. These machines are also described as constant flow controllers, constant flow generators, square flow generators, and rectangular flow ventilators.

In rectangular flow ventilators, inspiration is usually terminated by a preset time or volume which occurs well in advance of alveolar pressures reaching delivered pressure capabilities. The volume increases linearly with time owing to the constant flow rate, and inspiration is either time- or volume-cycled. Volume delivered by the ventilator during inspiration is constant.

With a constant gas flow, pressure at the mouth rises linearly, as does pressure in the alveoli. Pressure going to the conductive airways remains constant, owing to the constant flow of gas. During any one breath the airway resistance and gas properties are fairly stable. The pressure, volume, and flow curves produced during mechanical ventilation were reviewed in Chapter 2.

Figure 5–27 shows the points used to produce the curves on graphs which represent the function of a constant flow generator under normal lung conditions. Note that the flow rate ($\dot{V}$) is constant at 0.5 L/sec (Fig 5–27,A) In 0.5 second, 0.25 L is delivered; in 1 second, 0.5 L is delivered, and so on. The volume (V) can be calculated by multiplying flow by the time (t) ($V = \dot{V} \times t$) (Fig 5–27,B). Alveolar pressure can be determined if volume and lung compliance are known ($P_A = V/C$) (Fig 5–27,C). If the volume is 1 L at 2 seconds, and C is 0.1 L/cm H_2O, then $P_A = 1$ L/0.1 (L/cm H_2O) = 10 cm H_2O. Note that this curve has the same shape as the volume curve. In the clinical setting plateau pressure can be used to estimate alveolar pressure. The pressure lost to the airways during gas flow or transairway pressure is the product of flow and airway resistance (Raw). If Raw is 2 cm H_2O/(L/sec) and flow is 0.5 L/sec, then P_{TA} = flow × Raw; P = 0.5 L/sec × 2 cm H_2O/(L/sec); P_{TA} = 1 cm H_2O. Since flow is constant and resistance is assumed to remain the same, then P_{TA} will also be unchanged (Fig 5–27,D). The upper airway pressure is the sum of alveolar pressure (P_A) and the pressure lost to the airways ($Pawo = P_A + P_{TA}$). Figure 5–27,E shows these values graphed together. This is the pressure that is observed on a ventilator manometer as it delivers a breath.

To summarize the curves in Figure 5–27, it can be seen that with constant flow, the curves for flow and pressure lost to the airways are constant. The curves for volume, P_A, and mouth pressure increase linearly (ascending ramps).

Most currently used commercial ventilators have the capability of being constant flow controllers and are usually time- or volume-cycled, i.e., inspiration ends after a predetermined volume or time has been reached. These ventilators have a pressure-limiting feature which prevents upper airway pressure from exceeding a preset value. This prevents extremely high pressures from reaching the lungs. If the preset pressure limit is reached before the machine either time-cycles or volume-cycles out of inspiration, then the volume will *not* be delivered as described. Reaching the preset pressure limit will prevent a constant volume delivery. This can occur if the patient's lungs are much stiffer (less compliant) and if the airway resistance is increased significantly. Examples include the Puritan Bennett 7200 and the Servo 900C.

Effects of Changes in Lung Characteristics on Pressure Curves with Constant Flow

As patient's lungs become stiffer (less compliant) or their airway resistance increases, these changes can affect some of the features achieved during mechanical ventilation. In this section we deal with how changing lung characteristics affect the P_A, P_{TA}, and Pawo during mechanical ventilation. We use a constant flow ventilator as an example since it is the easiest to follow. It should be kept in mind, however, that similar factors affect curves for P_A, P_{TA}, and Pawo in other types of ventilators. For example, nonconstant flow ventilators and nonconstant pressure ventilators experience similar changes in these curves with changes in compliance and resistance.

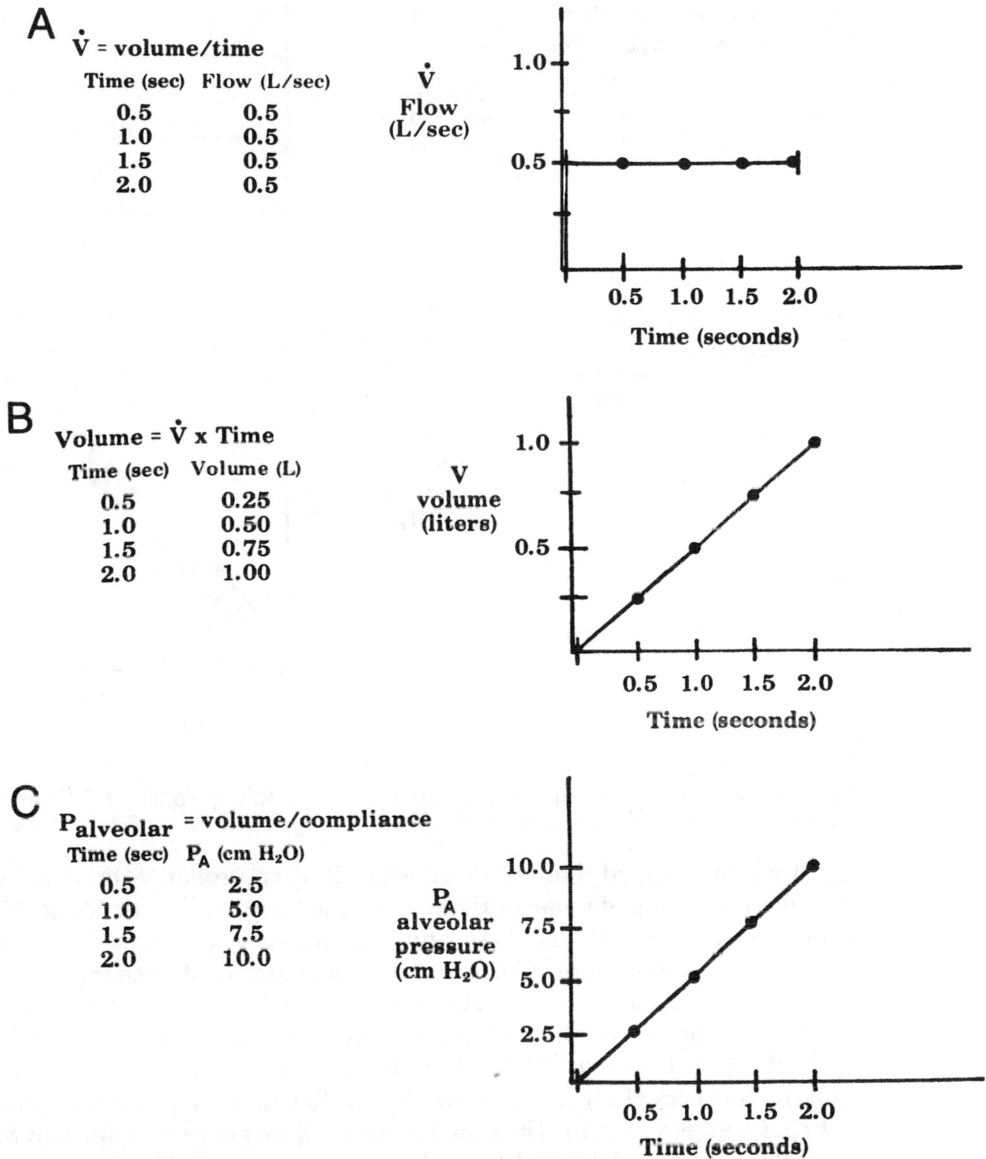

FIG 5–27.
Curves of constant or rectangular flow under normal lung conditions (C = 0.1 L/cm H_2O; Raw = 2 cm H_2O/L/sec). Inspiratory time is 2 seconds. **A**, the flow rate is constant at 0.5 L/sec. **B**, the volume increases at a constant rate during inspiration, achieving a tidal volume of 1 L. **C**, Alveolar pressure *(PA)* increases at a constant rate, as does the volume, to a maximum of 10 cm H_2O.

(Continued.)

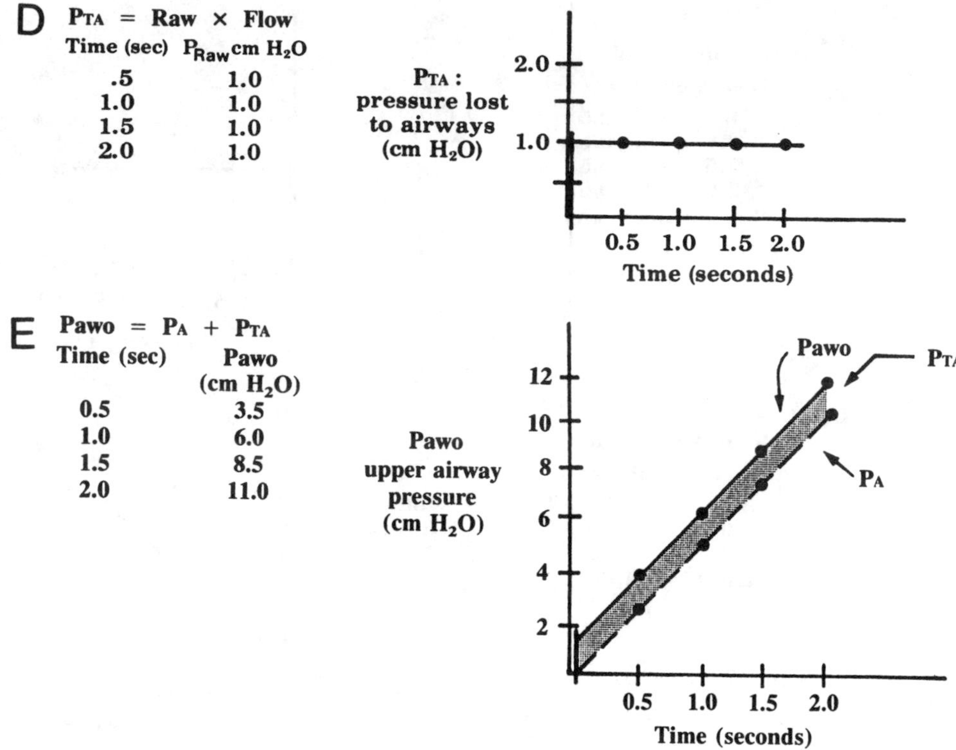

FIG 5–27 (cont.).
D, since the flow is constant, the pressure lost due to Raw is constant. This assumes that resistance and flow do not change. PTA is 1.0 cm H_{2O}/L/sec. PTA = flow × Raw.

It was mentioned that with a constant flow controller, volume delivery and flow were unchanged regardless of changes in lung characteristics in this type of ventilator. As a result, the flow and volume curves remain the same under changing lung conditions. However, as lung characteristics change the pressure curves change. As an example, let compliance be decreased (stiff lung condition). With the compliance half of the previous value (0.05 L/cm H_2O vs. 0.1 L/cm H_2O), the PA will double (20 cm H_2O) (Fig 5–28,A). Paow reaches 21 cm H_2O, the sum of PA (20 cm H_2O) and pressure lost to Raw (PTA = 1.0 cm H_2O) which has not changed (Fig 5–28,B). Thus, in a constant flow generator, one can anticipate a constant volume delivered from the ventilator even with changes in compliance as long as the ventilator is time- or volume-cycled. An example of this type of ventilator is the Monaghan 225/SIMV.

Let us consider what changes will occur with this type of ventilator if flow, inspiratory time, and compliance remain constant at 0.5 L/sec, 2 seconds, and 0.1 L/cm H_2O, respectively, but the Raw increases to twice its previous value, i.e., from 2 to 4 cm H_2O/(L/sec). Again, flow and volume delivery are constant. Since

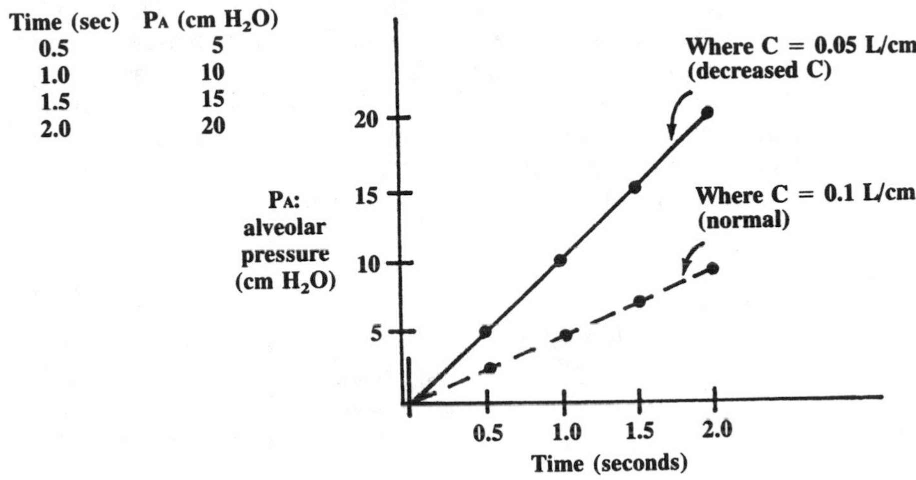

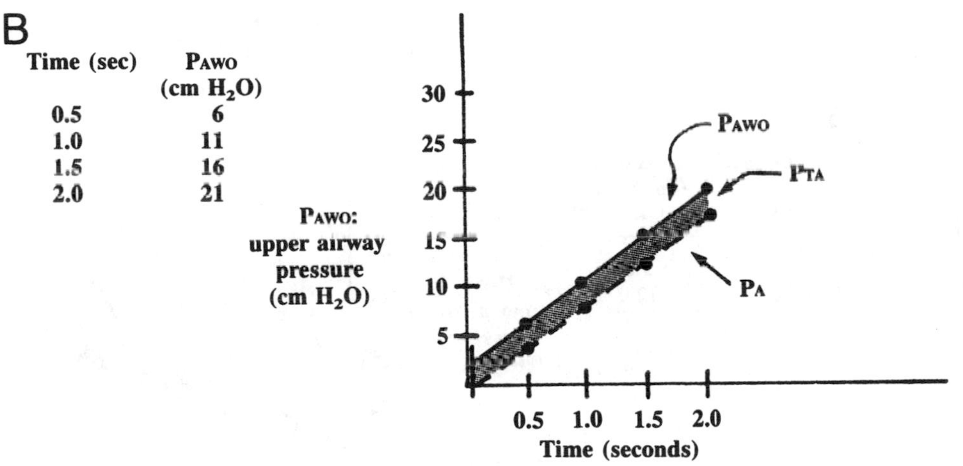

FIG 5–28.
A, flow is constant at 0.5 L/sec. Inspiratory time is 2 seconds. The volume coming from the ventilator remains the same at 1 L even though compliance *(C)* is reduced. This is a situation of constant flow, time-limited ventilation. Alveolar pressure *(PA)* is doubled at 20 cm H_2O in this situation since the compliance is half of its previous value. This figure shows the curve for normal compliance (C = 0.1 L/cm H_2O) as a *dashed line* and the curve for reduced compliance (C = 0.05 L/cm H_2O) as a *solid line.* **B,** since flow is constant and the airway resistance is constant, the pressure lost to the airways is constant (PTA = 1.0 cm H_2O). PTA is the *shaded area.* Upper airway pressure will be much higher than normal since compliance is reduced.

compliance does not change, the PA does not change, but the Raw is increased, so the pressure lost to the airway increases from 1 cm H_2O when Raw was 2 cm H_2O/(L/sec) to 2 cm H_2O/(L/sec) (Fig 5–29,A). The pressure at the upper airway will also increase slightly and reach a peak of 12 cm H_2O (Fig 5–29,B).

Clinically, an increase in Raw will result in increased peak pressures with PA (plateau pressures) remaining fairly constant or decreasing slightly. Therefore, the difference between the two increases. The volume delivered will remain constant as inspiratory time is the same. Again, with any type of ventilator, the PA curve resembles the volume delivery curve. Transairway pressure resembles the flow curve. Pawo is the sum of PA and PTA.

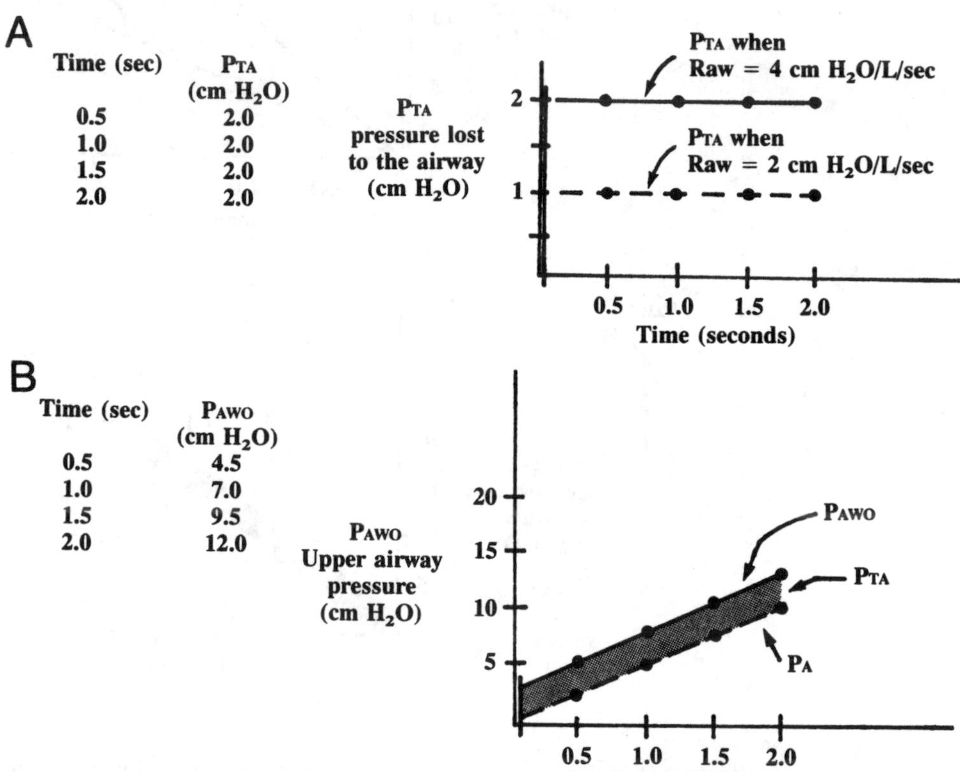

FIG 5–29.
Constant flow ventilator. The following inspiratory curves are produced when airway resistance is increased to 4 cm H_2O/L/sec and compliance is normal (C = 0.1 L/cm H_2O). **A,** pressure lost to the airways *(PTA)* is the product of flow and airway resistance (flow × Raw). With an increase in Raw, PTA increases to 2 cm H_2O *(solid line)* compared to normal at 1 cm H_2O *(dashed line).* **B,** upper airway pressure *(Pawo),* the sum of alveolar pressure *(PA)* and PTA, increases to a maximum of 12 cm H_2O since PTA is increased *(shaded area).* The difference between the peak and the plateau or PA increases.

Constant Flow Controller With Low to Moderate Pressure Drive Mechanism

A constant flow ventilator with a low to moderate working pressure, i.e., between 40 and 120 cm H_2O, creates a constant flow waveform under normal lung conditions (Fig 5–30,A). Normally, adequate V_T can be delivered well before P_A nears the generating pressure. The flow remains constant throughout inspiration since the generating pressure under normal conditions remains well above the pressure in the lungs.

Unfortunately, worsening of the patient lung characteristics will create a different appearance in the flow waveform. When compliance is significantly reduced and resistance increased, flow decreases during inspiration. This is because of the decrease in the pressure gradient between the ventilator and the alveoli. An example of this type of ventilator is the MA-1. Clinically, a decrease in compliance will be reflected as an increase in peak pressure at the upper airway. When the driving mechanism can no longer generate a pressure at least five times the Pawo, the ventilator no longer functions as a constant flow ventilator.

Along with the rise in peak pressure, the plateau pressure will rise as the

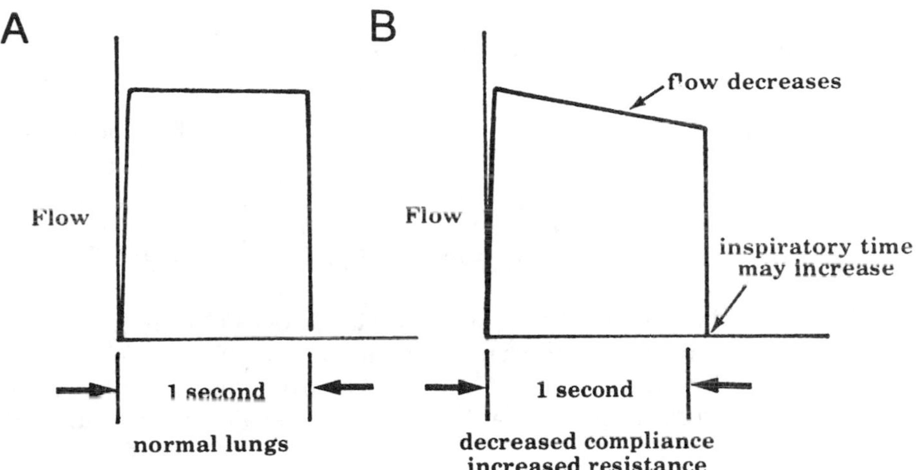

FIG 5–30.
Inspiratory curves represent the changes in flow that can occur using a constant flow ventilator with moderate-to-low pressure–generating drive mechanism. Under normal conditions, flow is constant **(A)**. As compliance decreases significantly and resistance increases, the flow decreases slightly **(B)**. This type of curve has been called a tapered square, a modified square wave, or a modified descending ramp. If the ventilator is volume-limited, the volume will be delivered from the ventilator, but inspiratory time may increase **(B)**. This can affect the inspiratory-expiratory ratio. Reduced compliance will cause an increase in alveolar and upper airway pressures as long as the ventilator is not pressure-limited out of inspiration. Increased airway resistance will increase the pressure lost due to airway resistance and the upper airway pressure as long as the ventilator is not pressure-limited.

static compliance decreases. The difference between the peak pressure and the plateau pressure will remain nearly constant as long as Raw is not also changing. If the ventilator is volume-cycled, as in the MA-1, the inspiratory time will increase. This will affect the I/E ratio (Fig 5–30,B). If the ventilator is time-cycled out of inspiration, as in the Servo 900 series, then the V_T delivered will be lower than the previous volume under normal conditions. If the ventilator is pressure-cycled, the inspiratory gas flow delivery to the patient will stop before all the volume is delivered. This might also shorten the inspiratory time. This will occur with the MA-1 and the Servo if they are pressure-cycled.

In summary, with the constant flow ventilator with a drive mechanism that only produces a moderate to low generating pressure, inspiratory flow decreases slightly in a linear fashion during inspiration. With a large decrease in lung compliance and an increase in airway resistance, it can result in increased inspiratory time when volume is constant as a result of volume cycling. When compliance decreases in this type of ventilator, P_{TA} and P_A are increased. When Raw alone is increased, Pawo and P_{TA} are increased, but P_A remains approximately the same.

Nonconstant Flow Controllers (Generators)

A nonconstant flow controller has a flow pattern that is not square or rectangular. The flow pattern may be shaped like the sinusoidal pattern commonly called a sine wave (Fig 5–31). It may have a pattern that is shaped like an ascending ramp (Fig 5–32) or like a descending ramp (Fig 5–33). In nonconstant flow, the flow pattern is dependent upon the mechanism that produces it. The characteristics of a nonconstant flow generator are:

1. Its flow waveform, whatever it is, does not change shape during inspiration, even with changes in lung characteristics.
2. The waveform remains the same from one breath to the next.
3. Pressure patterns at the upper airway vary with relation to compliance and Raw.

One very common flow wave is the half-cycle of the sinusoidal or sine wave ventilator. A rotary wheel drive piston produces this pattern, as in the IMV Emerson. But because the volume in the piston cylinder can be measured, this ventilator is really *volume-controlled.* The microprocessor ventilators can also produce this pattern. The precise control of solenoid valves or similar output control valves makes this possible. Since flow and not volume is measured in this ventilator, these are correctly classified as nonconstant flow ventilators when these flows are selected.

In the half-cycle sine flow pattern shown in Figure 5–31 the typical curve patterns are illustrated. At the beginning of a breath, the inspiratory flow is slow.

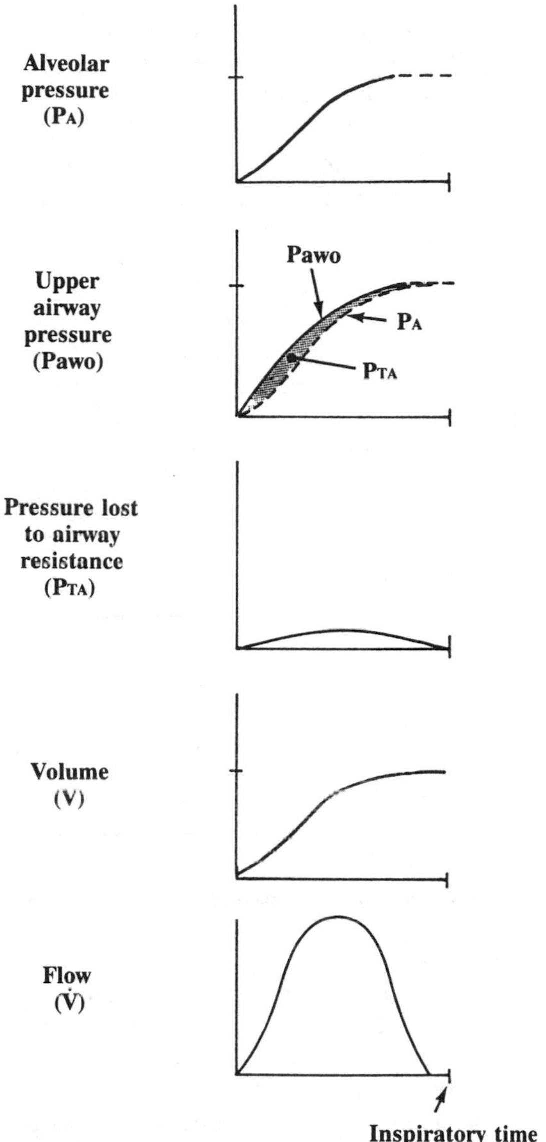

FIG 5–31.
Inspiratory curves represent a nonconstant flow controller, the IMV Emerson. This example shows a sinusoidal curve. Because of the force behind the volume delivery, the flow, volume, and time remain constant even with changes in lung characteristics. The upper airway pressure will increase if compliance decreases or airway resistance increases. When compliance is reduced the pressure in the lung *(PA)* will increase. When resistance increases the pressure lost to airway resistance increases. The volume delivery from the ventilator will not decrease unless a pressure limit is reached during inspiration before the volume delivery is completed.

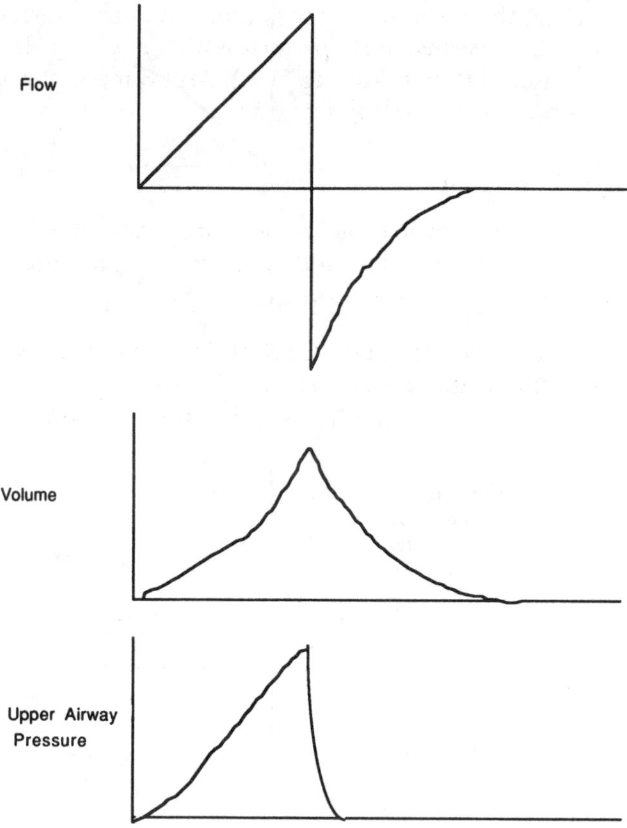

FIG 5–32.
Curves represent an ascending ramp flow waveform.

This eliminates any abrupt rise in mouth pressure as seen in several other types of ventilating modes. The flow rate rises, peaks at midinspiration, and then tapers off gradually. Pressure and volume curves also vary in patterns that resemble portions of the sine curve.

Regardless of changes in lung compliance and Raw, the flow pattern remains the same in a nonconstant flow ventilator. If compliance decreases, the P_A rises, as does Pawo. Changes in lung compliance do not result in a reduction of the flow rate or V_T. The Veolar and 7200a are ventilators which can operate in this way. If resistance increases, the volume accumulation and flow rate (peak value) are the same. The Pawo and P_{TA} increase owing to greater pressure being lost to the airways. The difference between Pawo and P_A increases.

In other nonconstant flow ventilators the pattern is basically sinusoidal or exponential, but the flow may stop abruptly at some point in the inspiratory cycle of the wave so that only a portion of the curve results. One example of this is an accelerating flow pattern which rises rapidly and is cut off sharply to an inflation hold pattern (Fig 5–34). An example of a ventilator which can produce this pattern is the Engström 30.

Pressure Controllers

The two basic types of pressure controllers for positive pressure ventilators are constant pressure and nonconstant pressure ventilators. These used to be called pressure generators.

Constant Pressure Controllers.—When a ventilator provides a constant pressure at the upper airway it is called a *constant pressure controller (generator).* This type of machine has four important characteristics:

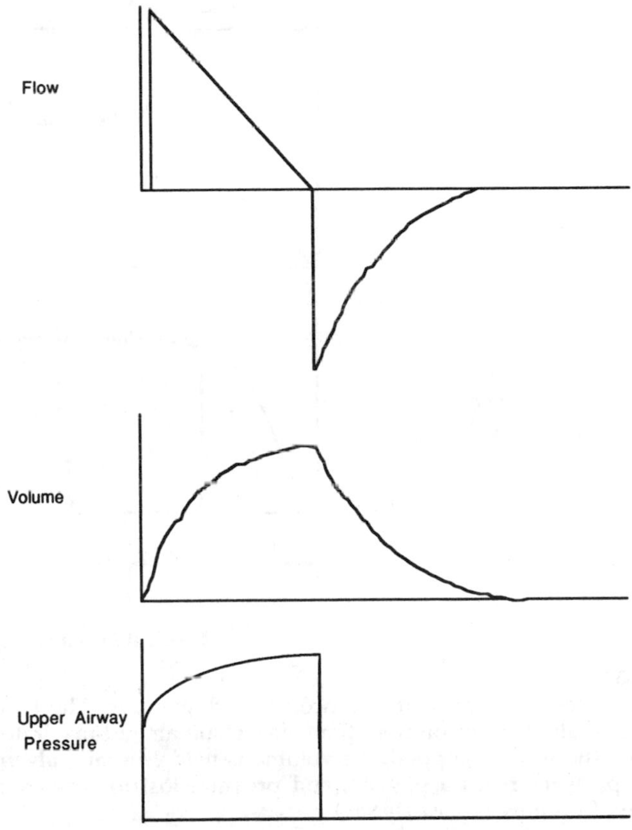

FIG 5–33.
Inspiratory curves represent a descending ramp flow pattern.

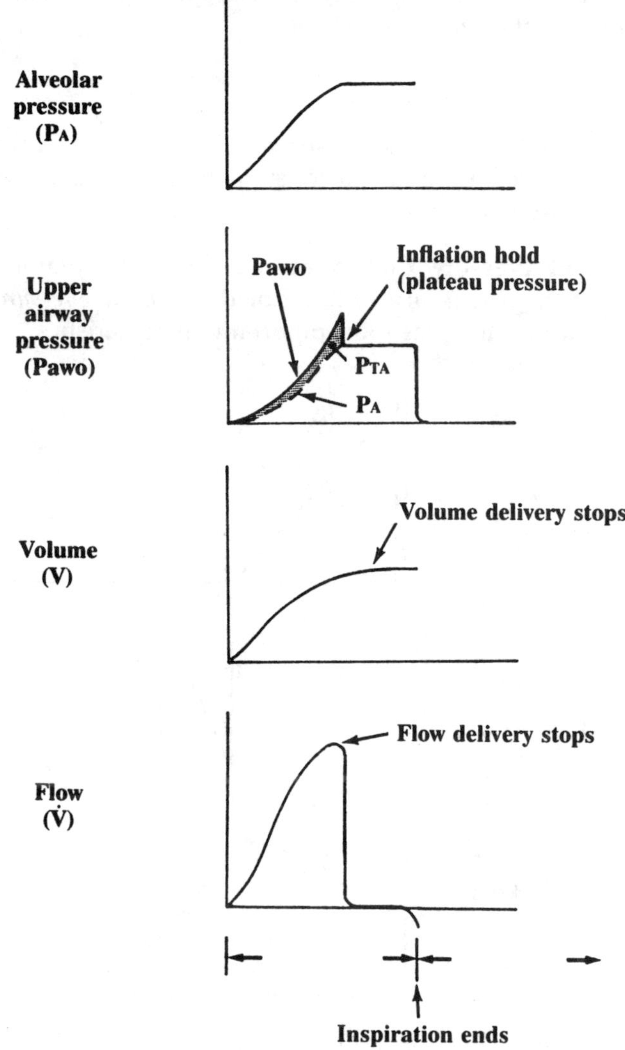

FIG 5–34.
Inspiratory curves represent a nonconstant flow curve. The tidal volume delivery may not require all of the inspiratory time. As a result an end-inspiratory pause or hold occurs in which the flow is stopped, the volume is held constant, alveolar pressure and upper airway pressure reach a plateau, and pressure lost to airway resistance drops to zero because of no flow *(shaded portion)*.

1. It provides a rectangular or constant waveform.
2. The waveform and pressure are not affected by changes in the patient's lung characteristics (compliance and resistance).
3. The rate of flow delivery varies depending on the patient's lung characteristics.
4. The flow waveform starts at a high rate and decreases during inspiration (descending ramp flow pattern).

An example of a constant pressure ventilator is depicted in Figure 5–9. A weight is placed on top of a bellows and is connected to the patient. Microprocessor ventilators that use the modes called pressure support or pressure control also act as constant pressure ventilators. They use output control valves such as solenoids to achieve this.

A constant pressure ventilator is usually one in which the drive mechanism or output control valve produces a pressure that is less than five times the pressure at the upper airway at the end of inspiration. Patterns for mouth, alveolar, and airway resistance pressures, volume, and flow delivery are shown in Figure 5–35 for normal lung conditions. Theoretically, the source pressure will equal only the pressure needed to ventilate the patient. The end of inspiration may be determined by a preset cycling pressure or a premeasured flow value. The final volume delivery will depend on lung characteristics and preset pressure. Examples are the Mark 7 or 8 on air/mix. Other, newer examples are the microprocessor ventilators like the Advent and Servo 300. When these are programmed to use pressure control or pressure support modes they function as constant pressure ventilators. During pressure support, inspiration normally ends at a predetermined flow rate of gas. During pressure control, inspiration usually ends at a preset inspiratory time.

Most constant pressure ventilators function as follows: At the beginning of inspiration there is no pressure in the lungs. Gas flow from the ventilator reaches the upper airway and is at its highest flow rate. It is here that the pressure gradient between the ventilator and the lung is the highest. The pressure exerted at the upper airway causes the Pawo readings to rise rapidly at the beginning of inspiration. The gas flow begins to traverse the conductive airways and enter the lungs. As the lungs begin to fill, the P_A begins to rise and approach the generating pressure. The closer they approach in value, the less the gradient of pressure between the ventilator and the alveoli. As the gradient becomes smaller, the rate of flow decreases. The resulting flow waveform is called an exponential decay. The rate of volume filling also decreases until inspiration is ended. As flow rate decreases, assuming Raw is constant, the pressure lost to the airways (P_{TA}) decreases throughout inspiration. The volume of gas in the lungs at any point in the cycle will equal the product of lung compliance and P_A.

The changes in pressure, flow, and volume given as examples in Table 5–2

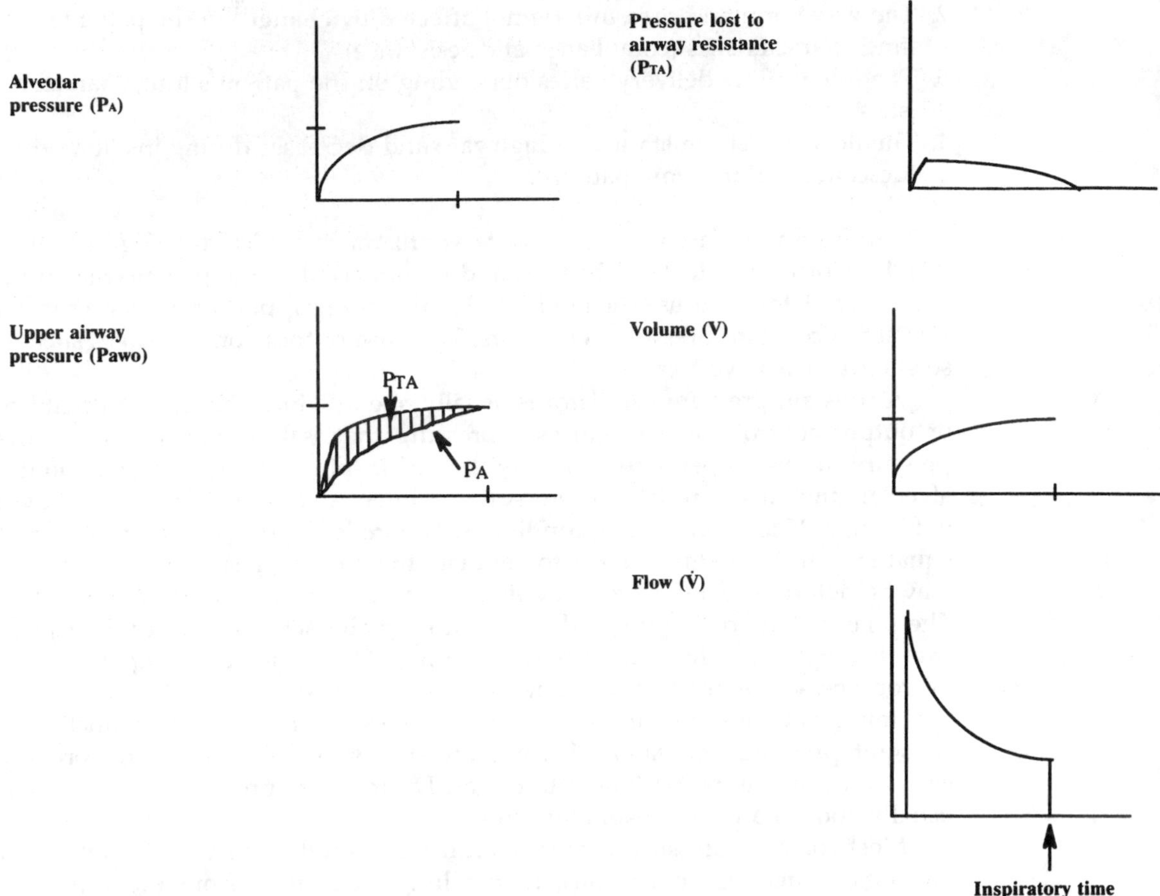

FIG 5–35.
Inspiratory curves represent the changes in volume, flow, and time when using a constant pressure ventilator that is pressure-cycled out of inspiration. As compliance decreases or resistance increases, the flow is reduced. In the clinical situation the pressure limit is usually reached prematurely. This shortens inspiratory time and reduces the delivered volume compared to normal conditions. If the flow is low enough that the pressure is not reached early, the inspiration could be prolonged and potentially the desired tidal volume would be delivered. The *shaded portion* of the curve of airway pressure *(PTA)* represents pressure lost to airway resistance (PRAW or PTA).

can be seen to parallel what happens in Figure 5–35, with normal lung conditions. When lung conditions change, the patterns also change. If the compliance is halved in value to 25 mL/cm H_2O (0.025 L/cm H_2O) and all other factors are kept constant, then the initial flow is unaltered; however, as the flow reaches the alveoli, the PA rises at twice the normal rate because of the greater elastance (lower compliance) of the alveoli. Pressure begins to approach its maximum much sooner while only half of the volume is delivered. This occurs because the pressure gradient falls so rapidly between the ventilator and the alveoli that inadequate flow is delivered. In other words, the flow rate falls off very rapidly and the preset pressure is reached sooner.

Suppose that PA is again 14 cm H_2O, and compliance is now 0.025 L/cm H_2O. The delivered volume will be 0.35 L (see Table 5–2, Reduced compliance). In this situation, the amount of pressure lost to the airways due to resistance will be approximately the same since the generating pressure is the same and the Raw has not changed. To correct clinically for the decreased compliance and lower volume delivery, the preset pressure is increased until the desired measured exhaled VT is achieved.

Consider the example in Table 5–2 for increased resistance. At the beginning of inspiration, let the flow be 0.75 L/sec (less than normal). With a resistance of 12 cm H_2O/L/sec, the PTA will be 0.75×12, or 9 cm H_2O. At midinspiration, the flow will be lower and loss to the airways will decrease. At the end of inspiration, the flow will eventually stop. The PA will not approach generator pressure. The desired volume will not be delivered. Inspiratory time is decreased. The preset pressure limit is often reached early and less volume is delivered.

When a patient has an increase in Raw, and the flow rate decreases, sometimes the flow is low enough so that the pressure limit is not reached prema-

TABLE 5–2.

Changes in Function in a Constant Pressure Ventilator with Alteration in Lung Characteristics*

	Generating Pressure (cm H_2O)	PA	Pawo	Flow (L/sec)	PTA	Volume Delivery (L)
Normal characteristics (C = 0.05 L/cm H_2O, Raw = 6 cm H_2O/(L/sec)						
Begin inspiration	15	0	6	1.0	6	0.00
Mid-inspiration	15	5	8	0.5	3	0.25
End-inspiration	15	14	14	0.0	0	0.70
Reduced compliance (C = 0.025 L/cm H_2O)						
Begin inspiration	15	0	6	1.0	6	0.00
Mid-inspiration	15	7	11	0.5	3	0.17
End-inspiration	15	14	14	0.0	0	0.35
Increased resistance (R = 12 cm H_2O/(L/sec)						
Begin inspiration	15	0	9	0.75	9	0.00
Mid-inspiration	15	5	11	0.50	6	0.25
End-inspiration (with increased inspiratory time)	15	7	14	0.00	0	0.35

*C = compliance; PA = alveolar pressure; Pawo = pressure at the mouth; PTA = transairway pressure.

turely. If the inspiratory time is prolonged, potentially the desired V_T could be delivered with this type of ventilator. This, however, would also affect the respiratory rate and the $\dot{V}_E$.

When a ventilator is used as a constant pressure ventilator in the pressure support mode, the flow, volume, and pressure curves will be similar to those pictured in Figure 5–33. Most of these microprocessor ventilators terminate inspiration when the flow rate reaches some predetermined flow rate. For example, on the Servo 900C, inspiration will normally end when the flow is 25% or less of the value measured as the peak flow. If the ventilator measures a peak inspiratory flow produced by the patient's active inspiration of 100 L/min, then it will cut off the constant pressure breath when the inspiratory flow drops to 25 L/min. In the 7200a ventilator, the pressure support ends when the flow drops to 5 L/min.

Ventilators that can be set to provide pressure-controlled ventilation become constant pressure generators in this mode with the same characteristic curves. Pressure-controlled ventilation is normally terminated when a preset time has been reached. Most of the microprocessor ventilators now offer the pressure control mode. The operator sets the desired pressure and can generally control rate and inspiratory time. As with pressure support, the volume delivered to the patient will depend on the patient's lung characteristics and may also change with active inspiratory effort.

Nonconstant Pressure Controllers.—The *nonconstant* pressure controller (generator) has a pressure waveform that is not rectangular or constant during inspiration. The waveform may be an accelerating or ascending ramp or be sinusoidal or exponential depending on the type of mechanical device that generates the curve. *Nonconstant* pressure controllers have three distinct characteristics:

1. The pressure curve has a pattern that is nonrectangular.
2. The waveform of the pressure curve is the same regardless of changes in the patient's lung characteristics.
3. Flow and volume delivery vary with the type of pressure waveform, the lung characteristics, and the inspiratory time allowed. If the pressure pattern decreases at the end of inspiration, flow is a descending ramp. If the pressure pattern increases during inspiration, and the flow pattern starts out low and progressively increases, flow is an ascending ramp.

An example of a ventilator with a nonconstant pressure curve is one with a spring-loaded bellows. When the bellows is full, spring pressure is high. As the bellows empties during inspiration, spring tension drops. Thus, the pressure curve descends during inspiration. Flow will also decrease (Fig 5–36). An example of this is the Servo 900C. When working pressure is set low, it operates as a

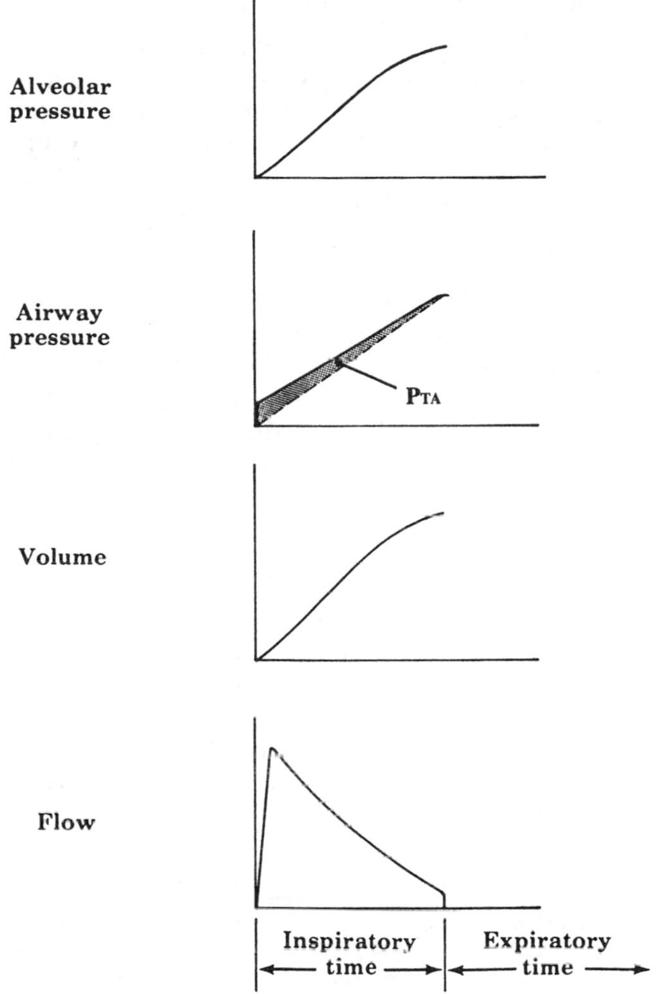

FIG 5–36.
Inspiratory curves represent a nonconstant pressure waveform.

nonconstant pressure generator. However, in actual clinical practice with the working pressure set high, any pressure drop is usually insignificant. This ventilator, under normal conditions, operates as a constant flow ventilator.

Another nonconstant pressure curve is the ascending pressure curve. Some microprocessor ventilators can function in this way when the operator selects an accelerating or ascending ramp–type flow curve. Examples are the Veolar and the BEAR 5. To produce a progressive increase in flow throughout inspiration, the pressure must increase progressively (see Fig 5–32).

Summary

The various operating modes for the delivery of the inspiratory phase of ventilation have been reviewed. These have included flow controllers, constant and nonconstant, and pressure controllers, constant and nonconstant. It should be kept in mind that these various types of ventilators are generalized examples of theoretical waveform patterns. Many ventilators in clinical use vary slightly in some way from these models but resemble them in principle. Some ventilators have more than one mode of operation during the inspiratory phase that can be selected as desired. The advantage of being familiar with these functional modes is that it allows the practitioner to understand how the ventilator functions during the inspiratory phase when it is interfaced with a patient whose lung characteristics vary from time to time. While recognition and use of the waveform patterns is not necessary for clinical evaluation, newer monitoring techniques allow for viewing the waveform patterns. This expands the clinician's ability to understand the ventilator-patient interaction. Table 5–3 summarizes these concepts.

Limiting Inspiration

During the inspiratory phase the operator can set on the ventilator a limit on the value of one of the variables of pressure, volume, or flow. For example, in the Emerson 3-PV ventilator, the cylinder which contains the piston has a very specific volume which can be set. The volume cannot exceed that amount. It might, for some reason, be less. But it cannot be more. A limiting characteristic or a parameter is the maximum value a variable (pressure, volume, or flow) can

TABLE 5–3.
Chatburn's Guide to Ventilator Classification*

To determine whether the ventilator in question is a pressure, time, or flow controller, use the following guide.

From the operator's manual, experiments, and previous knowledge, answer the following questions:

1. Does the pressure waveform at the upper airway change when the patient's resistance or compliance change?
   If not, the ventilator is a pressure controller (stop here)
   If yes, go to no. 2
2. Does the volume waveform stay constant when the patient's lung characteristics change?
   If not, the ventilator is a time controller (stop here)
   If yes, go to no. 3
3. Is the volume measured directly by either a volume displacement device or by a flow transducer?
   If not, the ventilator is a flow controller (stop here)
   If yes, the ventilator is a volume controller (stop here)

*Data from references 6 and 7.

attain. This limits the variable during inspiration, but does not end the inspiratory phase.

Pressure Limiting.—Let us look again at the example of the rotary piston of the Emerson 3-PV ventilator (see Fig 5–6). The ventilator will push the volume out of the ventilator to the patient circuit. If the patient has very stiff lungs (decreased compliance), then the peak pressure will rise during inspiration. The operator sets a high pressure limit to prevent excessive peak pressures. With the Emerson device, the ventilator does *not* cycle out of inspiration when it reaches the set pressure limit. The excess pressure is vented through a spring-loaded pop-off valve. The excess gas pressure issues into the room like steam from a pressure cooker.

The Baby Bird and the Sechrist IV-100B also pressure-limit the inspiratory phase, but these are time-cycled out of inspiration, as is the Emerson. Other examples of pressure limiting are the modes called pressure support and pressure control. When a value is preset in either of these two modes, the pressure that can go to the airway is limited.

Volume Limiting.—Volume-limiting ventilators have a prefixed volume contained in a bag, bellows device, or piston cylinder. These represent volume-limiting devices where the volume in the bag or bellows is the amount set by the operator. This actually limits, to a maximum value, the amount of volume that can be delivered. Reaching that volume does not necessarily end inspiration. The same is true of a piston. Volume is limited to what is contained in the piston cylinder. It cannot be higher. The forward movement of the piston rod or arm controls the *time* of inspiration (time-cycled). The volume in the piston cylinder limits the volume. Ventilators can have more than one limiting feature at a time. The Emerson is both pressure-limited (by the pop-off valve) and volume-limited (by the cylinder housing).

Flow Limiting.—If the flow reaches a constant value before the end of inspiration, then a ventilator is considered to be flow-limited. The flow provided is limited to a certain amount. For example, the constant forward motion of a linear-drive piston (see Fig 5–5) provides a constant rate of gas delivery over a certain period of time. Remember that volume delivery is determined by the rate of gas flow (L/min or L/sec) and the length of inspiration. In this example, the ventilator is time-cycled. This is determined by the length of time it takes the piston rod to move forward. It is also volume-limited to the volume inside the piston cylinder. It is also flow-limited. The flow will not exceed what is needed to give the volume in the designated time.

Pressure Limiting vs. Pressure Cycling.—All ventilators on which a volume or a minute ventilation can be set have a knob or control called a *pressure limit.* This control is used to prevent excessive pressure from going into a patient's lungs. We normally set this at 10 cm H_2O above the peak inspiratory pressure (PIP). In most volume ventilators, when the set pressure is reached it will end the inspiratory phase. If this occurs, it means the machine was pressure-cycled for that breath. By definition, a cycling mechanism ends inspiration. One should keep this in mind when considering how to classify the function of a ventilator. Examples of ventilators which provide pressure cycling when the preset pressure limit control is set are the MA-1, and the 7200a in the controlled mechanical ventilation (CMV) mode.

TERMINATION OF INSPIRATORY PHASE: CYCLING MECHANISM

The way in which a ventilator marks the end of inspiratory gas flow and the beginning of expired gas flow is called the *cycling* method or the cycling mechanism. The end of inspiration is achieved by a specific mechanism inside the ventilator. There are four parameters the ventilator can control to cycle out of inspiration: pressure, flow, volume, and time. For any single breath only one of the four can be operating. A ventilator breath may be pressure-cycled, time-cycled, volume-cycled, or flow-cycled. Most ventilators have more than one mode in which they can be cycled.

Pressure-Cycled Ventilation

When a preset pressure threshold (limit) is reached at the mouth or upper airway, a ventilator in the pressure-cycled mode will terminate inspiration. The volume delivered to the patient depends on the flow pattern delivered, the length of inspiration, and the patient's lung characteristics. Let us first consider an example of a constant flow ventilator that is pressure-cycled.

A clinician must first decide what pressure to use to achieve an adequate V_T.

TABLE 5–4.

Tidal Volume (V_T) Determination During Pressure-Cycling Ventilation in Normal Lungs Using a Constant Flow Ventilator*

Let C = 50 mL/cm H_2O and Raw = 6 cm H_2O/L/sec, and flow = 0.5 L/sec (constant)
If P_A = 15 cm H_2O
then,

$$V_T = C \times P_A = 50 \text{ mL/cm } H_2O \times 15 \text{ cm } H_2O \text{ and } V_T = 750 \text{ mL}$$
$$P_{TA} = Raw \times flow = 6 \text{ cm } H_2O/(L/sec) \times 0.5 \text{ L/sec}$$
$$P_{TA} = 3 \text{ cm } H_2O$$
$$Pawo = P_A + P_{TA}$$
$$Pawo = 15 \text{ cm } H_2O + 3 \text{ cm } H_2O = 18 \text{ cm } H_2O$$

*C = compliance; Raw = airway resistance; P_A = alveolar pressure; P_{TA} = transairway pressure; Pawo = upper airway pressure.

TABLE 5–5.
Tidal Volume (VT) Determination During Pressure-Cycled Ventilation in Lungs With Decreased Compliance (C) on a Constant Flow Ventilator*

Let C = 25 mL/cm H_2O, Raw = 6 cm H_2O/(L/sec), and flow = 0.50 L/sec (constant)
Cycling pressure is preset at 18 cm H_2O

$$P_{TA} = 3 \text{ cm } H_2O \ (\text{Raw} \times \text{flow} = P_{TA})$$
$$P_A = 15 \text{ cm } H_2O \ (P_A = \text{Pawo} - P_{TA})$$

$$V_T = C \times P_A = 25 \text{ mL/cm } H_2O \times 15 \text{ cm } H_2O$$
$$V_T = 375 \text{ mL (decreased)}$$

To achieve V_T = 750 mL, the PA needed is:

$$V_T = C \times P_A$$
$$P_A = V_T/C$$
$$P_A = 0.75 \text{ L/(25 mL/cm } H_2O) = 750 \text{ mL/(25 mL/cm } H_2O) = 30 \text{ cm } H_2O$$
$$\text{Pawo} = P_A + P_{TA} \ (P_{TA} \text{ remains constant at 3 cm } H_2O)$$
$$\text{Pawo} = 30 \text{ cm } H_2O + 3 \text{ cm } H_2O$$
$$\text{Pawo} = 33 \text{ cm } H_2O$$

*For abbreviations, see footnote, Table 5–4.

To make this determination, consideration must be given to the lung characteristics of the patient. Cycling pressure or pressure at the upper airway will be the sum of both PA and pressure lost due to Raw. Table 5–4 shows an example of a patient with normal lung conditions in whom a preset pressure of 18 cm H_2O is determined to be adequate for achieving a desired V_T of 750 mL.

Noncompliant lungs with normal Raw will require more pressure to deliver the same V_T. Table 5–5 shows how a reduction in compliance reduces delivered volume during pressure cycling and how cycling pressure must be increased to 33 cm H_2O to achieve the previous V_T of 750 mL.

Patients with increased Raw and normal compliance also need an increase in the preset pressure to compensate for increases in Raw. Table 5–6 gives an example of a patient whose Raw has increased to 12 cm H_2O/(L/sec) and describes how the V_T delivered with a constant flow ventilator is reduced.

In these situations of decreased compliance or increased resistance, the inspiratory time is shortened with a constant flow generator that is pressure-cycled. Since the mouth pressure (cycling pressure) rises rapidly under conditions of increased resistance or decreased compliance, a preset cycling pressure would probably be reached before the desired V_T had been delivered, and delivery time would be shortened. To correct for this, the cycling pressure is increased. It may also be desirable to readjust the flow rate where Raw has increased to achieve a desirable inspiratory time.

Pressure-cycled ventilators have the disadvantage of delivering a lower V_T when decreases in compliance and increases in resistance occur. They have the advantage of limiting peak pressure which may be damaging to the lungs. For the short-term ventilation of patients with fairly stable lung conditions, such as the postoperative patient, these ventilators are adequate. One possible advantage with most pressure-cycled machines using low generating pressures and decelerating flow patterns is the distribution of ventilation. Theoretically, as the flow decreases, the amount of turbulence in the airways is reduced. This helps contribute to better distribution of air into airways with varying resistance levels. One example of a pressure-cycled ventilator is the Mark 7. Others are the Servo 900C, the MA-1, the 7200a, and the Veolar when the pressure limit is reached and the ventilator ends inspiration. Many microprocessor ventilators with pressure support and pressure control have a safety pressure valve that will end inspiration during pressure support (or pressure control). For example, on the Servo 900C a pressure support breath will cycle into exhalation if the peak pressure is 3 cm H_2O above the preset pressure support value. On the 7200a it will do this at 1.5 cm H_2O.

System Leaks in Pressure-Cycled Ventilation

If a leak is present in the patient circuit on a ventilator that is pressure-cycled, then two possible situations can occur: (1) the leak will be large enough so that the preset pressure is never reached, or (2) the leak will be small enough so that the preset pressure is eventually reached.

In the first situation, there will be inadequate pressure going to the patient's lungs and an adequate VT will never be delivered. Some pressure-cycled venti-

TABLE 5–6.

Tidal Volume (VT) Determination During Pressure-Cycled Ventilation With Increased Airway Resistance (Raw) Using a Constant Flow Ventilator*

Let C = 50 mL/cm H_2O, Raw = 12 cm H_2O/(L/sec), and flow = 0.5 L/sec (constant)
Cycling pressure is preset at 18 cm H_2O

$$P_{TA} = Raw \times flow = 12 \text{ cm } H_2O \text{ (L/sec)} \times 0.50 \text{ L/sec} = 6 \text{ cm } H_2O$$
$$P_A = P_{TA} - P_{TA} = 18 - 6 = 12 \text{ cm } H_2O$$

$$V_T = C \times P_A = 50 \text{ mL/cm } H_2O \times 12 \text{ cm } H_2O$$
$$V_T = 600 \text{ ml}$$

To achieve VT = 750 mL

$$P_A = V_T/C$$
$$P_A = 750 \text{ mL/(50 mL/cm } H_2O)$$
$$P_A = 15 \text{ cm } H_2O$$

$$Pawo = P_A + P_{TA}$$
$$Pawo = 15 + 6 = 21$$
$$Pawo = 21 \text{ cm } H_2O \text{ (will achieve a } V_T \text{ near 750 mL)}$$

*For abbreviations, see footnote, Table 5–4.

lators have a time-limiting device on them so that even with a large leak present, the ventilator will actually cycle into the expiratory phase. PR-2 has a time-limiting device when the rate control is used. Most microprocessor ventilators also have a inspiratory time-limiting device when pressure support is used. Others have no time limit. The Mark 7 will remain in the inspiratory phase if a large circuit leak is present.

If the leak is small enough so that the preset pressure is finally achieved, then the inspiratory time will be increased. The leak reduces the net flow of gas to the patient. V_T will still be delivered as long as the preset pressure is reached and compliance and resistance have not changed in the meantime. With an increase in the inspiratory time, the rate will be slower. The result is a reduction in the $\dot{V}_E$ caused by a reduction in the respiratory rate.

Volume-Cycled Ventilation

When a ventilator terminates the inspiratory phase after the desired volume has been delivered from the ventilator, then it is referred to as a volume-cycled ventilator. The amount of volume is preset by the operator. In most cases, the volume delivered from the ventilator will remain constant with changes in patient lung characteristics. The pressures required to deliver the volume and flow rates of gas, however, will change with compliance and resistance changes (Table 5–6).

The volume delivered from the ventilator is not the volume that enters the patient's lungs. During inspiration the build-up in positive pressure in the circuit results in expansion of the patient circuit and compression of some of the gas. This gas never reaches the patient's lungs. The best way to evaluate the actual volume delivered to the patient is to measure the exhaled volume at the endotracheal or tracheostomy tube. If the volume is measured at the exhalation valve, then it must be corrected for tubing compliance (compressible volume). This is reviewed in Chapter 8.

In a volume-cycled ventilator like the MA-1, for example, the inspiratory cycle is usually terminated when a preset volume is achieved. If a patient were to develop an increased Raw and a decreased compliance, the flow rate would drop off slightly. With lower flows, the inspiratory time increases even though the desired volume is being delivered from the ventilator (see Fig 5–30). In addition, with increased resistance and decreased compliance, the pressures generated at the mouth and in the ventilator circuit are higher than under normal conditions. As a result, more volume is lost to the tubing with less actually being delivered to the patient.

In flow controllers, the preset inspiratory time and flow rate do not change with alterations in patient lung characteristics. These ventilators are useful for delivering a fixed $\dot{V}_E$ since the rate and volume coming out of the ventilator remain the same. The volume compressed in the circuit results in some loss of volume to the patient. Volume is lost due to leaks in the circuit and around the endotracheal tube.

Some microprocessor ventilators, like the 7200a, have computers which can correct for volume lost to the tubing. The volume displayed on this ventilator indicates what is intended for the patient's lungs, having corrected for tubing compliance loss.

Time-Cycled Ventilation

A ventilator can be considered time-cycled if the inspiratory phase ends when a predetermined time has elapsed. This is controlled by a timing mechanism within the ventilator which is not affected by conditions in the patient's lungs. The time remains fixed. Examples are the Sechrist IV-100, and the Servo 900C.

If a pressure controller is being used, and the inspiratory time is set, both the volume delivered and the flow will vary. Ventilators of this type are not often used in this cycling mode because of limited variability and uncertainty of V_T and $\dot{V}_E$ delivery. When V_T and $\dot{V}_E$ can be monitored, as in the newer microprocessor ventilators, modes such as pressure-controlled ventilation are time-cycled. Volume delivery will depend on lung compliance, Raw, patient effort (if present), and the particular ventilator in use.

If a flow controller (either constant or nonconstant) is being time-cycled, any increases in Raw or decreases in compliance will not affect the flow rate. As a result, the volume delivery in a fixed time frame will be the same while the pressures change (see Table 5–6). Pressure support also has a safety back-up maximum inspiratory time on most ventilators. Usually a lapsed time of about 5 seconds will end inspiration, if it is not ended normally by flow.

Flow-Cycled Ventilation

While not a common parameter, flow can be used to determine the end of the inspiratory phase. Once a predetermined flow has been achieved, the ventilator cycles into the expiratory phase. Volume and time vary according to changes in patient lung characteristics. The Puritan Bennett ventilators which employ the Bennett valve (PR-1 and 2, AP series, and PV-3P) may be considered flow-cycled ventilators since the valve switches from the inspiratory phase to the expiratory phase when the flow rate to the patient has dropped to a certain level. This low flow is achieved when the pressure gradient between the alveoli and the ventilator is small and the pressures are nearly equal. Since pressure is nearly being achieved, as well as a low flow rate, these ventilators are sometimes considered to be pressure-cycled. However, since the predetermined pressure is never actually reached, they are truly flow-cycled ventilators. When the rate control is used, they can function as time-cycled ventilators as long as flow or pressure limits are not reached first. Microprocessor ventilators that provide pressure support are normally flow-cycled out of inspiration. Volume and flow delivery vary with patient effort and lung characteristics.

EXPIRATORY PHASE

During the early development of mechanical ventilatory techniques, many believed that it was as essential to assist the expiratory phase as it was the inspiratory phase. This was accomplished in one of two ways. First, expiration could be assisted by applying a negative pressure to the upper airway to draw air out of the lungs. This was done either with a bellows device or a Venturi entrainer positioned at the mouth or upper airway. This technique was later termed *negative end-expiratory pressure (NEEP)*. The second method for assisting expiration was to apply positive pressure to the abdominal area, below the diaphragm, and to try to force the air out of the lungs by pushing the visceral organs up against the diaphragm. With the use of IPPV, expiration is now usually passive and depends upon the recoil of the elastic tissues in the lung to move air out of the alveoli and into the ambient air. There are several methods of changing what occurs during exhalation. These exhalation techniques, such as NEEP, PEEP, and CPAP, are discussed below.

Time-Limited Exhalation

The BEAR Cub ventilator is an example of an expiratory time limit ventilator. It limits the low end of the expiratory time. The ventilator monitors machine-delivered times and breaths. If the expiratory time between one delivered breath and the next is less than 0.25 seconds the ventilator signals an I time display and will not permit the time to be less than 0.25 second. It time-limits exhalation.

Continuous Flow Exhalation

Flow-by or bias flow are options available on some ventilators (the 7200a and Newport Wave, respectively). These provide gas flow between machine-delivered breaths. They are used with SIMV (7200a) to provide fresh gas flow to the patient and with pressure support (Newport Wave) to assist with spontaneous breathing and with triggering the pressure support breath.

Negative End-Expiratory Pressure

Most of the hazards associated with positive pressure ventilation are associated with the pressures exerted in the lungs and transmitted throughout the

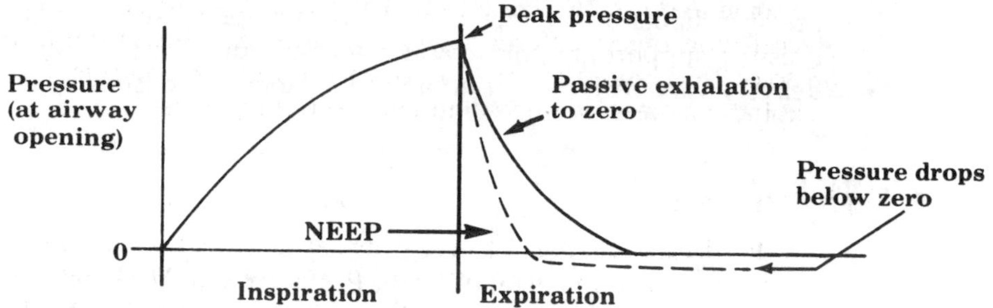

FIG 5–37.
Negative end-expiratory pressure *(NEEP)*. Expiration occurs more rapidly and the pressure drops below baseline (negative) compared with a normal passive exhalation to zero end-expiratory pressure.

thoracic cavity. To reduce these problems, a method of exhalation was devised to reduce the mean or average airway pressure. It was called negative end-expiratory pressure. The intent of NEEP was to help facilitate expiration by providing negative pressure at the proximal airway at the end of exhalation (Fig 5–37). It was advocated in shock as a means of increasing venous return to the heart. In neonates it allowed for faster respiratory rates. However, used with some patients, especially those with chronic obstructive airway disease, it proved dangerous. NEEP increased the risk of airway collapse and air trapping in the alveoli. The use of NEEP is also associated with reduced lung volumes below functional residual capacity (FRC) which could increase Raw and cause pulmonary collapse. Since the benefits are not significant and the hazards are high, NEEP is now seldom used. It is mentioned here lest we forget and make the same mistake again.

High-frequency oscillators assist inspiration and expiration. Basically, they push air in and then pull it back out at extremely high frequencies. Their function is similar to a speaker system on a stereo. If the mean airway pressure is set to equal ambient pressure, then the airway pressure oscillates above and below the zero baseline. During exhalation it actually creates a negative transrespiratory pressure. This technique is currently used most often in the ventilation of infants.

Expiratory Hold

Expiratory hold or expiratory pause is accomplished by allowing the patient to exhale and then having the ventilator pause prior to delivering the next machine breath. The purpose of this maneuver is to see if there is any pressure from trapped air still in the lungs before the next positive pressure breath. It has been found that high minute ventilation in adults can result in air remaining in the lungs at the end of exhalation. This trapped air, called auto-PEEP, can lead to some undesirable side effects. The gas may go undetected during mechanical ventilation unless an end-expiratory pressure is measured (see Chapter 7). The Servo 900C and the Advent have buttons or controls for measuring end-expiratory pressure during an end-expiratory pause.

Expiratory Retard

In diseases that lead to early airway closure, such as emphysema, the spontaneously breathing patient often has a prolonged expiratory phase and uses pursed lip breathing. Unfortunately, with an endotracheal tube in place, a mechanically ventilated patient cannot use this technique. To mimic this phenomenon, some mechanical ventilations used to provide a method of exhalation called *expiratory retard.* This adds a certain amount of resistance to expiration (Fig 5–38), which theoretically prevents early airway closure and improves ventila-

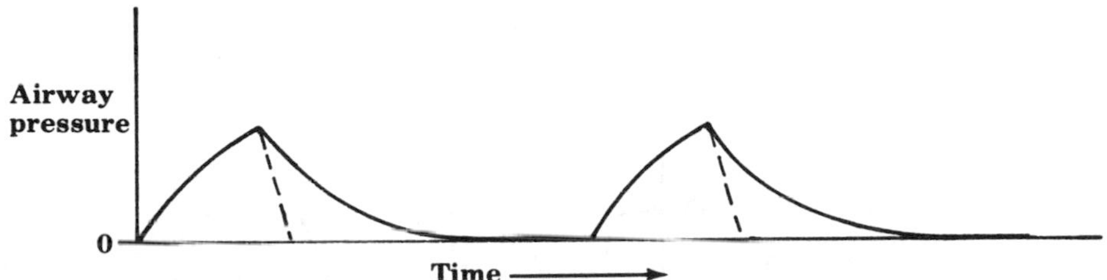

FIG 5–38.
Intermittent positive pressure ventilation (IPPV) with expiratory retard denoted by the *solid line,* and passive expiration to zero baseline noted as the *dashed line.* Expiratory retard does not change expiratory time, but increases the amount of pressure in the airway during exhalation.

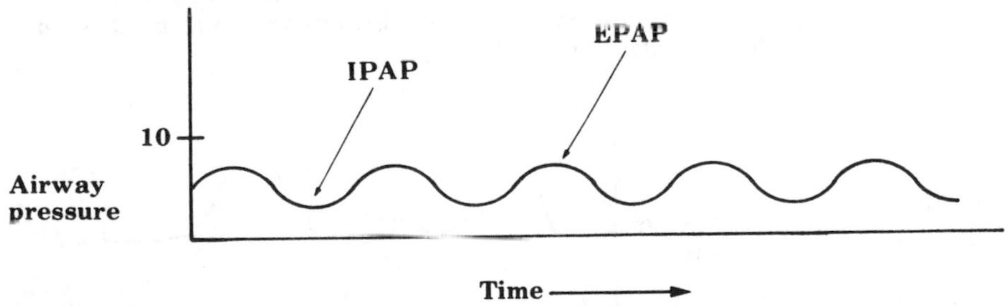

FIG 5–39.
Continuous positive airway pressure (CPAP). Breathing is spontaneous when inspiratory positive airway pressure *(IPAP)* and end-expiratory positive airway pressure *(EPAP)* are present. This is also referred to as continuous positive pressure breathing (CPPB) and continuous airway pressure (CAP). Pressures do not come back to zero baseline. The baseline is now positive.

tion. While popular in the early 1970s, the method has lost its popularity for some unknown reason. Some practitioners now use low levels of PEEP ($\leq +5$ cm H_2O) for the same purpose (see Chapter 10).

Positive End-Expiratory Pressure and Continuous Positive Airway Pressure

In the early 1900s, European anesthesiologists tried applying continuous positive pressure to patients' airways during thoracic surgery. They managed to successfully maintain survival of patients during surgery by this method. Barach readapted this technique of mechanical ventilatory support in the United States during the 1930s. He called this mode of ventilation continuous positive pressure breathing (CPPB). It was sometimes referred to as continuous (constant) positive pressure ventilation (CPPV).

This concept was not used clinically until the 1960s when it was readapted for use in critically ill patients. It eventually was modified. The result was two

(Text continued on p. 160.)

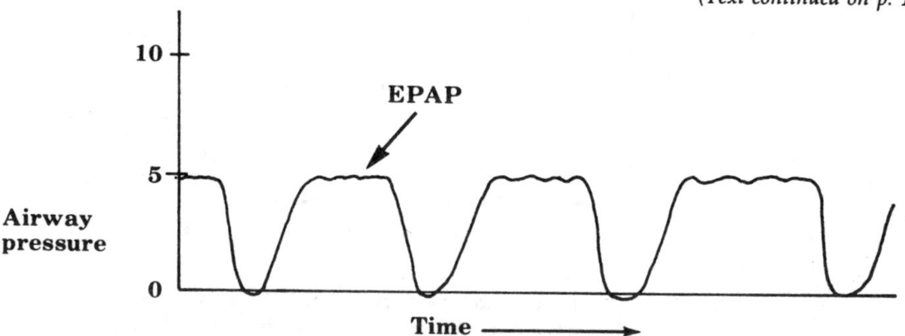

FIG 5–40.
End-expiratory airway pressure *(EPAP).* Ventilation is spontaneous. Positive pressure is exerted at the upper airway during expiration and pressures are at ambient or below ambient during inspiration. This is also referred to as positive end-expiratory pressure (PEEP) or spontaneous PEEP (sPEEP).

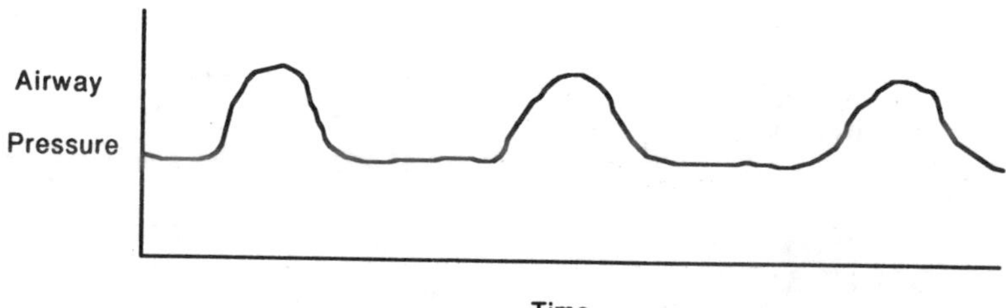

FIG 5–41.
IPAP plus EPAP. Inspiratory positive airway pressure (IPAP) is usually higher than end-expiratory positive airway pressure (EPAP) when this method of continuous airway pressure is applied to patients. It is used for nasal continuous positive airway pressure (CPAP) in the home and as a technique in home ventilation.

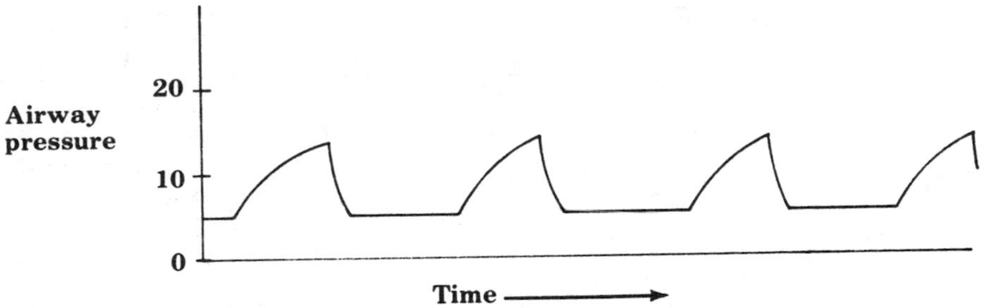

FIG 5–42.
Positive end-expiratory pressure (PEEP) during controlled positive pressure ventilation. There are no spontaneous breaths between machine breaths and no negative deflections of the baseline, which is above zero. This is sometimes called continuous positive pressure ventilation (CPPV).

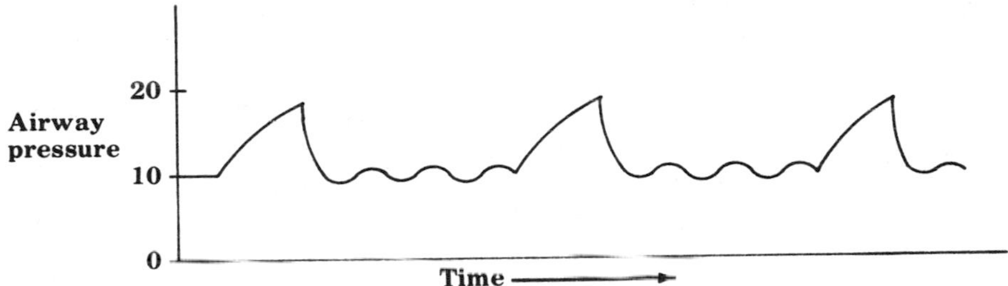

FIG 5–43.
Continuous positive airway pressure (CPAP) or positive end-expiratory pressure (PEEP) with intermittent mandatory ventilation (IMV). There are spontaneous breaths between machine breaths. The baseline is above zero. The machine breaths are an equal distance apart and occur regardless of what phase of the respiratory cycle the patient is in during the spontaneous breath. CPAP or PEEP can also be achieved with synchronized intermittent mandatory ventilation (SIMV) on some ventilators, so that the patient still triggers the machine breath and the baseline remains above ambient.

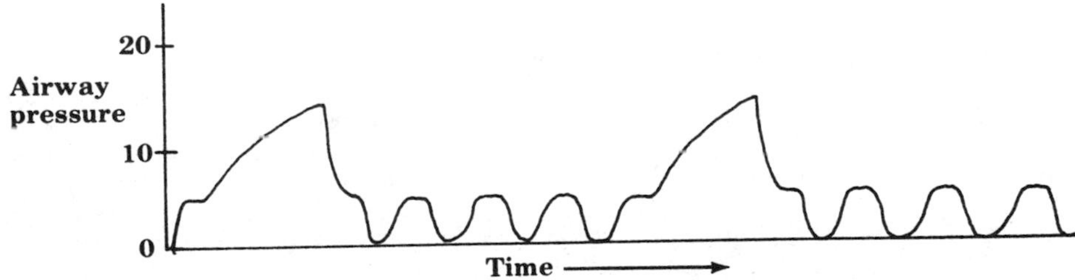

FIG 5–44.
Another way in which positive end-expiratory pressure (PEEP) is used with intermittent mandatory ventilation (IMV). Here the expiratory pressures are always positive (EPAP) and the inspiratory pressure on spontaneous breaths is below zero. This is also called IMV with EPAP.

TABLE 5–7.
Ventilator Classification Examples*†

Ventilator	Power Source	Circuitry	Control Mechanism	Control Variable
Infant				
BEAR BP-200	Pneumatic	Single	Electronic	P ⎍ Flow ⎍
Bear Cub (BP-2001)	Pneumatic	Single	Electronic	P ⎍ Flow ⎍
Baby Bird	Pneumatic	Single	Pneumatic	P ⎍ Flow ⎍
Sechrist IV-100B	Pneumatic	Single	Fluidic/electronic	P ⎍ Flow ⎍
Pediatric/adult				
Adult Star	Pneumatic	Single	Electronic	P ⎍ Flow ⟍ ⎍ ⟋ ∩
Bear 1	Pneumatic	Single	Electronic	Flow ⎍ ⟍
Bear 2	Pneumatic	Single	Electronic	Flow ⎍ ⟍
Bear 5	Pneumatic	Single	Electronic	P ⎍ Flow ⎍ ⟍ ⟋ ∩
Puritan Bennett MA-1	Electric	Double	Electronic	Volume ⟋
Puritan Bennett MA-2	Electric	Double	Electronic	Volume ⟋
Puritan Bennett 7200ae	Pneumatic	Single	Electronic	P ⎍ Flow ⎍ ⟍ ∩
Bird Mark 7 and 8	Pneumatic	Single	Pneumatic	Flow ⎍ 100% O_2 ⟍ on air mix
Bird 6400	Pneumatic	Single	Electronic	P ⎍ Flow ⟍ ⎍
Emerson 3-PV	Electric	Single	Electronic	P ∫ Flow ∩
IMV Emerson	Electric	Single	Electronic	P ∫ Flow ∩
Engström Erica	Pneumatic	Single	Electronic	Flow ⎍ ⟍ ⟋
Hamilton Veolar	Pneumatic	Single	Electronic	P ⎍ Flow ⎍ ⟍ ⟋ ∩
Irisa (PPG Biomedical)	Pneumatic	Single	Electronic	P ⎍ Flow ⎍ ⟍
Newport Wave E200	Pneumatic	Single	Electronic	P ⎍ Flow ⟍ ⎍
Siemens Servo 900C§	Pneumatic	Single	Electronic	P ⎍ Flow ⎍ ⟍
Siemens Servo 300§	Pneumatic	Single	Electronic	P ⎍ Flow ⎍ ⟍

*Data from reference 4, 6, 15.
†T = time; P = pressure; V = volume; C = control; AC = assist-control; IP = inspiratory pause; PS = pressure support; PC = pressure control; IMV = intermittent mandatory ventilation; SIMV = synchronized intermittent mandatory ventilation; APRV = airway pressure release ventilation; MMV = mandatory minute ventilation; PEEP = positive end-expiratory pressure; CPAP = continuous positive airway pressure;
‡CMV = controlled mechanical ventilation; sigh = periodic deep breaths.
§Neonates to adults.

Trigger Initiating Inspiration	*Limit* Inspiratory Phase Limit	*Cycle* Ending Inspiration	Modes
T	P/flow	T	IMV, PEEP, CPAP, IP
T	P/flow	T	IMV, PEEP, CPAP
T	P/flow	T	IMV, PEEP, CPAP
T	P/flow	T	IMV, PEEP, CPAP
P/T	P/flow/V/T	P/T/flow	C, AC, SIMV, PEEP, CPAP, IP, sigh, PS, PC
P/T	V/flow	V/P/T	C, AC, SIMV, PEEP, CPAP, IP
P/T	V/flow	P/V/T cycled	C, AC, SIMV, PEEP, CPAP, IP
P/T	P/V/flow	P/V/flow, T	C, AC, SIMV, PEEP, CPAP, IP, sigh, PS, MMV
T/P	V/flow	V	C, A, C, PEEP, sigh
T/P	V/flow	V	C, AC, SIMV, PEEP, CPAP, sigh
T/P/F	P/V/T/ flow	V/P/T/flow	C, AC, SIMV, PEEP, CPAP, sigh, IP, PS, PC, flow-by
P/T	P/flow	P	C, AC
P/T	P	V/flow/T/P	C, AC, SIMV, sigh, CPAP, IP, PS
T	P/V/flow	T	Simple CMV
P/T	P/V/flow	T	IMV, PEEP, CPAP
F/T	Flow	V/P/T	C, AC, SIMV, PEEP, CPAP, IP, sigh, PS, MMV
P/T	P/V/flow	P, flow, V, T	C, AC, SIMV, sigh, PEEP, CPAP, PS, PC, IP, MMV
P/T	P/flow/V	P/T/flow	C, AC, SIMV, PEEP, CPAP, IP, PS, PC, APRV, MMV
P/T	P/V/flow	P/T/flow	C, AC, SIMV, PEEP, CPAP, IP, PS, PC, SIMV with PC and PS, bias flow, sigh
P/T	P/V/flow	P/flow/T	C, AC, SIMV, PEEP, CPAP, IP, sigh, PS, PC
P/T/flow	P/V	T/P/flow/V	C, AC, SIMV, PEEP, CPAP, IP, PS, PC, volume support, pressure-regulated volume control

separate methods or modes, both of which help to improve oxygenation in patients with refractory hypoxemia. One method is referred to as continuous positive airway pressure (CPAP), which is continuous spontaneous breathing at pressures above ambient to improve oxygenation (Fig 5–39). Another form of CPAP is expiratory positive airway pressure (EPAP) (Fig 5–40). A third is bilevel positive end-expiratory pressure (PEEP), sometimes is referred to as BiPAP, which was named after a device that can deliver bilevel PEEP (Fig 5–41).

The second mode, PEEP, is pressure at the airway above ambient at the end of expiration. While its purest definition states that the use of PEEP can be either during spontaneous or mechanical ventilation, the more popular usage of the term PEEP implies its use with a mechanical ventilator (Figs 5–42, 5–43, and 5–44). CPAP and PEEP theoretically help to prevent early airway closure or alveolar collapse, or both, at the end of expiration by increasing the FRC of the lungs. This allows for better oxygen exchange at the alveolar-capillary membranes.

It is important to point out here that none of these techniques provide "ventilation." They can only be used to improve oxygenation.

Summary

The discussion on cycling mechanisms and the functional operating modes in various mechanical ventilators has relied heavily on theoretical descriptions. The assumption is also made that resistance and compliance in a patient do not change during a breathing cycle although this is not always true in clinical situations. This material attempts to summarize and simplify some of the characteristics of ventilators and how their function relates to patient lung compliance and airway resistance changes. It is hoped, this will help improve the understanding of the patient-ventilator interaction as the discussion turns to some of the practical problems related to the effects of positive pressure ventilation. Table 5–7 gives the classification of several types of ventilators.

STUDY QUESTIONS

Match the drive mechanism with the ventilator at the right.

1. ____ Spring-loaded bellows.	a. Emerson.
2. ____ Blower (compressor).	b. PR-2.
3. ____ High pressure gas source.	c. Bird Mark 7 on air mix.
4. ____ Venturi entrainer.	d. Monaghan 225/SIMV.
5. ____ Pressure-reducing valve.	e. MA-1.
6. ____ Weighted bellows.	f. Servo 900.
7. ____ Rotary piston.	g. Gill 1.
8. ____ Linear drive piston.	h. Bourns LS-104

9. Define the function of an output control valve.
10. Name two examples of different types of output control valves.
11. What are the primary functional parts of a patient or external circuit?
12. List the three most frequently used methods of triggering inspiration.
13. Describe APRV.
14. Define a pressure controller.
15. What are the five basic waveforms used for flow delivery?
16. In a constant flow controller, what would happen to PIP, P_{TA}, and P_A if a patient's lung compliance were to decrease?
17. In a ventilator with a low to moderate driving pressure, like the MA-1, what would happen to the flow waveform if a patient's lung compliance were to decrease significantly and the Raw were to increase significantly?
18. What effect would reaching a pressure limit have on a time-cycled ventilator?
19. Define PEEP.
20. Classify the BEAR 2 ventilator.

ANSWERS TO STUDY QUESTIONS

1. f.
2. e.
3. d.
4. c.
5. b.
6. g.
7. a.
8. h.
9. The output control valve interacts with the drive mechanism to determine the pattern of flow delivery.
10. Resistance-type or high resistance valve; proportional valve; stepper motor with valve; solenoid valve.
11. Main inspiratory line, patient airway connector with adapter (wye-connector), main expiratory line, expiratory valve, expiratory valve line.
12. Pressure, time, flow.
13. APRV, or airway pressure release ventilation, is a spontaneous breathing mode at a positive baseline with time-cycled release to lower pressure levels that allows the lungs to passively deflate.
14. A pressure controller keeps the same pattern of pressure at the mouth regardless of changes in patient lung conditions. It can be constant or nonconstant.
15. Rectangular, sinusoidal, ascending ramp, descending ramp, and exponential.

16. PIP would increase, P_{TA} would stay the same, and P_A would increase.
17. The flow would decelerate slightly.
18. The ventilator would not deliver all the volume intended because the pressure limit would be reached, and excess pressure would vent to the room until the ventilator were finally time-cycled into exhalation.
19. PEEP, or positive end-expiratory pressure, is a positive pressure exerted during exhalation which results in a baseline pressure above zero.
20. The BEAR 2 is a pneumatically powered, single-circuit, electronically controlled ventilator. Flow waves can be rectangular or in the shape of a descending ramp. It can be pressure- or time-triggered, flow- or volume-limited, and pressure-, volume-, or time-cycled. It offers PEEP, CPAP, and inspiratory pause.

REFERENCES

1. Bendixon HH, Egbert LD, Hedley-Whyte J: *Respiratory Care.* St Louis, Mosby–Year Book, Inc, 1965.
2. Bone RC: Monitoring respiratory function in the patient with adult respiratory distress syndrome. *Semin Respir Med.* 1981; 2–140.
3. Branson RD: Enhanced capabilities of current ICU ventilators: Do they really benefit patients? *Respir Care* 1991; 36:362–376.
4. Burton GG, Hodgkin JE, Ward JJ: *Respiratory Care: A Guide to Clinical Practice.* Philadelphia, JB Lippincott Co, 1991.
5. Chatburn RL: Dynamic respiratory mechanics. *Respir Care* 1986; 31:703–711.
6. Chatburn RL: *Classification of Mechanical Ventilators.* Dallas, American Association for Respiratory Care, 1988.
7. Chatburn RL: A new system for understanding mechanical ventilators. *Respir Care* 1991; 36:1123–1155.
8. Demers R: Mechanical ventilation wave patterns. *Curr Rev Respir Ther* 1980; 2:80–81.
9. Desautels D: Ventilator classification: A new look at an old subject. *Curr Rev Respir Ther* 1979; 1:81–88.
10. Dupuis YG: *Ventilators. Theory and Clinical Application.* St Louis, Mosby–Year Book, Inc, 1986.
11. Freeman C, Cicerchia E, Demers RR, et al: Static compliance, static effective compliance, and dynamic effective compliance as indicators of elastic recoil in the presence of lung disease. *Respir Care* 1976; 21:323–326.
12. Fuleihan SF, Wilson RS, Pontoppidan H: Effect of mechanical ventilation with end-inspiratory pause on blood-gas exchange. *Anesth Analg* 1976; 55:122–130.
13. Kirby RR, Banner MJ, Downs JB: *Clinical Applications of Ventilatory Support.* New York, Churchill Livingstone Inc, 1990.
14. Lindahl S: Influence of an end inspiratory pause on pulmonary ventilation, gas distribution and lung perfusion during artificial ventilation. *Crit Care Med* 1979; 7:540–545.

15. McPherson SP, Spearman CB. *Respiratory Therapy Equipment,* St Louis, Mosby–Year Book, Inc, 1990.
16. Mushin WW, Rendell-Baker L, Thompson PW, et al: *Automatic Ventilation of the Lungs.* Philadelphia, FA Davis Co, 1980.
17. Scanlan CL, Spearman CB, Sheldon RL: Egan's Fundamentals of Respiratory Therapy, ed 5. St Louis, Mosby–Year Book, 1990.
18. Spearman CB, Sheldon RI, Egan DH: *Egan's Fundamentals of Respiratory Therapy,* ed 4. St Louis, Mosby–Year Book, Inc. 1982.
19. Sullivan M, Saklad M, Demers RR: Relationship between ventilator waveform and tidal-volume distribution. *Respir Care* 1977; 2:386–393.

Chapter 6

Selecting Modes and Initial Settings

On completion of this chapter the reader will be able to:

1. Select the appropriate type of ventilator and mode or method of ventilation for a patient.
2. Calculate initial tidal volume, rate, minute ventilation, and F_{IO_2} settings.
3. Choose an appropriate flow rate and pattern.
4. Determine the I/E ratio from total cycle time and inspiratory time.
5. Calculate the expiratory time from the total cycle time and inspiratory time.
6. Determine the inspiratory time from tidal volume and flow.
7. Determine tidal volume from inspiratory time and flow.
8. Calculate flow from tidal volume and inspiratory time.
9. Estimate appropriate alarm settings.
10. List the considerations necessary in preparing the final ventilator setup.
11. Describe the steps in beginning ventilatory support.

SELECTING MODES AND INITIAL SETTINGS

With a basic understanding of the functional capabilities of various mechanical ventilators, we now discuss initiating ventilatory support on a patient in acute respiratory failure. The decisions that need to be made are:

1. What type of ventilator to select—positive or negative pressure?
2. Which mode or method of ventilation is appropriate?
3. How should minute ventilation ($\dot{V}_E$), tidal volume (V_T), and rate be set?

4. What other parameters are important?
5. How can the patient be prepared for the experience?

VENTILATOR SELECTION

In picking the appropriate type of ventilator, one must consider negative vs. positive pressure and high-frequency ventilation vs. normal rates.

Negative Pressure Ventilators

Negative pressure ventilators, such as the iron lung, have the advantage of being durable, easy to use, and dependable. They also can provide ventilation to a patient without requiring an artificial airway. Some of the other advantages are that patients can speak, eat, and drink. Complications associated with artificial airways are also avoided. Tank ventilators have several disadvantages. They are cumbersome, large, and make bronchial drainage and intravenous therapy difficult to accomplish. In some patients, negative pressure applied to the abdominal area, as well as the thorax, results in a pooling of blood in the abdominal vasculature. This leads to a reduction in venous return to the heart and subsequent reduction in cardiac output. If a patient has excessive secretions or has a depressed (obtunded) epiglottic reflex response, then airway management becomes a problem and requires an artificial airway.

Since most tank ventilators are controllers, they do not allow for spontaneous breathing efforts from the patient. Tidal volume is predetermined by the amount of negative pressure applied over the thoracic area as well as the compliance and resistance characteristics of the lung. Tidal volume must be measured on the patient during setup and monitoring. Regulation of V_T and rate allows for little or no physiologic adjustment to the patient's spontaneous efforts or needs.

The chest cuirass type of negative ventilator partially compensates for some of these problems. The cuirass is a rigid shell that is placed over the patient's chest and also touches the upper abdomen. There is a space between the shell and the chest wall. The design restricts most of the negative pressure to the thoracic area. Some models have an assist mode that functions by sensing a patient's flow or pressure pattern at the nostrils. Slight changes in airflow during a patient's inspiratory effort are sensed or detected by the ventilator and an assist breath is accomplished.

Problems of leaking around the chest used to occur with older sealing materials. The use of plastic wrapping around the shell (cuirass) has helped to eliminate this problem. In addition, specially designed shells have been developed for ventilator patients with severe kyphoscoliosis.[100] The chest cuirass is still used in some patients with respiratory failure caused by neurologic problems, but whose lungs are otherwise normal.[41] Negative pressure ventilators are also used as night ventilation in cases where the primary cause of alveolar hypoventilation is due to the absence of a central drive to breathe, leading to nocturnal apnea.[67] This nighttime use is also beneficial to some patients with chronic obstructive pulmonary disease (COPD).[22]

For patients with normal lungs who are hypoventilating as a result of neurologic causes, particularly during the night, the negative pressure ventilator may be the ventilator of choice for maintaining adequate gas exchange.[41, 101]

Positive Pressure Ventilators

The greatest selection of ventilators by far are those which provide inspiration through positive pressures at the upper airway. There are two basic types. First, there are those that control volume. In general, these operate as flow generators. Second, there are the simple pressure-cycled ventilators, such as the Bird Mark 7, which are usually used for intermittent positive pressure breathing (IPPB) aerosol treatments.

Flow Generators.—The constant flow or nonconstant flow generators have the advantage of being able to provide a constant V_T regardless of changes in patient lung characteristics. These types of ventilators are usually volume-cycled or time-cycled. Ventilation, oxygenation, and compliance are better maintained in constant V_T ventilators as compared to pressure-cycled ventilators. They are usually very sophisticated and have extensive alarm systems and additional options. These are recommended for use in all types of patient situations. These ventilators generally require an electrical source and at least one compressed gas source, if not two. Sometimes they can be purchased with a built-in compressor that provides the compressed gas source.

The most recent generation of microprocessor ventilators can operate as flow or pressure generators. They can provide not only assist-control ventilation, synchronized intermittent mandatory ventilation (SIMV), positive end-expiratory pressure (PEEP) or continuous positive airway pressure (CPAP), and inflation hold, but some also have pressure support, pressure control, and mandatory minute ventilation (MMV). Many also provide a variety of flow patterns including constant flow, sine wave, and descending and ascending ramps.

Pressure Generators.—The constant pressure, pressure-cycled machines such as the Mark 7, have generating pressures that are approximately equal to the pressure that is finally delivered to the patient. As a result, the amount of volume that is delivered during each breath is dependent upon the characteristics of the patient's lungs, and the patient's inspiratory demand. Volume can change breath by breath. This should be kept in mind when selecting this type of ventilator for continuous use. In addition, most descending flow ventilators that are pressure-cycled, like the Mark 7, do not have accessories for PEEP, inflation hold, sigh modes, intermittent mandatory ventilation (IMV), adjustments for fractional concentration of oxygen in inspired gas (F_{IO_2}), or alarm systems. All of these capabilities must be added.

There are some distinct advantages in using the descending flow pattern present in most constant pressure, pressure-cycled ventilators. In patients with obstructed airways, a descending flow pattern is more likely to deliver set V_T at a lower pressure and provide for better distribution of air throughout the lung than a ventilator with a constant flow or an ascending flow. This is especially true if the ventilator has a flow-sensitive valve (like the Bennett valve) that adjusts automatically to changes in lung characteristics. Some studies have shown that one drawback to the pressure-cycled descending flow ventilator is that the mean airway pressure is likely to be higher than the mean airway pressure in a constant flow ventilator delivering a small volume.[7] This may increase the risks of complications associated with positive pressure ventilators.

Additional advantages of these ventilators are that they tend to be small and portable, require no electricity, operate from compressed gas, and have leak-compensating mechanisms. They are of value in patient transport and for use in ambulatory patients who are dependent on continuous ventilator support. The pressure-cycled ventilator is most appropriate for use during emergency situations or for short-term ventilation in the postoperative patient who is slow to recover from anesthesia, or for short-term transport situations.

High-Frequency Ventilators

Reports suggest that this modality may be beneficial during intraoperative procedures such as laryngoscopy and bronchoscopy, as well as for ventilation in patients with interrupted airway disease such as bronchopleural fistula. Use of high-frequency ventilation in adults has been limited primarily to research or experimental situations. This mode of ventilation is used most often in infants.

FULL (TOTAL) VENTILATORY SUPPORT AND PARTIAL VENTILATORY SUPPORT

Full ventilatory support (FVS) and partial ventilatory support (PVS) are terms that can be used to describe the extent of mechanical ventilation that is being provided. FVS was defined by Shapiro and Cane.[95] FVS is represented by two components. First, the ventilator provides all the energy necessary to maintain effective alveolar ventilation. Second, since ventilator rates of 8 or more breaths/min and V_T values of 12 to 15 mL/kg will result in partial pressure of carbon dioxide in arterial blood ($Pa{CO_2}$) values of less than 45 mm Hg in almost all patients, we can define mechanical rates of 8 or more breaths/min and V_T of 12 to 15 mL/kg as FVS. PVS is any amount of mechanical ventilation less than this in which the patient is participating in the work of breathing that helps maintain effective alveolar ventilation.

FVS is provided by use of the control mode, assist-control, IMV or SIMV, or pressure control. These modes must be set so that the patient will receive adequate alveolar ventilation regardless of whether or not he or she breathes spontaneously.[83] PVS can also use any mode of ventilation, but the patient, by definition, will be actively participating in ventilation to adequate levels of $Pa{CO_2}$.

SELECTING MODES AND METHODS OF VENTILATION

The various methods by which a patient can be ventilated are discussed in Chapter 5. This section deals with how to decide which method is best for the particular clinical situation. In acute respiratory failure, the initial goal is to supply all the necessary ventilation (FVS) while allowing the ventilatory muscles time to rest.[64, 65] After 3 to 4 days the patient will hopefully be stabilized and beginning to recover. Maintaining complete rest after reasonable recovery can result in muscle wasting or atrophy. At this time the patient can begin doing part of the work of breathing (PVS), other factors being stable.[64, 65]

Controlled Ventilation

The use of controlled ventilation (time cycling into inspiration) is appropriate only when a patient is making no effort at ventilating. It is probably never appropriate to "lock out" a patient by making the ventilator totally insensitive to patient effort.[53] Patients that are obtunded because of drugs, cerebral malfunction, spinal cord or phrenic nerve injury, or motor nerve paralysis may have no voluntary ventilations. Controlled ventilation may be used to support these patients.

In other types of patients, controlled mechanical ventilation is difficult to use unless the patient is paralyzed or sedated with medications or is being deliberately hyperventilated to suppress ventilation. On controlled ventilation, an inspiratory effort will *not* produce a machine-delivered breath. The patient will not be breathing in synchrony with the ventilator. To prevent the patient from "fighting the machine," mild respiratory alkalosis must be maintained or spontaneous ventilation must be suppressed with medications. This is not usually indicated.

In rare situations it may be appropriate to paralyze and sedate a patient and use control if seizure activity or sustained contractions, as occur with tetanus, cannot be prevented. Deliberate hyperventilation and controlled ventilation may be needed to induce respiratory alkalosis to decrease intracranial pressure (ICP), e.g., in patients with closed head injury or after neurosurgery where ICP is elevated. Paralyzing a patient has the risk that if the patient becomes disconnected he or she will be totally apneic. It is essential that these patients have adequate alarms and monitors connected to them.

Perhaps the safest use of controlled ventilation is in the IMV mode. The IMV mode is similar to the control mode in that the time-triggering mechanism from the ventilator determines the mandatory ventilator breath. The desired volume and rate can be set, but the patient will be able to breathe spontaneously if the ventilatory drive returns. Technically, if the ventilator is doing all the work of breathing, even if the IMV mode is dialed in, the patient is on FVS.

Assisted and Assist-Control Ventilation

If the patient is making some effort to breathe, then an assist mode of ventilation can be used. Assist triggering occurs because the ventilator is sensitive to pressure changes when the patient attempts to take in a breath. When the slightly negative pressure is sensed by the ventilator (usually set at approximately -1 to -2 cm H_2O), the inspiratory cycle begins. If a patient must initiate all breaths, it is called assisted ventilation.

One of the hazards of assisted ventilation is that the patient might not make an inspiratory effort. By setting a minimum control rate on the ventilator, this guarantees a minimum minute ventilation ($\dot{V}_E$) and the patient can breathe additionally if desired. This mode is referred to as assist-control. With assisted or assist-control ventilation, every breath is a positive pressure breath.

It was previously thought that with assisted ventilation, the ventilator provided nearly all the work of breathing. It is now known that the patient must do 33% to 50% of the work of inspiration.[60,70] If inspiration is active and the preset flow rate does not match that of the patient's, then the work of breathing will be even higher.

Another problem is sensitivity. If the machine is overly sensitive to patient effort, rapid machine cycling will result. This can be corrected by making the machine less sensitive to patient effort, i.e., having a more negative pressure required to trigger a machine-delivered breath. Conversely, if an inspiratory effect gives a manometer reading of -3 to -10 cm H_2O or more below the baseline, the machine is too insensitive to the patient's effort and the sensitivity must be increased. If auto-PEEP or trapped air is present (see Chapter 7), the patient may have to take a deep inspiration to overcome undetected PEEP levels plus the -1 cm H_2O of set sensitivity to trigger the machine breath. Under these conditions, it is even more difficult to adjust sensitivity and the cause of the problem can go undetected unless auto-PEEP is measured.

Without respiratory depressants, muscle relaxants, or sedatives, it is hard to prevent respiratory alkalosis on assist-control ventilation. During assisted ventilation with large V_T values, the Pa_{CO_2} will be close to the apneic threshold and alkalosis cannot be avoided.[27] In humans, Pa_{CO_2} levels of 32 mm Hg are considered the apneic threshold. Above 32 mm Hg, respirations are likely to occur.[26]

Assisted or assist-control ventilation is widely used as a primary mode of support. It is often selected in patients who have spontaneous effort. However, as further research investigates the benefits of pressure support, pressure control, and IMV or SIMV, these modes may become more frequently used.

Intermittent (IMV) and Synchronized Intermittent Mandatory Ventilation (SIMV)

The IMV or SIMV mode of ventilation may be selected if it is desirable for the patient to be able to breathe spontaneously without receiving a positive pressure breath. This mode can be set at either full support or partial support. The advantage is that the patient may be able to retain a certain amount of ventilatory muscle strength, since not all breaths are supported by the ventilator. When supported by PVS, patients also tend to maintain a Pa_{CO_2} near normal as they gradually begin to take over some of the work of breathing.

During SIMV, the patient breathes spontaneously between positive pressure breaths. Mandatory (volume- or pressure-controlled) breaths are triggered after a certain time has passed and when the patient makes an inspiratory effort (pressure triggering). If the patient never breathes in, a mandatory breath is delivered.

The IMV and SIMV modes of ventilation have the potential for fewer cardiovascular side effects since portions of the $\dot{V}_E$ may occur at ambient pressure. IMV and SIMV can also be used in weaning patients from mechanical ventilation (see Chapter 12). As the mandatory rate is reduced, the patient assumes a greater part of the work of breathing.

All the modes of ventilation mentioned so far (assisted, controlled, IMV/SIMV) are useful in treating respiratory acidosis and can help to provide adequate alveolar ventilation. With assisted or assist-control ventilation, patients are more likely to breathe spontaneously and trigger the ventilator until Pa_{CO_2} values approach the apneic threshold and are maintained at this level.[26] The IMV and SIMV modes of ventilation can provide needed mechanical support while allowing patients to breathe without assistance and maintain their own Pa_{CO_2}. This can help avoid mild respiratory alkalosis without medications. However, breathing through a ventilator circuit and an endotracheal (ET) tube during a spontaneous breath will add to the work of breathing. Thus, both modes require that the patient continue to do some work of breathing.

PRESSURE CONTROL AND PRESSURE SUPPORT

History

Since the mid 1960s and up to the 1990s there has been basically one mode of ventilation preferred for adults—volume-cycled or volume-controlled ventilation. In the late 1980s the introduction of microprocessor ventilators paralleled two new modes of ventilation: pressure-supported (PSV) and pressure-controlled ventilation (PCV).

Pressure Control.—The first use of pressure-control or pressure-limited ventilation began in the early 1970s. It was used at that time as a means of improving oxygenation in neonates with infant respiratory distress syndrome and was used with an inverse inspiratory-expiratory (I/E) ratio.[90] In the 1980s pressure-controlled inverse ratio ventilation (PCIRV) was made available on the Siemens Servo 900C ventilator for adult use. Since that time, PCV has received some attention in the literature. Other adult ventilators now have it as an added feature, e.g., the Hamilton Veolar and the Puritan Bennett 7200ae.

Pressure Support.—PSV originally appeared in 1981 as part of the Engström Erica and the Servo 900C ventilators before any articles had appeared in the literature about its use.[45, 49, 50] Two of the earliest reports in the North American literature were by MacIntyre in 1986.[61, 62] PSV is very similar to the flow-cycled, pressure-limited ventilation seen with the PR-2 ventilator.[12] In fact, the respiratory and hemodynamic effects of the two modes are very similar.[73]

Technology

Ventilators set for pressure support or pressure control function as pressure generators. PCV and PSV provide a constant pressure at the airway. The operator sets the desired pressure limit for either mode and the inspiratory time and rate for pressure control. The resulting flow curve is a descending ramp (Fig 6–1). This is an advantage since this flow curve has been shown to improve gas distribution.[2, 7, 45, 49, 50]

In PCV, V_T delivery varies with compliance, resistance, PIP (pressure limit), inspiratory time, and probably auto-PEEP levels.[48] With PSV, V_T varies with compliance, resistance, PIP, and the degree of patient effort.

PCV is time-cycled. Inspiration ends at a predetermined time. PSV is flow-cycled, that is, inspiration ends at a certain flow rate. In addition, PSV is always an assist mode of ventilation, pressure-triggered by the patient into inspiration. PCV is usually a control mode (time-triggered) with a set rate and inspiratory time determined by the operator. It can also be an assist mode when the patient is allowed to breathe spontaneously and sensitivity is set.

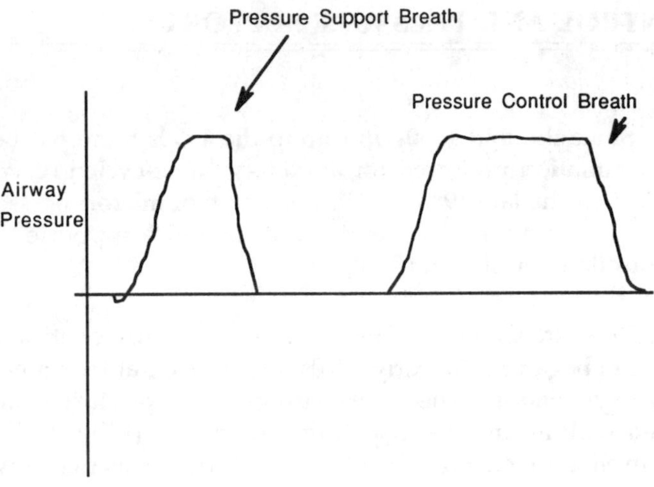

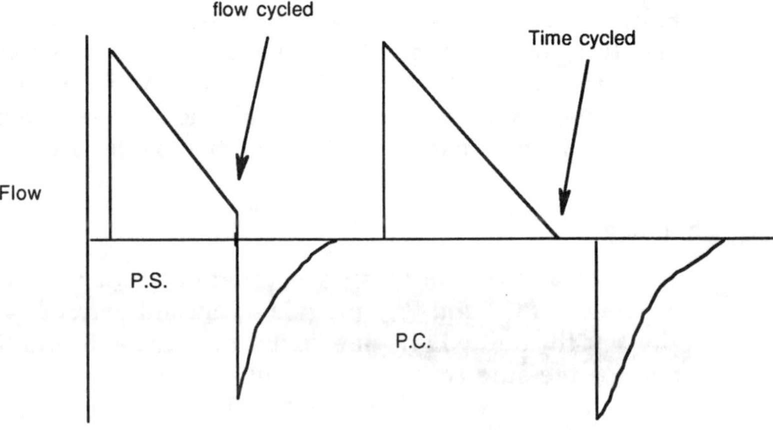

FIG 6–1.
Comparison of a pressure-supported *(P.S.)* breath and a pressure-controlled *(P.C.)* breath showing airway pressure and flow curves and cycling mechanism.

One of the advantages of PSV or PCV is that flow to the patient is not preset. The patient can vary the inspiratory flow of gas on demand. In conventional volume-controlled ventilation, if the patient actively inspires, there is a noticeable drop of the pressure curve during inspiration. This increases the patient's work of breathing. The patient is actively breathing in, but the flow to the patient is predetermined by the set flow rate (Fig 6–2). PSV and PCV technology allow a demand flow to occur as the patient actively inspires. The ventilator does this in order to maintain the preset pressure. Some ventilators, like the Engström Erica, provide for adjustable flow rates with PSV or PCV. This may be an advantage for patients with high or low flow demands and may help improve patient-ventilatory synchrony and reduce the work of breathing[13] (Fig 6–3).

Pressure Support Ventilation (PSV)

Indications.—Since PSV is a fairly new mode of ventilation, indications for its use have not yet been established by scientific investigation. Its use, on the other hand, is very widespread. For this reason, the current acceptable indications are reviewed. PSV is discussed in greater detail in Chapter 12. PSV is used for three basic functions. First, it may be used with CPAP or in any spontaneously breathing patient with an ET tube in place. In this case it is used to overcome the work of demand valve systems, and the resistance of the ventilator circuit and endotracheal tube. Second, PSV can be used with IMV or SIMV for the spontaneous breaths to eliminate the same system resistance. This allows

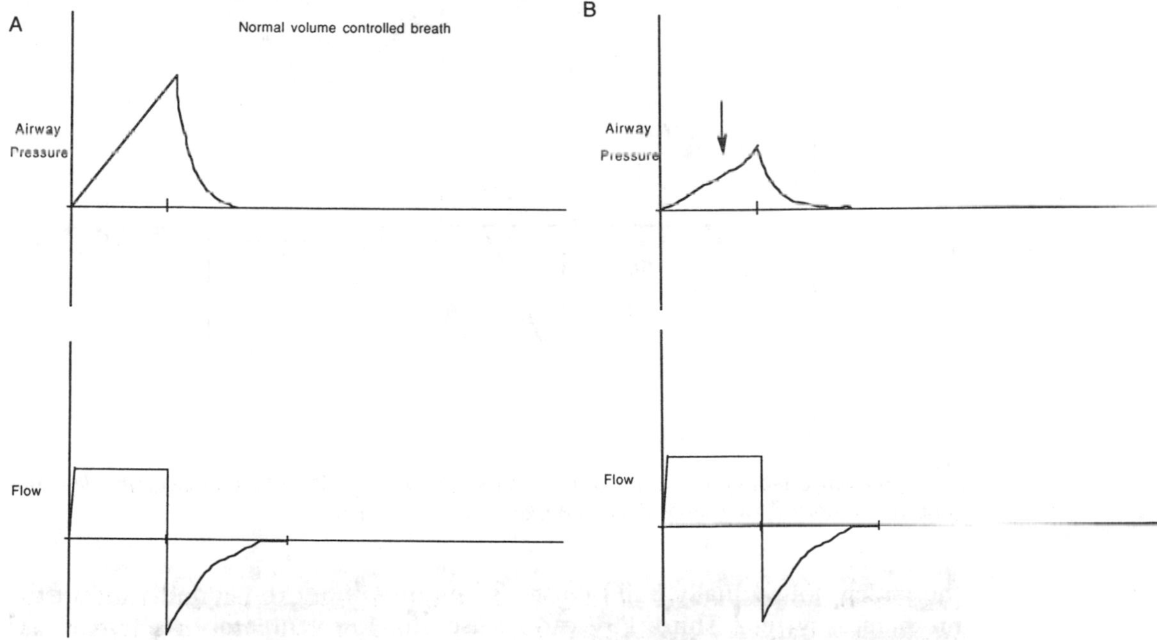

FIG 6–2.
A, a normal volume-controlled breath showing airway pressure and flow curves. **B,** a volume-controlled breath in which flow is inadequate to meet the patient's demands.

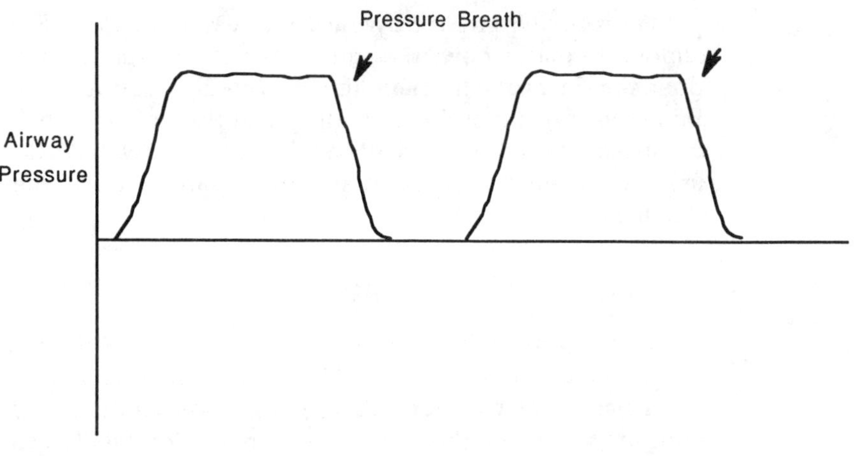

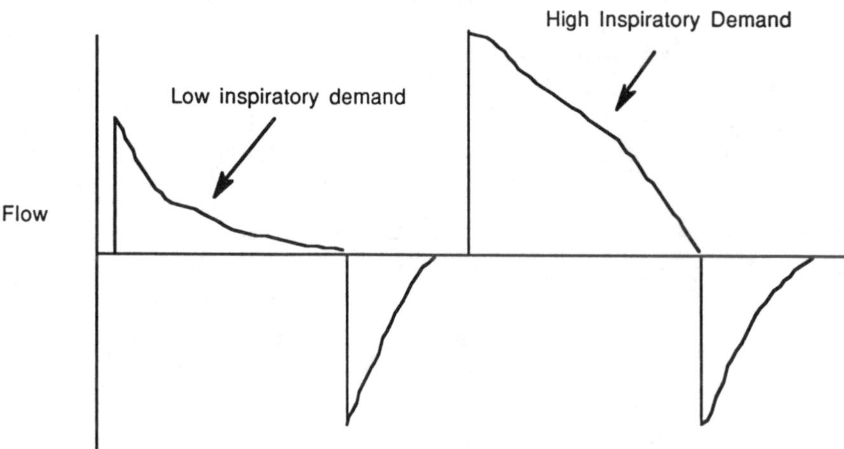

FIG 6–3.
Pressure-controlled ventilation showing low inspiratory flow demand on the *left* and high inspiratory flow demand on the *right.*

the patient to gradually build muscle strength without the added work of the mechanical system. Third, PSV can be used for full ventilatory support in the assist mode where each patient breath is a pressure-supported breath. In this use the patient must have a dependable and intact respiratory center and fairly stable lung condition, or V_T can vary. This is referred to as PSVmax.[64, 65]

When used as partial ventilatory support, IMV plus PSV can effectively remove the added work of breathing of the demand valve system, ventilator circuit, and ET tube. For a patient on CPAP or one who just needs the tube in for airway management, again, the pressure support level can be adjusted to a level to overcome the ET tube resistance. At full ventilatory support, PSVmax is used only in patients with active ventilatory drive and stable, if abnormal, lung conditions.

A patient with absent or depressed respiratory drive or a patient with impaired neuromuscular respiratory function may be able to perform little or no spontaneous ventilatory work without going into respiratory failure. Controlled ventilation is appropriate in these cases[54] and PSV is *not.*

Setting PSV With IMV or SIMV or With CPAP With Spontaneous Breathing.—When PSV is used with IMV or SIMV or with CPAP with spontaneous breathing through an ET tube, pressure support is set at a level required to prevent a fatiguing workload on the respiratory muscles. Some recommend calculation of pressure support from bedside estimation of total ventilatory system resistance (R) (patient plus circuit): R = Ppeak − Pplateau/flow during intermittent positive pressure ventilation (IPPV) with constant flow.[45, 49, 50]

Setting PSVmax.—For PSVmax the pressure is set at a level high enough to provide a V_T of 10 to 12 mL/kg. This may reach as high as 40 cm H_2O, but rarely exceeds 50 cm H_2O.

Additional information about PSV, including technical aspects and complications, are presented in Chapter 12.

Pressure Control Ventilation (PCV)

Use of PCV.—PCV is used as a control mode with a normal I/E ratio, as a control mode with inverse I/E ratios (Fig 6–4), or as an assist mode or in combination with PSV. In the last, mandatory timed machine breaths are pressure-controlled breaths. In between these timed breaths, patient effort receives a pressure-supported breath. At present, the primary indication for pressure control is for ventilatory support of patients with adult respiratory distress syndrome (ARDS) in whom conventional IPPV with PEEP does not seem to be effective.[5, 35, 37] Some institutions are also beginning to select pressure control as an option when PIP on IPPV is very high ($>$60 cm H_2O). PCV at normal I/E ratios has been shown to be able to improve oxygenation of patients when all other ventilating variables are kept constant.[1] Further studies are needed to confirm these findings.

Selection Criteria.—Specific criteria generally include patients on an F_{IO_2} of 1.0, a PIP of 50 cm H_2O or higher, PEEP levels of 15 cm H_2O or higher, high

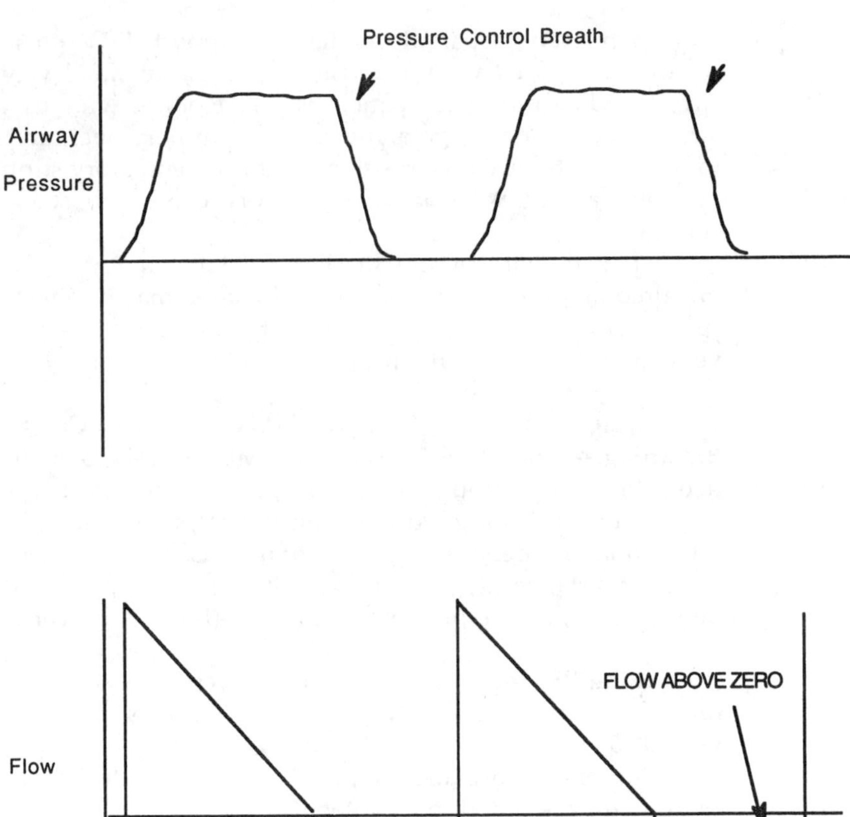

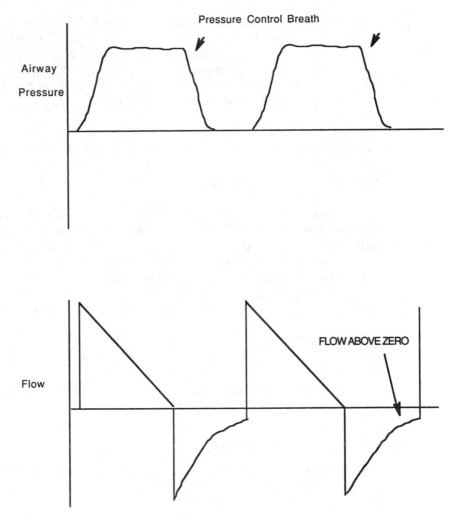

FIG 6–4.
Pressure-controlled ventilation with inverse ratio. The expiratory flow does not return to zero at the end of exhalation. The breath is time-cycled. As a result, air trapping (auto-PEEP) is present in the patient's lungs.

assist-control rates ($\geq$16 breaths/min) with low partial pressure of oxygen (Pa_{O_2}) values and low lung compliance.[5, 36, 37, 56]

Initial Settings.—At present there is not enough well-established research to provide information on what are appropriate initial settings for PCV. Those that are most frequently used include the following: (1) an F_{IO_2} of 1.0, (2) a PIP of about one-half that on IPPV before starting PCV (readjust as needed), and (3) no

PEEP if it was less than 8 cm H_2O before PCV. If a PEEP of more than 8 cm H_2O was used before PCV, then about one-half the PEEP level is selected.[56] The starting PEEP needs to be lower since PCV with inverse I/E may add auto-PEEP. Some practitioners start the I/E ratio on PCV at conventional levels of 1:2 or less. Others start at 1:1 and increase the level progressively to as high as 4:1.[5, 37, 56]

Most patients on PCIRV are paralyzed and sedated because this mode of ventilation may be uncomfortable for the patient.[46] On the other hand, if PCV is not used with an inverse I/E ratio and the patient is permitted to assist, then paralysis and sedation may not be necessary.[1] Since PCV is a pressure-limited mode, exhaled VT may vary significantly. For this reason exhaled VT as well as rate need to be monitored. Most new ventilators have low exhaled volume and high rate settings which can be helpful.

Another consideration with PCIRV is that since intrinsic PEEP (auto-PEEP) will develop, alveolar pressures will rise. This is not detectable as an elevated baseline on the ventilator and must be measured specifically (see Chapter 7). Higher alveolar pressures will increase the driving pressure for exhalation. This can shorten expiratory time, which is not true with PEEP that is selected by the operator. Shorter expiratory times allow for longer inspiratory times. PCIRV will show a progressive drop in $\dot{V}$E as the more intrinsic PEEP is present. This is the reverse of volume-controlled ventilation, where PIP will rise and volume will stay constant as auto-PEEP increases. If the patient is in the assist mode with PCIRV, an additional workload is placed on the patient. It becomes more difficult to inhale deeply enough to trigger the sensitivity.

Results.—Pressure control, especially when used with an inverse I/E ratio, has been shown to increase oxygenation, improve gas exchange, reduce PIP, increase mean airway pressure, reduce the required applied PEEP, and reduce $\dot{V}$E.[1, 36, 37, 56, 104] PCIRV may also reduce the risk of barotrauma and cardiovascular side effects compared to IPPV with PEEP.[56]

PCIRV may also result in auto-PEEP when the inspiratory time is increased to a significant level.[6, 39, 40, 46] This is usually at an I/E level of more than 2:1.[68–70] Usually the presence of ARDS helps prevent air trapping at low I/E ratios. Under normal conditions an expiratory time of three to four times the patient's time constant for his or her lungs is required to avoid air trapping. ARDS usually results in short time constants so the lungs tend to empty quickly. Thus, shorter expiratory times can be used.

Auto-PEEP may be difficult to measure by routine clinical techniques. It can have grave clinical consequences when it goes unnoticed. Like all forms of positive pressure in the thorax, it can reduce venous return and cardiac output. Auto-PEEP may also increase the risk of barotrauma.[48]

Auto-PEEP during PCIRV can be detected by monitoring expiratory waveform curves (see Fig 6–4). Expiratory flow does not return to zero before another breath starts. Other methods of evaluating auto-PEEP are discussed in Chapter

7. If auto-PEEP is not measured, it will result in errors in the calculation of compliance.[93] It can also cause errors in reading hemodynamic data and affect cardiovascular pharmacologic treatment.[80] Auto-PEEP will also increase the amount of effort or pressure it takes for a patient to initiate a breath if he or she is assisting. This may be one reason why PCIRV is uncomfortable for the patient and requires paralysis and sedation.[48]

Assessment.—PCV, particularly PCIRV, is still experimental. For this reason, monitoring during PCV needs to be extensive. To evaluate the effectiveness and the effects of PCV the clinician needs to monitor V_T, respiratory frequency (f), $\dot{V}_E$, PIP, mean airway pressure, auto-PEEP and added (extrinsic) PEEP, lung compliance, end-tidal P_{CO_2} and the arterial-to-end-tidal P_{CO_2} gradient, arterial oxygen saturation (Sa_{O_2}) by oximetry, mixed venous partial pressure of oxygen ($P\bar{v}_{O_2}$), blood gases, heart rate, cardiac output, central venous pressure, pulmonary artery pressure, pulmonary capillary wedge pressure, systemic blood pressure, pulmonary vascular resistance, and urine output.

Mandatory Minute Ventilation (MMV)

MMV was first introduced in 1977. It is a method of ventilation that allows the operator to set a guaranteed $\dot{V}_E$ on the ventilator. Whatever part of the $\dot{V}_E$ that the patient does not complete, the ventilator provides for the patient. This need for ventilation can be provided either as a pressure-supported breath or in a preset volume breath, depending on the ventilator. At present it is not being extensively used. It is usually used in weaning patients and is discussed in Chapter 12.

PEEP AND CPAP

When a patient is in need of oxygenation, the clinician has the obvious choice of increasing the patient's F_{IO_2}. When the patient has refractory hypoxemia, stiff lungs, low functional residual capacity (FRC), and increased shunting in both lungs, then PEEP or CPAP offers another method to improve oxygenation. PEEP and CPAP were defined in Chapter 2 and are discussed extensively in Chapter 10.

AIRWAY PRESSURE RELEASE VENTILATION (APRV)

This method of ventilation is relatively new. At present it is only available on the Irisa ventilator. It is similar in the waveforms it creates to PCIRV. APRV requires a lower PIP but produces higher mean airway pressure ($\overline{P}aw$) than

PCIRV, other factors, such as arterial blood gas results and hemodynamic data, being equal.[15] Its use at the present time is experimental.

CYCLING OR LIMITING THE INSPIRATORY PHASE

Volume control ventilators have a pressure-limiting feature. If one wants to pressure-cycle rather than volume-cycle the machine into the expiratory phase, then this mode of ventilation can be selected simply by adjusting the pressure limit control. This prevents the pressure delivered from exceeding the preset amount. The more common practice, however, is to use the pressure-limiting feature as a safety mechanism so that a certain pressure cannot be exceeded during the inspiratory phase as the VT is being delivered. This reduces the risk of barotrauma. The pressure limit is usually set at 5 to 10 cm H_2O higher than is required to deliver the VT. Once the pressure limit is reached, the ventilator either ends the inspiratory phase or the excess pressure is vented into room air, depending on the type of ventilator used.

Another method of ending inspiration is by time cycling. When a ventilator is time-cycled, both volume or pressure, or both, can change during the preset time depending on changes in the compliance or resistance characteristics of the patient's lungs. In ventilators that are flow generators, the volume is constantly delivered so that a given volume is delivered in a specific timed interval. Time cycling in a flow generator will not interfere with volume delivery but pressure may vary under these circumstances with changes in lung characteristics. Time-cycled ventilators can also be pressure-limited to prevent undesirable high pressure during inspiration.

DETERMING INITIAL VENTILATOR SETTINGS

The patient setup of a mechanical ventilator requires several considerations. These include: $\dot{V}E$ settings (VT and rate), inspiratory gas flow, I/E ratio, pressure limit, oxygen concentration, sigh volumes and rates, inflation hold, expiratory retard, PEEP, humidity, gas temperature monitoring, and alarms.

Minute Ventilation and Tidal Volumes

Achieving a desired $\dot{V}E$ is a primary goal when establishing initial ventilator settings. Selecting the desired volumes and pressures depend on the type of ventilator selected. Tidal volume and rate are the primary determining factors in establishing the $\dot{V}E$ in most volume ventilators. Set pressure is the determining factor in establishing VT in pressure-limited ventilators.

Tidal Volume.—Studies have shown that with pressure-cycled ventilators like the PR-2, delivery of an acceptable VT (11–18 mL/kg) can be achieved in adults with preset pressures of about 20 to 25 cm H_2O.[32] Pressures in this range can be used as initial settings; values less than 40 cm H_2O are desirable. Once the patient has been connected to the ventilator, then VT and rate can be monitored to determine the patient's actual $\dot{V}E$. Arterial blood gas evaluation is required to further substantiate the adequacy of ventilation.

With volume-cycled ventilation, many institutions use a clinical guideline for VT of 10 to 15 mL/kg of ideal body weight (IBW) for adults and 6 to 10 mL/kg for infants and children.[17,51,72] IBW in pounds in men is equal to 106 + 6 (H − 60), where H is height in inches. For example, if a man is 66 in. tall, his IBW is 106 + 6 (66 − 60) = 106 + 6 (6) = 142 lb. For women the formula is: 105 + 5 (H − 60). Therefore, 105 + 5(66 − 60) = 105 + 5(6) = 135 lb is the IBW for this woman. Dividing weight in pounds by 2.2 will convert the value to kilograms.

A VT of more than 15 mL/kg is not recommended because of the high peak pressures which result and the accompanying risk of barotrauma and other complications.[51] Because 10 to 15 mL/kg represents a large VT, a sigh mode is not generally used with this range.

A lower VT can also be calculated by multiplying IBW by 4 (about 9 mL/kg) or using the range of 5 to 7 mL/kg of IBW. A VT in the lower range for a man 5 ft 6 in. tall would be 4 × 142 = 569 mL or, at 65 kg (142/2.2), a range of 325 to 455 mL. The estimated VT for a woman of the same height will be 4 × 135 = 540 mL or, at 61 kg (135/2.2), a range of 305 to 425 mL. The Radford nomogram (Fig 6–5) uses volumes in this range and provides a rapid method for obtaining approximate ventilator settings.

The advantage of low VT is that lower peak pressures are generated. Low VT may be appropriate when using a PEEP mode on patients to avoid high pressures.[86] Low VT in conjunction with PEEP on postsurgical patients has been shown to be as effective as the higher volume settings.[58]

Minute Ventilation.—Minute ventilation is normally equal to four times the body surface area (BSA) in men and 3.5 times the BSA in women. BSA can be estimated using the DuBois formula: $BSA = 0.007184H^{0.725}W^{0.425}$, where BSA = body surface area in square meters, H = body height in centimeters, and W = body weight in kilograms. Figure 6–6 is a nomogram for BSA based on this formula. This calculation assumes normal conditions and must be changed if the patient is hyperthermic or hypermetabolic.

For every degree Fahrenheit above 99°F, the $\dot{V}E$ should be increased 5%. For every degree Celsius above 37°C, the $\dot{V}E$ is increased 9%; for metabolic acidosis it should be increased 20%. For every 2,000 ft above sea level, the $\dot{V}E$ should be increased 5% (Fig 6–5, Table 6–1). If the patient is hypermetabolic due to the stress of illness, the $\dot{V}E$ should be increased equivalently. Burn victims, for example, may have metabolic rates ($\dot{V}O_2$) twice as high as normal and $\dot{V}E$ would

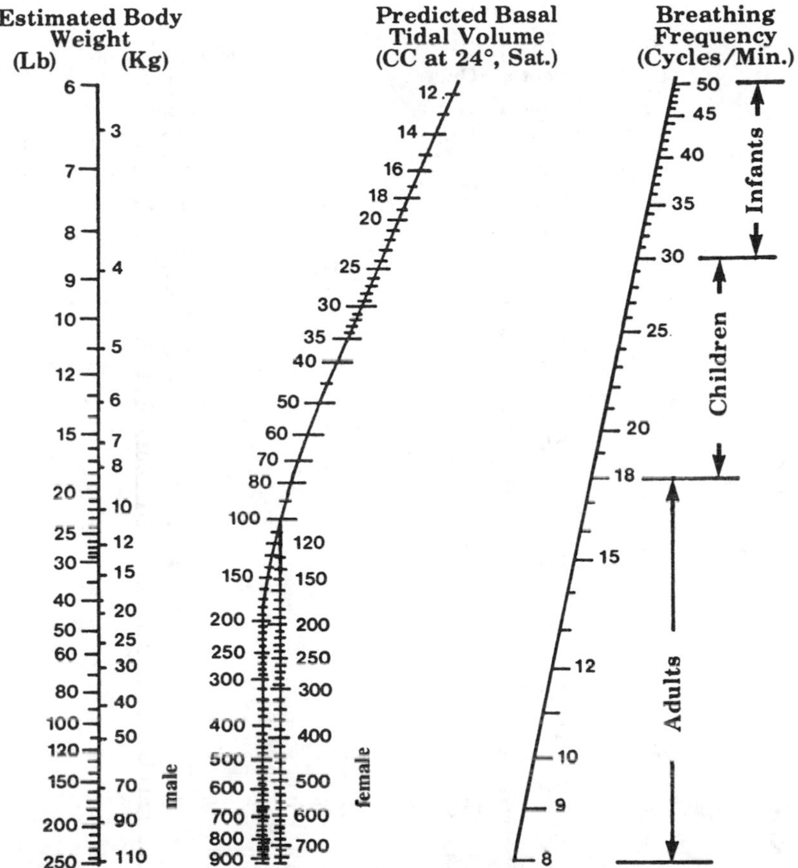

FIG 6–5.
(Radford's nomogram): Breathing nomogram predicted tidal volumes and rates. Corrections to be applied to predict basal (minimum) tidal volume: daily activity (patient not in coma): add 10%; fever: add 5% per degree Fahrenheit above 99° F (rectal), or add 9% per degree Celsius above 37° C (rectal); altitude: add 5% for every 2,000 ft above sea level; artificial airway: subtract the volume equal to one-half the body weight in pounds or subtract 1 cc/kg of body weight; add equipment dead space volume; metabolic acidosis: add 20%. (From Radford EP, Ferris BG, Jr, Driete BC: *N Engl J Med* 1954; 21:877–884. Used by permission.)

have to be doubled to compensate. Lung disorders that increase physiologic dead space will also require an increased $\dot{V}_E$.

There are many factors which will affect the $\dot{V}_E$ setting and these should be kept in mind when an initial $\dot{V}_E$ is estimated. The minimum setting for $\dot{V}_E$ is represented by the unaltered calculation based on sex and BSA (4 × BSA for males and 3.5 × BSA for females). Tidal volume can be determined by using

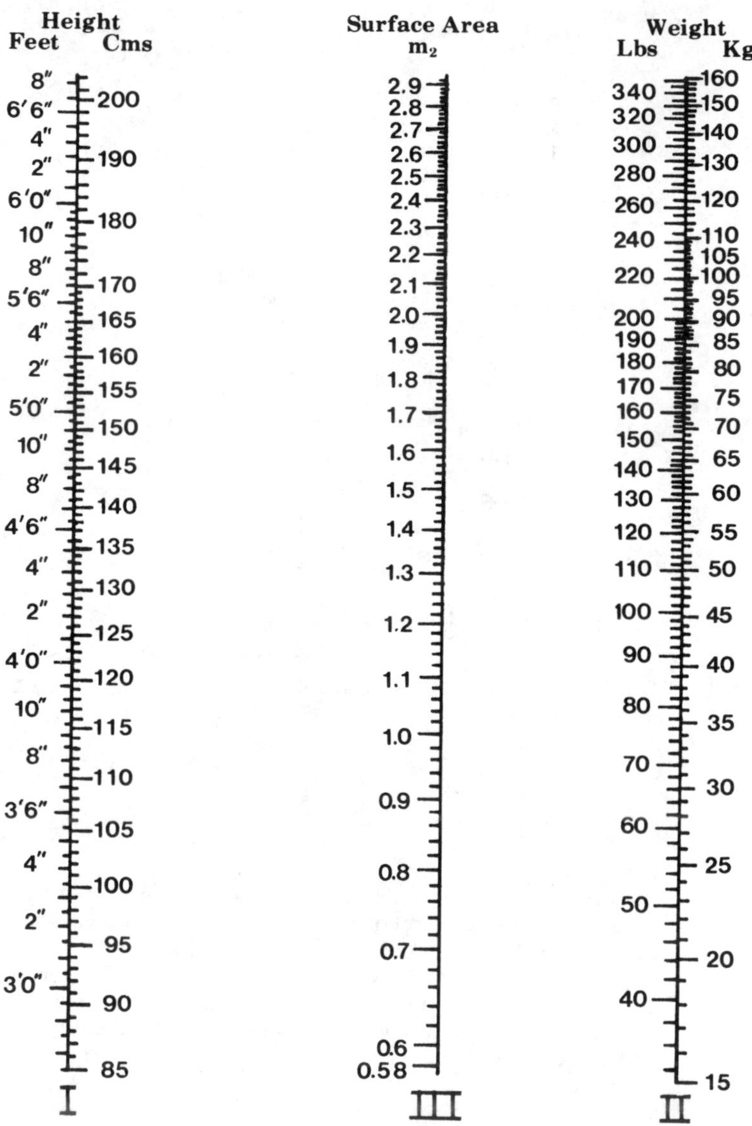

FIG 6–6.
DuBois body surface chart. To determine body surface area (BSA), locate the patient's height in inches or centimeters on scale *I* and the weight in pounds or kilograms on scale *II*. Place a straight edge between these two points. Where the straight edge intersects scale *III* will determine the patient's BSA in square meters (m^2). (From Boothby WM, Sandiford RB: *Boston Med Surg J* 1921; 185:337–354.)

TABLE 6–1.

Determination of Pressure, Tidal Volume, Respiratory Frequency, and Minute Ventilation to Establish Initial Ventilator Settings

Pressure-cycled ventilation
Tidal volume achieved = 11–18 mL/kg
Preset pressure = 20–25 cm H_2O
Rate = 10–15 breaths/min

Volume-cycled ventilation
Minute ventilation ($\dot{V}_E$)
  Men = 4 × BSA
  Women = 3.5 × BSA
  Increase this by:
    5%/F° >99°F or 9%/C° >37°C
    20% for metabolic acidosis
    5%/2,000 ft above sea level
    50%–100% if resting energy expenditure is equally increased
Tidal volume (V_T)
  Minimum of 4 mL/lb IBW (requires sigh mode)
  Maximum of 15 mL/kg IBW (does not require sigh mode)
Frequency (f)
  ($f = \dot{V}_E/V_T$)

either of the two methods previously described: 10 to 15 mL/kg, or 4 × IBW (lb). For example, a 6-ft-tall man has an IBW of 178 lb, or 81 kg, assuming he has a normal metabolism, temperature, and acid-base status, and has a BSA of 2.0 m^2. What are his ventilator settings? If we use a V_T of 12 mL/kg in the 81-kg patient, the V_T is about 975 mL. Minute ventilation is 4 × 2.0, or 8 L/min. It is simple from this point to determine the respiratory rate by dividing the $\dot{V}_E$ by the V_T ($f = \dot{V}_E/V_T$). Respiratory rate is (8 L/min)/(0.975 L), or about 8 breaths/min.

The V_T set on the ventilator control panel represents a close estimate of volume to be delivered into the patient circuit. Not all this volume reaches the patient; some will be lost to leaks and tubing compliance.

Tubing Compliance

The tubing compliance or system compressibility reflects the amount of gas, in milliliters, compressed in the ventilator circuit for every centimeter of H_2O pressure generated by the ventilator during the inspiratory phase. As the pressure begins to build in the ventilator circuit during inspiration, this pressure exerts force against the circuit and causes it to expand. A certain amount of volume that was internally set in the ventilator and intended for the patient's lungs goes into expanding the circuit and is unable to reach the patient's lungs. As expiration begins, the volume of gas trapped under pressure in the patient circuit now flows out the expiratory valve. This is referred to as the *compressible volume,* or the volume lost as a result of tubing compliance. The compressible volume will vary depending on the type of circuit and ventilator in use and should be determined for each ventilator system prior to its use on a patient. This calculation is especially important in infants, children, and very small patients. Tubing compliance for a patient circuit will change with temperature. As the inspired gas temperature increases, tubing compliance also increases. This is not clinically significant since the change would not dramatically alter the delivered volume in most patients.

Ventilator or tubing compliance can be determined during the initial setup by setting a low V_T (100–200 mL), setting the pressure limit as high as possible so that the cycle is not pressure-limited, manually cycling the ventilator into the inspiratory phase, occluding the patient connection, recording the peak pressure that is reached on the manometer as the low V_T is completely compressed in the patient circuit, and finally, measuring the volume at the exhalation valve.

Tubing compliance will equal the volume measured divided by the pressure reached. For example, if the volume was 200 mL and the pressure reached was 70 cm H_2O, then the tubing compliance will equal 200 mL/70 cm H_2O = 2.9 mL/cm H_2O. Once the ventilator is connected to the patient, the amount of volume lost to the circuit will equal the peak pressure reached during a V_T delivery times the tubing compliance factor (2.9 mL/cm H_2O). If an average peak pressure is 30 cm H_2O during V_T delivery, the amount of volume lost to the tubing will be 2.9 times 30, or 87 mL. This amount must be added to the V_T setting in order for it to be more accurate. Tubing compliance is very important when V_T settings are very low (< 300 mL) since a substantial part of the desired V_T can be lost due to tubing compressibility. Correcting for tubing compliance is especially important in babies if the patient circuit is not made of low-compliance tubing.

For example, if the estimated V_T for a male was 1,000 mL, and his peak pressure reading during inspiration was 30 cm H_2O, then his V_T of 1,000 mL would have to be increased to 1,000 + 87 mL (2.9 × 30), or 1,087 mL, in order to take into account the volume lost to the circuit. Tidal volume, then, will equal the initial estimation, plus volume lost due to tubing compliance.

Mechanical Dead Space Considerations

One final consideration in the setting of V_T is the use of ET tubes. Since the ET tube bypasses the upper airway, it effectively reduces the anatomic dead space and contributes to better alveolar ventilation per V_T of machine setting. For this reason, the initial V_T setting is sometimes reduced by that amount. Reduction in dead space is equal to about 1 mL/kg of IBW. For example, if the patient weighs 70 kg, then the V_T setting can be reduced by 70 mL. If the initial V_T was 500 mL, then the new setting, after taking ET intubation into account, would be 500 − 70, or 430 mL. This type of maneuver is unnecessary in most clinical situations as mechanical dead space between the ventilator and the patient adds about 75 mL of dead space; hence, the two factors cancel each other out.

Selecting Rates and Tidal Volumes Based on Patient Lung Characteristics

Selecting which V_T and rate in the ranges provided can be decided based on patient history. In patients with normal lungs a large V_T (12–15 mL/kg) and a slow rate (8–12 breaths/min) is appropriate. Flow rate (see below) should be set high enough (50–80 L/min) to match patient inspiratory demand[51] so that work of breathing is low regardless of the mode.

In patients with chronic lung disease in which compliance and airway resistance are high, it is best to use low rates (<8–10/min) and V_T in the moderate range (10–12 mL/kg). This may provide adequate time for both volume delivery and for exhalation without air trapping.[51] In chronic restrictive disorders such as fibrosis, smaller V_T (<10 mL/kg) and faster rates (12–20/min) may be beneficial. In severe acute lung injury, such as ARDS, the lungs are not homogeneous. Compliance tends to be low and resistance varies. These patients often require high levels of PEEP. Tidal volumes may need to be decreased, sometimes to less than 10 mL/kg.[51] Volumes need to be readjusted as PEEP is increased.[102] Frequency may need to be very high, but this will depend on the individual patient's response to mechanical ventilation.

Inspiratory Flow Rates and Patterns

Flow Rates.—The flow rate setting on a mechanical ventilator gives an estimated mean delivered flow of inspired gas. High flow rates of more than 40 L/min shorten inspiratory time and may result in high peak pressures and poor gas distribution.[31] Slow flow rates may reduce peak pressures and improve gas distribution, but only at the expense of increasing the I/E ratio, which may increase $\bar{P}aw$ and cardiovascular side effects. Unfortunately, long inspiratory times will also shorten expiratory times and this can lead to air trapping.

In general, it is probably best to get the air into the lungs in the shortest time possible. This is not hard to achieve with normal lungs. Varying lung conditions, however, require different rates. Slow inspiratory times of three to four time constants ($t = C \times R$) have been shown to improve ventilation in nonhomogeneous lungs like those seen in ARDS.[7] Fast flow rates (using fewer time constants) may benefit patients with low lung compliance and increased airway resistance, as in COPD. This provides longer expiratory time and prevents air trapping.[21]

As a beginning point, flow rate is normally set to deliver an I/E ratio of 1:2 or less, e.g., 1:4. Flows are set to meet the patient's inspiratory demand so that the patient is not breathing in without the ventilator supplying adequate gas flow. With adults, this probably requires a range of 50 to 80 L/min.

Flow Patterns.—A constant flow pattern provides a flow at the value selected. Using any other flow pattern will change the peak flow rate for a set V_T and inspiratory time. Sine, descending, and ascending flow patterns will have higher *peak* flows than the square wave.

In ventilators that have a sine flow pattern, the tapered flow at the end of the inspiratory phase contributes to a more even distribution of gas in the lungs compared to the constant flow ventilator.[25] Volume-controlled ventilators with descending flow patterns may be even better. Studies have shown that the descending flow pattern may improve the distribution of gas in the lungs. This can reduce dead space and increase oxygenation.[2, 7]

Ascending flow patterns have a lower $\overline{P}aw$ than a descending pattern, but result in higher peak pressures.[89] $\overline{P}aw$ and peak pressures are about the same for sine and square wave patterns. Peak pressures will be higher with the sine wave than with the square flow when airway resistance (Raw) is high.[89]

In selecting a waveform one considers if $\overline{P}aw$ or PIP is of more importance to the patient. High peak pressures are not always bad and not always associated with barotrauma. When Raw and flows are high and accelerating flow patterns are used, then peak pressures will be high. Much of this pressure is overcoming the Raw and never reaches alveolar level. So high peak pressures are not always going to increase the risk of barotrauma in lung parenchyma.

Conversely, high $\overline{P}aw$ is not always bad. It may improve oxygenation in some patients and the distribution of ventilation. It is best to match the pattern and rate of gas flow to the patient. *No* set prescribed pattern or rate of flow is best for all patients.

Relationship Between Tidal Volume, Flow, Cycling Time, and the I/E Ratio

We have discussed methods for determining the $\dot{V}_E$ to use on a patient requiring mechanical ventilation using V_T and frequency. Not all ventilators have V_T and rate controls to easily establish these two parameters. Some ventilators have inspiratory flow control, inspiratory time, total cycle time (TCT), I/E ratio settings, and so on. These are used to establish the patient's $\dot{V}_E$. Therefore, an understanding of the interrelation of these variables will help the practitioner to ventilate a patient regardless of the type of equipment in use.

Volume (V_T) is delivered as a result of a gas flow over a period of time. The concept of flow is expressed in volume per unit of time. On adult ventilators this is read as liters per minute. The flow is delivered during inspiration. The positive pressure applied during inspiration is important since it can lead to hemodynamic complications in the cardiopulmonary system. When inspiration equals or exceeds expiratory time, complications are more likely to result. $\overline{P}aw$ increases significantly. This can lead to increases in physiologic dead space, decreases in venous return to the thorax, and decreased cardiac output.

For this reason, I/E ratios are usually set at 1:2 (or at a smaller fraction such as 1:3 or 1:4), so that expiration is substantially longer than inspiration and the effects of positive pressure are reduced. Long expiratory times also help prevent auto-PEEP (air trapping) (see Chapter 7).

There are some rare situations where inspiratory times exceed expiratory times for the purpose of improving oxygenation. These situations are usually restricted to very specific conditions, such as in infants with idiopathic respiratory distress syndrome or adults with ARDS. I/E ratios of 2:1 or 3:1 are referred to as inverse I/E ratios.

Calculation of Total Cycle Time and Frequency.—Many ventilators have dials for setting the respiratory rate without making calculations. Some, however, use inspiratory time (T_I) and expiratory time (T_E) or TCT to determine ventilator frequency. To determine the frequency for the patient, one needs to determine the length of the respiratory cycle (TCT = $T_I + T_E$) and see how many cycles can occur in 1 minute. For example, if $T_I = 2$ seconds and $T_E = 4$ seconds, TCT = $T_I + T_E = 2 + 4 = 6$ seconds. Since a minute is 60 seconds long, there is the possibility of 10 breaths/min: 60 sec/6 sec = 10 (60 sec/TCT = rate) (Table 6–2).

TABLE 6–2.

Interrelation of Tidal Volume, Flow, Inspiratory Time, Expiratory Time, Total Cycle Time, and Respiratory Frequency

Total cycle time (TCT) = inspiratory time (T_I) plus expiratory time (T_E)

$TCT = T_I + T_E$

Respiratory frequency (f) = 1 min (60 sec) divided by TCT

$$f = \frac{1 \text{ min}}{TCT} = \frac{60 \text{ sec/1 min}}{TCT \text{ (sec)}} = \text{breaths/min}$$

Calculate *TCT* from f; $TCT = \frac{60 \text{ sec}}{f}$

Inspiratory-expiratory (I/E) ratio = T_I/T_E

Given TCT and T_I calculate I/E

$TCT = T_I + T_E$, $TCT - T_I = T_E$

Calculate T_E from f and T_I

$$f = \frac{60 \text{ sec}}{TCT} \text{ and } TCT = T_I + T_E$$

$T_E = TCT - T_I$

Reducing the *I/E ratio* to its *simplest form*

Divide the numerator and denominator by T_I

$I/E = (T_I/T_I)/(T_E/T_I)$

Calculating T_I, T_E, and TCT when given I/E and f

$TCT = T_I + T_E$; f = 60 sec/TCT

f = 60 sec/(I + E)

$T_I + T_E = 60$ sec/f

Calculating T_I when tidal volume (V_T) and flow rate ($\dot{V}$) are known

$T_I = V_T/\dot{V}$

Calculating V_T from T_I and flow rate

$V_T = \dot{V} \times T_I$

Calculating flow rate from V_T and T_I

$\dot{V} = V_T/T_I$

Calculating I/E.—Knowing either the T_I or the T_E and the rate, the I/E ratio can be calculated. To do this, one divides 60 seconds by the rate to determine the respiratory cycle time. If the rate is 12 breaths/min the respiratory cycle time will be 60 sec/12 = 5 seconds. Since the respiratory cycle is the sum of T_I and T_E, then T_I or T_E can be determined by subtracting one or the other from the TCT. In this case, let T_I be 1 second. The T_E will equal 5 − 1 = 4 seconds (TCT − T_I = T_E, TCT − T_E = T_I). The I/E ratio is then determined by T_I/T_E (1:4) (see Table 6–2).

Usually the I/E ratio is expressed so that T_I = 1. If the I/E ratio were calculated as 2:3 seconds, the I/E ratio would be expressed as 1:1.5. This can be determined by dividing the numerator and denominator by the T_I (see Table 6–2). When I/E ratios are inverse (I > E), then T_E takes on the value of 1. For example, if T_I = 3 seconds and T_E = 2 seconds, I/E = 3:2 or 1.5:1.

Inspiratory Time Calculated from Tidal Volume and Flow.—Inspiratory time can be determined when the V_T and flow rate are known. If the V_T setting on a ventilator were 1,000 mL (1 L) and flow was set at 2 L/sec, T_I would equal 1,000 mL/2 L/sec, T_I = 0.5 second. Often, the flow rate knob is calibrated in liters per minute so that the value for flow needs to be converted to liters per second. If the flow is 30 L/min, this is the same as 30 L/60 sec. The flow rate is 3 L/6 sec or 1 L/2 sec, or 0.5 L/1 sec (see Table 6–2).

Conversely, V_T can be determined when inspiratory time and flow ($\dot{V}$) are known ($V_T = \dot{V} \times T_I$). Using the above example, if T_I were 2 seconds and $\dot{V}$ = 0.5 L/sec, V_T would be 2 seconds × 0.5 L/sec, or 1 L (see Table 6–2).

Calculating Tidal Volume From Inspiratory Time and Flow.—Tidal volume can be determined if flow rate and T_I are known. If the set flow rate is 54 L/min, this is the same as 54 L/60 sec, or 0.9 L/sec. V_T = 900 mL and T_I = 1 second ($V_T = \dot{V} \times T_I$).

Calculating Flow From Tidal Volume and Inspiratory Time.—To calculate flow, simply divide V_T by T_I. For example, if $\dot{V}$ = 900 mL/1 sec, this is 0.9 L/(min/60), or 54 L/min (multiply the numerator by 60 to convert to minutes) (see Table 6–2). Again, these examples assume that flow is constant.

Initial Settings on Some Ventilators

The following are examples of setting the $\dot{V}_E$ on some commercially available ventilators:

Puritan Bennett MA-1.—To set a $\dot{V}_E$ on the MA-1, the operator dials in the appropriate rate and V_T (see Table 6–2). Inspiratory time depends on the flow rate set on the flow control knob. The faster the flow, the shorter the T_I for a given V_T. A ratio light comes on in the control mode if T_I exceeds one half or more of the set TCT. To correct this situation and keep the same $\dot{V}_E$, one increases the inspiratory flow rate.

A special situation needs to be described that sometimes occurs on the MA-1 or similar ventilators, like the BEAR 2 or 3, where the I/E alarm measures set TCT. For example, suppose the machine rate is set at 10 breaths/min, $\dot{V}$ is 30 L/min (0.5 L/sec), and V_T is 1 L. The T_I will be 2 seconds ($T_I = V_T/\dot{V} = 1$ L/(0.5 L/sec). $T_E = 4$ seconds. On these settings the I/E ratio alarm will *not* sound.

Suppose, however, that the patient begins to assist breaths and the actual rate is 20 breaths/min. The T_I will not change. It is still 2 seconds. TCT will change. It is now 3 seconds. T_E is only 1 second long. The alarm will *not* sound because T_I (2 seconds) has not exceeded half the *set* TCT which is unchanged at 6 seconds. Remember the set machine rate is still 10 breaths/min, even though the patient is breathing faster.

Sechrist IV-100.—This is an infant ventilator and represents an interesting example of ventilator control settings. Rather than a rate control, the Sechrist uses a T_I and a T_E control. These set the TCT ($T_I + T_E$) and establish a ventilatory rate [$(T_I + T_E)/60$]. The gas power source is 50 psig (pounds per square inch gauge) and has the potential for creating a constant flow rate. To determine an estimated V_T delivery the following equation can be used:

$$\text{Estimated } V_T = \frac{T_I \times \dot{V} \text{ (L/min)}}{60}$$

Since it is difficult to obtain an exact flow rate value and to ensure the constant flow pattern, this calculation is only an estimate.

IMV Emerson.—On this time-cycled machine, T_I and TCT are set by the operator. Frequency is determined by $f = 60/(\text{TCT})$. Tidal volume is a separate setting. Inspiratory flow rate can be estimated from T_I and V_T ($\dot{V} = V_T/T_I$). This is only an estimate since the Emerson is a sine wave (nonconstant) and not a square wave (constant) flow generator.

Siemens Servo 900C.—On this ventilator there is a $\dot{V}_E$ inspiratory percent time, and a rate setting. Tidal volume is determined by $\dot{V}_E$ and f ($V_T = \dot{V}_E/f$). Inspiratory flow will equal V_T/T_I. In the Servo 900B and C the inspiratory time can be calculated by determining TCT (TCT = 60/f) and multiplying this by the percent indicated on the inspiratory time percent (T_I%) control. This determines the percent of cycle time spent in inspiration. Expiratory time becomes TCT minus T_I ($T_E = \text{TCT} - T_I$). Suppose, for example, that the $\dot{V}_E$ is set at 10 L/min and the frequency is set at 12. The V_T will equal (10 L/min)/12 or 833 mL. The cycle time will equal 60/12, or 5 seconds. If T_I% is set at 20%, then 0.20×5

seconds or 1 second will be spent in inspiration. T_E will equal 5 − 1, or 4 seconds. The I/E ratio will be 1:4.

When inspiratory flow is set on the constant flow pattern, then the flow rate of gas can be estimated ($\dot{V} = V_T/T_I$). Or it can be determined by dividing $T_I\%$ into 100 and multiplying the quotient by the $\dot{V}_E$ setting [$\dot{V} = \dot{V}_E \times (100/T_I\%)$].

Special Considerations in Setting the Minute Ventilation

Practical considerations in setting a desired $\dot{V}_E$ for patient use have been discussed, but there are a few precautions that should be considered before implementing these procedures.

Values for I/E ratios are normally set so that expiratory time, in general, exceeds inspiratory time. In most cases this provides an optimal pattern of ventilation and reduces the potential side effects of positive pressure ventilation. Alterations in the I/E ratio, while maintaining the same $\dot{V}_E$, usually require changes in the inspiratory flow rate. To shorten inspiration and allow a greater time for exhalation, the inspiratory flow rate is increased. It has been shown that an optimal inspiratory flow rate exists for each individual patient and no set value can be applied to ensure the best patient care. An optimal inspiratory flow rate and pattern will improve Pa_{O_2} without significantly affecting Pa_{CO_2}.[69, 79]

In some instances, it is a rapid flow rate that provides the best method of ventilation. There are also cases where a slower flow rate is necessary to obtain the best arterial blood gas results with the least physiologic side effect. The variability in results is related to the condition of the patient's lungs and conductive airways. The lung in various pathologic conditions does not behave as a homogeneous mechanical unit. Some regions differ from others in their compliance and resistance characteristics. Because of this, the pattern of ventilation imposed by the mechanical ventilator must establish a compromise between the different regional gas flows and the pressure requirements necessary to provide optimal ventilation. It is for this reason that I/E ratios, flow patterns, and optimal flow rates for ventilation and oxygenation will vary from situation to situation.

If Pa_{O_2} values begin to decrease and the Pa_{CO_2} values to increase while one increases the $\dot{V}_E$ on a ventilated patient, something is definitely wrong. Possibilities include the presence of auto-PEEP, poor ventilation-to-perfusion ($\dot{V}/\dot{Q}$) matching in the nonhomogeneous lung, and changes in venous return. This situation may require a change in flow rate, V_T, respiratory rate, flow pattern, or I/E ratio. Use of spontaneous modes of ventilation such as SIMV plus PSV might also be of benefit. This would allow the spontaneously breathing patient to have some control over ventilation. There is no bottom line, no easy prescription. Management of the patient on mechanical ventilation is both an art and a science. It requires sound judgment.

Inspiratory Hold

Inspiratory or inflation hold (also called end-inspiratory pause) is a maneuver that occurs as part of the inspiratory phase. It is accomplished by preventing the expiratory valve from opening for a short time at the end of inspiration. It has been shown that inflation hold helps to improve the distribution of air throughout the lungs regardless of the type of flow pattern used[24, 25, 43] and provide optimum $\dot{V}/\dot{Q}$ matching and reduce physiologic dead space–tidal volume (V_D/V_T) ratios. In addition to aiding gas distribution in the lung, it can also be used to calculate the static compliance (Cs) in the ventilated lung.

Newer methods of ventilation have taken the place of inflation hold in recent years. These include changing flow patterns or rates of flow, shortening inspiration time, or switching modes of ventilation.

Expiratory Retard

During normal expiration, gas flow out of the lung can be described as follows. (The numeric values are used only as examples for simplicity and are not representative of actual values.) The elastic recoil of the alveolus (+2 cm H_2O) plus the forces from the intrathoracic area (+3 cm H_2O) acting on alveolar gas volume provide the energy which allows for the flow of gas out of the lungs (Fig 6–7,A). The total pressure (+5 cm H_2O) at the alveolar level is greater than that at the mouth, and the air moves out of the lung. As the exhaled air moves across the conductive airways, some of the driving pressure is lost to the resistance of the airways (−1 cm H_2O). In the normal lung, this pressure loss is small. While the intrathoracic forces exert pressure on the alveoli, they also exert force on the conductive airway. In normal airways, the resilience of the airway combined with the pressure of the gas in the lumen of the airway prevents airway collapse during most phases of the respiratory cycle, and in most regions of the lung. The pressure in the alveolus minus the pressure drop across the airway equals the pressure in the airway lumen (+5 cm H_2O − 1 cm H_2O = +4 cm H_2O intraluminal pressure).

In patients with weakened airways caused by loss of supportive connective tissue, as occurs with aging or in patients with emphysema, the pattern changes. Figure 6–7,B shows an example of an alveolus with elastic recoil forces lower than normal because of disease changes (+ 1 cm H_2O). The intrathoracic forces will not be affected (+3 cm H_2O). But the total force providing airflow out of the lungs is lower (+4 cm H_2O). When air flows along the resistance airways, pressure is lost to a greater extent than in normal airways (−2 cm H_2O). As a result, the intraluminal pressure is lower (+4 cm H_2O − 2 cm H_2O = +2 cm H_2O). Since thoracic pressures are greater than the intraluminal pressures, the small airways, weakened by disease, tend to collapse. The maneuver, known as

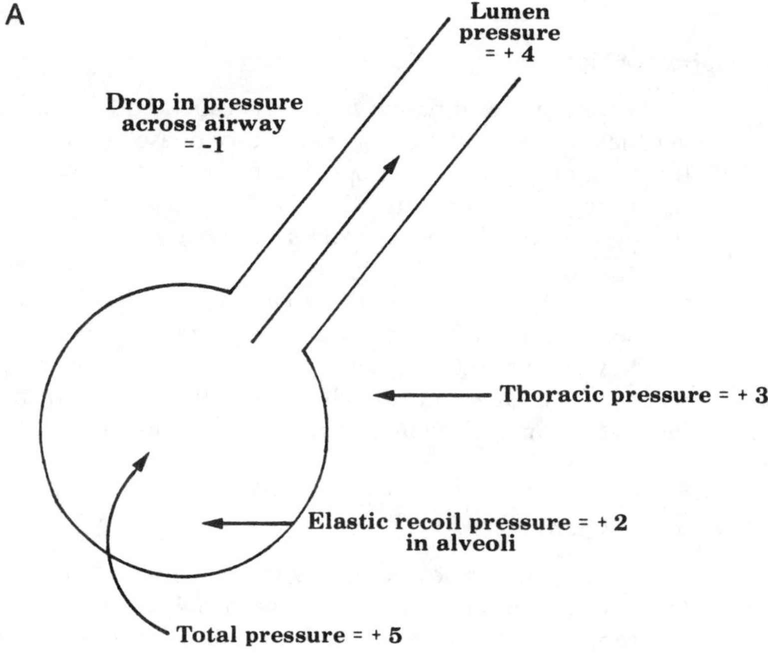

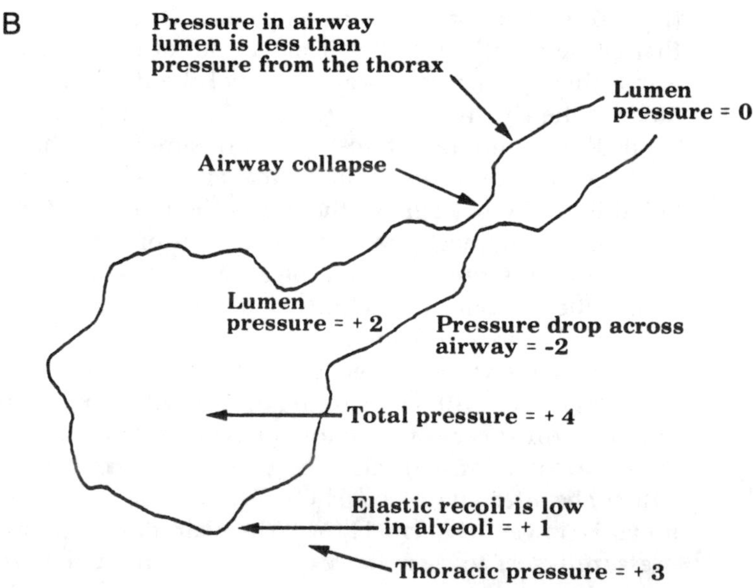

FIG 6–7.
A, alveolar, thoracic, and airway dynamics during exhalation in a patient with normal lungs (units in cm H_2O pressure). **B**, alveolar, thoracic, and airway dynamics during exhalation in a patient with chronic obstructive lung disease (units in cm H_2O pressure).

pursed lips breathing, helps to keep the intraluminal pressure higher and prevent airway collapse by offering resistance to expiration, thus raising pressures across the entire length of the airway.

For the patient with emphysema or a similar pulmonary disease, one maneuver that can be accomplished during mechanical ventilation is expiratory retard. This maneuver slows the rate of exhalation by applying resistance to expired gas flow in much the same way as pursed lips breathing. The resistance can be applied by using an orifice of restrictive diameter at the exhalation port. Used with careful observation of the cardiovascular condition of the patient, this modality may be beneficial in preventing air trapping in patients with known early airway closure.

Newer microprocessor ventilators do not provide an expiratory retard knob. Practitioners now use low levels of PEEP (≤ 5 cm H_2O) which provides the same effect. Many expiratory and PEEP valves actually increase resistance to exhalation whether it is desired or not.

Periodic Hyperinflation or Sighing

In 1963, a study by Bendixon et al.[9] demonstrated that anesthetized and intubated postsurgical patients developed increased shunting as well as decreased Pa_{O_2} values and reduced compliance following artificial ventilation. These changes were attributed to microatelectasis associated with the use of constant low V_T. When subjects were given periodic deep breaths (sighs), these changes were reversed. The use of periodic sighing or hyperinflation remains controversial as other studies have not entirely supported the findings of Bendixon et al.[10, 20, 42, 57, 59] The drop in lung compliance and drops in Pa_{O_2} seen in postsurgical patients may actually be due to loss of FRC in the supine position and to the effects of anesthesia, muscle relaxants, and similar medications on the diaphragm and intercostal muscles.[20]

Because the sigh or deep breath was a popular idea during the 1960s, many ventilators commercially developed since that time have sigh modes which can be used selectively. These sigh modes offer the capability of giving one or more deep breaths at periodic timed intervals, such as three or four times per hour or once every 10 minutes, depending on the machine in use. Since a normal sigh in a spontaneously breathing nonintubated person occurs every 6 minutes,[9] sighs are set to occur with a similar frequency. Volumes are set at 1.5 to 2.0 times the regular low V_T setting.[9]

Besides the sigh mode, other investigators find that large V_T settings (10–15 mL/kg) in anesthetized patients reduce atelectasis.[103, 107] For patients in acute respiratory failure, these volumes also reduced intrapulmonary shunting.[38] The most widely used choice is the higher V_T range (10–15 mL/kg) rather than the sigh mode.

If low V_T settings are provided (≤ 8 mL/kg), the sigh mode is generally used. Use of an occasional sigh breath with low V_T settings is probably not harmful. Until further studies can help determine the real need to sigh or not to sigh at low V_T, we are probably best advised to follow convention.

There are three options available for the prevention of potential microatelectasis in ventilated adult subjects. First, for patients on pressure-cycled ventilation, such as the PR-2, periodic deep breaths to increase ventilating pressures for a breath or two or use of manual ventilation with a resuscitator bag is recommended. These breaths should be given at least every 30 minutes. Most of the pressure-cycled ventilators do not have a mechanical device for accomplishing this task. Second, for patients on volume-cycled ventilation where V_T settings (<8–10 mL/kg) are used, the sigh mode is recommended with several sigh breaths (1.5–2.0 times the V_T setting) given every 10 to 15 minutes.[9] Third, for patients on high V_T settings (10–15 mL/kg), periodic hyperinflation of the lungs is not necessary, but these patients should be carefully observed to be sure atelectasis, reduced compliance, and increased shunting do not occur.[84]

Selection of F_{IO_2}

The goal in selecting a specific F_{IO_2} is to try to achieve clinically acceptable Pa_{O_2} values between 60 and 100 mm Hg. Before a patient is mechanically ventilated, an initial arterial blood gas report is usually available. This information is helpful for the determination of an F_{IO_2} setting on the ventilator. If the Pa_{O_2} of the patient is within the desired range prior to ventilatory support, then the same F_{IO_2} can be used when ventilation is started. If the Pa_{O_2} is not in the desired range, then the following equation can be used to estimate F_{IO_2}:

$$\text{Desired } F_{IO_2} = \frac{Pa_{O_2}\text{ (desired)} \times F_{IO_2}\text{ (known)}}{Pa_{O_2}\text{ (known)}}$$

This relationship is based on the assumption that the patient's cardiopulmonary function will not change radically from the time of the known arterial blood gas report to the time the F_{IO_2} is placed on its new setting.[75,76] Obviously, some changes will occur because the hypoventilated patient will now be normoventilated. Also, the employment of positive pressure ventilation may also affect cardiopulmonary status. On the other hand, at least the initial F_{IO_2} setting on the ventilator can be made with some basis of patient need.

If a baseline arterial blood gas assessment is not available, it is advisable to select a high initial F_{IO_2} setting (0.50–1.0). This is beneficial for patients with severe hypoxemia since it can provide a way of restoring normal oxygenation and repleting tissue oxygen stores where oxygen debt and lactic acid accumulation has occurred. It may also be helpful in estimating the magnitude of right-to-left shunt.

Some clinicians are skeptical in using high F_{IO_2} values in patients breathing on a hypoxic drive. As long as the $\dot{V}_E$ settings are adequate to meet the patient's need, removal of the hypoxic drive need not be a concern. The F_{IO_2} can then be adjusted after ventilation has begun and an arterial blood sample is collected. Use of high F_{IO_2} values is especially helpful in patients with COPD and acute respiratory failure. A large alveolar-arterial difference in partial pressure of oxygen [$P(A - a)O_2$] in this type of patient might indicate a new, acute lung disease such as pneumonia or pulmonary edema. A low $P(A - a)O_2$ suggests an acute reversible lung disease.[31]

After the first 15 minutes of mechanical ventilation, an arterial blood gas sample is obtained to assess the adequacy of ventilation and oxygenation. Appropriate ventilation changes based on arterial blood gas results are considered in Chapter 8. Suffice it to say that at this point the F_{IO_2} should be readjusted. If an F_{IO_2} greater than 0.60 is required to maintain oxygenation, then PEEP may be indicated (see Chapter 10). An F_{IO_2} maintained above this level increases the risk of oxygen toxicity and increased intrapulmonary shunting.[96] The above equation for desired F_{IO_2} can be used to calculate an appropriate F_{IO_2}.

In most ventilators an F_{IO_2} or oxygen percentage dial is available for giving the desired F_{IO_2} settings. If it is not, an oxygen blender is used. On ventilators where the IMV mode is not governed by the F_{IO_2} dial, a separate adjustment must be made to the gases used to power the IMV reservoir. An oxygen analyzer placed in the main inspiratory line of the patient circuit is necessary to check the accuracy of the F_{IO_2} setting.

Mechanical Support for Oxygenation Without Ventilation

In addition to the modalities and parameters discussed, sometimes support is needed for the patient who requires only an improvement in oxygenation, but for whom the use of oxygen therapy by mask or cannula is not adequate. The most popular method for improving oxygenation is CPAP. This procedure increases the transpulmonary pressure by the continuous application of positive pressure to the respiratory system. CPAP at the upper airway provides the force to increase the transpulmonary pressure and the FRC. It is necessary with CPAP that the patient be breathing spontaneously and that the work of breathing not be excessive; otherwise, it may be necessary to augment ventilation. CPAP is beneficial in the treatment of refractory hypoxemia and may decrease the $P(A - a)O_2$, the percentage shunt, and increase FRC and arterial oxygenation.

ALARMS

Alarms are ways of warning of possible dangers. On ventilated patients these dangers are so numerous that Chapter 7 is devoted to the problem. This section reviews the most common alarms and how they are set by most institutions.

Low pressure alarms are usually set about 10 cm H_2O below PIP and are used to detect patient disconnection events and leaks in the system. High pressure alarms are set about 10 cm H_2O above PIP and usually end inspiration. They indicate events such as coughing, increased secretions, drops in compliance, tube kinking, and so on. Low PEEP and CPAP alarms are usually set about 5 cm H_2O below the baseline. They sound when the PEEP or CPAP level has dropped. This can be due to leaks.

Apnea alarms can be used to monitor ventilator and spontaneous breaths depending on the machine. They are usually set so that the patient will not miss two consecutive machine breaths ($>$TCT and $<$TCT $\times$ 2). For spontaneous breaths, they are preset on some ventilators to sound after a 20-second apnea period. This time can be adjusted on other ventilators.

A ratio alarm or indicator is present on some ventilators and indicates when the inspiratory time exceeds more than half the set TCT (see discussion on I/E ratios). Some ventilators, such as the Bird 6400, will automatically end inspiration if the expiratory time gets so short the patient will not have time to exhale. In the Bird, the shortest possible expiratory time is 0.25 seconds. This can either be activated or deactivated.

Low source gas alarms inform the operator that the available high pressure gas source is no longer functional. For the newer microprocessor ventilators this can be critical. If they do not come with a built-in compressor, there may not be another source of gas and these ventilators rely on high pressure gas to function. Many of these ventilators automatically sound this alarm and the alarm cannot be silenced if the gas is critical to the operation of the ventilator.

Volume alarms monitor low V_T, low and high $\dot{V}_E$, and low and high rates. There are no real predetermined levels for these settings. Operators must use their judgment in placing alarm settings to alert them to possible changes in the patient's condition. Alarms need not be so sensitive, however, that they are constantly sounding and frightening the patient. Other alarms warn of a low battery, an inoperative ventilator, ventilator circuit malfunction, an exhalation valve leak, settings that are inappropriate or outside the range of what is available, etc. There are so many alarms, buzzers, beeps, tweets, and honks that you begin to ignore them after a while. Maybe we would be better off with fewer alarms.

FINAL CONSIDERATIONS IN VENTILATOR SETUP

A final check must be given to the ventilator selected for final use. These steps include the following:

1. Check ventilator function to be sure it operates correctly and there are no significant leaks present.

2. Fill the humidifier with sterile water and set the humidifier temperature so that final air temperature at the airway will be approximately 32 to 37 °C and no higher.
3. Place a temperature monitoring device near the patient connector.
4. Check the F_{IO_2}.
5. Turn on and check the alarms: the apnea or low pressure alarm, the high pressure alarm, the I/E ratio monitor or alarm, the failure-to-cycle alarm, the loss of 50-psig gas source alarm, the F_{IO_2} alarm, and the temperature alarm. Set alarm limits for V_T, $\dot{V}_E$, and frequency, if available.
6. Be sure an electrocardiogram (ECG) monitor is connected to the patient.
7. Have an emergency airway tray available should the patient's airway be removed or damaged.
8. Provide airway suctioning equipment.
9. Select a volume monitoring device and an oxygen analyzer if they are not part of the ventilator.
10. Keep a resuscitation bag with the ventilator.

STEPS IN BEGINNING VENTILATORY SUPPORT

Once the decision has been made to connect the patient to a ventilator, several steps are taken. These include: preparing the patient, establishing an airway, manually ventilating the patient, stabilizing the cardiovascular system, meeting ventilatory needs, and treating the cause of respiratory failure.[72, 94]

Patient Preparation

If the patient is conscious, it is necessary to prepare him or her for what is about to occur. This includes an explanation of how ventilators work and why one is being used. The patient should be told that the use of an artificial airway will inhibit communication. This is an obvious step in preoperative preparation of patients undergoing open heart surgery where postoperative ventilatory support is likely. It should also be done in emergency elective intubation to reduce the patient's level of anxiety and discomfort.

If the patient is not conscious, then the situation should be explained as soon as the patient has regained consciousness. This is critical since these patients are unable to speak and may be completely unaware of what has occurred.

Establishing an Airway

An airway should be established. The three most commonly used types of artificial airways are orotracheal, nasotracheal, and tracheostomy tubes. Orotracheal tubes are used for emergencies and are generally kept in for 12 to 18 hours, but they may be used for as long as several days. Nasotracheal tubes offer better patient comfort and can be kept in for up to a week or more but require more time for insertion and usually have a smaller lumen than orotracheal tubes. Tracheostomy tubes require a surgical procedure for insertion but can be used for extended periods of time. They also allow for easier pulmonary toilet, are apparently more comfortable for the patient, and in some cases even allow the patient to talk.

Artificial airways provide an airtight seal between the patient and the mechanical ventilatory support, and are essential in continuous artificial ventilation. Additionally, they protect the airway from the possibility of aspiration. New soft sealing masks are also available. These are usually limited to use in spontaneous CPAP or for night ventilation in patients at home. Some masks seal the mouth and nose area. Others seal the nose only. These are usually used for nasal CPAP in the adult patient on home care (see Chapter 14).

In preparation for intubation, all the necessary equipment should be assembled. Appendix C lists some of the basic equipment needed for this procedure and Appendix D gives examples of ET and tracheostomy tube sizes and laryngoscopy blade sizes.

Manual Ventilation

Once the airway has been established, it is then possible to support the patient's ventilatory requirements by using a manual resuscitation bag. These devices are accessible, easy to operate, provide immediate ventilatory assistance, and allow the operator to closely monitor the patient's own breathing efforts and respond to changes in airway resistance or lung compliance.

Cardiovascular Stabilization

The stress of acute or impending respiratory failure combined with that of ET intubation can lead to cardiovascular complications. They may be present already. The patient might suffer from myocardial hypoxia and develop cardiac dysrhythmias. The interaction of intubation with the effect of any of the pharmacologic agents used to assist in intubation (topical anesthetics, sedatives, narcotics, muscle paralyzing agents) might lead to hypotension and a condition of relative hypovolemia. This can result in reduced venous return. Appropriate cardiovascular support should be provided as necessary.

Ventilatory Needs

Once the patient's cardiovascular status is stabilized and the primary ventilatory needs are being met, there is time to select the appropriate ventilatory equipment and choose the initial ventilator settings to be used.

Treating the Cause of Respiratory Failure

Once the patient is on ventilatory support and a life-threatening situation no longer exists, attention can be turned to treating the initial problems that resulted in the patient being placed on mechanical ventilatory support. Artificial ventilation is not curative; the underlying problem must be overcome whether it be due to central nonresponsiveness, neuromuscular problems, or increased work of breathing caused by trauma, ARDS, COPD with complications, or other disorders. It makes little sense to be aggressive with these palliative methods if the underlying pathologic condition is irreversible.

SPECIFIC VENTILATORS

Selection of a specific ventilator depends not only on theoretical considerations but on practical considerations as well. The equipment available within an institution will limit selection. The familiarity of personnel with the available equipment is another determining factor in ventilator selection.

It is not the intention of this text to describe all of the available ventilators and their features. This is done well in other sources.[16, 48, 54, 60, 74, 78, 95] Appendix E contains a description of some of the ventilators currently available and their characteristics.

In considering what type of positive pressure ventilator (PPV) to select, it is helpful to consider each ventilator and what it can provide for the patient. A brief overview of flow generators vs. pressure generators, the basic capabilities of PPVs, and an assessment of ventilator performance are provided here.

Basic Capabilities

Spearman[99] describes a variety of parameters and alarms that outline the essential components for adult ventilators for use in the intensive care unit (ICU). Volume control is a primary feature. Tidal volume range needs to be between 200 and 2,000 mL. Respiratory rate should range from 1 to 60 breaths/min. Higher rates are rarely used.

Pressure-generating capabilities need to be between 0 and about 100 cm H_2O. Drive pressure should be high enough to maintain the gas flow pattern through inspiration regardless of how high peak pressures climb. Flow rates between 10 and 120 L/min are desirable for this V_T range. Controls for V_T, respiratory frequency, and flow rate are preferable to controls for $\dot{V}_E$, inspiratory time, and expiratory time. An I/E ratio display is beneficial. Demand valves, patient circuits, exhalation valves, and PEEP valves should all be designed to reduce the work of breathing and the resistance to inspiration and expiration. Oxygen controls must be available at a range of room air to 100% with incremental changes of 1% to 2%. PEEP or CPAP should be available in the range of 0 to 30 cm H_2O.

Available modes of ventilation might include assist-control, IMV or SIMV, inflation hold for static compliance measurements, expiratory pause for auto-PEEP measurements, and PEEP and CPAP. Pressure-controlled modes like pressure control and pressure support are possible additions. The humidification system needs to provide 100% relative humidity at a range of about 32 to 37 °F for all available flow rates up to minute ventilations of 20 to 30 L/min. It also needs a servo-controlled heater with a temperature readout and a temperature alarm. The ventilator requires a nebulizer system that operates during mechanical or spontaneous inspiration. This system should not alter V_T or oxygen delivery or alarm function. It also needs to provide sufficient operative pressure to adequately nebulize medications. If no nebulizer control is provided, the ventilator should be adaptable to an add-on external micronebulizer powered by an external compressed gas source. This add-on system must not interfere with ventilator function regardless of what mode is in use. Alarms include a pressure limit and a low and high pressure alarm, a power failure alarm, and an oxygen system alarm. High and low rate and V_T alarms are desirable extras.

While the above give the basic needs for an adult ventilator, they do not describe an ideal ventilator. The newer-generation microprocessor ventilators are capable of many more modes and features. These were only provided here as fundamentals.

Performance Evaluation

A performance evaluation must be made of every brand of ventilator prior to purchase and to every ventilator in use prior to connecting it to a patient.

Before purchasing a new ventilator the department needs to consider its specific needs. What types of patients are most often ventilated in the institution? How many ventilators are needed? What type of respiratory care staff is available? How much in-service training is required? How well does the staff adapt to the device? How well can the device be adapted to the ICU setting and the patients? How much money is available?

In addition, a bench test or performance test is made of every ventilator prior to purchase. Forms are available for doing these tests and for looking at lung analogues, both in other texts[54] and through the Joint Commission on Accreditation of Hospitals[44] and the American National Standards Institute.[3] A bench test requires the use of a lung analogue which can simulate lung characteristics, and instruments for measuring volume, pressure, flow, and time. The bench test examines the ventilator's performance during changes in compliance and resistance and leak conditions. It checks classification, general features, parameter ranges, and alarm systems. The test must also include a variety of simulated conditions such as very low and very high $\dot{V}_E$ needs, causes of air trapping (auto-PEEP), function during added nebulization, function of the CPAP system, and so on.

Regular maintenance and testing programs are also mandatory for every ventilator prior to use on a patient. Requirements for maintenance and calibration are usually outlined in the manufacturer's maintenance program. Hospitals might add additional cleaning and testing procedures. This is especially the case if the department has modified the ventilator in any way. Records must be kept of the testing and maintenance programs for each ventilator. A department's policies and procedures regarding ventilator maintenance, testing, quality control, and monitoring are vital to function and patient safety. All employees that will operate the equipment need to be trained in its use and periodically given refresher courses. Documentation of this training is also an essential part of a department's records.

During use, a ventilator may malfunction. When this occurs, the initial assessment is to ensure that the patient is being ventilated. Troubleshooting follows. When in doubt, disconnect the patient from the ventilator, manually ventilate the patient, silence the alarms, and get help. If another practitioner cannot correct the problem, the operating manuals provided with the ventilators usually have troubleshooting sections to solve most situations. The final resort is to call the local maintenance representative from the company.

CASE STUDY

An example of respiratory failure associated with increased work of breathing is the patient with chronic CO_2 retention who suffers some additional stress such as a respiratory infection. The following case study is provided to give the reader some practice on making initial basic ventilator setting selections. Study questions at the end of the chapter provide additional practice.

A 73-year-old man with a history of COPD has developed an upper respiratory infection. Upon admission his respiratory rate is 39 breaths/min, pulse is 145 beats/min, temperature is 102 °F and spontaneous V_T is 225 mL. His estimated $\dot{V}_E$ is 10.1 L/min. Alveolar ventilation is estimated to be: $(V_T - V_D) \times f = (225 - 150) \times 39 = 2.93$ L/min. Arterial blood gas results on room air are: $Pa_{O_2} = 35$ mm Hg, $Pa_{CO_2} = 97$ mm Hg, and pH = 7.24.

Oxygen by a 28% Venturi tube is begun. The patient is given IPPB with albuterol. Despite continued and aggressive therapy, the patient does not improve. The pH continues to fall and work of breathing remains high. The decision is made to intubate and begin respiratory support.

The patient is 5 ft 8 in. tall and weighs 148 lb. His BSA is 1.78 m^2. IBW is calculated at 70 kg. The SIMV mode is selected since the patient is breathing spontaneously. Initial V_T is selected at 12 mL/kg, or 840 mL. Since this patient has a history of COPD, the risk of barotrauma is reduced with the lower V_T setting. Minute ventilation is set at 8 L/min: $4 \times BSA = 4 \times 1.78 = 7$ L/min; $\dot{V}_E$ is increased by 5% per degree Fahrenheit. If temperature = 102 °F, increase by 1.05 L/min. Respiratory rate is set at 10 breaths/min ($\dot{V}_E/V_T$ = f). Flow is set at 60 L/min. F_{IO_2} is set at 0.5 to begin.

After initiating ventilation, the following values are noted: PIP = 33 cm H_2O, $P_{Plateau}$ = 25 cm H_2O, P_{TA} = 33 − 25 = 8 cm H_2O. The patient is spontaneously breathing an additional 10 breaths/min with a V_T of 200 mL. The decision is made to add pressure support for the spontaneous breaths to overcome the work of breathing imposed by the artificial airway. Resistance is estimated at P_{TA}/flow or 8 cm H_2O/60 L min, or 8 cm H_2O/(1 L/sec). Pressure support is set at 8 cm H_2O.

This is an example of initiating ventilatory support in a patient with COPD. Of note are the use of a lower V_T setting, increasing the $\dot{V}_E$ because of the patient's temperature, and the use of pressure support for spontaneous breaths which are set only enough to overcome the resistance imposed by the airway.

STUDY QUESTIONS

1. A patient being ventilated on a BEAR 2 has progressively developed very stiff lungs (C = 18 mL/cm H_2O) and increased Raw. The V_T was set at 1,000 mL, the respiratory rate at 12 breaths/min on the assist-control mode. The patient is initiating another 3 breaths/min so the total rate is 15 breaths/min. What is the patient's total actual $\dot{V}_E$?
   a. 12 L/min.
   b. 15 L/min.
   c. 18 L/min.
   d. 12,000 L/min.
2. If the flow rate is set at 30 L/min, what is the flow in liters per second?
   a. 1 L/sec.
   b. 0.5 L/sec.
   c. 500 L/sec.
   d. You cannot calculate this from this information.
3. What is the TCT based on the set machine rate of 12 breaths/min?
   a. 5 seconds.
   b. 3 seconds.
   c. 6 seconds.
   d. 10 seconds.
   e. 4 seconds.
4. What is the TCT based on the actual machine rate of 15 breaths/min?
   a. 5 seconds.
   b. 3 seconds.
   c. 6 seconds.

d. 10 seconds.
e. 4 seconds.

5. What is the inspiratory time based on a flow of 30 L/min and a VT of 1,000 mL?
   a. 0.5 second.
   b. 1 second.
   c. 2 seconds.
   d. 3 seconds.
   e. 4 seconds.
6. On the BEAR 2, the respiratory rate is 10 breaths/min, the inspiratory time is 2 seconds, the VT is 1,000 mL, and the peak pressure is 30 cm H_2O. What is the I/E ratio?
   a. 1:3.
   b. 2:6.
   c. 1:2.
   d. 1:4.
7. What is the $\dot{V}E$?
   a. 6 L/min.
   b. 30 L/min.
   c. 10 L/min.
   d. 2 L/min.
8. What is the TCT?
   a. 6 seconds.
   b. 10 seconds.
   c. 8 seconds.
   d. 2 seconds.
9. Which of the following would you use for mechanical ventilation of a patient in the recovery room for about 20 minutes?
   a. Negative pressure ventilator.
   b. Pressure-cycled ventilator (e.g., Bird Mark 7).
   c. Volume-cycled ventilator (e.g., Puritan-Bennett 7200a).
   d. Manual resuscitation bag.
10. Which would you use for a trauma victim with crushed chest injuries?
    a. Negative pressure ventilator.
    b. Pressure-cycled ventilator (e.g., Bird Mark 7).
    c. Volume-cycled ventilator (e.g., Puritan-Bennett 7200a).
    d. Manual resuscitation bag.
11. Which would you use for a patient with permanent respiratory muscle paralysis due to polio?
    a. Negative pressure ventilator.
    b. Pressure-cycled ventilator (e.g., Bird Mark 7).
    c. Volume-cycled ventilator (e.g., Puritan-Bennett 7200a).
    d. Manual resuscitation bag.

12. Which would you use while transporting a patient from the emergency room to the ICU?
    a. Negative pressure ventilator.
    b. Pressure-cycled ventilator (e.g., Bird Mark 7).
    c. Volume-cycled ventilator (e.g., Puritan-Bennett 7200a).
    d. Manual resuscitation bag.
13. A patient with hiccups is being ventilated on the MA-1 ventilator with an IMV circuit added to it. What mode of ventilation would you select?
    a. Paralyze and control the patient.
    b. Assist-control.
    c. Pressure control.
    d. IMV.
    e. Pressure support.
14. A patient with severe tetanus (a rigid paralysis) needs ventilatory support. Which of the following modes would you select?
    a. Paralyze, sedate, and control ventilation.
    b. Assist-control.
    c. SIMV.
    d. Pressure control with inverse I/E ratio.
    e. Pressure support.
15. In which of the following circumstances is it appropriate to select pressure-supported ventilation?
    I. As a method of weaning.
    II. To reduce the work of breathing around the ET tube and the circuit.
    III. For a patient with ARDS.
    IV. For long-term support of permanently paralyzed patients.
    a. I and III.
    b. II only.
    c. III only.
    d. IV only.
    e. I and II.
16. In which of the following conditions would it be appropriate to use pressure control?
    I. ARDS.
    II. When the patient is capable of doing most of the work of breathing.
    III. COPD.
    IV. When peak pressures exceed 60 cm H_2O.
    a. I only.
    b. II and III.
    c. III only.
    d. I and IV.
    e. IV only.

17. A male patient has a BSA of 1.5 m^2, is 5 ft 8 in. tall, and weighs 175 lb. The patient has a history of lung damage due to old tuberculosis scars. What $\dot{V}_E$ setting would you select for this patient?
    a. 5.25 L/min.
    b. 1.5 L/min.
    c. 6.0 L/min.
    d. 2.25 L/min.
    e. 4.2 L/min.
18. What V_T setting would you select?
    a. 550 ml.
    b. 660 ml.
    c. 840 ml.
    d. 1,100 ml.
    e. 1,500 ml.
19. A patient at 10,000 ft altitude must have the initial $\dot{V}_E$ adjusted on the ventilator. You
    a. Increase it by 25%.
    b. Decrease it by 9%.
    c. Decrease it by 10%.
    d. Increase it by 10%.
    e. Do not change.
20. A patient on the BEAR 2 is being ventilated with the assist-control mode. The flow rate is set at 30 L/min. V_T is 1,000 mL. The machine rate is set at 10 breaths/min, but the actual assisted rate is 20 breaths/min. You notice that the peak pressure has been rising progressively over the last several breaths. Pressure does not go back to zero at the end of exhalation and seems to be rising. The pressure limit alarm starts sounding. To correct this situation, what would you do?
    a. Decrease the rate.
    b. Increase the pressure limit.
    c. Increase the flow.
    d. Decrease the flow.
    e. Increase the sensitivity.

ANSWERS TO STUDY QUESTIONS

1. b	6. c	11. a	16. d
2. b	7. c	12. d	17. c
3. a	8. a	13. d	18. d
4. e	9. b	14. a	19. a
5. c	10. c	15. e	20. c

REFERENCES

1. Abraham E, Yoshihara G: Cardiorespiratory effects of pressure controlled inverse ratio ventilation in severe respiratory failure. *Chest* 1989; 96:1356–1359.
2. Al-Saady N, Bennett ED: Decelerating inspiratory flow waveform improves lung mechanics and gas exchange in patients on intermittent positive-pressure ventilation. *Intensive Care Med* 1985; 11:68–75.
3. American National Standards Institute: *American National Standard for Breathing Machines for Medical Use.* New York, American National Standards Institute. 1976 (Jan 26); 7:no. 279.
4. Andersen J: Ventilatory strategy in catastrophic lung disease: Inversed ratio ventilation (IRV) and combined high frequency ventilation (CHFV). *Acta Anaesthesiol Scand* 1989; 33:145–148.
5. Arnold JS, Summer JL, Tipton RD, et al: Inverse ratio ventilation in hypoxic respiratory failure (abstract). *Chest* 1989; 2:150S.
6. Baldwin E, Cournard A, Richards DW Jr: Pulmonary insufficiency: Methods of analysis, physiologic classification, standard values in normal subjects. *Medicine (Baltimore)* 1948; 27:243–278.
7. Banner MJ, Boysen PG, Lampotang S, et al: End-tidal CO_2 affected by inspiratory time and flow waveform – time for a change. *Crit Care Med* 1986; 14:374.
8. Beaty CD, Ritz RH, Benson MS: Continuous in-line nebulizers complicate pressure support ventilation. *Chest* 1989; 96:1360–1363.
9. Bendixen HH, Hedley-White J, Laver MB: Impaired oxygenation in surgical patients during general anesthesia with controlled ventilation: A concept of atelectasis. *N Engl J Med* 1963; 269:991–996.
10. Bergman NA (ed): Concerning sweet dreams, health and quiet breathing. *Anesthesiology* 1970; 32:297–298.
11. Boothby WM, Sandiford RB: Nomographic charts for the calculation of the metabolic rate by the gasometry method. *Boston Med Surg J* 1921; 185:337–354.
12. Boysen PG, McGough E: Points of view: Pressure support. *Respir Care* 1989; 2:129–134.
13. Branson RD: Enhanced capabilities of current ICU ventilators: Do they really benefit patients? *Respir Care* 1991; 36:362–376.
14. Branson RD, Campbell RS, Davis K, et al: Altering flowrate during maximum pressure support ventilation (PSV_{max}): Effects on cardiorespiratory function. *Respir Care* 1990; 35:1056–1064.
15. Burton GG, Gee AN, Hodgkin JE: *Respiratory Care – A Guide to Clinical Practice.* Philadelphia, JB Lippincott Co, 1977.
16. Burton GG, Hodgkin JE, Ward JJ: *Respiratory Care – A Guide to Clinical Practice,* ed 3. Philadelphia, JB Lippincott Co, 1991.
17. Bushnell SS, Bushnell LS, Reichle MJ, et al: *Respiratory Intensive Care Nursing.* Boston, Little, Brown & Co, 1973.
18. Ciszek TA, Modanlou HD, Owings D, et al: Mean airway pressure – significance during mechanical ventilation in neonates. *J Pediatr* 1981; 99:121–126.
19. Cole AGH, Weller SF, Sykes MK: Inverse ratio ventilation compared with PEEP in adult respiratory failure. *Intensive Care Med* 1984; 10:337–339.

20. Colgan FJ, Marocco PP: Cardiorespiratory effects of constant and intermittent positive-pressure breathing. *Anesthesiology* 1970; 36:444–448.
21. Connors AF, McCaffree DR, Gray BA: Effect of inspiratory flow rate on gas exchange during mechanical ventilation. *Am Rev Respir Dis* 1981; 124:537–543.
22. Cropp A, DiMarco AF: Effects of intermittent negative pressure ventilation on respiratory muscle function in patients with severe chronic obstructive pulmonary disease. *Am Rev Respir Dis* 1987; 135:1056–1061.
23. Czervinske MP, Shreve J, Lester KB, et al: Effects of pressure on respiratory pattern and airway pressure during pressure support ventilation (PSV) in infants with chronic lung disease (abstract). *Respir Care* 1988; 33:930.
24. Dammann JF, McAslan TC: Optimal flow pattern for mechanical ventilation of the lungs—evaluation with a model lung. *Crit Care Med* 1977; 5:128.
25. Dammann JF, McAslan TC, Maffeo CJ: Optimal flow for mechanical ventilation of the lungs. 2. The effect of a sine versus square wave flow pattern with and without an end-inspiratory pause on patients. *Crit Care Med* 1978; 6:293–310.
26. Downs JB: Ventilatory patterns and modes of ventilation in acute respiratory failure. *Respir Care* 1983; 28:586–591.
27. Downs JB, Douglas ME, Ruiz BC, et al: Comparison of assisted and controlled mechanical ventilation in anesthetized swine. *Crit Care Med* 1979; 7:5–8.
28. Duncan SR, Rizk NW, Raffin TA: Inverse ratio ventilation: PEEP in disguise? (editorial) *Chest* 1987; 92:390–391.
29. Egan DF: *Fundamentals of Respiratory Therapy.* St Louis, Mosby–Year Book, Inc, 1973.
30. Ershowsky P, Krieger B: Changes in breathing pattern during pressure support ventilation. *Respir Care* 1987; 32:1011–1016.
31. Feeley TW: Mechanical ventilatory support: Current techniques and recent advances. Chicago, American Society of Anesthesiology Refresher Courses, 1983; 202:1–7.
32. Fleming WH, Bowen JC: A comparative evaluation of pressure limited and volume limited respiration for prolonged postoperative ventilatory support in combat casualties. *Ann Surg* 1972; 176:49–53.
33. Forrette TL, Cairo JM: Changes in ventilatory dynamics during mechanical ventilation with pressure support (abstract). *Respir Care* 1988; 33:930.
34. George B, Jerurski W, Plummer A: A physiological approach to patients requiring mechanical ventilation. *Respir Care* 1978; 23:71–78.
35. Graves TH, Gordon M, Cramolini M, et al: Inverse ratio ventilation in a 6-year-old with severe post-traumatic adult respiratory distress syndrome. *Crit Care Med* 1989; 17:588–589.
36. Gurevitch MJ, VanDyke J, Young ES, et al: Improved oxygenation and lower peak airway pressure in severe adult respiratory distress syndrome: Treatment with inverse ratio ventilation. *Chest* 1986; 89:211–213.
37. Hastings D, Sabo J: Pressure-controlled inverse ratio ventilation for adult respiratory distress syndrome (abstract). *Respir Care* 1988; 33:957.
38. Hedley-White J, Pontoppidan H, Morris MJ: The relation of alveolar to tidal ventilation during respiratory failure in man. *Anesthesiology* 1966; 27:218–219.
39. Hess D, Ruppert T, Kemp T: A bench evaluation of pressure-controlled ventilation (PCV) (abstract). *Respir Care* 1989; 34:1045–1046.

40. Hoffman RA, Ershowsky P, Krieger BP: Determination of auto-PEEP during spontaneous and controlled ventilation by monitoring changes in end-expiratory thoracic gas volume. *Chest* 1989; 96:613–616.
41. Holtakers TR, Loosborck LM, Gracey DR: The use of the chest cuirass in respiratory failure of neurologic origin. *Respir Care* 1982; 27:271–275.
42. Housley E, Louzada N, Becklake MR: To sigh or not to sigh. *Am Rev Respir Dis* 1970; 101:611–614.
43. Jansson L, Jonson B: A theoretical study on flow patterns of ventilators. *Scand J Respir Dis* 1972; 53:237–246.
44. Joint Commission of Accreditation of Hospitals: *Accreditation Manual for Hospitals.* Chicago, Joint Commission on Accreditation of Hospitals, 1984.
45. Kacmarek RM: The role of pressure support ventilation in reducing work of breathing. *Respir Care* 1988; 33:99–120.
46. Kacmarek RM: Points of view: Pressure support. *Respir Care* 1989; 34:136–138.
47. Kacmarek RM, Dimas S, Mack CW: *The Essentials of Respiratory Therapy.* St Louis, Mosby–Year Book, Inc, 1982.
48. Kacmarek RM, Hess D: Pressure-controlled inverse-ratio ventilation: Panacea or auto-PEEP (editorial). *Respir Care* 1990; 35:945–948.
49. Kacmarek RM, McMahon K, Staneck K: Pressure support level required to overcome work of breathing imposed by endotracheal tubes at various peak inspiratory flowrates (abstract). *Respir Care* 1988; 33:933.
50. Kacmarek RM, Stoller JK (eds): *Current Respiratory Care,* Philadelphia, BC Decker, Inc, 1988.
51. Kacmarek RM, Venegas J: Mechanical ventilatory rates and tidal volumes. *Respir Care* 1987; 32:466–478.
52. Kirby RR: Weaning from mechanical ventilation. *Curr Rev Resp Ther* 1985; 6:lesson 10.
53. Kirby RR: Modes of mechanical ventilation, in Kacmarek RM, Stoller JK (eds): *Current Respiratory Care.* Philadelphia, BC Decker, Inc, 1988, pp 128–131.
54. Kirby RR, Banner MJ, Downs JB: *Clinical Applications of Ventilatory Support,* ed 2. New York, Churchill Livingstone Inc, 1990.
55. Lachman B, Danzman E, Haendly B, et al: Ventilator settings and gas exchange in respiratory distress syndrome, in Prakash O (ed): *Applied Physiology in Respiratory Care,* Boston, Martinus Nijhoff, 1982, pp 141–176.
56. Lain DC, DeBenedetto R, Morris SL, et al: Pressure control inverse ratio ventilation as a method to reduce peak inspiratory pressure and provide adequate ventilation and oxygenation. *Chest* 1989; 95:1081–1088.
57. Laver MB, Morgan J, Bendixen HH, et al: Lung volume, compliance, and arterial oxygen tensions during controlled ventilation. *J Appl Physiol* 1964; 19:725–733.
58. Lee PC, Helsmoortel CM, Cohn SM, et al: Are low tidal volumes safe? *Chest* 1990; 97:425–429.
59. Levine M, Gilbert R, Auchincloss JH Jr: A comparison of the effects of sighs, large tidal volumes, and positive end expiratory pressure in assisted ventilation. *Scand J Respir Dis* 1972; 53:101–108.
60. Lough MD, Chatburn R, Schrock WA: *Handbook of Respiratory Care.* St Louis, Mosby–Year Book, Inc, 1983.

61. MacIntyre NR: Respiratory function during pressure support ventilation. *Chest* 1986; 89:677–683.
62. MacIntyre NR: Pressure support ventilation. *Respir Care* 1986; 31:189.
63. MacIntyre NR: Pressure support ventilation: Effects on ventilatory reflexes and ventilatory-muscle workloads. *Respir Care* 1987; 32:447–457.
64. MacIntyre NR: Weaning from mechanical ventilatory support: Volume-assisting intermittent breaths versus pressure-assisting every breath. *Respir Care* 1988; 33:121–125.
65. MacIntyre NR: Pressure support:inspiratory assist, in Kacmarek RM, Stoller JK (eds): *Current Respiratory Care,* Philadelphia, BC Decker, Inc, 1988, pp 144–147.
66. MacIntyre NR, Leatherman NE: Ventilatory muscle loads and the frequency-tidal volume pattern during inspiratory pressure-assisted (pressure-supported) ventilation. *Am Rev Respir Dis* 1990; 141:327–331.
67. Man GCW, Jones RL, McDonald GF, et al: Primary alveolar hypoventilation managed by negative-pressure ventilators. *Chest* 1979; 76:219–220.
68. Marini JJ, Capps JS, Culver BH: The inspiratory work of breathing during assisted mechanical ventilation. *Chest* 1985; 87:612.
69. Marini J, Crooke P, Truwit J: Determinants and limits of pressure-preset ventilation: A mathematical model of pressure control. *J Appl Physiol* 1989;67:1081–1092.
70. Marini JJ, Rodriguez RM, Lamb V: Bedside estimation of the inspiratory work of breathing during mechanical ventilation. *Chest* 1986; 89:56.
71. Marks A, Bogles J, Morganti L: A new ventilatory assister for patients with respiratory acidosis. *N Engl J Med* 1963; 268:61–68.
72. Martz KV, Joiner J, Shepherd RM: *Management of the Patient-Ventilator System: A Team Approach,* ed 2. St Louis, Mosby–Year Book, Inc, 1984.
73. McGough EK, Banner MJ, Boysen PG: Pressure support and flow-cycled, assisted mechanical ventilation in acute lung injury. *Chest* 1990; 98:458–462.
74. McPherson SP: *Respiratory Therapy Equipment.* St Louis, Mosby–Year Book, Inc, 1981.
75. Mithoefer JC, Holford FD, Keighley JFH: The effect of oxygen administration on mixed venous oxygenation in chronic obstructive pulmonary disease. *Chest* 1974; 66:122–133.
76. Mithoefer JC, Keighley JF, Karetzkey MS: Response of the arterial PO_2 to oxygen administration in chronic pulmonary disease. *Ann Intern Med* 1971; 74:328–335.
77. Moomjian AS, Schwartz JG, Shutack JG, et al: Use of external expiratory resistance in intubated neonates to increase lung volume. *Arch Dis Child* 1981; 56:869–873.
78. Mushin WW, Rendell-Baker L, Thompson PW, et al: *Automatic Ventilation of the Lungs.* Philadelphia, FA Davis Co, 1980.
79. Owen-Thomas JB, Ulan OA, Swyer PR: The effect of varying inspiratory gas flow rate on arterial oxygenation during IPPV in the respiratory distress syndrome. *Br J Anaesth* 1968; 40:468–502.
80. Pepe PE, Marini JJ: Occult positive end-expiratory pressure in mechanically ventilated patients with airflow obstruction. *Am Rev Respir Dis* 1982; 126:166–170.
81. Perel A: Newer ventilatory modes: Temptations and pitfalls (editorial). *Crit Care Med* 1987; 15:707–709.

82. Perlman ND, Schena J, Thompson JE, et al: Effects of ET tube-size, working pressure and compliance on pressure support ventilation (abstract). *Respir Care* 1988; 33:928.
83. Peruzzi WT: Full and partial ventilatory support: The significance of ventilator mode (editorial). *Respir Care* 1990; 35:174–175.
84. Pierson DJ: Indications for mechanical ventilation in acute respiratory failure. *Respir Care* 1983; 23:570–578.
85. Primiano FP, Chatburn RL, Lough MD: Mean airway pressure: Theoretical considerations. *Crit Care Med* 1982; 10:378–383.
86. Quan SF: A ghost from the past. Low tidal volume mechanical ventilation revisited (editorial). *Chest* 1990; 97:261–262.
87. Radford EP, Ferris BG, Kriete BC: Clinical use of a nomogram to estimate proper ventilation during artificial respirations. *N Engl J Med* 1954; 251:877–884.
88. Rarey KP, Youtsey JW: *Respiratory Patient Care.* Englewood Cliffs, NJ, Prentice-Hall, Inc, 1981.
89. Rau JJ, Shelledy DC: The effect of varying inspiratory flow waveforms on peak and mean airway pressures with a time-cycled volume ventilator: A bench study. *Respir Care* 1991; 36:347–356.
90. Reynolds EOR: Effect of alterations in mechanical ventilatory settings on pulmonary gas exchange in hyaline membrane disease. *Arch Dis Child* 1971; 46:152–159.
91. Ritz R, Bishop M, Robinson C: Guidelines for choosing the appropriate level of pressure support (PS) with a BEAR 5 to overcome imposed work of breathing (WOBi) (abstract). *Respir Care* 1988; 33:933.
92. Robinson C, Bishop M, Ritz R: Guidelines for choosing the appropriate level of pressure support with a Servo 900C to overcome imposed work of breathing (WOBi) (abstract). *Respir Care* 1988; 33:933.
93. Rossi A, Gottfried SB, Zocchi L, et al: Measurement of static compliance of the total respiratory system in patients with acute respiratory failure during mechanical ventilation. The effect of intrinsic positive end-expiratory pressure. *Am Rev Respir Dis* 1985; 131:672–677.
94. Scanlan CL, Spearman CB, Sheldon RL: *Egan's Fundamentals of Respiratory Care,* ed 5. St Louis, Mosby–Year Book, Inc, 1990.
95. Shapiro BA, Cane RD: The IMV-AMV controversy: A plea for clarification and redirection. *Crit Care Med* 1984; 12:472–473.
96. Shapiro BA, Cane RD, Harrison RA, et al: Changes in intrapulmonary shunting with administration of 100 percent oxygen. *Chest* 1980; 77:138–141.
97. Shelledy DC, Mikles SP: Newer modes of mechanical ventilation; part 1: Pressure support. *Respiratory Management* July/Aug, 1988, pp 14–20.
98. Slonim N, Balfour L, Hamilton H: *Respiratory Pharmacology.* St Louis, Mosby–Year Book, Inc, 1971.
99. Spearman CB: Appropriate ventilator selection, in Kacmarek RM, Stoller JK: *Current Respiratory Care.* Philadelphia, BC Decker, Inc, 1988, pp 123–127.
100. Spearman J, Sheldon R, Egan DF: *Fundamentals of Respiratory Therapy.* St Louis, Mosby–Year Book, Inc, 1982.
101. Splaingard ML, Frates RC, Jefferson LS, et al: Home negative pressure ventilation: Report of 20 years of experience in patients with neuromuscular disease. *Arch Phys Med Rehabil* 1985; 66:239–247.

102. Suter PM, Fairley HB, Isenberg MD: Effect of tidal volume and positive end-expiratory pressure on compliance during mechanical ventilation. *Chest* 1978; 73:158–162.
103. Sykes MK, Young WE, Robinson BE: Oxygenation during anesthesia with controlled ventilation. *Br J Anaesth* 1965; 37:314–325.
104. Tharratt RS, Allen RP, Albertson TE: Pressure controlled inverse ratio ventilation in severe adult respiratory failure. *Chest* 1989; 94:755–762.
105. Tokioka H, Saito S, Kosaka F: Effect of pressure support ventilation on breathing patterns and respiratory work. *Intensive Care Med* 1989; 15:491–494.
106. Trevino MD, Walters PR: The effects of working pressure on tidal volume and inspiratory flow during pressure support ventilation with the Siemens 900C (abstract). *Respir Care* 1988; 33:926.
107. Visick WD, Fairley HB, Hickey RE: The effects of tidal volume and end-expiratory pressures on pulmonary gas exchange during anesthesia. *Anesthesiology* 1973; 19:285–290.
108. Walker K, Parker JR: Effect of inspiratory flow pattern on peak and mean airway pressures with the Veolar ventilator (abstract). *Respir Care* 1988; 33:905.
109. Whitten CE: *Anyone Can Intubate.* San Diego, Medical Arts Press, 1989.
110. Wissing DR, Romero MD, George RB: Comparing the newer modes of mechanical ventilation. *J Crit Illness* 1987; 2:41–49.

Chapter 7

Effects and Complications of Mechanical Ventilation

On completion of this chapter the reader will be able to:

1. Explain the effects of positive pressure ventilation on cardiac output and venous return to the heart.
2. Discuss the three factors affecting cardiac output during IPPV.
3. Describe how IPPV increases intracranial pressure.
4. Summarize the effects of IPPV on renal response and humoral response in the body.
5. Describe the effects of abnormal arterial blood gases on renal function.
6. Explain the effects of IPPV on gas distribution and pulmonary blood flow in the lungs.
7. List the effects of mechanical ventilation on ventilatory status.
8. Define auto-PEEP and list its complications.
9. Name three physiologic factors which lead to the occurrence of auto-PEEP.
10. Describe the procedures for measuring auto-PEEP.
11. List three potential methods for reducing auto-PEEP.

12. Discuss one benefit of auto-PEEP.
13. Explain the three primary hazards of oxygen therapy with mechanical ventilation.
14. List and describe four types of barotrauma associated with mechanical ventilation.
15. Summarize the risks of artificial airways during mechanical ventilation.
16. Discuss the problems of infections in intubated patients.
17. Define the following terms: work of breathing, intrinsic work, extrinsic work, and system-imposed work of breathing.
18. From a graph, explain the components of work of breathing.
19. List the steps to take to reduce the work of breathing in mechanically ventilated patients.
20. From a description of a malfunction on a ventilator, determine the possible cause of the malfunction.
21. Name five ways of assessing a patient's nutritional status.
22. Describe techniques that can be used to reduce some of the complications associated with mechanical ventilation.

EFFECTS AND COMPLICATIONS OF MECHANICAL VENTILATION

Artificial ventilation is an invasive technique. There are many complications and hazards that can occur whenever one's normal balance is interrupted by outside factors. The benefits will outweigh the complications since failure to support ventilation is likely to result in death. Intermittent positive pressure ventilation (IPPV) has been in general use for many years. Most of the time it is without significant side effects. When used safely and effectively, IPPV continues to be the primary tool for maintaining ventilation in patients with acute respiratory failure.

The effective use of mechanical ventilation requires thorough understanding of its effects on both normal body function and on the functional physiology of the diseased patient. What these effects are and how adverse effects can be minimized are the focus of this chapter. Much of the research concerning the side effects of positive pressure ventilation also includes studies on PEEP. Where appropriate, the findings of these studies are included.

CARDIOVASCULAR EFFECTS OF MECHANICAL VENTILATION

The primary cardiovascular complication of mechanical ventilation, reduction of cardiac output (CO), has been known for several decades. This phenomenon can be understood by comparing normal spontaneous ventilation to positive pressure breathing.

Decreased Cardiac Output

The Normal Thoracic Pump Mechanism (Fig 7–1).—During spontaneous ventilation, the fall in intrathoracic pressure that draws air into the lungs also draws blood into the major thoracic vessels and heart. With the return of blood to the right heart and the stretching and enlargement of the right heart volume, the right ventricular preload is enhanced. As a result, the stroke volume, or the amount of blood pumped per beat, also increases from the right heart. During spontaneous exhalation the return of blood to the left heart temporarily increases as blood from the right heart passes through the pulmonary circulation. This increase in left ventricular preload then transiently increases left ventricular stroke volume.

The right ventricle receives less blood during passive spontaneous exhalation since the intrathoracic pressure is less negative. As the right heart output decreases, the left heart output decreases at the end of passive exhalation. The cycle then repeats itself with each breath.

The Thoracic Pump Mechanism During IPPV and PEEP.—During inspiration with positive pressure ventilation the increased pressures are transmitted to the vessels and other structures in the thorax (Fig 7–2). The major blood vessels

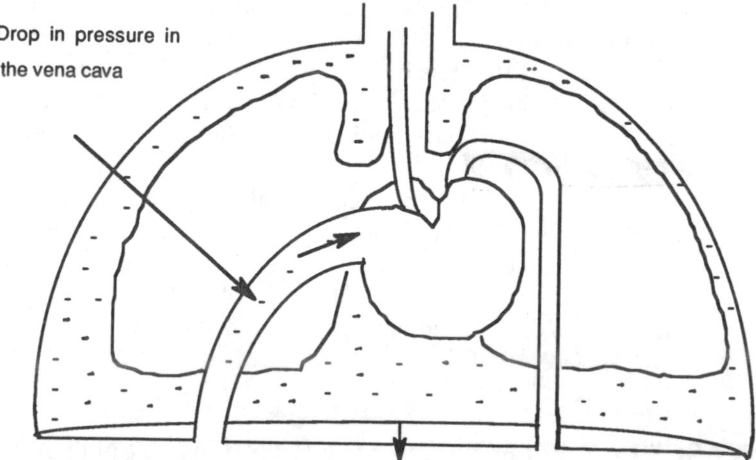

FIG 7–1.
The negative intrapleural pressures that occur during spontaneous inspiration are transmitted to the intrathoracic vessels. A drop in pressure in the vena cava increases the pressure gradient back to the heart and venous return increases.

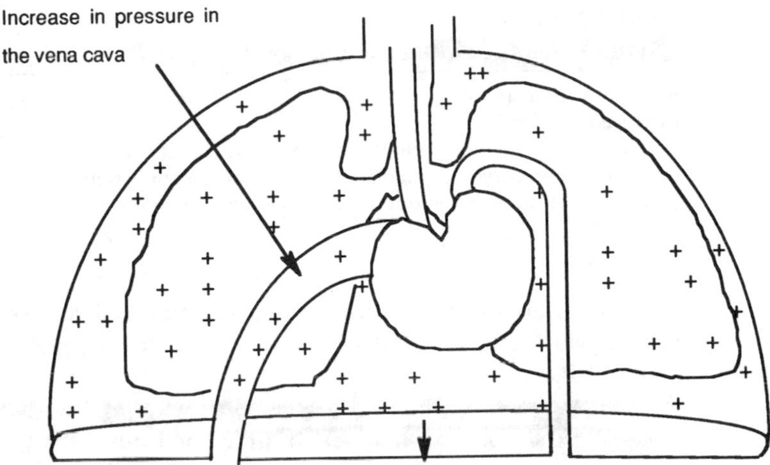

FIG 7–2.
Positive pressure breath (IPPV) increases lung and intrapleural pressures. This positive pressure is transmitted to the intrathoracic vessels. A rise in pressure in the vena cava reduces venous return to the heart.

are compressed, and the central venous pressure increases. As a result the pressure gradient for blood flow back to the heart is reduced so less blood returns to the thorax. The decrease in venous return causes a lowering of right ventricular filling (preload) and right heart stroke volume.[31] At the same time, the pulmonary capillaries which interlace the alveoli are stretched and narrowed. This squeezes the blood into the left heart causing a brief increase in the left ventricular stroke volume. The left ventricular output then falls as a result of lower right heart output.[19, 50] This can bring about a drop in systemic blood pressure, especially in hypovolemic patients.

Right heart output can also drop as high positive end-expiratory pressure (PEEP) levels increase the resistance of blood flow through the pulmonary system. This results in a rise in the resting volume of the right ventricle. This forces the interventricular septum to the left. As a result, left ventricular volume may decrease since its ability to fill is limited. This may also affect CO, but is not as important as the reduction in venous return to the thorax.[50] In addition, lower CO may be due to reduced perfusion to the myocardium and result in myocardial ischemia. The lower perfusion could be a result of low CO and blood pressure or it may be a direct effect of the positive pressure on the outside of the heart. This would reduce the blood supply to the heart.

Left ventricular output may also decrease as a result of changes in afterload and changes in the ability of the heart to contract. Contractility of the heart may be affected by chemicals produced by the body that are actually negative inotropic agents. It may also be affected by abnormal neural reflexes. But the effect

TABLE 7–1.
Factors Reducing Cardiac Output During IPPV and PEEP

Reduced venous return
Increased afterload
Possible decrease in contractility from myocardial ischemia
Circulating normally produced agents that reduce contractility
Low left ventricular filling due to right ventricular volume increase and septal shifting

of these endogenous humoral agents and neural reflexes is modest.[50] Table 7–1 lists the factors that tend to decrease CO during positive pressure ventilation and PEEP.

During the inspiratory phase of controlled ventilation, the heart is compressed between the expanding lungs. The longer the inspiratory phase and the greater the peak pressure, the less the CO. This tamponade effect occurs when venous return to the thorax is reduced. It is questionable whether the decrease in CO is due to lower venous return from increased intrapleural pressure, or compression of the heart and subsequent alteration of its function.

Compensation in Normal Persons.—In normal patients a fall in blood pressure rarely occurs as a result of compensatory mechanisms. The decrease in stroke volume rapidly leads to the development of tachycardia and an increase in systemic vascular resistance and peripheral venous pressure due to sympathetic arterial and venous constriction. Some peripheral shunting of blood away from the kidneys and lower extremities also occurs.[127] The net effect is a maintenance of blood pressure even with a decrease in CO.[127]

The ability of the compensating mechanisms to perform their function depends on the integrity of normal reflexes. These reflexes can be blocked or impaired in the presence of sympathetic blockade, spinal anesthesia, moderate levels of general anesthesia, spinal cord transection, or severe polyneuritis.[30] In a patient in whom IPPV is being started or the ventilatory mode is being changed, the blood pressure is measured to ensure that the normal vascular reflexes are intact. A normal response shows that the patient is in no danger of a significant drop in CO and blood pressure.

Factors Affecting Decreased Cardiac Output

Lung Compliance.—The degree of depression in CO with mechanical ventilation depends on several factors. Modest increases in intrapleural pressure will not alter the CO as much as high increases in intrapleural pressure.[12–14] Also, patients with very stiff lungs, such as those with adult respiratory distress syndrome (ARDS), are less likely to experience hemodynamic changes with high ventilating pressures. With stiff lungs, less of the alveolar pressure (P_A) is transmitted to the intrapleural space. On the other hand, patients with compliant lungs and stiff (noncompliant) chest walls are more likely to have higher intrapleural pressures during IPPV.

Lower Positive Pressures.—One way to lessen the decrease in CO is to reduce the amount of positive pressure exerted in the thorax. It is known that minimal changes in CO occur during mechanical ventilation when relatively rapid inflation, rapid deflation, and inspiratory-expiratory (I/E) ratios of 1:2 or less are used.[31] The type of flow patterns used to deliver the breath, e.g., square wave vs. sine wave vs. decelerating flow wave, are less important than the I/E ratio.[30]

Increased Airway Resistance.—With patients who have increased airway resistance (Raw), the peak inspiratory pressure (PIP) during mechanical ventilation may be very high. Much of the pressure, however, is lost to the resistive airways and less pressure actually reaches the alveolar level and the intrapleural space.[30] So high PIP does not always mean that CO will be affected.

EFFECTS OF PEEP AND IPPV

The effects of PEEP on normal heart function are more significant than with IPPV alone. PEEP plus IPPV decreases CO more than PEEP with intermittent mandatory ventilation (IMV) or continuous positive airway pressure (CPAP) with no mechanical breaths. The complications of PEEP and its effect on cardiac function are covered in Chapter 10.

EFFECTS OF MECHANICAL VENTILATION ON INTRACRANIAL PRESSURE AND CEREBRAL PERFUSION

The amount of flow of blood to the brain is determined by the cerebral perfusion pressure (CPP). CPP is calculated by subtracting the intracranial pressure (ICP) from the mean systemic arterial blood pressure (MAP).[100] Since mechanical ventilation with or without PEEP can decrease CO and MAP, this can potentially decrease CPP. For example, if MAP drops from 100 to 70 mm Hg and the ICP was 15 mm Hg, then the CPP would decrease from 85 mm Hg (100 − 15 = 85) to 55 mm Hg (70 − 15 = 55).

Since mechanical ventilation increases central venous pressure, this may decrease venous return from the head, increase ICP, and decrease CPP. Clinically, this could be observed by an increase in jugular vein distention. The net result is a potential for cerebral hypoxemia from a reduced perfusion to the head and an increase in cerebral edema from increased ICP.

The greatest clinical risk related to cerebral perfusion is for patients who already have an increased ICP and who may develop cerebral edema. Patients with head injuries, cerebral tumors, and postneurosurgery patients fall into this category. With normal intracranial dynamics, patients do not seem to develop increased ICP with positive pressure ventilation,[127] while those with abnormal cerebral function do appear affected by changes in cerebral perfusion and pressures. These patients are often mechanically hyperventilated to reduce cerebral perfusion by lowering arterial carbon dioxide partial pressure ($Paco_2$) to 25 to 30 mm Hg. Alkalosis from low $Paco_2$ can constrict cerebral vessels. This reduces ICP and augments cerebral perfusion.

Some patients with head injury or cerebral dysfunction require PEEP for the treatment of refractory hypoxemia due to increased shunting and decreased functional residual capacity (FRC). PEEP, as shown previously, can increase ICP. On the other hand, if PEEP is needed to maintain oxygenation, it may be lifesaving and should be used. It is important to monitor ICP in this patient group.[50]

RENAL EFFECTS OF MECHANICAL VENTILATION

It has been known for more than four decades that pressurized breathing can induce changes in renal function.[40] These changes can be broken down into three areas:

1. Renal responses to hemodynamic changes resulting from high intrathoracic pressures.
2. Humoral responses including antidiuretic hormone (ADH), atrial natriuretic peptide (ANP), and renin-angiotensin-aldosterone changes occurring with positive pressure breathing and later renal functions.
3. Abnormal pH, $Paco_2$ and arterial oxygen partial pressure (Pao_2) abnormalities affecting the kidney.

Renal Response to Hemodynamic Changes

The decreased CO following positive alveolar pressure tends to decrease renal blood flow and glomerular flow rates, and as a result, to decrease urinary output.[106, 108] The decreased urine production, however, is not entirely due to the decreased CO, since returning CO to adequate levels is not accompanied by parallel increases in urinary output.

The following phenomena support the idea that decreased urinary output with IPPV is not due entirely to a decreased CO. When the kidneys are not affected by neural or humoral factors, renal blood flow and glomerular flow rate stay fairly constant over a wide range of arterial pressures. As a result, urinary output stays fairly constant. MAP must drop below 75 mm Hg before renal blood flow decreases. As the glomerular capillary pressure decreases, glomerular flow rate is reduced and urinary flow decreases. In profound hypotension, urinary outflow may stop.[108]

Since the arterial blood pressure is usually compensated where IPPV is used, decreased blood pressure is probably not a significant factor leading to decreased urinary output during mechanical ventilation. The redistribution of blood inside the kidney, on the other hand, may be responsible for cardiovascular-induced changes in kidney function during mechanical ventilation.[8, 40, 57]

Total renal blood flow has been found to remain nearly constant in dogs even when continuous positive pressure breathing (CPPB) of +10 cm H_2O is used. What occurs is a redistribution of intrarenal blood. Flow to the outer cortex decreases, while flow to the inner cortex and outer medullary tissue (juxtamedullary nephrons) increases (Fig 7–3).[53] The net result is that urinary output decreases by 40%. Less creatinine (23%) and less sodium (63%) are excreted by the kidneys. This occurs because the juxtamedullary nephrons are more efficient at reabsorbing sodium than the nephrons at the outer cortex. As a result of this shift in blood flow, more sodium is reabsorbed and this is accompanied by a reabsorption of water.

This same type of event also occurs with congestive heart failure, hemorrhage, stimulation of renal sympathetic nerves, and low sodium diets.[57] Since the total renal flow is relatively unchanged with positive pressure ventilation, the

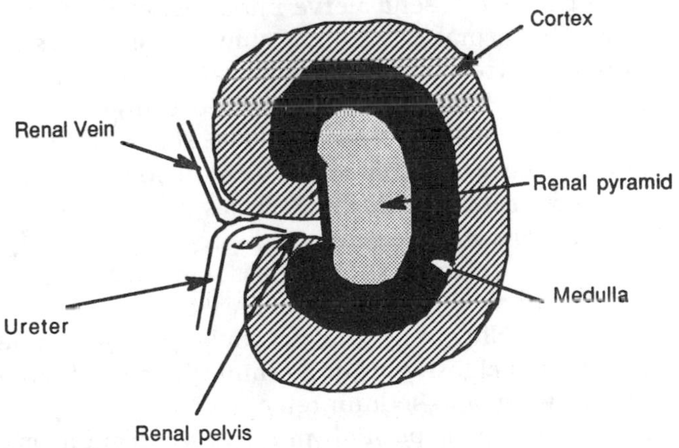

FIG 7–3.
Schematic representation of the kidney.

redistribution of blood in the kidney may be a response to some sympathetic stimulation, such as an increase in catecholamines, vasopressin, or angiotensin. Another possible explanation for this may be related to the renal venous pressure. When the inferior vena cava is constricted or when the right ventricular end-diastolic pressure is increased, as in congestive heart failure, blood flow to the renal cortex decreases. Glomerular flow rate and sodium excretion decrease. This increased sodium retention leads to increased water retention. This effect is reversed when renal perfusion is increased.[108] What this implies is that even if inferior vena cava pressures and renal venous pressures increase due to decreased venous return to the heart as a result of IPPV or CPPB, the effect is reversed if the arterial pressure is maintained.

The importance of this for patients on IPPV is that as long as arterial blood pressure is maintained, one would not expect water retention to occur. If arterial pressures are not maintained, however, water retention may result. This would increase plasma volume and might contribute to the formation of pulmonary edema. Thus the use of dopamine can improve the renal dysfunction that occurs with PEEP in some patients.[50, 127]

Effects of Mechanical Ventilation on Antidiuretic Hormone Activity and Atrial Natriuretic Peptide

Urinary output during mechanical ventilation is believed to decrease as a result of still other mechanisms. For one, the increased release of antidiuretic hormone (ADH), or vasopressin, from the posterior pituitary may reduce urine production. As its name implies, ADH inhibits urine secretion. The higher the level of ADH that is circulating in the blood, the lower the formation of urine, and the greater is the body's fluid volume. Within the left atrium are volume receptors which send nerve impulses over a vagal pathway to the hypothalamus. This neural activity can stimulate increases or decreases in ADH production and secretion. The baroreceptors in the carotid bodies and along the aortic arch sense changes in pressure and can also raise or lower the ADH levels.[94] Since both of these areas are exposed to changes in intrathoracic pressures, blood volume, and blood pressure, it follows that they might respond to mechanical ventilation or PEEP. It has been found that negative pressure ventilation inhibits ADH release and produces diuresis, whereas positive pressure ventilation enhances ADH release and results in oliguria. As IPPV and PEEP reduce atrial filling pressure, this reduces the secretion of atrial natriuretic peptide (ANP). ANP is a naturally produced diuretic agent. It also inhibits secretion of aldosterone and renin. When levels are low from IPPV, this contributes to water and sodium retention.[50]

The effect of positive pressure ventilation on urinary output is probably more a result of cardiovascular changes than a result of increase in plasma ADH or ANP. It is difficult to demonstrate significant changes in these agents. Thus, urinary output changes with mechanical ventilation are probably related to changes in blood pressure, CO, and intrarenal perfusion or mechanisms other than hormonal changes.[8, 108]

Arterial Blood Gases and Kidney Function

Pao_2 and $Paco_2$ changes contribute to the effects of ventilation on the kidneys. Decreasing Pao_2 values in patients with respiratory failure have been known to result in a decreased urinary flow and renal function. With pressures below 40 mm Hg (severe hypoxemia), kidney function was dramatically decreased again. Similarly, $Paco_2$ of greater than 65 mm Hg also decreased renal function and increased ADH.[108]

Effects of Mechanical Ventilation on Other Body Systems

Some patients on IPPV and PEEP show evidence of liver malfunction as reflected by a rise in serum bilirubin (> 2.5 mg/100 mL) even when no evidence of preexisting liver disease is present.[57] This may be a result of a downward movement of the diaphragm against the liver, a decrease in portal venous flow, or an increase in splanchnic resistance, leading to possible ischemia in the liver, or other factors which may lead to impaired liver function.[50]

Positive pressure ventilation increases splanchnic resistance, decreases splanchnic venous outflow, and may contribute to gastric mucosal ischemia. This is one of the factors leading to increased incidence of gastrointestinal bleeding and gastric ulcers which are frequently seen in critically ill patients. These changes are associated with increased permeability of the gastric mucosal barrier. Use of antacid therapy may reduce the incidence of gastrointestinal bleeding from acute stress ulceration.[57]

Mechanical ventilation, especially with PEEP, may increase the release of plasminogen activating factor from the lungs.[89] This activator is responsible for the conversion of plasminogen to plasmin which is an enzyme active in clot dissolution (fibrinolysis).[109] The increase in fibrinolysis may be beneficial to patients on mechanical ventilation who have disorders where increased intravascular coagulation may occur. In other patients on mechanical ventilation, the effect of this increased clot digestion is probably of no clinical significance.

EFFECTS OF MECHANICAL VENTILATION ON GAS DISTRIBUTION AND PULMONARY BLOOD FLOW

Ventilation to Nondependent Lung

Mechanical ventilation alters ventilation-perfusion ($\dot{V}/\dot{Q}$) ratios by directing the greatest amount of gas flow to the nondependent lung regions. During spontaneous ventilation in the upright or supine position, the greatest volume of gas moves toward the diaphragm during inspiration. Thus, the dependent lung areas receive a higher portion of ventilation as well as perfusion. In mechanically ventilated subjects, gas moves through the nondependent regions, taking the path of least resistance.[46] This is due in part to nonmovement of the diaphragm which becomes less compliant than the chest wall and anterior part of the lungs in the supine patient. Unfortunately, this results in areas of $\dot{V}/\dot{Q}$ mismatching and increased dead space ventilation.

During spontaneous ventilation, the distribution of gas not only favors the dependent lung areas but also appears to favor the periphery of the lung closest to the moving pleural surfaces. The peripheral areas receive more ventilation than the central areas.[59, 131, 132] During positive pressure breathing with passive inflation of the lung, the central, upper airway, and peribronchial portions of the lung are preferentially filled with air.[59] This may be another mechanism by which $\dot{V}/\dot{Q}$ mismatching occurs during a positive pressure breath.

During a positive pressure breath, the conductive airways increase in size. This increases dead space ventilation. Additionally, if normal alveoli overexpand with IPPV at the expense of adjacent perfusion vessels, this will also increase dead space. If an increased tidal volume (VT) is delivered and IPPV improves ventilation distribution with respect to perfusion, on the other hand, then IPPV will decrease dead space.

Redistribution of Pulmonary Blood Flow

Normal pulmonary blood flow favors the gravity-dependent areas and the central or core areas of the lungs. Mechanical ventilation with PEEP both decreases CO and redistributes pulmonary perfusion to the lung periphery rather than the center.[56] The clinical significance of this is unknown at this time, but it might alter $\dot{V}/\dot{Q}$ matching.

The increased volume during a positive pressure breath or PEEP squeezes the blood out of nondependent zones, particularly in areas of normal lung. This further contributes to $\dot{V}/\dot{Q}$ mismatching and physiologic dead space by sending more blood into dependent areas where ventilation is now lower, or into disease-affected areas of the lung where lung volumes are not substantially increased. This can lead to increased shunting and decreased Pa_{O_2}.[20, 127]

Conversely, improvement in $\dot{V}/\dot{Q}$ matching occurs when positive pressure is applied to patients who have refractory hypoxemia secondary to a decreased FRC and increased shunting.[35] With PEEP, shunting decreases and Pa_{O_2} increases.[35] This implies improvement in $\dot{V}/\dot{Q}$ matching.

It seems that under this set of circumstances a classic and predictable response of gas distribution and pulmonary perfusion does not exist.

Effects of Positive Pressure on Pulmonary Vascular Resistance

PVR and IPPV.—As described previously, pulmonary perfusion may be compromised during the positive pressure phase of artificial ventilation. In-

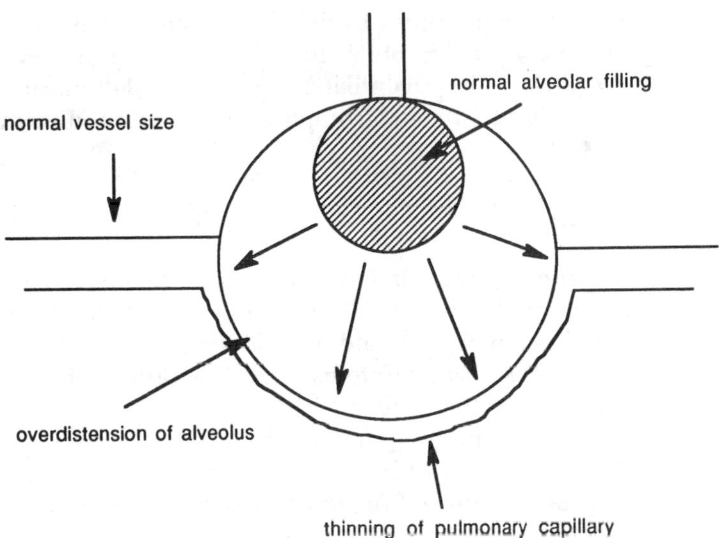

FIG 7–4.
Overfilling of an alveolus. The result is thinning and compression of the pulmonary capillary. Pulmonary vascular resistance is increased.

creased airway and PA leads to thinning and compression of pulmonary capillaries (Fig 7–4). This can result in decreased perfusion and increased pulmonary vascular resistance (PVR). Fortunately, if expiration is prolonged and unimpeded, i.e., if no PEEP or expiratory resistance is used, the decreased pulmonary perfusion may be offset by normal flow back to the thorax during expiration with no net effect on PVR.[108]

In most patients, severe hypoxemia leads to increased PVR. This is caused by constriction of the pulmonary vessels and subsequent pulmonary hypertension. When mechanical ventilation improves oxygenation in these patients by opening up the capillary beds, pulmonary perfusion and PVR may actually improve.

PVR and PEEP.—At low lung volumes, wherein FRC is decreased, the addition of PEEP can potentially open up collapsed alveoli, recruiting intraparenchymal vessels.[60] This improves the $\dot{V}/\dot{Q}$ relationships of the lungs. If volumes become very high, overdistention reduces lung compliance and increases vascular resistance.[65]

EFFECTS OF MECHANICAL VENTILATION ON VENTILATORY STATUS

The primary goal of maintaining normal ventilatory status for a patient on assisted ventilation is not achieved when the ventilator is mismanaged or when it causes abnormalities to the patient such as air trapping. The patient's blood gases end up being abnormal. Causes of ventilatory problems associated with IPPV include hypoventilation, hyperventilation, air trapping, body position, gastric distention, and complications associated with oxygen therapy during IPPV.

Hypoventilation

Acute hypoventilation can occur in patients receiving ventilatory assistance if adequate alveolar ventilation is not provided. This results in a $Paco_2$ above the patient's normal level and an acidotic pH, from the rising $Paco_2$. Evaluation of clinical signs and symptoms as well as arterial blood gas analysis will lead to recognition of the problem.

Acidosis causes a shift to the right in the oxygen dissociation curve and reduces the ability of hemoglobin to bind and carry oxygen. In addition, rises in $Paco_2$ lead to proportionate decreases in Pao_2 and contribute to hypoxemia. If the patient already had hypoxemia, these factors may further reduce oxygenation. Severe acidosis can also lead to cellular damage. Rising $Paco_2$ and a falling pH can lead to coma. Elevated hydrogen ion content contributes to high plasma potassium levels (hyperkalemia) which affect cardiac function and can lead to cardiac dysrhythmias (Table 7–2). Hypercarbia increases cerebral perfusion and can lead to increased ICP. This can be detrimental to patients with cerebral trauma, cerebral hemorrhage, or similar disorders.

Normally the kidneys can compensate for respiratory acidosis within 18 to 36 hours. Obviously, it is more desirable to correct the cause of the problem by increasing alveolar ventilation than it is to wait for renal compensation. This can

TABLE 7–2.
Clinical and Cardiac Changes Associated With Respiratory Acidosis, Hypoxia, and Hyperkalemia

Clinical signs and symptoms
Hypertension (mild to moderate acidosis)
Hypotension (severe acidosis)
Anxiety
Agitation
"Fighting the ventilator"
Dyspnea
Attempts to increase minute ventilation
Headaches
Hot moist skin (associated with increased $Paco_2$)
Cardiac changes associated with hyperkalemia
Elevated and peaked T waves
ST segment depression
Widened QRS complex
Long PR interval

be done by increasing VT or rate. When respiratory acidosis is present in patients on controlled ventilation, the patient may try to override the ventilator and take in a breath. The patient might not be able to trigger the machine and will appear to be fighting the ventilator. Increasing the sensitivity will allow the patient to trigger the ventilator and receive a machine breath (assist mode). Placing the patient on IMV allows for spontaneous ventilation between machine breaths. Still, a minimum effective VT and rate should be set regardless of what mode of ventilation is used in order to correct respiratory acidosis. Use of descending flow rate patterns and use of pressure support are two other possibilities to help relieve the problem.

Hyperventilation

Just as hypoventilation is inappropriate in mechanically ventilated patients, so is hyperventilation in most situations. Hyperventilation results in a lower-than-normal $Paco_2$ and a rise in pH. Evaluation of the patient's clinical picture and arterial blood gases will reveal the problem. Alkalosis causes a shift to the left in the oxygen dissociation curve which enhances the ability of hemoglobin to pick up oxygen in the lungs, but makes it less available at the tissue level. This is known as the Haldane effect. Low hydrogen ion concentrations in the blood are accompanied by hypokalemia (low potassium) which can lead to cardiac arrhythmias (Table 7–3).

Sustained severe hypocarbia can lead to tetany and also reduces cerebral perfusion which may contribute to increased cerebral hypoxia. In patients with increased ICP and cerebral edema, however, this reduced perfusion may be beneficial in reducing abnormally high ICPs. Normally functioning kidneys can help to restore blood pH by retaining hydrogen and excreting bicarbonate over an 18- to 36-hour period. This can compensate for and restore normal acid-base status.

Hyperventilation in mechanically ventilated patients reduces the drive to breathe and leads to apnea.[35] This has the advantage of preventing the patient from trying to fight the ventilator, or from experiencing feelings of dyspnea.[17] The disadvantage is that weaning becomes more difficult if the patient is kept in respiratory alkalosis for a prolonged period of time.[17] The reason for this is related to the central chemoreceptors which respond to changes in Pco_2 and pH. In situations of respiratory alkalosis, carbon dioxide diffuses out of the cerebrospinal fluid (CSF). The hydrogen ion concentration in the CSF then drops and respirations are not stimulated. As long as this condition exists, apnea will remain until the Pao_2 drops low enough to stimulate the peripheral chemoreceptors. If chronic hyperventilation and respiratory alkalosis persist, renal compensation begins. The kidneys remove bicarbonate from the plasma and excrete it in the urine. At the same time, bicarbonate is actively transported out of the CSF so that CSF balances with the plasma bicarbonate. The pH is restored to

TABLE 7–3.
Clinical and Cardiac Changes Associated With Respiratory Alkalosis and Hypokalemia

Clinical signs and symptoms
Cool skin (decreased $Paco_2$ and decreased Pao_2)
Twitching
Tetany
Cardiac changes associated with hypokalemia
Prolonged QT interval
Low rounded T waves
Depressed ST segment
Negative T waves
Inverted P waves
Atrioventricular block
Premature ventricular contractions
Paroxysmal tachycardia
Atrial flutter

normal in both the plasma and the CSF. The bicarbonate and Pco_2 levels will be lower than normal.

Following prolonged hyperventilation, weaning becomes more difficult. As the respiratory rate of the ventilator is reduced, the $Paco_2$ rises. This causes the pH to fall. The patient tries to maintain a high alveolar ventilation to keep the $Paco_2$ at the level at which it has been equilibrated. The patient may tire and be unable to do so. As a result, the $Paco_2$ continues to rise. The carbon dioxide also diffuses into the CSF where the pH will fall. This stimulates the central receptors to increase ventilation, but the patient may not be able to increase ventilation. Thus, weaning becomes a problem until the patient's normal bicarbonate and $Paco_2$ levels are reestablished and the pH is back to the patient's normal value. Interestingly, normalization of $Paco_2$ can result in increased Pao_2, increased oxygen transport, and increased CO.[17] Because of this it is believed that hyperventilation, low $Paco_2$, and high pH may actually affect the patient's oxygenation.

Uneven Ventilation

All lung units are not created equal. As a result of this lack of homogeneity of compliance and resistance components in a diseased lung, the distribution of air is not uniform. Parts of the lung having high resistance or low compliance, or both, will have less of a tendency to receive an even portion of air during a mechanical or spontaneous breath. Those with normal compliance and resistance receive a greater portion of the air. This results in increased dead space and $\dot{V}/\dot{Q}$ mismatching.

In many cases of uneven ventilation with IPPV, especially in patients with bullous emphysema, the added risk of barotrauma exists. High volumes and flows of gas force air under pressure into areas of the lung where alveoli may rupture and result in the formation of a pneumothorax. On the other hand, there are lung conditions where IPPV or PEEP may open up atelectatic areas and improve $\dot{V}/\dot{Q}$ matching. It is wise, then, to monitor the physiologic dead space–tidal volume ratio (V_D/V_T) and shunt changes and to try to establish inspiratory flow rates, I/E ratios, and expiratory maneuvers that can improve gas exchange.

Body Position and Mechanical Ventilation

Hospitalized patients, especially those on mechanical ventilatory support, are often immobilized. It is important to turn these patients frequently during the day to help prevent such pulmonary complications as atelectasis and hypoxemia.[128] Body position is also important in patients with certain types of pulmonary disorders to ensure that optimal ventilation and oxygenation is maintained. It has been found that when one lung is affected by some pathologic process such as atelectasis, consolidation, or infiltrates, and the affected lung is in the dependent position, this is usually associated with a lower Pa_{O_2} than when the normal lung is in the dependent position.[44, 111] This same concept holds true in thoracotomy patients. In most cases, oxygenation is best when the unaffected side is down.[111]

Normally, the dependent portion of the lung receives a better part of the perfusion. When the affected lung is in the dependent position, the blood flow is greatest to the dependent area while ventilation to that lung is not increased appropriately. The relative decrease in ventilation to the dependent area could be due to the disease process itself, i.e., the alveoli could be filled with exudate.[111] It could also be due to increased distribution of ventilation to the nondependent areas if the patient is on positive pressure ventilation.[46, 128]

It should also be pointed out that the Pa_{O_2} in the supine position is usually closer to the value noted when the affected lung is down. Thus, the supine position may be less than optimal due to $\dot{V}/\dot{Q}$ mismatching.[46]

A variety of different disorders can affect either ventilation or perfusion to isolated areas of the lung. It is important to try to position the patient so that $\dot{V}/\dot{Q}$ and V_D/V_T are optimal[97] when an arterial blood sample is drawn so that changes that occur in Pa_{O_2} can be evaluated in relation to body position as well as fractional concentration of oxygen in inspired gas ($F_{I_{O_2}}$) and pulmonary pathologic changes.

Auto PEEP: Air Trapping During Mechanical Ventilation

When airway resistance is increased in spontaneously breathing persons, both inspiratory and expiratory flows are impeded. This can occur in patients with severe chronic obstructive pulmonary disease (COPD), status asthmaticus, and similar problems. Small or medium airways close off or collapse during exhalation and the air in the lung does not empty completely. This trapping of air in the alveoli can occur if expiration is not long enough.

Auto-PEEP (air trapping during IPPV) has received a lot of attention in the literature recently. It is defined as an unintentional PEEP that occurs with mechanically ventilated patients when a new inspiratory breath is delivered before expiration has ended. It is a complication that may not be apparent unless it is looked for.[18] Auto-PEEP differs from PEEP, which is a preselected value at the end-expiratory gas flow.[74] Auto-PEEP is also called occult PEEP, inadvertent PEEP, gas trapping, breath stacking, and intrinsic PEEP.

Complications.—Auto-PEEP is more likely in patients who lose the structural quality of the conductive airways. In patients with COPD, the phenomenon of air trapping is well known. Severe airflow obstruction increases the time needed for exhalation. These patients have increased time constants. Their increased Raw reduces their ability to exhale in a normal amount of time.

When air trapping occurs, the increased P_A is transmitted to the intrapleural space like an artificial PEEP (auto-PEEP) effect. This reduces venous return and CO. Artificially high intravascular pressures may be measured, such as an increase in pulmonary capillary wedge pressure (PCWP) which normally reflects left heart function. Some clinicians mistakenly interpret the increased PCWP as an increase in left atrial pressure and left heart failure. It should be kept in mind that these are artificially high readings. If these patients are given diuretics and vasoactive agents to treat the supposed left heart failure, their condition gets worse rather than better.[65, 101] Auto-PEEP can also lead to barotrauma. The level of volume in the lung at the end of exhalation on a ventilated patient may be more important than peak pressures in causing barotrauma.[126] Pulmonary hyperinflation may be life-threatening in patients with acute severe asthma on ventilatory support. The risk of tension pneumothorax and circulatory depression is increased in these patients.[126] Since air trapping is not normally measured or detectable, it makes its occurrence even a greater threat to patients. When it occurs in spontaneously breathing, intubated patients, it can add to their work of breathing (WOB). Trapped air makes it more difficult for patients to breathe in.

How It Occurs.—An expiratory time of at least three to four time constants is needed for the lungs to empty completely (98% of the inspired volume). When expiratory time is less than this, it prevents complete emptying of the lungs to their normal resting lung volume (FRC). Lung volumes and lung pressures at the end of exhalation start to build with each breath. As higher volumes are reached, tissue recoil increases so the force pushing air out of the lungs increases. This keeps the airways open. This is also true in obstructed airways. As a result, the airway resistance to exhaled flow gets progressively lower. Within a few breaths the lung volumes stabilize. At this point the venti-

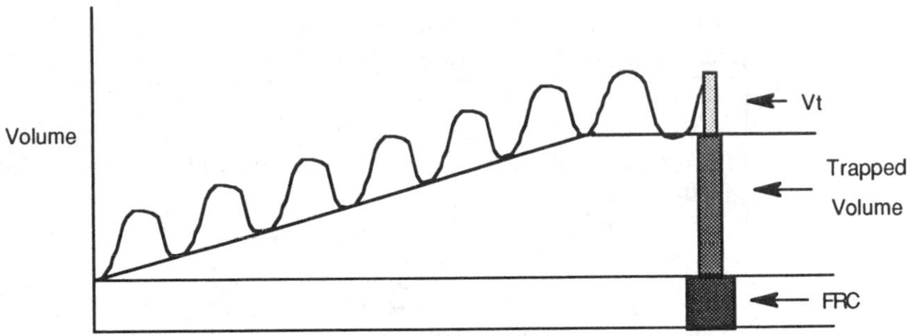

FIG 7–5.
Volume of trapped air above the functional residual capacity *(FRC)* due to auto-PEEP. The gradual rise in volume shows the progressive trapping of air in the lungs. *Vt* = tidal volume. (Redrawn from Tuxen DV: *Am Rev Respir Dis* 1989; 140:5–9.)

lator V_T delivered can be exhaled.[101] The result, however, is a higher FRC than normal and higher P_A (Fig 7–5). Alveolar pressure is greater than ambient pressure at end-exhalation.

Physiologic Factors.—There are three distinctive forms of auto-PEEP[82, 83]:

1. Auto-PEEP occurs because the expiratory muscles are actively contracting during exhalation. This raises P_A at end-exhalation. It does not increase the volume at end-exhalation. This is auto-PEEP without lung distention.
2. Auto-PEEP can occur in patients who do not have airway obstruction. In these patients with normal Raw, air trapping can occur in the presence of high $\dot{V}_E$, long inspiratory times, and factors that increase resistance to exhalation, such as small endotracheal (ET) tubes, expiratory valves, and PEEP devices which increase expiratory resistance above normal. Total expiratory resistance across the lungs, ET tube, and exhalation line and valve is normally less than 4 cm H_2O/L/sec.[82, 83]
3. Auto-PEEP also occurs in patients with airflow obstruction that tend to have airway collapse during exhalation and flow limitation during normal tidal breathing. In these patients, an increased expiratory effort only increases the P_A and does not improve the expiratory flow rate.

The level of auto-PEEP cannot be accurately predicted. Factors that increase its risk of occurring are listed in Table 7–4.

Detection.—When you measure exhaled gas flow during the regular expiratory phase, if the measuring respirometer shows continuous flow up to the point when the next inspiration started, you would know the patient had not com-

TABLE 7–4.
Factors That Increase the Risk of Auto-PEEP*

1. COPD[74, 101]
2. A $\dot{V}_E$ of ≥ 10 L/min (39% incidence[39]; with $\dot{V}_E$ > 20 L/min, the incidence is 100%[18])
3. Increased age, particularly patients aged >60 yr (the $\dot{V}_E$ requirement for auto-PEEP decreases with age[18])
4. Decreases in ET tube size[115, 116]
5. Increases in compliance
6. As respiratory frequency increases, the risk of gas trapping increases, particularly as inspiratory time approaches expiratory time in value[10] (in adult volume ventilation,[10] and infant pressure-limited, time-cycled ventilation[21])
7. Reduced inspiratory flow leading to a shorter expiratory time, even though peak pressures decrease[126]
8. Increases in V_T, particularly in patients with airway obstruction[126]

*COPD = chronic obstructive pulmonary disease; $\dot{V}_E$ = minute ventilation; V_T = tidal volume.

pletely exhaled. If you were using a volume spirometer, such as the Bennett spirometer, and the spirometer continued to fill slowly through exhalation until it was interrupted by the start of the next breath, you could suspect auto-PEEP.[101] Air trapping can be detected with volume ventilation by observing an increase in peak and plateau pressures, a transient reduction in exhaled volumes, a reduction in breath sounds, a decrease in compliance, and an increase in resonance on percussion of the chest wall. It can also be detected by measuring the auto-PEEP levels (see below). Chest radiographs may reveal increased radiolucency.[110]

Measurement.—The amount of auto-PEEP present in the patient's lungs at end-exhalation is not registered on the ventilator manometer. During regular mechanical ventilation, the pressure on the manometer during exhalation in most ventilators is measured internally on the inspiratory side of the machine (see Fig 5–25, Chap 5). The machine is measuring pressure in the circuit. Normally, during exhalation, the expiratory valve is open to the atmosphere (Fig 7–6).[101] Pressure in the circuit is zero and the manometer measures this pressure. But air may still be actively flowing out of the patient's lungs. The exhaled flow does not return to a zero value prior to the next breath. Monitoring expiratory flow waveforms can be used to detect air trapping. Some of the gas volume remains in the patient's lungs and remains trapped there. This adds to the resting FRC, but it remains undetected because the ventilator manometer during exhalation just reads ambient pressure.

Some ventilators have end-expiratory pause buttons. These are usually microprocessor ventilators that can time the closing of the exhalation valve. They close the valve just prior to the time when the next positive breath would occur. They then delay the next breath and measure the pressure in the circuit. The

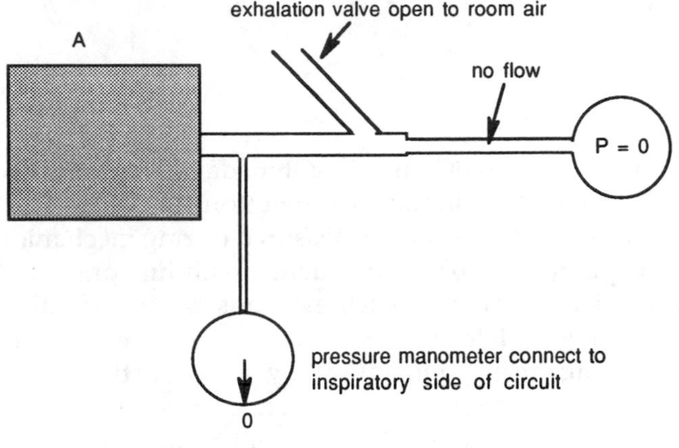

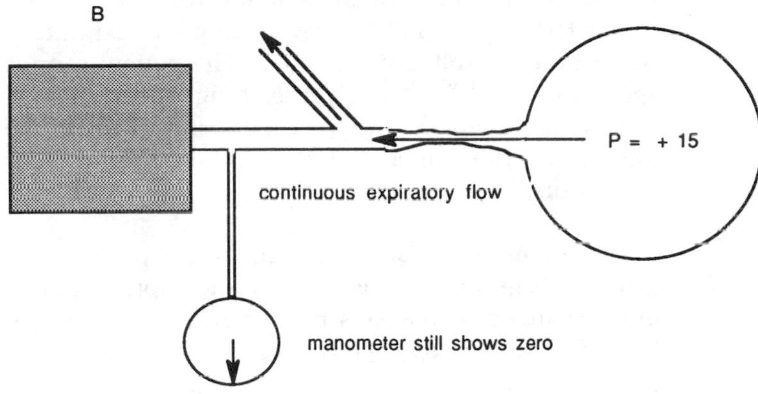

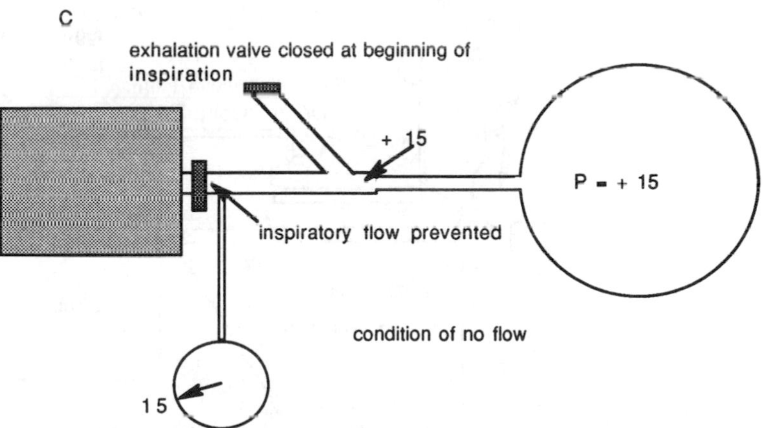

FIG 7–6.
A mechanical ventilator connected to a lung under normal conditions and when auto-PEEP is present. **A,** ventilator system during normal exhalation with no air trapping, no auto-PEEP, and with the manometer reading zero. **B,** during exhalation with auto-PEEP present, the manometer still reads zero (ambient) because the exhalation valve is open to room air but there is 15 cm H_2O of air trapped in the lung. **C,** when the exhalation valve is closed and inspiratory flow stopped at end-exhalation and prior to the next breath, a manometer will be able to read the approximate auto-PEEP level in the lungs and circuit. (**A–C** redrawn from references 80 and 101.)

Siemens Servo 900C and the Ohmeda Advent are two examples of ventilators that have end-expiratory pause buttons or controls.

Auto-PEEP can also be measured during mechanical ventilation by occluding the expiratory limb of the patient circuit just prior to the next positive pressure breath. Delivery of the next breath must be slowed either by delaying the breath or by slowing its delivery. This can be done by reducing the respiratory rate[101, 126] or by slowing the inspiratory flow. By occluding the exhalation valve the manometer measures the pressure in the patient's airway as the pressure equilibrates with the circuit (Figs 7–7 and 7–8). This will actually be an underestimation since the trapped gas must equilibrate with the ventilator circuit.[78]

Detecting auto-PEEP by measuring end-expiratory pressure requires a quiet patient on controlled ventilation.[18] The patient cannot be assisting or breathing spontaneously. An actively breathing patient may forcibly inhale or exhale during measurement and alter the results. Brown and Pierson[18] provide examples of how this can be performed on the Puritan Bennett MA-1 and Servo 900B ventilators.[126]

Effect on Ventilator Function.—The presence of auto-PEEP will actually slow the beginning of gas flow during inspiration. Flow from the ventilator will only begin when the pressure generated exceeds the pressure at the alveolar level. Remember, for gas flow to occur there must be a pressure gradient. If P_A is

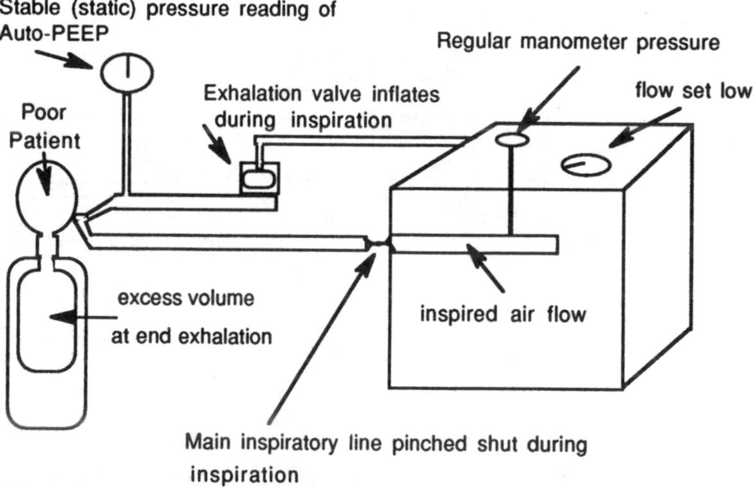

FIG 7–7.
Schematic drawing of a ventilator and the conditions that must exist to measure auto-PEEP. When a ventilator cycles into inspiration the exhalation valve closes. The manometer will read the pressure in the circuit. Inspiratory flow must be prevented or it will interfere with this reading.

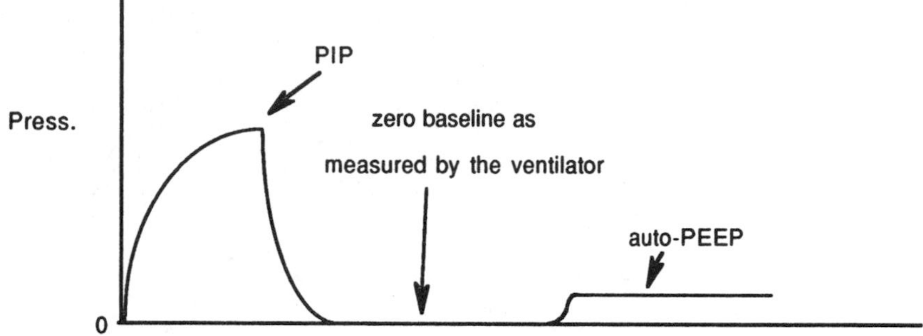

FIG 7–8.
Airway pressure graphed over time when measuring auto-PEEP. Note that following normal exhalation the manometer will read zero pressure. When the exhalation valve is closed, the manometer needle rises and the auto-PEEP level can be seen. *PIP* = peak inspiratory pressure.

higher than ambient at the end of exhalation (auto-PEEP), flow delivery will not start until mouth pressure exceeds this value.[112]

Measuring Static Compliance With Auto-PEEP.—Static compliance values are normally calculated as V_T divided by plateau pressure minus PEEP. For this calculation to be accurate, the PEEP value must include the PEEP applied by the ventilator and any auto-PEEP that might be present in the alveoli before the next inspiration begins.

Inability to Trigger Ventilator.—Sometimes patients appear weak, hyperpneic, and breathless. The patient may be unable to trigger the ventilator even though the set sensitivity level is very sensitive and the patient is making an obvious effort. This inability to trigger an assisted breath may be due to auto-PEEP. To trigger the ventilator the patient's inspiratory effort must equal the set end-expiratory pressure plus the auto-PEEP level[80] (Fig 7–9). One way to overcome this problem is to set a PEEP level (extrinsic PEEP) just below the intrinsic PEEP level. This will reduce the pleural pressure swings needed to trigger the ventilator.[78] Extrinsic PEEP has no effect on expiratory flow during dynamic airway collapse. It only acts to keep airway pressure nearly equal to P_A. Thus the next patient inspiratory effort is easier for the ventilator to detect.[78]

Methods of Reducing Auto-PEEP.—To reduce auto-PEEP, use higher inspiratory flow rates to shorten inspiratory time and allow a longer time for exhalation. Longer expiratory times can also be accomplished by using smaller V_T settings and low respiratory rates. Using a low compressible volume (less compliant) ventilator patient circuit may reduce auto-PEEP in adult patients.[116] Use of low resistance exhalation valves and large ET tubes may also reduce air

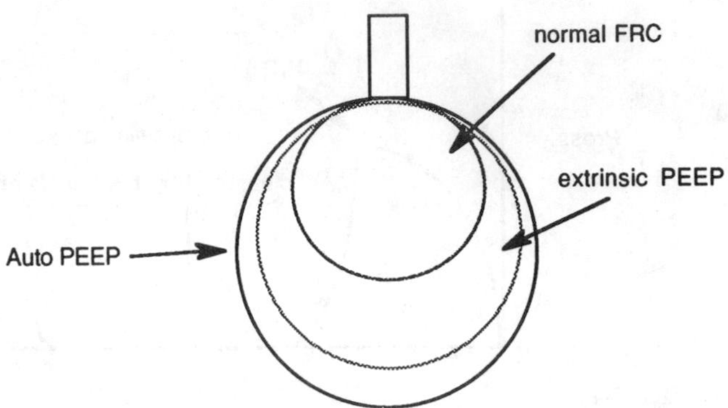

FIG 7–9.
Alveolar filling. The smallest circle represents resting FRC under normal conditions. The second circle represents the addition of extrinsic PEEP. The third and largest circle shows the resting lung volume with auto-PEEP present as well. (Redrawn from references 83–86.)

trapping. The use of bronchodilators in patients with reactive airways may also be beneficial. PEEP devices may also help reduce this risk.[85]

Alternatives When Auto-PEEP Is Present.—Normally, the goal of mechanical ventilation is to achieve a normal pH range and a normal Pa_{CO_2} for the patient. Sometimes severe airway obstruction or high $\dot{V}_E$ demands make this impossible as they result in high levels of air trapping. Some researchers recommend hypoventilation under these circumstances. The patient essentially acquires mild respiratory acidosis. Sometimes this may be preferable to the complications that occur with high $\dot{V}_E$ and auto-PEEP in patients with severe airflow obstruction.[33, 126] Another alternative is to use methods of ventilation that allow as much spontaneous ventilation to occur as the patient can tolerate. IMV or SIMV, pressure support, and CPAP may be beneficial in these situations.

Benefits of Auto-PEEP.—Inverse ratio ventilation causes air trapping. The use of inverse I/E ratios on both adults and babies has been found to improve oxygenation in most patients. It may be that the auto-PEEP in these instances is beneficial. There have been a few reported cases of patients with acute hypoxemic respiratory failure that had improvements in oxygenation when external PEEP was discontinued and inverse ratios were used to produce intrinsic PEEP.[130]

Gastric Distention With Mechanical Ventilation

When masks are used for ventilation rather than ET tubes or tracheostomy tubes, air can be forced into the stomach from the positive ventilating pressures.

This occurs when mask pressures exceed 20 cm H_2O.[97] Increased gas volume in the stomach can cause upward pressure on the left hemidiaphragm and restrict ventilation. Air swallowing or air forced into the stomach during ventilation can also lead to colonic ileus, distention, and cecal perforation.[48] Some clinicians recommend the use of nasogastric suction if gastric distention is occurring. Caution is advised with gastric suction since it can alter acid-base balance by reducing normal acid levels.

HAZARDS OF OXYGEN THERAPY WITH MECHANICAL VENTILATION

Oxygen-Induced Bradypnea

In patients who are breathing on a hypoxic drive, such as those with COPD and chronic CO_2 retention, high O_2 levels can suppress the drive to breathe. This is a problem with mechanically ventilated patients only if an adequate alveolar ventilation is not provided by the ventilator.

Absorption Atelectasis

High O_2 concentrations (> 70%) often lead to rapid absorption atelectasis in hypoventilated lung units.[88] This increases intrapulmonary shunt. In mechanically ventilated patients this is especially a problem if low V_T settings or pressure-cycled ventilators with low cycling pressures are used.

Oxygen Toxicity

When the F_{IO_2} is greater than 0.6 in the adult for prolonged periods (> 48 hours) complications may result. If the Pa_{O_2} is more than 80 mm Hg in a newborn or premature infant, then pulmonary O_2 toxicity becomes a potential hazard.[45] The higher the concentration of O_2, the higher the ventilating pressures, and the more prolonged the use, the greater the risk of damage to the pulmonary tissues or to the eyes. If adequate O_2 therapy is withheld, however, death may result from hypoxia, so O_2 therapy should always be provided as needed.

The use of high O_2 concentrations (F_{IO_2} = 1.0) can induce pulmonary changes in humans in as little as 6 hours. Pulmonary changes associated with high O_2 concentrations include the following: decreased tracheal mucus flow, decreased macrophage activity, decreased vital capacity, endothelial cell damage and accompanying increased lung water, progressive formation of absorption atelectasis, decreased surfactant production, decreased compliance, increased alveolar-arterial oxygen partial pressure difference [$P(A-a)_{O_2}$], decreased diffusing capacity, decreased pulmonary capillary blood volume, capillary injury, and platelet aggregation in the pulmonary vasculature.[45, 66] Exposure for more than 72 hours causes development of a pattern similar to ARDS.[66]

In acute respiratory failure most patients already have abnormal chest radiographs because of their underlying lung disorder. As a result, it is difficult to assess the onset of O_2 toxicity. The lowest possible F_{IO_2} that maintains oxygenation should be administered. If an F_{IO_2} of greater than 0.5 to 0.6 is required, then other modes such as PEEP or CPAP should be instituted.[66] The improvement in oxygenation with CPAP or PEEP often allows the F_{IO_2} to be reduced. In general, use of F_{IO_2} values less than 0.4 is considered safe. The maximum amount that can be given safely for long periods of time in mechanically ventilated patients is not known. It probably differs from patient to patient.[45]

METABOLIC ACID-BASE IMBALANCES AND MECHANICAL VENTILATION

With adequate and appropriate alveolar ventilation, Pa_{CO_2} and pH can be expected to be near the patient's normal levels. If the Pa_{CO_2} is near the patient's normal level but the pH is not, the cause is a metabolic problem and this needs to be corrected. Severe metabolic acidosis may require the administration of bicarbonate. The bicarbonate requirement will equal one third of the body weight in kilograms times the base excess, with the product of these being divided by two:

$$HCO_3^- \text{ required} = \frac{1/3 \text{ kg} \times \text{BE}}{2}$$

where kg = body weight in kilograms and BE is base excess. Bicarbonate administration is only given to patients with adequate ventilation.[69] If a patient is not ventilated, the additional bicarbonate will combine with plasma hydrogen ions and increase CO_2 production. If this CO_2 is retained, the acidosis may increase.

TABLE 7–5.
Blood Chemistry in Metabolic Acidosis and Alkalosis*†

	Serum Sodium	Serum Chloride	Serum Potassium	Arterial Blood pH	Pa_{CO_2}
Alkalosis	→ or ↓	↓	→ or ↓	↑	→ or ↑
Acidosis	→ or ↑	↑	→ or ↑	↓	↓

*↑ = increase; ↓ = decrease; → = no change.
†Normal values: sodium = 135–145 mEq/L; chloride = 98–106 mEq/L; potassium = 3.5–5.0 mEq/L; pH = 7.35–7.45; Pa_{CO_2} = 35–45 mm Hg.

Normally, metabolic alkalosis can correct itself in most cases if the cause is removed. On the other hand, if the alkalosis is severe, prompt action is needed. Administration of ammonium chloride or potassium chloride may be considered for treatment.[49] Abnormalities in blood chemistry associated with metabolic acidosis and alkalosis are summarized in Table 7–5.

BAROTRAUMA IN MECHANICAL VENTILATION

Barotrauma is a term used to describe several conditions that occur due to pressure or volume damage in the lung. In normal lungs, the possibility of damaging lung tissue or barotrauma is probably higher than we expect. Animal studies have shown that lungs may be damaged at pressures as low as 40 cm H_2O.[113] In lungs where blebs may be present, or in patients with chest wall injury, the risk of rupture to the lung is much greater. Types of conditions that predispose a patient to barotrauma are listed in Table 7–6. The incidence of barotrauma in patients on IPPV and PEEP can be as high as 15%.[12,14,113] The rupture of lung tissue leads to such complications as pneumothorax, pneumomediastinum, subcutaneous emphysema, pneumoperitoneum, and damage at the cellular level.

The site where the pressure effects and resulting injury is most commonly seen is the distal noncartilaginous airway.[113] Damage to peripheral airways and alveoli during mechanical ventilation may result in gas under pressure proceeding along perivascular sheaths toward the hilum and mediastinum causing pneumomediastinum.[13,113] Air can then break through the pleural surface of the mediastinum into the intrapleural space causing pneumothorax.[97,113] This may be unilateral or bilateral. Additionally, air in the mediastinum may dissect along tissue planes producing subcutaneous emphysema. Pneumoperitoneum may follow pneumomediastinum and occurs when air dissects initially into the retroperitoneum. Air under the diaphragm may interfere with effective ventilation.[113]

TABLE 7–6.
Conditions Predisposing to Barotrauma

High peak airway pressures with low end-expiratory pressures
Bullous lung disease (e.g., emphysema and history of tuberculosis)
High levels of PEEP with high tidal volumes[113]
Aspiration of gastric acid
Necrotizing pneumonias
ARDS[113]

Subcutaneous Emphysema

Detection of subcutaneous emphysema is not difficult. It may be visible as a puffing of the skin in the patient's neck, face, and chest. It may even be present in distal areas like the feet and abdomen.[113] The skin is crepitant to the touch. Subcutaneous emphysema usually occurs without complication and tends to clear without treatment. If it is present with dyspnea, cyanosis, and increased PIPs, it may be accompanied by pneumothorax or tension pneumothorax.

Pneumomediastinum

Pneumomediastinum may lead to compression of the esophagus, great vessels, and the heart, and can be observed on the chest radiograph. Treatment depends on the severity of the problem and its effect on adjacent structures. If severe, the air has to be removed, especially if tamponade of the heart is present.

Pneumothorax

Pneumothorax may lead to lung collapse on the affected side and mediastinal shifting away from the affected side. This can compress the unaffected lung and the heart. Pneumothorax can be detected by a hyperresonant percussion note and absence of breath sounds on the affected side. Treatment may require the use of chest drainage through a chest tube if it is severe. Another way of detecting a pneumothorax in patients on mechanical ventilation is to observe progressive changes in PIP. Increases in PIP occurring within a short period of time, such as a few minutes to a few hours, may signal the presence of pneumothorax of either rapid onset or slow insidious leak. Physical examination and chest film confirm the diagnosis.

A simple pneumothorax can develop into a tension pneumothorax in a patient on mechanical ventilation, so careful monitoring is required. Since positive pressure ventilation may aggravate the presence of air in the pleural space, it may be advisable to manually assist ventilation in the patient, using a resuscitation bag on 100% O_2 until the problem can be treated.[13]

A tension pneumothorax needs to be treated immediately since it is life-threatening. Tension pneumothorax occurs when air can enter the pleural space, but cannot leave. This gradually builds up pressure collapsing the affected lung. It also puts pressure on the heart and the unaffected lung. Tracheal deviation and neck vein distention are possible signs. Breath sounds are absent and the percussion note is tympanic.

Treatment for tension pneumothorax is placement of a 14-gauge needle (or one of similar size) into the anterior second-to-third intercostal space on the affected side, in the midclavicular line, with the patient in the head-up position. This maneuver can be lifesaving.[57] While waiting for trained personnel to be summoned to perform this procedure, it is advisable to decrease mean airway pressures ($\overline{P}aw$) as much as possible while still supporting ventilation and oxygenation with manually assisted ventilation on high O_2 concentrations.

Current ventilators are capable of delivering up to 120 cm H_2O and potentially even higher PIPs. To help avoid barotrauma it is desirable to keep PIP as low as possible, and V_T low where high PIPs occur, and maintain good ventilation (see Table 7–6). The potential for overinflation of alveoli also exists with high PEEP levels. When a large V_T is added to an already overinflated lung, the risk of barotrauma is very high. When PEEP levels of 25 to 44 cm H_2O are used, the incident of pneumothorax may be as high as 14%. The use of lower V_T can reduce the risk of barotrauma.[12–14] The damage seen in the lung is probably due not so much to the pressures, but to the elastic expansion of the alveoli beyond their limits by the volumes that accompany these pressures.[25]

Cellular Injury

Early in the development of positive pressure ventilation it was known that positive pressures could cause lung trauma by rupture of lung tissue. But many are unaware of the damage that can occur at the cellular level. We know that ventilation can contribute to fluid retention in the lung and pulmonary edema. Pressures of 30 to 80 cm H_2O in normal dogs, rats, and sheep produced interstitial emphysema associated with perivascular and alveolar hemorrhage, alveolar rupture, reduced compliance, severe hypoxemia, and death (Fig 7–10).[37, 38, 72, 99, 133] Death occurred as quickly as within an hour.[37, 38] Some animals survived as long as 35 hours, but eventually died.[72] Apparently, when high PIP is accompanied by PEEP, the PEEP seems to offer some protection from tissue damage.[37, 38, 45] What is amazing is the rapidity of this damage and the pressures at which it occurred. What is disturbing is how many times human subjects are regularly ventilated at these pressures in our hospital intensive care units. As many as 21% of patients diagnosed with ARDS may require ventilating pressures of 80 cm H_2O or greater.[15] We have already seen what high PIP can do to what remains of normal lung in animal models. It is no wonder that survival for ARDS is only about 50%. The damage caused by our treatment may actually be indistinguishable from the underlying disease process.[113] It is no wonder that because of this physicians are looking at alternative forms of ventilation that can accomplish oxygenation and ventilation of the patient without requiring high peak airway pressures.

Ideally, for the patient with acute lung injury or ARDS, we want to provide augmented ventilation, perhaps with PEEP, but without causing high PIPs and volumes which damage lung tissue, or high mean airway pressures which can reduce CO. Such a system might allow the patient to breathe spontaneously without a high WOB and without having to be paralyzed. Newer alternatives to mechanical ventilation might provide such an option. They include such modes

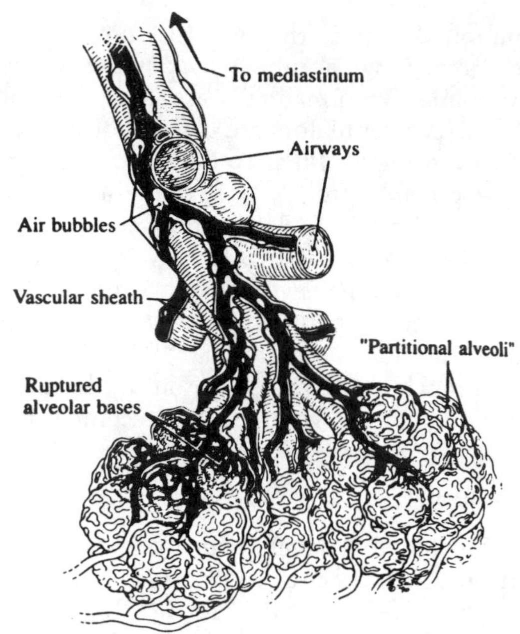

FIG 7–10.
Artist's conception of the development of interstitial emphysema. (From Samuelson WM, Fulkerson WJ: Barotrauma in mechanical ventilation, in Fulkerson WJ, MacIntyre NR: *Problems in Respiratory Care: Complications of Mechanical Ventilation.* Philadelphia, JB Lippincott Co, 1991, p 58. Used by permission.)

as pressure-controlled ventilation, pressure control with inverse I/E ratio, airway pressure release ventilation, liquid ventilation of the lung, low-frequency ventilation with extracorporeal CO_2 removal, intravascular oxygenating devices, and high-frequency ventilation. In situations where only one lung is affected, the independent ventilation of each lung may be the treatment of choice.

In summary it is important to again point out that PIP may not be the guilty party in this discussion, but rather the overexpansion of alveoli beyond their limit owing to the volume that accompanies these pressures.[25] Remember, too, that part of the PIP is pressure that goes to overcoming airway and ET tube resistance never reaches the alveolar level. In monitoring the ventilator, be sure to consider P_A, lung compliance, and volumes delivered when thinking about the potential for lung damage.

COMPLICATIONS OF ARTIFICIAL AIRWAY

The use of artificial airways provides a variety of ways in which problems can arise. These include complications associated with the artificial airway itself, infection of the patient's airway, excessive heat to the airway from humidification systems, and inadequate or excessive humidification from the humidification system. A comprehensive review of airway complications and methods of insertion and airway care techniques are available in other texts and are not covered in detail here.[107, 108, 117] Appendix F provides a summary of the major complications associated with artificial airways.[107, 108, 117, 121]

Care must be employed in the use, insertion, maintenance, and removal of artificial airways. High volume and low pressure cuffs of good quality used by qualified and knowledgeable practitioners for as short a time as possible will reduce the incidence of complications. All suctioning of the airway should be done using sterile technique and with the utmost care to avoid mucosal damage and the risk of infection. Invasion of the upper airway with an artificial device bypasses normal defense mechanisms. This is amplified by being in a hospital environment where the type and amount of infecting agents are increased. This, combined with poor nutrition, stress, and the use of immunosuppressive agents increases the chance of infection in patients with artificial airways.

In addition to invading the upper airway, tubes also bypass the normal filtration, warming, and humidification system that is provided by the body. Warmed filtered and humidified air must be supplied whenever mechanical ventilation is used. If inadequate amounts of water are supplied, there is mucosal drying, slowing of ciliary movement, drying of secretions, potential airway occlusion, and increased risk of infection and atelectasis. Adequate humidity (60%–100% relative humidity at near body temperature, 33°C ±1°) must be provided.[23] If the output from the humidifying device or the temperature of the air is too low, adequate humidification will not occur. Selection of appropriate equipment and understanding of its use is essential. A device that produces warm water vapor poses less risk of infection than one which nebulizes and provides the potential for carrying infecting organisms with it. Use of a heated cascade-type bubble humidifier, a pass-over, or a heated wick-type humidifier can provide the needed humidification with a lower chance of infection. A heated water reservoir provides an excellent growth medium for bacteria; therefore, sterile water is used to fill the reservoir. The humidifying device and patient circuit are usually changed every 24 to 48 hours.[51] When draining water condensate from the corregated tubing, always drain away from the patient to avoid contaminating the airway.

While inadequate humidity is a problem, so is too much water. Excessive water from heated nebulizers can create fluid overload when used with small patients, particularly if renal function is compromised. This can be recognized as an unexplained weight gain and possible edema formation in the lungs. Use of an ultrasonic nebulizer with a large reservoir or a Babbington-type nebulizer should be avoided during continuous ventilation.

It is not unusual for heated reservoirs of water to reach 45°C or more. A reservoir temperature that is too high can cause thermal burns of the upper airway, and this can lead to swelling, increased airway resistance, and elevation in body temperature. For this reason it is essential that a thermometer measure in-line temperatures at the patient's upper airway. Some temperature-sensing devices provide not only measurement capabilities but also alarms which detect high or low temperature limits, and servo-control devices to regulate the temperature in the humidifier reservoir to the desired level.

If complications occur as a result of inappropriate inspired air humidification or temperature, it might be reflected in clinical signs such as unexplained increases in body temperature, unexplained weight gain, increased airway resistance, crusting of secretions, edema of the airway, increased white blood cell count reflecting a potential infection, and the presence of a pathogenic organism in the sputum.

INFECTIONS

Intubated patients on mechanical ventilation are usually very ill and at high risk for nosocomial infections and pneumonias.[32, 123] Their chances of infection are increased by both invasive catheters and monitoring devices (Table 7–7) and predisposing illnesses or disorders (Table 7–8). The most common organisms

TABLE 7–7.

Invasive Devices That Increase Risk for Nosocomial Infections*
Nasotracheal or ET tubes
Intravenous lines
Central venous lines
Arterial monitors
Pulmonary artery catheters
Intracranial pressure monitors
Indwelling urinary catheters

*Data from Rossi A, Gottfried SB, Zocchi L, et al: *Am Rev Respir Dis* 1985; 131:672–667.

TABLE 7–8.

Factors Predisposing Patients to Nosocomial Infections and Pneumonias*
Severe illness
Long duration of hospital stay
Increased age and disability
Use of antibiotics
Use of invasive devices (see Table 7–7)
Major surgery

*Data from references 22, 123.

TABLE 7–9.
Commonly Isolated Pathogenic Organisms From Nosocomial Pneumonias*

Gram-negative aerobes
Pseudomonas aeruginosa
Klebsiella pneumoniae
Escherichia coli
Enterobacter sp.
Serratia marcescens
Acinetobacter calcoaceticus
Proteus mirabilis
Haemophilus influenzae
Gram-positive aerobes
Staphylococcus aureus
Streptococcus pneumoniae
Gram-negative anaerobes
Bacteroides fragilis
Others
Legionella pneumophila
Fungi
Candida sp.

*Data from references 22, 79, 122, 123.

associated with nosocomial pneumonias are listed in Table 7–9. Colonization of the oropharynx with bacteria ranges in incidence from 16% to 75%.[32] Nosocomial pneumonias occur with about 20% frequency in intubated patients.[123] The fatality rates in mechanically ventilated patients with pneumonia range from 50% to 70% compared with 25% to 29% in those without pneumonias.[123]

The usual clinical features that occur with pneumonias are cough, sputum production, fever, elevated white blood cell count, and infiltrates on chest film. Infiltrates may not be present in some patients. For example 36% of patients with gram-negative pneumonias and low granulocyte counts will initially not have infiltrates on chest film.[123] Elderly patients, patients with liver or kidney failure, or patients on corticosteroid therapy may not develop fever.[123]

One of the common causes of nosocomial pneumonias is aspiration of oropharyngeal organisms. This can even occur in patients with cuffed ET tubes in place.[32, 123] Many patients in medical intensive care units are colonized with gram-negative bacteria in the oropharynx. As many as 22% of these patients are colonized the first day they are in the unit. The occurrence of bacterial colonization can be as high as 73%.[32] Other possible causes of infection are poor suctioning techniques, and accidental contamination of the ET tube with water from the ventilatory circuit. Other factors that can predispose a patient with an ET tube in place to nosocomial pneumonia are injury of the nasopharynx and tracheal surface, decreased effectiveness of the cough mechanism, passage of bacteria into the trachea, bypassing the upper airway defense mechanisms, and

TABLE 7–10.

Conditions Predisposing to Oropharyngeal Colonization*

Alcoholism	Underlying illness (pulmonary disease)
Diabetes mellitus	Antibiotic therapy
Coma	Hypoxemia
Hypotenson	Intubation
Acidosis	Nasogastric tubes
Azotemia	Nutritional status
Leukocytopenia	Viral infection
Leukocytosis	Surgery

*Data from references 22, 122, 123.

TABLE 7–11.

Methods to Reduce Risk for Nosocomial Pneumonias in Mechanically Ventilated Patients*

Extubate and remove nasogastric tube as clinically indicated
Reduce the risk of aspiration
- Maintain patient in the upright position to reduce reflux and aspiration of gastric organisms
- Avoid CNS depressants
- Change ET tubes periodically
- Consider selective decontamination of the oropharynx and stomach with antibiotics in certain patient groups

Related to respiratory equipment
- Careful removal and disposal of ventilator circuit condensate
- Single patient use of respirometers, O_2 analyzers, resuscitation bags, etc.
- Careful use of in-line micronebulizers
- Careful use of heat-moisture exchangers
- Consider use of expiratory-line gas traps or filters

Infection control
- Change ventilatory circuits and humidifiers every 48 hr
- Sterile suction technique
- Handwashing between patients
- Use of gloves when contacting patients
- Appropriate disinfection and sterilization techniques

Methods to improve host immunity
- Maintain nutritional status
- Avoid agents that impair pulmonary defenses (aminophylline, anesthetics, antibiotics, corticosteroids, sedative narcotics, antineoplastic agents)
- Minimize use of invasive procedures
- Remove or treat disease states that affect host defenses (acidosis, dehydration, hypoxemia, ethanol intoxication, acid inspiration, stress, thermal injury, diabetic ketoacidosis, liver failure, kidney failure, heart failure)

*Data from references 22, 24, 122, 123.

reduced healing if nutrition is poor. Table 7–10 lists factors that increase the chances of colonization. Another common infection in intubated patients is nosocomial sinusitis that may occur in as many as 94% of patients with nasotracheal tubes in for more than 8 days.[123] Responsible organisms are very similar to those that infect the lungs.

Nosocomial pneumonias are common. The infecting organism needs to be identified and treated with appropriate antibiotic therapy. Table 7–11 lists ways in which hospital personnel can reduce the risk of nosocomial pneumonias. The best we can do at the present time is to be as careful as possible when using invasive devices, be aware of the risk of pneumonia, and treat the infections appropriately.

WORK OF BREATHING AND MUSCLE FATIGUE

Respiratory muscle fatigue is another common complication of the use of artificial airways and mechanical ventilation systems. This fatigue is usually brought on by an increase in the work of breathing (WOB). This work is both intrinsic and extrinsic.[68]

Intrinsic Work

Intrinsic work is a result of work to overcome the normal elastic and resistive forces of the lung and thorax and work to overcome a disorder or disease process affecting normal respiratory muscle workloads. The normal WOB is related to elastic tissues in the thorax, nonelastic forces from gas moving through the airway, and inertial forces to move structures in the thorax. Abnormal intrinsic work occurs, e.g., in chronic bronchitis. This disorder increases the resistance of gas flow through the conductive airways. This increased resistance impedes gas flow and increases WOB. In fibrotic diseases of the lung, compliance is reduced and alveolar movement is restricted. This reduced movement impedes the ability of the lungs to expand and bring in air. This impedes gas movement into the lung.

Extrinsic Work

Extrinsic work is work imposed (WOBi) by systems that are added to the patient. Common examples that increase WOBi are the ET tube, the sensitivity systems that must be triggered to initiate a breath with the assist mode or with pressure-supported ventilation (PSV), the demand valve systems which must be opened during IMV or SIMV, the humidifier, and the patient circuit. Expiratory work is increased by the exhalation valve or PEEP valve. It is unfortunate that

WOB during ventilation occurs most frequently in the patient least able to handle it. These are patients with hyperinflated lungs, low nutritional status, and heart problems.

Definition

By definition WOB is the integral of pressure and volume (WOB = $\int PV$), i.e., the amount of pressure that must be generated to move a certain volume of gas. It is sometimes described by the amount of O_2 consumed by the working respiratory muscles, although this is difficult to measure. Normally the respiratory muscles use 1% to 4% of the total oxygen consumption ($\dot{V}O_2$) or 0.35 to 1.0 mL/L of ventilation.[79, 80] Oxygen consumption by the respiratory muscles may be as high as 35% to 40% of total $\dot{V}O_2$ in patients with COPD.[70]

System-Imposed WOB

Until IMV became a popular mode of ventilation, not much was said about WOB. Most people assumed that with a patient on control or assist-control that the ventilator did most or all of the WOB. It is now known that WOB on the assist mode can be greater than that required for other modes.[86] This is due to poorly designed circuits, inadequate flow, and insensitive triggering devices. IMV and SIMV systems can be equally imposing because of inadequate demand valves or regulators, high-resistance circuits and humidifiers on the inspiratory side, and high-resistance expiratory or PEEP valves on the exhalation side.

When patients are being weaned from ventilation on IMV or SIMV they have longer periods during which they spontaneously breathe. During spontaneous ventilation periods the WOB through a ventilator may be very high and fatigue the patient. WOBi can be almost eliminated with low levels of PSV (about 10 cm H_2O).[61]

Unfortunately, some poorly designed demand flow valve CPAP systems on some ventilators actually increase WOB.[61, 70] This can result from poor response in demand flow valves, circuits and humidifiers with high resistance, and low flow oxygen blenders. These, along with expiratory resistance from some PEEP and CPAP exhalation valves, can all lead to fatigue in the patient. Newer, threshold resistor PEEP and CPAP values offer lower resistance to exhalation (see Chapter 10). Clinical studies have shown that CPAP or PEEP can decrease the total WOB in patients with acute lung injury.[61] The use of PSV with CPAP can reduce the WOB through many ventilator systems.[61] These results suggest that if a patient needs CPAP or PEEP through a ventilator system, it may be advisable to use low levels of PSV to overcome the WOBi imposed by the ventilator design and the circuitry. Freestanding CPAP systems have low WOBi when they use low flow resistance PEEP valves, such as the Emerson water column and the Vital Signs CPAP valve, and have appropriate continuous flow rates set.[61, 70]

Graphic Representation of WOB

The literature on this subject often includes graphic representations of what the WOB looks like on ventilated patients. Figure 7–11 shows a controlled breath during IPPV on constant flow with the ventilator doing the resistive and elastic work of breathing for the patient. Figure 7–12 shows WOB during CPAP. Figure 7–13 shows the components of a spontaneous breath and a ventilator breath. It distinguishes those parts of the breath that the patient must perform and those parts which the ventilator provides. Figure 7–14 shows curves representing a normal spontaneous breath, a spontaneous breath with high impedence to breathing, and a machine-delivered breath. Newer monitoring equipment comes with display screens that can provide pressure-volume curves representative of the WOB of the patient.

Work of Breathing During Weaning

There is still controversy as to whether patients in respiratory failure should rest completely during ventilatory support or be allowed to breathe at a level they can manage. Allowing patients to do some work may prevent muscle atrophy. With total support, muscle atrophy can occur in 72 to 96 hours.[70] On the other hand, imposed work along with intrinsic work can lead to fatigue. A balance must be achieved. This is still unresolved, but common sense needs to prevail. In the severely ill unstable patient, it may be better to rest the patient completely until the patient is stabilized. Once improvement is seen, it is probably in the patient's best interest to allow him or her to begin to assume some

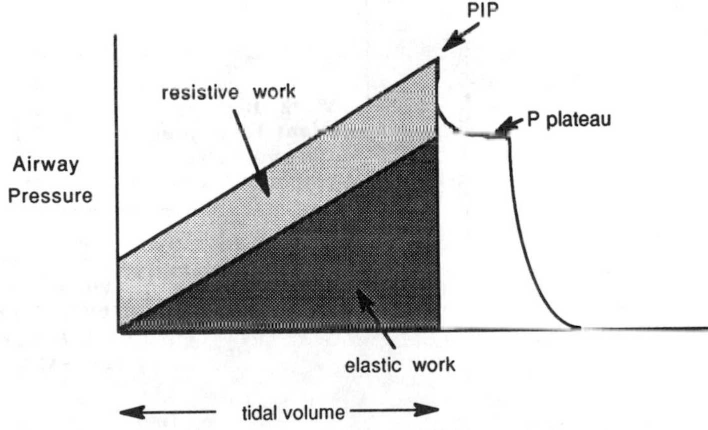

FIG 7–11.
Airway pressure over volume during controlled ventilation with a constant flow of air. The work due to airway resistance (resistive work) and elastic recoil (elastance) of the lung and thorax are the work of breathing that occurs during inspiration. *PIP* = peak inspiratory pressure. (Redrawn from references 70 and 81.)

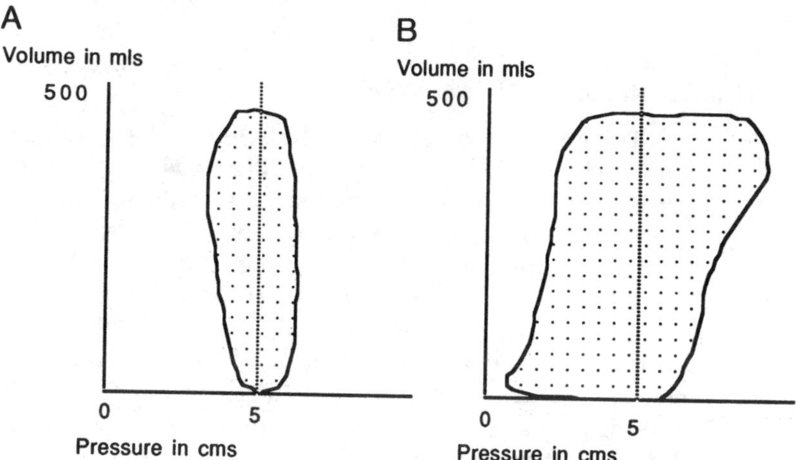

FIG 7–12.
Work of breathing (WOB) is the integral of airway pressure and tidal volume. The greater the area of the loop, the greater the work. Loop **A** is of a freestanding continuous positive airway pressure (CPAP) system. Spontaneous breaths read clockwise, inspiration to expiration. Loop **B** is CPAP through a demand flow ventilator system and shows an increase in imposed WOB (WOBi). The *area to the left of the ventrical lines* (baseline pressure of 5 cm H_2O) is the WOBi during inspiration. The *curve to the right of the lines* represents expiration. The *area to the right* is the WOBi of exhalation. (Redrawn from references 61, 68, 70.)

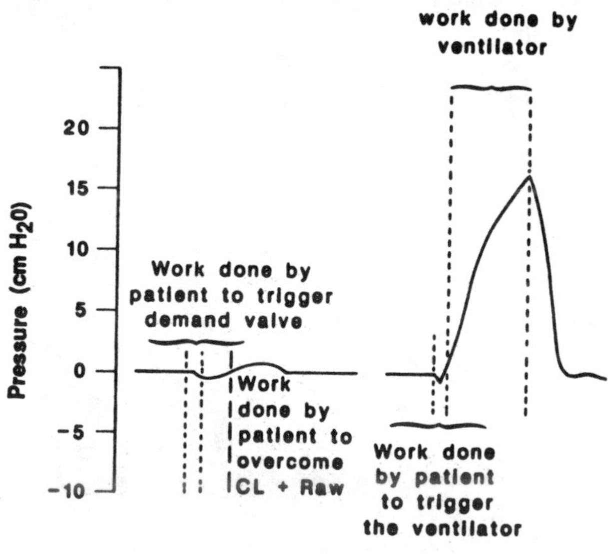

FIG 7–13.
Spontaneous *(left)* and assisted *(right)* breath during mechanical ventilation. In both, imposed work of breathing (WOBi) can occur during triggering of the breath. In the spontaneous breath, once the breath is initiated, the patient continues to perform work to overcome elastic *(CL)* and resistive *(Raw)* forces, while in the assisted breath, the ventilator provides the work. (From Branson RD: *Respir Care* 1991; 36:365–369. Used by permission.)

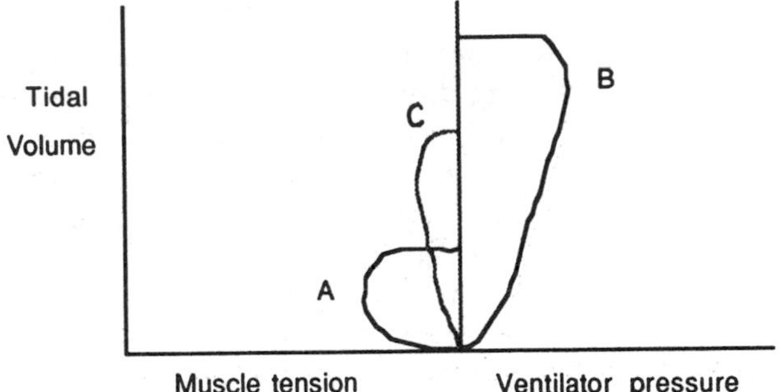

FIG 7–14.
In this figure, a spontaneous breath under normal conditions is represented by curve *C*. Curve *A* represents breathing through an ET tube on a patient with increased impedance (increased airway resistance or decreased compliance, or both). This occurs during T-tube trials for ventilation or during spontaneous breathing through an IMV continuous flow system. Curve *B* represents the work done by the ventilator during a controlled volume breath. In this the ventilator does all the work. (Redrawn from references 70 and 77.)

WOB. The clinician needs to be sure that progressive increases in patient work are not causing fatigue.

Retraining of the muscles involves a program that improves both endurance and strength. Endurance training requires progressively increasing the duration of exercise with low workloads. The principle is similar to aerobics. Strength training requires short periods with high workloads and long periods of rest between. This is similar to weight training. Rest and nutrition are important to both.

Steps to Reduce Work of Breathing During Mechanical Ventilation

Reducing the WOBi during ventilation procedures can be accomplished in several ways.[81] First, the largest possible ET tube is recommended. Long and narrow tubes significantly increase resistance. The tube needs to be kept free of secretions, kinks, or other types of constrictions. The use of PSV and PEEP can offset the work imposed by the tube.

Machine sensitivity must be at its most sensitive without leading to autocycling. Flow rates need to match patient demand. Flows of 60 to 80 L/min are usually adequate. The patient and ventilator need to be synchronized. This will depend on not only flow and sensitivity but possibly also on flow pattern and mode. If the goal is the least amount of patient work, then an assist mode is needed. Pressure support may also be beneficial if the patient has an intact respiratory center. One needs to use threshold resistor expiratory or PEEP valves to reduce the resistance to exhalation. Scissor valves and balloon-type valves have a higher flow resistance quality. Resistance to exhalation increases as flow increases. This increases the PEEP levels during expiratory flow.

Anything that can reduce the patient's Raw or improve compliance will also help. This might mean suctioning of the airway or the use of bronchodilators to reduce Raw using diuretics to reduce lung water, pleural drainage to eliminate pleural fluid or air, and positioning the patient in Fowler's position to keep the diaphragm in a downward position without visceral organs impeding its movement. Perhaps the single most important factor is $\dot{V}_E$. If $\dot{V}_E$ requirements can be reduced, this will decrease the overall work of breathing. Specifically, this means reducing fever, agitation, shivering, seizures, and any other factors that are elevating metabolic rate.[81]

Careful attention to the patient's WOB and consideration of all possible methods to reduce this work can be beneficial in the recovery of mechanically ventilated patients.

VENTILATOR MECHANICAL AND OPERATIONAL HAZARDS

One problem with artificial life support systems is failure in the device or failure of personnel to adequately monitor and care for the device. Mechanical ventilators are no exception. Some of the mechanical failures that can occur are listed in Table 7–12.

A comprehensive study by Zwillich and associates[138] covered 354 episodes of mechanical ventilation on 314 patients. Four hundred individual complications or potential complications were observed, some of which were associated with increased morbidity and mortality. Table 7–13 summarizes the findings in the study of Zwillich et al.

Abramson et al.[1] evaluated complications during mechanical ventilation. They found 145 adverse occurrences over a 5-year period. Fifty-three (37%) were

TABLE 7–12.

Potential Mechanical Failures With Mechanical Ventilation

Disconnection from power source
Failure of power source
Failure of ventilator to function due to equipment manufacturing problems or improper maintenance
Failure of alarms to work due to mechanical failure or failure of personnel to turn them on or use them properly
Failure of heating or humidifying devices
Failure of pressure relief valve to open
Disconnection of patient wye connector
Leaks in the system resulting in inadequate pressure or tidal volume delivery
Failure of expiratory valve to function causing a large system leak or a closed system with no exit for exhaled air
Inappropriate assembly of patient circuit

TABLE 7–13.
Potential Complications of Mechanical Ventilation*

	No. of Cases	Incidence (%)
Complication attributed to intubation, extubation, or tube malfunction		
Prolonged intubation attempts	46	30
Intubation of right mainstem bronchus	34	10
Premature extubation	21	7
Self-extubation	30	9
Tube malfunction	21	6
Nasal necrosis	6	2
Complication attributed to operation of the ventilator		
Machine failure	6	2
Alarm failure	13	4
Alarm found off	32	9
Inadequate nebulization or humidification	45	13
Overheating of inspired air	7	2
Medical complications		
Alveolar hypoventilation	35	10
Alveolar hyperventilation	39	11
Massive gastric distention	5	2
Atelectasis	16	5
Pneumonia	13	4
Hypotension	16	5

*Data from Zwillich CW, Pierson DJ, Creagh IE, et al: *Am J Med* 1974; 57:161–169.

the result of mechanical failure and 92 (63%) were the result of human error. Harm to the patient occurred in 45% of the incidence reports; this percentage is 72% when patients who were unattended are included.

Ventilater Disconnection

A common mechanical problem is ventilator disconnection. Table 7–14 summarizes the situations in which ventilator disconnections can occur. Table 7–15 shows how these disconnection situations may go undetected.[129] While dependable equipment, good alarm systems, and sophisticated surveillance systems are beneficial, they do not replace careful monitoring by trained personnel. By standardizing procedures and familiarizing all essential members of the health care team with equipment function, human error can be kept to a minimum.

Unexpected Ventilator Responses Associated With Newer Ventilators

Problems can occur with some microprocessor-controlled ventilators that stem from inappropriate use of the machine or idiosyncrasies associated with the machine. These include: unseating of the exhalation valve, excessive CPAP

TABLE 7–14.
Reasons for Accidental Disconnections in Patient Circuit*

Environmental changes affecting connector performance (e.g., on the Conchapack, the tubing on the output side can soften and kink from the heat and disconnect/reconnect use)
Intentional loose assembly: weak connection at the ET tube and the wye connector
Inadequate connection force
Water traps, temperature probes, O_2 analyzers, humidification systems, capnographs act as circuit breakers
Incompatible components: nonstandard dimensions, dissimilar/inappropriate materials, reuse
High pressure within the circuit
Patient movement
Deliberate disconnection by patient

*Data from *Accidental Breathing Circuit Disconnections in the Critical Care Setting.* Rockville, Md, Food and Drug Administration, US Department of Health and Human Services, Publication No. FDA 90-4233.

TABLE 7–15.
Reasons Why Accidental Disconnections May Elude Detection*

Complacency due to reliance on alarms
Desensitization due to frequent false alarms
Inappropriate alarm settings
Inappropriate sensor location
Inadequate understanding of monitor/alarm function
Misinterpretation of alarms
Incompatible combination of monitors/alarms
Disabled alarms
Inaudible alarms
Malfunctioning alarms

*Data from *Accidental Breathing Circuit Disconnections in the Critical Care Setting.* Rockville, Md, Food and Drug Administration, US Department of Health and Human Services, Publication No. FDA 90-4233.

or PEEP levels, changes in sensitivity, inability to trigger a pressure-supported breath, low and high V_T delivery, and inadequate flow.

Unseating of Expiratory Valve.—This has been noted in the Bird 6400 ventilator, but needs to be watched for in any ventilator. Unseating of the valve can occur if you occlude the expiratory valve to get a static compliance reading. The cause is a pressure build-up making the exhalation valve disengage. During monitoring of a patient if you get a "vent in-op" alarm, a low pressure alarm, or a low CPAP or PEEP alarm, and the patient is struggling to breathe, this may be the cause. These same alarms can be caused by other things. To correct the problem, disconnect the patient and manually ventilate until the problem is found and corrected.

Excessive CPAP and PEEP Levels.—CPAP and PEEP levels above the set values can occur in certain situations. One potential problem of PSV is the sudden accidental delivery of high flow and pressure due to a leak in the breathing circuit. On the Bird 6400, during pressure support, a tracheal cuff leak can cause rises in PEEP. The ventilator attempts to correct for the leak by increasing flows. Sudden application of high flow to maintain PEEP or CPAP levels can result in sudden rises in these levels. The patient may develop dyspnea, tachypnea, and tachycardia.[11] If this occurs, removal of the leak will most likely solve the problem. Another example occurs with the Puritan Bennett 7200 ventilator. If a leak develops around the tube cuff and it is more than 5 L/min, the set PSV level is maintained thoroughout the cycle causing a CPAP in the circuit.[11] A drop of flow to 5 L/min is the normal mechanism that stops the PSV inspiratory phase in this ventilator. The ventilator finally ends inspiration after a short time interval or when a certain pressure is reached. The BEAR 3 has also been reported to cause excessive CPAP or PEEP levels from proximal line disconnections when PEEP is in use.[93] During a disconnection with CPAP or PEEP, the ventilator attempts to correct for the loss of PEEP by increasing flow. When the disconnection is the result of a leak that causes enough back pressure (e.g., the airway pressure line disconnection), pressure is held in the circuit and the baseline rises. The next breath may continue to the high pressure limit and give a high pressure alarm. This is a good reason to set the pressure limit no more than +10 cm H_2O above PIP. When this situation occurs, the proximal airway pressure display will read zero. The problem is easily corrected by reconnecting the line.

Altered Sensitivity.—Ventilators can become too sensitive or less sensitive in some situations. With the BEAR 3 in the pressure support mode, if the patient circuit traps gas, the effort required by the patient to trigger a breath to be delivered increases. For example, if 4.5 cm H_2O is trapped in the circuit and the sensitivity had been set at 1.5 cm H_2O, the patient must breathe in 6.0 cm H_2O to activate the breath. A patient with a weak effort, may activate the demand valve but not have enough effort to trigger pressure support on the BEAR 3. Apparently when inspiration is weak and shallow and inspiratory flow is low, it will open the demand valve but will not give a pressure-supported breath. Weak flow demands or gas trapped in the circuit (or lung) will result in an inability to meet the demand criteria. This is one reason why the third-generation BEAR ventilator (the BEAR 5) was developed. On the Servo 900C during ventilation of neonates, sensitivity can be an issue. When much higher rates are used, the ventilator can autocycle. To prevent autocycling, you only need to reduce the sensitivity.[102]

Inability to Trigger a Pressure-Supported Breath.—Patients in the pressure support mode must initiate the breath by creating a slight negative pressure in the circuit. When a continuous flow nebulizer is placed between the patient and the sensing device, it makes it more difficult for the patient to generate this negative pressure. These sensing devices are usually on the inspiratory side of the ventilator. Some patients will be unable to generate enough pressure to trigger the ventilator, especially aged patients with COPD and weak inspiratory efforts.[9] This occurred in two reported cases of patients on the Servo 900C ventilator, but the potential exists for this to affect any microprocessor ventilator when an external nebulizer is not accounted for. This is a potential problem for patients in the assist-control mode, but it is rarely seen clinically because of the set rate and volume that ensures an adequate $\dot{V}_E$ even if the patient does not trigger the breath. In the pressure support mode, no back-up rate exists. To correct this, use only the nebulizer provided by the ventilator, or switch to the assist-control mode for the duration of the treatment, or use a ventilator such as the Ohmeda Advent, which accounts for added flow in the circuit, or use an in-line metered-dose inhaler device.[9]

Low and High Tidal Volume Delivery.—Low or high V_T can occur under two notable circumstances. One is the use of external nebulizers. The other is idiosyncratic to microprocessor ventilators and results in low volume delivery. When externally powered nebulizers are used with ventilators they add extra flow. This can increase the V_T and also give artificially high readings of exhaled $\dot{V}_E$. While not significant in most adult situations, this can be very significant in neonates.

Low V_T delivery can occur in the 7200ae and perhaps in other microprocessor ventilators. The current programming in the 7200ae assumes that the delivery flow rate is perfect. For example, if you select the square waveform, the ventilator assumes that the flow goes instantly from zero to the set flow. Obviously, the flow cannot go instantly from zero to some value and there is a slight lag at the beginning of flow delivery where flow is slightly less than that set. Under most circumstances, this amount is so small as to be insignificant.[114]

On occasions when $\dot{V}_E$ requires delivery of a high V_T at a rapid rate (short inspiratory time), then a slightly greater error occurs. Because of the short time for flow, any delay in the immediate delivery of the set flow results in a greater volume loss. The ventilator calculates its output assuming that it will give the perfect square flow. As illustrated in Figure 7–15, the flow is not perfectly constant. So the actual output is less than desired.

The reading of exhaled V_T is done at the exhalation valve assembly. What it reads is the flow coming out of the patient and the ventilator circuit (patient volume plus volume lost to tubing compliance). The ventilator currently does not compare the set value to the exhaled value so it is never "aware" that there is a difference. Only the operator knows of this condition. During high V_T and high rate situations, the exhaled volume reading and the delivered volume will be lower than the set volume.

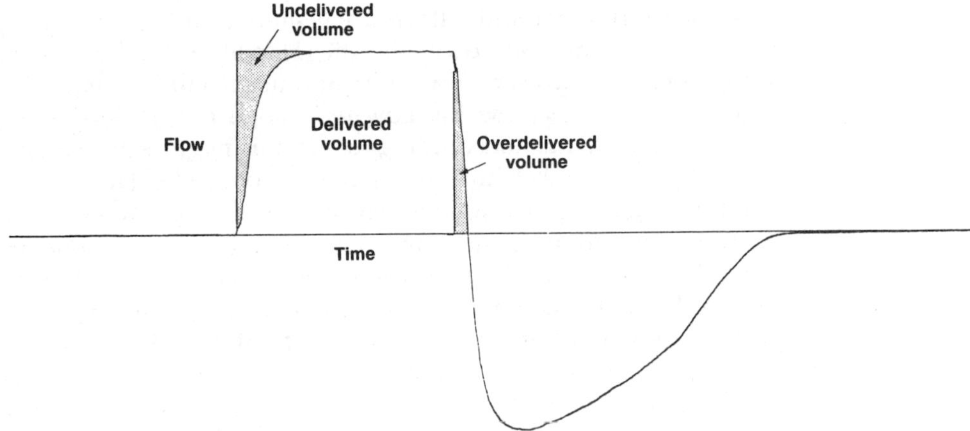

FIG 7–15.
Graph shows how the left-hand side of a constant flow curve can be "shaved off" with some ventilators when the tidal volume (V_T) is high and inspiratory time is short. This curve was produced with a 800-mL V_T at a flow of 40 L/min. The left-hand side of the curve shows a *shaded portion* of undelivered volume. This shows a rise of flow and its deviation from a true square shape. The *shaded portion* to the right of the curve shows a slightly overdelivered volume again since the flow does not stop in a perfect "rectangular" shape. (Courtesy of Warren Sanborn, Ph.D., Puritan Bennett Corp., Carlsbad, Calif.)

Remember that the set value is the volume you want to go to the patient's lungs. On the 7200ae, once the extended self-test (EST) is run, the ventilator will calculate the volume lost to the tubing compliance based on the peak pressure from the previous breath. The volume delivered from the ventilator is the volume desired plus that which is lost to the circuit. The digital display of the exhaled volume is a result of the measured flow at the exhalation valve assembly minus the volume that was lost in the circuit. Thus, it normally compensates for tubing compliance.

Under conditions of high volume and short inspiratory time, the monitored exhaled volume reading will be consistently lower than the set volume. This is because the ventilator cannot deliver the perfect square flow requested. This is a more accurate assessment of the volume the patient received. To correct for this difference, the operator needs only to increase the desired volume setting or lengthen the inspiratory time, if possible, until the exhaled volume reads the desired value of gas exhaled from the patient's lungs (excluding tubing compliance loss).

Inadequate Flow Delivery.—On most volume ventilators, when you set the V_T, flow, frequency, and inspiratory time, the flow rate to the patient is fixed using constant flow. If you are using the SIMV mode and the patient spontaneously inhales, the flow rate is limited to that which is preset by those parameters.[16] This can occur in the Hamilton Veolar as well as in other ventilators. The preset flow may not match the patient's inspiratory flow demand. If you increase the flow or change the flow pattern to match early inspiratory demands (descending wave), this might solve the problem. Another possibility is to switch to a pressure control mode. This allows the patient to pressure-trigger the breath and allow all of the flow demand he or she desires up to the maximum capacity of the ventilator and the resistance of the system. By setting the exhaled $\dot{V}_E$ (low $\dot{V}_E$) alarm, you can guard against drops in V_T due to changes in compliance or resistance. By selecting a high-frequency alarm you also guard against rises in the respiratory rate.

PSYCHOLOGICAL COMPLICATIONS IN PATIENTS IN INTENSIVE CARE

Critically ill patients who appear to be increasingly confused, lethargic, and less responsive as their stay in the intensive care unit is prolonged may be suffering from acute sleep deprivation. This is often brought on by high levels of noise and staff interferences. There is a higher morbidity and mortality rate associated with these patients when compared with patients who are disturbed less by noise and personnel.[108]

Patients on mechanical ventilation lose autonomy over a vital body function: breathing.[87] They also lose privacy, mobility, and speech as well as control over other bodily functions. These patients are under physical and psychological stress. Often, no one has explained the purpose of mechanical ventilation, ET tubes, blood sampling, monitoring devices and lines, or mentioned how long they will be used or why they are present. The patient becomes concerned over the reliability of the equipment and the personnel that handle it.

Patients need to know how to communicate and how to get help. They become disorientated as to time and place since there is often an absence of the normal environmental information systems such as clocks, calendars, newspapers, radios, and television. Many patients experience feelings of helplessness, loneliness, despair, and depression. Isolation from family members and familiar surroundings instills a feeling of helplessness and weakness.

Personnel and family often remain emotionally distant from the patient, giving mechanical responses and superficial answers to searching questions. For the family, it is a way to maintain an emotional distance so that they do not have to deal with illness and death. For hospital personnel, their own depersonalization saves them from grief and the guilt brought on by their treatment of the patient, which often causes the patient pain. These psychological problems complicate the patient's healing process and must be considered when planning a health program.

NUTRITIONAL COMPLICATIONS DURING MECHANICAL VENTILATION

The nutritional status of patients receiving ventilatory support is important if they are to successfully recover from their illness and be weaned from mechanical ventilation. Both medical and surgical patients have been reported to suffer from malnutrition during serious illness. This is often a result of inadequate intake and hypermetabolism (increased need for nutrition) which is associated with some major illnesses.[39] Many patients who develop respiratory failure already exhibit some form of malnutrition, usually caused by a preexisting chronic illness.[66] Patients on ventilatory support are generally unable to take in oral feedings because of the ET tube. Unless special routes for nutritional support are provided, such as nasogastric feedings or intravenous hyperalimentation, these patients develop malnutrition.

Nutritional depletion has several deleterious effects for the mechanically ventilated patient (Table 7–16).[104] Malnutrition contributes to infection, impaired wound healing, and inability to maintain spontaneous ventilation from weakened respiratory muscles. While adequate feeding is important, overfeeding can increase $\dot{V}O_2$, $\dot{V}CO_2$, and the need for increased $\dot{V}E$. This increases a patient's WOB. Feedings need to be of appropriate type and amount.[66, 104]

Assessment of a patient's resting energy expenditure (REE) provides information about the daily kilocalorie requirements. REE can be measured by indirect calorimetry. Assessment of nutritional status provides information regarding the patient's level of malnutrition. Table 7–17 lists parameters for assessing nutritional status. Once these have been evaluated, a correct feeding schedule can be instituted.

Nutritional supplements should always be delivered by the most natural route possible. This means that oral feedings are the first choice, nasogastric feedings second, and catheters into the gastrointestinal tract third. If enteral (through the gut) feedings are not possible, then parenteral (into a vein) nutri-

TABLE 7–16.
Effects of Malnourishment in Mechanically Ventilated Patients

Reduced response to hypoxia and hypercarbia
Muscle atrophy from prolonged bed rest and lack of use: this includes respiratory muscles, especially if the patient is on controlled ventilation
Muscle wasting from lack of nutrition including the respiratory muscles
Respiratory tract infections from impaired cell immunity and reduced or altered macrophage activity
Decreased surfactant production and development of atelectasis
Reduced ability of pulmonary epithelium to replicate, which slows healing of damaged tissue
Lower serum albumin levels which affect colloid oncotic pressures and can contribute to pulmonary edema formation (colloid oncotic pressures <11 mm Hg with normal left atrial pressure)

TABLE 7–17.
Assessment of Nutritional Status

Body composition
- Actual vs. predicted body weight
- Anthropometric measurements (limb circumference and skin fold measurements)
- Fat vs. lean muscle mass

Protein deficiencies
- Creatinine-height index*

Visceral protein malnutrition
- Serum albumin < 3.5 g/dL
- Transferrin < 300 mg/dL

Immunodeficiency
- Decreased skin test response to known recall antigens

*The ratio of 24-hour urine creatinine excreted in milligrams to height in centimeters. Less than 6.0 is considered a critical protein deficiency.

tion is provided. Intravenous feedings can use a peripheral vein or a central vein. Feedings must be given in adequate doses to restore the nutritional status of the patient without overfeeding. Intravenous feedings are associated with higher infection rates and need to be carefully handled.

MINIMIZING THE PHYSIOLOGIC EFFECTS AND COMPLICATIONS OF MECHANICAL VENTILATION

The harmful cardiovascular effects of IPPV are basically a result of high positive pressure within the lungs and the transmission of this pressure to the intrapleural space. Any methods that will reduce the intrapulmonary pressures will also reduce the pressure applied to the intrathoracic structures. Both the amount and the duration of the pressure are important. These two factors are combined in the term *mean airway pressure* ($\overline{P}aw$). The lower the $\overline{P}aw$, the less marked the cardiovascular effects. $\overline{P}aw$ is the area enclosed between the curve and the baseline for one respiratory cycle, divided by the duration of the cycle[97] (Fig 7–16). Areas enclosed below the baseline are negative and subtracted from the area of the pressure curve above the baseline.

$\overline{P}aw$ can be monitored using a variety of devices that use various algorithms to calculate and display the average value of $\overline{P}aw$ during mechanical ventilation of the subject.[7, 26, 120] It can also be manually calculated. In a constant flow, volume-cycled ventilator, the pressure rise is nearly linear with time and produces essentially a triangular pressure waveform (see Fig 7–16). $\overline{P}aw$ can be estimated by using the following equation: $\overline{P}aw$ = 1/2 [(Ppeak × (inspiratory time/total respiratory cycle)]. In this same ventilator mode with PEEP added, the

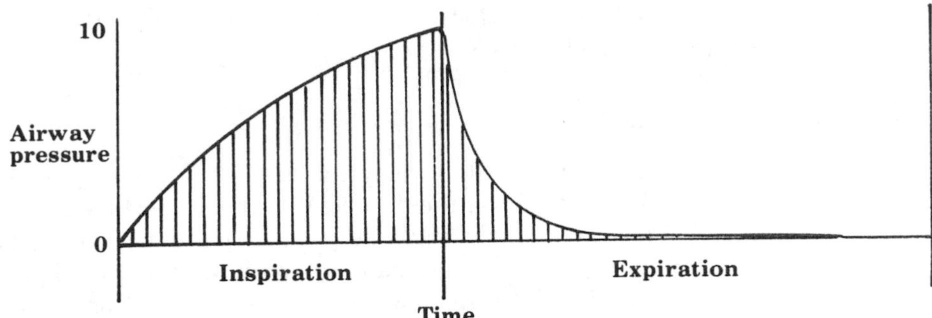

Positive pressure ventilation

FIG 7–16.
Vertical lines under the pressure curve represent frequent readings of pressure over the total respiratory cycle. The sum of these pressure readings, i.e., the area under the curve, divided by the cycle time will give the mean airway pressure.

equation is as follows: $\overline{P}aw = 1/2\ (Ppeak - PEEP) \times (inspiratory\ time/total\ cycle\ time) + PEEP$.[105]

The $\overline{P}aw$ generated during IPPV undergoes variations and may exhibit different waveforms (pressure curves) depending upon the types of ventilator employed, the mode of ventilation used, and the patient's pulmonary characteristics. For example, modes such as inflation hold, expiratory retard, pressure control, and PEEP have high $\overline{P}aw$ values compared to normal IPPV and zero end-expiratory pressure.

Mean Airway Pressure and Pao_2

$\overline{P}aw$ has clinical importance. For a specific V$_T$ it has been noted that Pao_2 may be predominantly affected by $\overline{P}aw$ and to a lesser extent the ventilator parameters used to achieve the $\overline{P}aw$.[27, 47] This is probably related to an increase in FRC with increased $\overline{P}aw$. Thus, changes in FRC are of importance to increased Pao_2.[35] The amount of $\overline{P}aw$ required to achieve a certain level of oxygenation may indicate the severity of a patient's lung disease[105]; however, a direct relationship between $\overline{P}aw$ and Pao_2 is still unproven.

Reduction in Mean Airway Pressure

Large values of $\overline{P}aw$ imply an increased intrapleural pressure and its associated problems. Positive pressure is never maintained higher or longer than is necessary to achieve adequate ventilation and oxygenation. Lower $\overline{P}aw$ can be achieved by changing inspiratory flow rates, the I/E ratio, inflation hold, PEEP, and expiratory retard. IMV or SIMV, and possibly modes such as pressure support, may also reduce $\overline{P}$aw.

Inspiratory Flow Rates

Rapid inspiratory flows may increase Ppeak but with normal conductive airways they can deliver the desired V_T in a shorter time and have a lower $\overline{P}$aw (Fig 7–17). Three things must be kept in mind with high flows. First, more pressure will be lost to the patient circuit with higher Ppeak. Second, more pressure will be lost to Raw (Raw = ΔP/flow). And third, uneven ventilation is more likely to occur with high flow rates. If, for example, the right bronchus is partially obstructed, most of the gas flow goes to the left lung. As flow increases, a greater proportion of gas goes to the left lung with less going to the right since gas flow takes the path of least resistance. As a result, a larger volume enters the left lung. The increased left lung volume increases left lung pressure compared to the right. This can do two things. The uneven distribution of gas may contribute to $\dot{V}/\dot{Q}$ mismatching. The higher pressure in the left lung may decrease left lung perfusion by compressing pulmonary capillaries and decreasing flow, and the increased left lung volume may have a dead space effect (more ventilation and less perfusion). Secondly, it may also increase the risk of alveolar rupture since more volume is going to one lung and creating greater pressures and alveolar stretch in that lung. In general terms, the goal is to use the highest

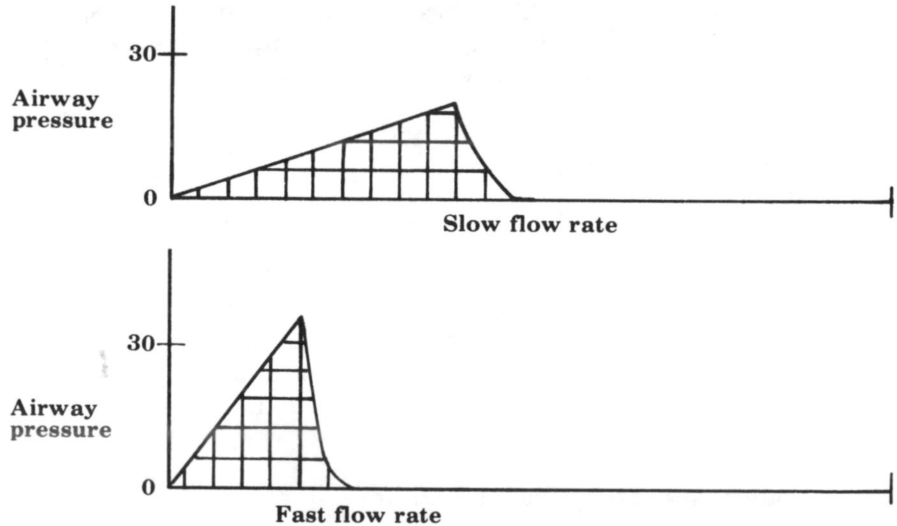

FIG 7–17.
Slower flow rate may reach a lower peak pressure compared to a rapid flow rate, but it may also produce a higher mean airway pressure. Note the number of boxes under each curve.

possible flow rates and carefully monitor the effects of the flow changes on volume delivery, V_D/V_T, $\dot{V}/\dot{Q}$, and P_{TA}.

I/E Ratio

Another point to consider is the duration of inspiration in relation to expiration. The shorter the inspiratory cycle and the longer the expiratory cycle, the more limited the effects of pressure with more time being spent in passive exhalation where intrathoracic physiology returns to normal. A range of I/E ratios of 1:1.5 to 1:4 or smaller in the adult is considered acceptable for mechanical ventilation. Values of 1:1, 2:1, and higher may result in significant increases in $\overline{P}aw$, air trapping, and significant hemodynamic complications unless the lung tissue is very stiff.

Values of 1:2, 1:3, 1:4, and smaller have a lower $\overline{P}aw$ and fewer associated hazards. In patients with poor airway conductance (increased resistance), a longer expiratory time also has the benefit of allowing better alveolar emptying. Short I/E ratios—1:6 or smaller in a nonspontaneously breathing patient where each breath is a machine breath—may increase physiologic dead space. This is due to rapid inspiratory flow rates with inspiratory time less than 0.5 second.[97] As a result, it is up to the practitioner to balance the patient's response to variations in I/E ratio and flow rates to achieve what is best for that patient.

Inflation Hold

To improve oxygenation and the distribution of gas in the lung, the maneuver referred to as inflation hold, or inspiratory pause, was at one time frequently used. Inflation hold is accomplished by a ventilator adjustment which holds the air in the lung at the end of inspiration for a brief period. This increases

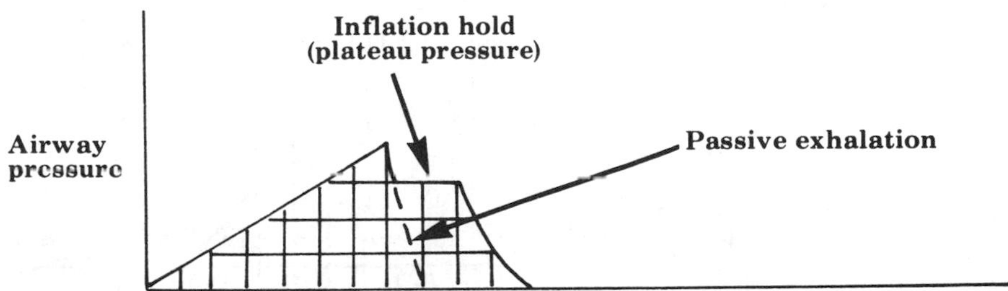

FIG 7–18.
Inflation hold or inspiratory pause may help to improve the distribution of gases in the lungs, but it also may increase mean airway pressure. The curve shows an inflation hold compared with a normal passive exhalation.

inspiratory time and also $\overline{P}aw$ (Fig 7–18). Expiration is allowed to continue passively and unimpeded. Employment of inflation hold can be detected by observing the upper (proximal) airway pressure manometer reading. End-inspiration occurs and the manometer needle peaks and then falls to a plateau pressure which is held for a fraction of a second before dropping to baseline, which is usually ambient or zero on the manometer.

Use of inflation hold is now primarily for the purpose of measuring plateau pressure for calculation of static compliance. It has been replaced by PEEP or CPAP for improving oxygenation. If inflation hold is used, it must be kept in mind that it will increase the $\overline{P}aw$ and may cause undesirable hemodynamic side effects.

PEEP

PEEP increases the FRC of the lungs and improves oxygenation but also increases $\overline{P}aw$ (Fig 7–19). The syndrome of the patients who require PEEP is decreased lung compliance. By virtue of a stiff lung, which is present in this patient group, increases in lung pressure by the use of PEEP do not always result in a significant portion of the pressure being transmitted through the alveoli to the intrathoracic space and the intrathoracic vessels. Thus, increased $\overline{P}aw$ with PEEP is not always accompanied by a decreased CO or decreased venous return.

Expiratory Retard

Varying the resistance to expiration is beneficial in patients who have increased risk of early small airway closure, and subsequently, air trapping. Expiratory retard does, however, increase $\overline{P}aw$ (Fig 7–20). The control marked "expiratory retard" no longer appears on newer-generation ventilators. On the other hand, we still employ techniques that do the same thing. For example, low levels of PEEP, particularly with the use of flow resistance PEEP valves, function the same way as expiratory retard. These also increase $\overline{P}aw$.

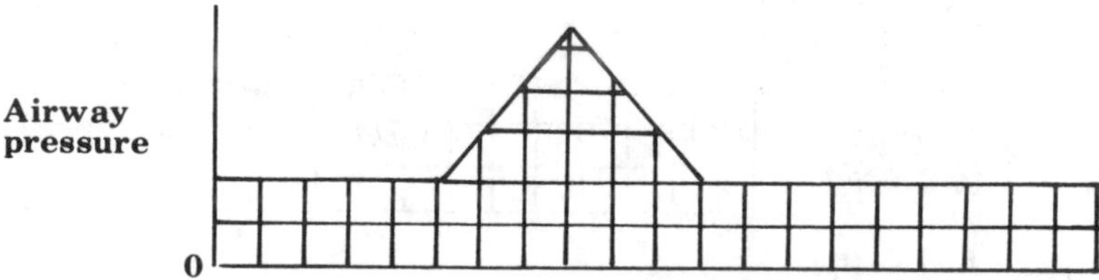

FIG 7–19.
PEEP during IPPV maintains a high baseline pressure and results in the increase of mean airway pressure.

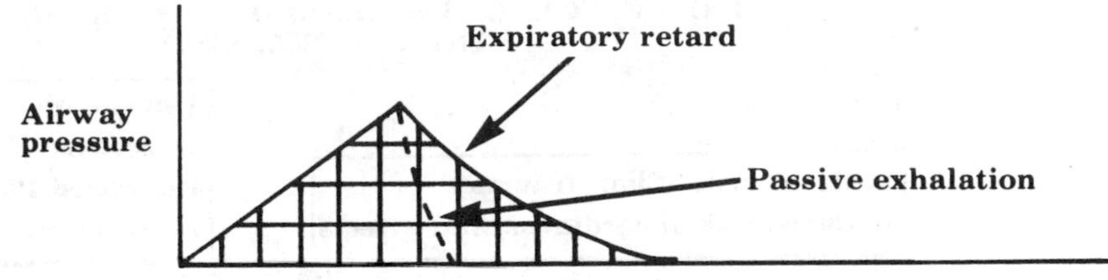

FIG 7–20.
Expiratory retard elevates mean airway pressure by extending the length of time that positive pressure is in the airways compared to passive exhalation. TE is the same.

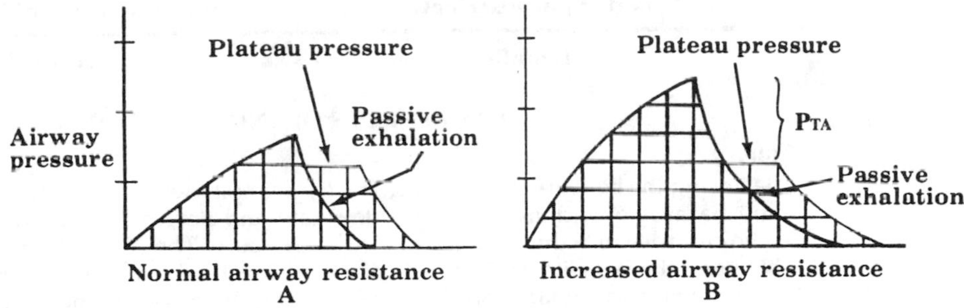

FIG 7–21.
A, normal pressure difference between peak and plateau pressure when airway resistance is normal. When airway resistance is increased, the difference between peak and plateau pressure is increased, i.e., more pressure is lost to the airways. **B,** note that peak pressure is also increased. PTA = transairway pressure.

High Peak Pressures From Increased Airway Resistance

While high peak airway pressure may be indicative of an increase in $\overline{P}$aw, there are some cases where this pressure is not transmitted to the intrapleural space. For example, patients with increased airway resistance caused by bronchospasm, mucous plugging, mucosal edema, or other airway problems have increased amounts of pressure lost to the airway that never reach the alveoli. Thus, high peak pressure detected at the upper airway will not be transmitted to the intrapleural space or the thoracic structures and plateau pressures will be low. However, if increased resistance leads to air trapping from inadequate expiratory time or from loss of normal expiratory resistance maneuvers such as pursed lips breathing, then hazardous cardiovascular effects will occur (Fig 7–21).

IMV and SIMV

Another mode of ventilation which can decrease $\overline{P}$aw of patients requiring IPPV is IMV. By reducing the frequency of machine positive pressure breaths

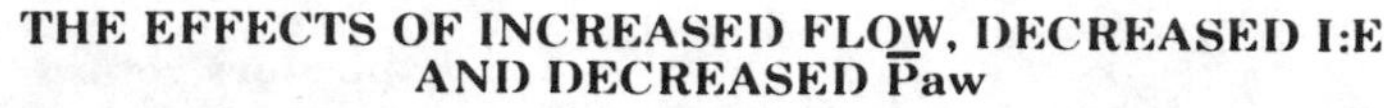

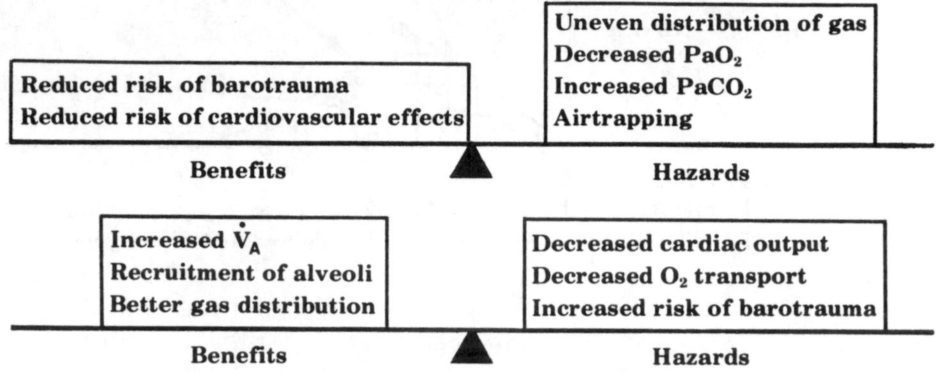

THE EFFECTS OF INCREASED $\overline{P}$aw

FIG 7–22.
Balancing the benefits and hazards. The *top figure* shows the balance between the benefits and hazards of increasing the gas flow rate and decreasing the inspiratory-expiratory ratio in order to reduce the mean airway pressure. The *bottom figure* shows the balance between the benefits and hazards of increasing the mean airway pressure in order to increase alveolar ventilation ($\dot{V}_A$) (by increasing $\dot{V}_A$ or respiratory rate), achieve alveolar recruitment with PEEP, and improve gas distribution (by using inflation hold or slowing inspiratory flow rates). All factors must be considered when treating patients on mechanical ventilatory support.

and allowing spontaneous breathing to occur against ambient pressure or with PEEP or CPAP in between these breaths, the cardiovascular complications of high $\overline{P}$aw are reduced. SIMV is beneficial in this regard since it prevents a machine breath from occurring simultaneously with a patient's end-inspiration (stacked breaths). IMV or SIMV, which requires that the patient assume a certain percentage of the WOB, must be used with caution. In attempting to decrease $\overline{P}$aw by decreasing the machine rate and increasing the patient's spontaneous breathing rate with the IMV mode, the clinician runs the risk of producing fatigue and adding stress to the patient who may need artificial respiratory support to allow recovery time from some exacerbating pulmonary problem.

If the patient's spontaneous respiratory rate between machine breaths is rapid and accompanied by low V_T, the patient's spontaneous breath may be ineffective. The patient's spontaneous $\dot{V}_E$ may be composed mostly of dead space ventilation and the patient's WOBi is probably leading to muscle fatigue.

If the patient's spontaneous respiratory rate is rapid and V_T is deep in the presence of normal $Paco_2$, the patient may have some underlying cause for an increased V_D/V_T ratio or increased CO_2 production. It is not uncommon for acutely ill patients such as those with sepsis, multiple organ failure, severe burns, or trauma to have metabolic rates that are higher than normal leading to increased $\dot{V}O_2$ and $\dot{V}CO_2$ and requiring an increased $\dot{V}E$. The clinician must ask if he or she wants the patient to continue to work this hard at maintaining adequate alveolar ventilation or if he or she wants to increase the machine rate and run the risk of causing cardiovascular and pulmonary complications from positive pressure ventilation (PPV). The answer lies in understanding each clinical situation and the personal requirements of the individual patient.

Of the many complications associated with PPV, the two most important are interference with cardiovascular function and interference with gas exchange.[97] Procedures which decrease $\bar{P}aw$ may decrease cardiovascular effects but contribute to uneven ventilation, and vice versa (Fig 7–22). The clinician must evaluate each aspect of the patient's problems and estimate a ventilation pattern which is as effective as possible.

STUDY QUESTIONS

1. Four days after being placed on ventilatory support, a post–open heart surgery patient has indications of low urine production and a weight gain of 1 kg. Which of the following might have caused these changes?
   I. Kidney failure.
   II. Positive pressure ventilation.
   III. Increased ADH levels in the blood.
   IV. Administration of furosemide (Lasix).
   V. High fluid outputs.
   a. I only.
   b. II only.
   c. I, II, and III.
   d. IV only.
   e. IV and V.
2. While listening to a patient's breath sounds during mechanical ventilation, the respiratory care practitioner (RCP) notices absence of breath sounds over the entire right hemithorax. Peak pressures have increased from 25 to 50 cm H_2O in the last 30 minutes. Percussion on the right is hyperresonant. The RCP should:
   a. Percuss over the left thorax.
   b. Disconnect the patient from the ventilator and let him or her spontaneously breathe.
   c. Increase the pressure limit to 60 cm H_2O.
   d. Request a chest film.
   e. Call a physician immediately.

3. Further evaluation of the patient reveals the following: chest film shows increased radiolucency and absence of vascular markings on the right side. The right chest is hyperresonant to percussion. The trachea is deviated to the left. The neck veins are distended. The patient is cyanotic, unconscious, and nonresponsive. What immediate action(s) should the RCP take at this time?
   I. Call a physician immediately.
   II. Disconnect the patient from the ventilator and manually support ventilation.
   III. Increase the pressure limit.
   IV. Increase the ventilator volume.
   V. Give +5 cm H_2O of PEEP.
   a. I and V.
   b. II only.
   c. III only.
   d. I and II.
   e. IV and V.
4. In a patient with pneumonia of the right lung receiving mechanical ventilation, the best position in which to place the patient for optimal oxygenation is the right lateral decubitus position. True or false?
5. Positive pressure ventilation can reduce perfusion to the renal cortex, and increase sodium and water retention. True or false?
6. Cardiovascular complications of mechanical ventilation include which of the following:
   I. Reduced venous return.
   II. Reduced cardiac output.
   III. Increased renal perfusion.
   IV. Increased ICP.
   V. Reduced blood pressures.
   a. I and III.
   b. II and IV.
   c. I, II, III, and IV.
   d. I, II, IV, and V.
   e. III and V.
7. Acidosis is associated with hyperkalemia. True or false?
8. Positive pressure ventilation causes air to go toward the dependent zones of the lungs in the supine patient. True or false?
9. Positive pressure ventilation can cause pulmonary blood flow to go to the periphery of the lung. True or false?
10. Hyperventilation and hypoventilation can be caused by mechanical ventilation. True or false?
11. A patient on ventilatory support has a Pao_2 of 101 mm Hg, $Paco_2$ of 60 mm Hg, and a pH of 7.30. The respiratory care practitioner should:

a. Increase $\dot{V}_E$.
b. Decrease $\dot{V}_E$.
c. Change the ventilation mode.
d. Very gradually, over several days, increase $\dot{V}_E$.
e. Very gradually, over several days, decrease the $\dot{V}_E$.

12. During mechanical ventilation, hyperventilation, particularly in patients with COPD, can cause which of the following:
    I. Muscle twitching and tetany.
    II. High pH values.
    III. Air trapping.
    IV. Spiked T waves.
    V. Cardiac arrhythmias.
    a. II only.
    b. I and III.
    c. II, III, and V.
    d. I, II, III, and V.
    e. I, II, III, IV, and V.
13. During mechanical ventilation on IMV of 4 breaths/min and V_T = 800 mL, a patient has a spontaneous rate of 34 breaths/min between machine breaths. The spontaneous V_T ranges from 175 to 325 mL. The patient is using accessory muscles to breathe. Arterial blood gas results are within the normal range. Which of the following might be appropriate?
    a. Increase the V_T from the ventilator.
    b. Increase the F_{IO_2}.
    c. Decrease the IMV rate.
    d. Add a pressure support of 10 cm H_2O.
    e. Switch to pressure control.
14. Reducing the WOBi can be accomplished by using which of the following?
    a. Increasing inspiratory flow rates.
    b. Increasing ventilator sensitivity.
    c. Putting the patient in the upright position so the visceral organs do not impede movement of the diaphragm.
    d. Ensuring patency of the ET tube.
    e. All of the above.
15. A patient has been on ventilatory support for several days. What should be done to see if any nosocomial pneumonias have begun to develop?
    I. Chest film for the presence of infiltrates.
    II. Chest film for the presence of pleural air leaks.
    III. White blood cell count.
    IV. Sputum examination for color, consistency, and odor.
    V. Patient temperature.
    a. I only.
    b. III and IV.

c. II, III, and V.
d. I, III, IV, and V.
e. II, III, IV, and V.

ANSWERS TO STUDY QUESTIONS

1. c.
2. b.
3. d.
4. False.
5. True.
6. d.
7. True.
8. False.
9. True.
10. True.
11. a.
12. d.
13. d.
14. e.
15. d.

REFERENCES

1. Abramson RS, Wald RS, Grenvik ANA, et al: Adverse occurrences in intensive care units. *JAMA* 1980; 244:1582–1588.
2. Al-Sady N, Bennett ED: Decelerating inspiratory flow waveform improves lung mechanics and gas exchange in patients on intermittent positive-pressure ventilation. *Intensive Care Med* 1985; 11:68–75.
3. Anderson J: Ventilatory strategy in catastrophic lung disease: Inversed ratio ventilation (IRV) and combined high frequency ventilation (CHFV). *Acta Anaesthesiol Scand* 1989; 33:145–148.
4. Arnold JS, Summer JL, Tipton RD, et al: Inverse ratio ventilation in hypoxic respiratory failure (abstract). *Chest* 1989; 96:150S.
5. Ashbaugh DG, Petty TL, Bigelow DB, et al: Continuous positive breathing in adult respiratory distress syndrome. *J Thorac Cardiovasc Surg* 1969; 57:31.
6. Ayres SM, Grace WG: Inappropriate ventilation and hypoxemia as causes of cardiac arrhythmias. *Am J Med* 1969; 46:495–504.
7. Banner MJ, Gallagher TJ, Bluth LJ: A new microprocessor device for mean airway pressure measurement. *Crit Care Med* 1981; 9:51–53.
8. Baratz RA, Philbin DM, Patterson RW: Plasma anti-diuretic hormone and urine output during continuous positive-pressure breathing in dogs. *Anesthesiology* 1971; 34:510–513.
9. Beaty CD, Ritz RH, Benson MS: Continuous in-line nebulizers complicate pressure support ventilation. *Chest* 1989; 96:1360–1363.
10. Bergman N: Intrapulmonary gas trapping during mechanical ventilation at rapid frequencies. *Anesthesiology* 1972; 37:626–633.
11. Black JW, Grover BS: A hazard of pressure support ventilation. *Chest* 1988; 93:333–335.
12. Bone RC: Complications of mechanical ventilation and positive end expiratory pressure. *Respir Care* 1982; 27:402–407.
13. Bone RC: Mechanical trauma in acute respiratory failure. *Respir Care* 1983; 28:618–623.

14. Bone RC, Francis PB, Pierce AK: Pulmonary barotrauma complicating positive end expiratory pressure. *Am Rev Respir Dis* 1976; 13:921.
15. Branson RD: Enhanced capabilities of current ICU ventilators: Do they really benefit patients? *Respir Care* 1991; 36:362–376.
16. Bray B: Personal communication, May 1991.
17. Breivik H, Grenvik A, Millen E, et al: Normalizing low arterial CO_2 tension during mechanical ventilation. *Chest* 1973; 63:525–531.
18. Brown DG, Pierson DJ: Auto-PEEP is common in mechanically ventilated patients: A study of incidence, severity, and detection. *Respir Care* 1986; 31:1069–1074.
19. Burton GG, Gee GN, Hodgkin JE: *Respiratory Care: A Guide to Clinical Practice.* Philadelphia, JB Lippincott Co, 1977.
20. Campbell EJM, Nunn JF, Peckett BW: A comparison of artificial ventilation and spontaneous respiration with particular reference to ventilation–blood flow relationships. *Br J Anaesth* 1958; 30:166–172.
21. Cartwright DW, Willis MM, Gregory GA: Functional residual capacity and lung mechanics at different levels of mechanical ventilation. *Crit Care Med* 1984; 12:422–427.
22. Carven DE, Goularte TA, Make BJ: Contamination condensate in mechanical ventilator circuits. *Am Rev Respir Dis* 1984; 129:625–628.
23. Chalon J, Loew DAY, Malebrache J: Effects of dry anesthetic gases on tracheobronchial ciliated epithelium. *Anesthesiology* 1972; 37:338–343.
24. Chatburn RL: Decontamination of respiratory care equipment: What can be done, what should be done. *Respir Care* 1989; 34:98–110.
25. Chatburn RL: Some possible misconceptions about airway pressures (letter). *Respir Care* 1991; 36:872–874.
26. Chatburn RL, Lough M, Primiano FP: Modification of a pressure monitoring circuit to permit display of mean airway pressure. *Respir Care* 1982; 27:276–281.
27. Ciszek TA, Modanlou HD, Owings D, et al: Mean airway pressure—significance during mechanical ventilation in neonates. *J Pediatr* 1981; 99:121–126.
28. Clark JM, Lambertsen CJ: Pulmonary oxygen toxicity: A review. *Pharmacol Rev* 1971; 23:37–133.
29. Cole AGH, Weller SF, Sykes MK: Inverse ratio ventilation compared with PEEP in adult respiratory failure. *Intensive Care Med* 1984; 10:337–339.
30. Conway CM: Hemodynamic effects of pulmonary ventilation. *Br J Anaesth* 1975; 47:761–766.
31. Cournand A, Motley HL, Werko L, et al: Physiological studies of the effects of intermittent positive pressure breathing on cardiac output in man. *Am J Physiol* 1948; 152:162–174.
32. Craven DE, Steger KA: Pathogenesis and prevention of nosocomial pneumonia in the mechanically ventilated patient. *Respir Care* 1989; 34:85–97.
33. Dariolo R, Perret C: Mechanical controlled hypoventilation in status asthmaticus. *Am Rev Respir Dis* 1984; 129:385–387.
34. DeWitt AL: Sunshine overloads detectors, some therapists discover. *Adv Resp Care Pract* July 16, 1990, p 14.
35. Downs JB: Ventilatory patterns and modes of ventilation in acute respiratory failure. *Respir Care* 1983; 28:586–591.
36. Downs JB, Mitchell LA: Pumonary effects of ventilatory pattern following cardiopulmonary bypass. *Crit Care Med* 1976; 4:295–300.

37. Dreyfuss DP, Basset G, Soler P, et al: Intermittent positive-pressure hyperventilation with high inflation pressures produces pulmonary microvascular injury in rats. *Am Rev Respir Dis* 1985; 132:880–884.
38. Dreyfuss D, Soler P, Basset G, et al: High inflation pressure pulmonary edema. *Am Rev Respir Dis* 1988; 137:1159–1164.
39. Driver AG, LeBrun M: Iatrogenic malnutrition in patients receiving ventilatory support. *JAMA* 1980; 244:2195–2196.
40. Drury DR, Henry JP, Goodman J: The effects of continuous pressure breathing on kidney function. *J Clin Invest* 1947; 26:945–951.
41. Emery MW, Gray BA, Carlile, PV: Effect of PEEP on lung injury due to positive pressure ventilation. *Chest* 1989; 96(Suppl):149s.
42. Fairley HB, Blenkarn GD: Effects on pulmonary gas exchange of variations in inspiratory flowrate during intermittent positive pressure ventilation. *Br J Anaesth* 1969; 38:320–328.
43. Fiastro JF, Habib MP, Quan SF: Pressure support compensation for inspiratory work due to endotracheal tubes and demand continuous positive airway pressure. *Chest* 1988; 93:499–502.
44. Fishman APL: Down with the good lung (editorial). *N Engl J Med* 1981; 304:537–538.
45. Fracica PJ: Oxygen toxicity, in Fulkerson WJ, MacIntyre NR (eds): *Problems in Respiratory Care. Complications of Mechanical Ventilation.* Philadelphia, JB Lippincott Co, 1991, pp 90–99.
46. Froese AB, Bryan AC: Effects of anesthesia and paralysis on diaphragmatic mechanics in man. *Anesthesiology* 1974; 41:242–255.
47. Gallagher TJ, Banner MJ: Mean airway pressure as a determinant of oxygenation. *Crit Care Med* 1980; 8:244.
48. Golden GT, Chandler JG: Colonic ileus and cecal perforation in patients receiving mechanical ventilatory support. *Chest* 1975; 68:661–664.
49. Grace WJ: *Practical Clinical Management of Electrode Disorders.* New York, Appleton-Century-Crofts, Inc, 1960.
50. Griebel JA, Piantadosi CA: Hemodynamic effects and complications of mechanical ventilation, in Fulkerson WJ, MacIntyre NR (eds): *Problems in Respiratory Care. Complications of Mechanical Ventilation.* Philadelphia, JB Lippincott Co, 1991, pp:25–35.
51. Griggs BM, Reinhardt DJ: *Fundamentals of Nosocomial Infections Associated With Respiratory Therapy.* New York, Projects in Health, Inc, 1975.
52. Guyatt GH: Positive pressure ventilation as a mechanism of reduction of left ventricular afterload. *Can Med Assoc J* 1982; 126:1310–1312.
53. Hall SV, Johnson EE, Hedley-Whyte J: Renal hemodynamics and function with continuous positive pressure ventilation in dogs. *Anesthesiology* 1974; 41:452–461.
54. Haynes JB, Carson SD, Whitney WP, et al: Positive end expiratory pressure shifts left ventricular diastolic pressure-area curves. *J Appl Physiol* 1980; 48:670–676.
55. Hedenstierna G: The anatomical and alveolar dead spaces during respiratory treatment: Influence of respiratory frequency, minute volume and tracheal pressure. *Br J Anaesth* 1975; 47:993–999.
56. Hedenstierna G, White FE, Wagner PD: Spacial distribution of pulmonary blood flow in the dog with PEEP ventilation. *J Appl Physiol* 1979; 47:938–946.
57. Hedley-Whyte J, Burgess GE, Feeley TW, et al: *Applied Physiology of Respiratory Care.* Boston, Little, Brown & Co, Inc, 1976.

58. Hedley-Whyte J, Pontoppidan H, Morris MJ: The relation of alveolar to tidal ventilation during respiratory failure in man. *Anesthesiology* 1966; 27:218–219.
59. Heironimus TW: *Mechanical Artificial Ventilation,* ed 2. Springfield, Ill, Charles C Thomas, Publisher, 1970.
60. Helmholz HF Jr: Statistical compliance and "best PEEP" (editorial). *Respir Care* 1981; 26:637–638.
61. Hirsch C, Kacmarek RM, Stankek K: Work of breathing during CPAP and PSV imposed by the new generation mechanical ventilators: A lung model study. *Respir Care* 1991; 36:815–828.
62. Hoffman RA, Ershowsky P, Krieger BP: Determination of auto-PEEP during spontaneous and controlled ventilation by monitoring changes in end-expiratory thoracic gas volume. *Chest* 1989; 96:613–616.
63. Holt JH, Branscomb BV: Hemodynamic responses to controlled 100% oxygen breathing in emphysema. *J Appl Physiol* 1965; 20:215.
64. Hooton TM: Protecting ourselves and our patients from nosocomial infections. *Respir Care* 1989; 34:111–115.
65. Hudson LD: Cardiovascular complications in acute respiratory failure. *Respir Care* 1983; 28:627–633.
66. Jenkinson SG: Nutritional problems during mechanical ventilation in acute respiratory failure. *Respir Care* 1983; 28:641–644.
67. Jenkinson SG: Oxygen toxicity in acute respiratory failure. *Respir Care* 1983; 28:614–617.
68. Kacmarek RM: The role of pressure support ventilation in reducing the work of breathing. *Respir Care* 1988; 33:99–120.
69. Kette F, Weil MH, von Planta M, et al: Buffer agents do not reverse intramyocardial acidosis during cardiac resuscitation. *Circulation* 1990; 81:1660–1666.
70. Kirby RR, Banner MJ, Downs JB: *Clinical Applications of Ventilatory Support.* New York, Churchill Livingstone Inc, 1990.
71. Kirby RR, Downs JB, Civetta JM, et al: High level positive end expiratory pressure (PEEP) in acute respiratory insufficiency. *Chest* 1975; 67:156–163.
72. Kolobow T, Moretti M, Fumagalli R, et al: Lung injury from oxygen in lambs: The role of artifical ventilation. *Am Rev Respir Dis* 1987; 135:312–315.
73. Kussin PS: Respiratory muscle fatigue and deconditioning. *Prob Respir Care* 1991; 4:68–89.
74. Lain DC, Chaudhary BA, Thorarinsson B, et al: Auto-PEEP and proximal airway pressure—Need for clarification. *Chest* 1990; 97:771.
75. Laver MB: Hemodynamic adjustment to mechanical ventilation: The role of coronary artery diseases, in *33rd Annual Refresher Course Lectures, American Society of Anesthesiology,* Chicago, no. 209, 1982, pp 1–7.
76. Liebman PR, Patten MT, Manny J et al: The mechanism of depressed cardiac output on positive end expiratory pressure (PEEP). *Surgery* 1978; 83:594–598.
77. MacIntyre NR: Weaning from mechanical ventilatory support: Volume-assisting intermittent breaths versus pressure-assisting every breath. *Respir Care* 1988; 33:121–125.
78. MacIntyre NR: Intrinsic positive end-expiratory pressure, in Fulkerson WJ, MacIntyre NR (eds): *Problems in Respiratory Care. Complications of Mechanical Ventilation.* Philadelphia, JB Lippincott Co. 1991, pp 44–51.

79. Malecka-Griggs B, Reinhardt DJ: Direct dilution sampling, quantitation, and microbial assessment of open-system ventilation circuits in intensive care units. *J Clin Microbiol* 1983; 17:870–877.
80. Marini JJ: The role of the inspiratory circuit in the work of breathing during mechanical ventilation. *Respir Care* 1987; 32:419–422.
81. Marini JJ: Work of breathing, in Kacmarek RM, Stoller JK (eds): *Current Respiratory Care.* Philadelphia, BC Decker, Inc, 1988, pp 188–194.
82. Marini JJ: Should PEEP be used in airflow obstruction (editorial). *Am Rev Respir Dis* 1989; 140:1–3.
83. Marini J, Crooke P, Truwit J: Determinants and limits of pressure-preset ventilation: A mathematical model of pressure control. *J Appl Physiol* 1989; 67:1081–1092.
84. Marini JJ, Culver BH, Butler J: Mechanical effects of lung distention with positive pressure on ventricular function. *Am Rev Respir Dis* 1981; 124:382–386.
85. Marini JJ, Culver BH, Kirk W: Flow resistance of exhalation valves and positive end-expiratory pressure devices used in mechanical ventilation. *Am Rev Respir Dis* 1985; 131:850–854.
86. Marini JJ, Rodriguez RM, Lamb V: The inspiratory workload of patient-initiated mechanical ventilation. *Am Rev Respir Dis* 1986; 134:902–909.
87. Martz IV, Joiner J, Shepherd RM: *Management of the Patient-Ventilator System.* St Louis, Mosby–Year Book, Inc, 1984.
88. McAslan TC, Matjasko-Chiu J, Turney SZ, et al: Influence of inhalation of 100% oxygen on intrapulmonary shunt in severely traumatized patients. *J Trauma* 1973; 9:811.
89. McLoughlin GA, Manny J, Grinklingen FA, et al: Pressure breathing and altered fibrinolytic activity. *Ann Thorac Surg* 1980; 29:156–165.
90. McPherson SP: *Respiratory Therapy Equipment.* St Louis, Mosby–Year Book, Inc, 1979.
91. Mithoefer JC, Holford FD, Keighley JFH: The effect of oxygen administration on mixed venous oxygenation in chronic obstructive pulmonary disease. *Chest* 1974; 66:122–133.
92. Mithoefer JC, Keighley JF, Karetzkey MS: Response of the arterial PO_2 to oxygen administration in chronic pulmonary disease. *Ann Intern Med* 1971; 74:328–335.
93. Monaco F, Goettel J: Increased airway pressures in Bear 2 and 3 circuits. *Respir Care* 1991; 36:132–134.
94. Moran WH: CPPB and vasopressin secretion (editorial). *Anesthesiology* 1971; 34:501–504.
95. Morgan BC, Martin WE, Hornbein TF, et al: Hemodynamic effect of intermittent positive pressure respiration. *Anesthesiology* 1966; 27:584.
96. Motley HL, Cournaud A, Werkö L, et al: Observations on the clinical use of positive pressure ventilation. *J Aviat Med* 1947; 18:417.
97. Mushin WW, Rendell-Baker L, Thompson PW, et al: *Automatic Ventilation of the Lungs.* Philadelphia, FA Davis Co, 1980.
98. Nichols CW, Lambertsen CJ: Effects of high oxygen pressures on the eye. *N Engl J Med* 1969; 281:25–30.
99. Ovensfors CO: Pulmonary interstitial emphysema. An experimental roentgen-diagnostic study. *Acta Radiol Suppl (Stockh)*1964; 1:224s.

100. Pearce L, Lilly K, Baigelman W: Effects of positive end expiratory pressure on intracranial pressure. *Respir Care* 1961; 26:754–756.
101. Pepe PE, Marini JJ: Occult positive end-expiratory pressure in mechanically ventilated patients with airflow obstruction. *Am Rev Respir Dis* 1982; 126:166–170.
102. Perry W: Personal communication, February 1991.
103. Pick RA, Handler JB, Friedman AS: The cardiovascular effects of positive end expiratory pressure. *Chest* 1982; 82:345–350.
104. Pilbeam SP, Head A, Grossman GD, et al: Undernutrition and the respiratory system. *Respir Ther* 1983; 12:65–69; 13:72–78.
105. Primiano EP, Chatburn RL, Lough MD: Mean airway pressure: Theoretical considerations. *Crit Care Med* 1982; 10:378–383.
106. Qvist J, Pontoppidan H, Wilson RS, et al: Hemodynamic responses to mechanical ventilation with PEEP. *Anesthesiology* 1975; 42:45–55.
107. Rarey KP, Youtsey JW: *Respiratory Patient Care.* Englewood Cliffs, NJ, Prentice-Hall, Inc, 1981.
108. Rattenborg C, Via-Reque E: *Clinical Use of Mechanical Ventilation.* St Louis, Mosby–Year Book, Inc, 1981.
109. Rau JL: Continuous mechanical ventilation. Part I. *Critical Care Update,* October 1981, pp 10–29.
110. Rau JL, Jr, Pearce DJ: *Understanding Chest Radiographs.* Denver, Multi-Media Publishing, Inc, 1984.
111. Remolina C, Khan AU, Santiago TV, et al: Positional hypoxemia in unilateral lung disease. *N Engl J Med* 1981; 304:523–525.
112. Rossi A, Gottfried SB, Zocchi L, et al: Measurement of static compliance of the total respiratory system in patients with acute respiratory failure during mechanical ventilation. *Am Rev Respir Dis* 1985; 131:672–677.
113. Samuelson WM, Fulkerson WJ: Barotrauma in mechanical ventilation, in Fulkerson WJ, MacIntyre NR (eds): *Problems in Respiratory Care. Complications of Mechanical Ventilation.* Philadelphia, JB Lippincott Co, 1991, pp 52–67.
114. Sanborn WG: Personal communication, August 1991.
115. Scott LR, Benson MS, Bishop MJ: Relationship of endotracheal tube size and auto-PEEP at high minute ventilations. *Respir Care* 1986; 31:1080–1082.
116. Scott LR, Benson MS, Pierson DJ: Effect of inspiratory flowrate and circuit compressible volume and auto-PEEP during mechanical ventilation. *Respir Care* 1986; 31:1075–1079.
117. Shapiro BA, Harrison RF, Trout CA: *Clinical Application of Respiratory Care.* St Louis, Mosby–Year Book, Inc, 1979.
118. Sladen A, Laver MB, Pontoppidan H: Pulmonary complications and water retention in prolonged mechanical ventilation. *N Engl J Med* 1968; 279:448.
119. Smith TC, Marini JJ, Lamb VJ: The inspiratory threshold load resulting from air-trapping during mechanical ventilation. *Am Rev Respir Dis* 1987; 135:A52.
120. Smyth JA, Volgyesi GA: Simple device for measurement of mean airway pressure. *Crit Care Med* 1983; 11:130–131.
121. Stauffer JL, Silvestri RC: Complications of endotracheal intubation, tracheostomy and artificial airways. *Respir Care* 1982; 27:417–434.
122. Summer WR, Nelson S: Nosocomial pneumonia: Characteristics of the patient-pathogen interaction. *Respir Care* 1989; 34:116–124.

123. Tapson VF, Fulkerson WJ: Infectious complications of mechanical ventilation, in Fulkerson WJ, MacIntyre NR, (eds): *Problems in Respiratory Care. Complications of Mechanical Ventilation.* Philadelphia, JB Lippincott Co, 1991, pp 100–117.
124. Thomas DV, Fletcher G, Sunshine P, et al: Prolonged respiratory use in pulmonary insufficiency in newborns. *JAMA* 1965; 193:183.
125. Tuxen DV: Detrimental effects of positive end-expiratory pressure during controlled mechanical ventilation of patients with severe airflow obstruction. *Am Rev Respir Dis* 1989; 140:5–9.
126. Tuxen DV, Lane S: The effects of ventilatory pattern on hyperinflation, airway pressures, circulation in mechanical ventilation of patients with severe air-flow obstruction. *Am Rev Respir Dis* 1987; 136:872–879.
127. Tyler DC: Positive end-expiratory pressure: A review. *Crit Care Med* 1983; 11:300–307.
128. Tyler ML: The respiratory effects of body position and immobilization. *Respir Care* 1984; 29:472–483.
129. US Department of Health and Human Services: *Accidental Breathing Circuit Disconnections in the Critical Care Setting.* Washington, DC, Public Health Service, *Food and Drug Administration,* Center for Devices and Radiological Health, US Department of Health and Human Services, Publication No. FDA 90–4233.
130. Walley KR, Schimidt GA: Therapeutic use of intrinisic positive end-expiratory pressure. *Crit Care Med* 1990; 18:336–337.
131. Watson WE: Observations on the dynamic lung compliance of patients with respiratory muscle weakness receiving intermittent positive pressure respiration. *Br J Anaesth* 1962; 34:690–695.
132. Watson WE: Observations on physiology deadspace during intermittent positive pressure respiration. *Br J Anaesth* 1962; 34:502.
133. Webb HH, Tierney DF: Experimental pulmonary edema due to intermittent positive pressure ventilation with high inflation pressures. Protection by positive end-expiratory pressure. *Am Rev Respir Dis* 1974; 110:556–565.
134. West JB: *Ventilation, Blood Flow and Gas Exchange,* ed 2. London, Blackwell Scientific Publishers, 1974.
135. West JB, Dollery CT, Naimark A: Distribution of blood flow in insolated lung: Relation to vascular and alveolar pressure. *J Appl Physiol* 1964; 19:713.
136. Woo SW, Hedley-Whyte J: Macrophage accumulation and pulmonary edema due to thoracotomy and lung overinflation. *J Appl Physiol* 1972; 33:14–21.
137. Zarins CK, Virgilio RW, Smith DE, et al: The effect of vascular volume on positive end-expiratory pressure–induced cardiac output depression and wedge–left atrial pressure discrepancy. *J Surg Res* 1977; 23:348.
138. Zwillich CW, Pierson DJ, Creagh CE, et al: Complications of assisted ventilation. *Am J Med* 1974; 57:161–169.

Chapter **8**

Patient Management and Stabilization

On completion of this chapter the reader will be able to:

1. Identify the parameters to be completed on a ventilator flow sheet.
2. Describe the procedure for measuring and calculating tidal volume, minute ventilation, alveolar ventilation, anatomic dead space, and tubing compliance.
3. Correct tidal volume and rate settings based on arterial blood gas results.
4. Select the sigh mode, pressure support mode, and pressure control mode based on patient findings.
5. Identify from a description the presence of a leak in a ventilator circuit.
6. Explain the procedure for finding a leak in a ventilator circuit.
7. Describe the minimum leak technique.
8. Describe the procedure for measuring cuff pressure and identify safe cuff pressures.
9. Identify changes in peak and plateau pressure and tidal volume and tell when changes in compliance or resistance have occurred.
10. Draw a pressure-volume curve.
11. Identify changes in compliance and resistance from a pressure-volume curve.
12. Change the F_{IO_2} based on arterial blood gas results.
13. List four ways in which the addition of an externally powered nebulizer to a mechanical ventilator circuit can affect the ventilator function or the patient.
14. Describe the findings in a ventilated patient with respiratory distress.
15. List the common causes of a patient's "fighting" the ventilator.
16. Give the first step in managing the ventilated patient in distress.

17. From changes in vital signs, laboratory data, and sputum characteristics, identify a patient that has a respiratory infection.
18. From changes in input and output data, body weight, and physical findings, identify a patient who has fluid retention during mechanical ventilation.
19. Describe the techniques for measuring vital capacity and maximum inspiratory pressure.

PATIENT MANAGEMENT AND STABILIZATION

The care of the critically ill patient requires the regular gathering, evaluating, and storing of information and data. This is particularly true in patients receiving mechanical ventilatory support. Continuous monitoring of cardiac and ventilatory data is required for patient safety. Periodic clinical assessment further guarantees patients' well-being and provides the opportunity to make changes in their care as needed. The simplest and most valuable method of evaluation is through the observation of well-trained and caring personnel.

Ventilator flow sheets are forms on which data are recorded for a patient receiving mechanical ventilatory support (Fig 8–1). The top of the sheet holds basic patient information: name, diagnosis, physician, hospital number, admitting date, age, weight, height, ideal body weight, body surface area (BSA), initial ventilator settings, endotracheal (ET) tube size and the centimeter marking at the teeth, corner of the mouth, or nares, the date mechanical ventilation was initiated, and the current date.

There are also spaces for filling in current information on patient and ventilator parameters: time, mode of ventilation, minute ventilation ($\dot{V}_E$), alveolar ventilation ($\dot{V}_A$), rate, tidal volume (V_T), peak and plateau pressures, static and dynamic compliance, fractional concentration of oxygen in inspired gas (F_{IO_2}), sigh volume, sigh rate, sigh frequency, inspired temperatures, inspiratory-expiratory (I/E) ratio, continuous positive airway pressure (CPAP) or positive end-expiratory pressure (PEEP), arterial blood gases the physiologic dead space–tidal volume ratio (V_D/V_T), the alveolar-arterial oxygen tension difference [$P(A - a)O_2$], the ratio of partial pressure of arterial oxygen (Pa_{O_2}) to alveolar oxygen (P_{AO_2}), shunt, vital capacity (VC), maximum inspiratory pressure (MIP), vital signs, and alarm settings. Volumes, pressures, temperature, vital signs, and F_{IO_2} are measured every hour or two. Alarms are activated to ensure that the patient is being ventilated. Arterial blood gases, shunt, V_D/V_T, $P(A - a)O_2$ and Pa_{O_2}/P_{AO_2} are determined when there is a major change in the patient's condition or in the ventilator settings. The way these parameters are measured and how they are changed is the focus of the following section.

Patient Name Jane Doe **Physician** DR. Bone **Ventilator** MAG-3 **Start Date** 6-21-92
Diagnosis Myasthenia Gravis **Age** 36 **Ht.** 5'4" **Wt.** 113#
IBW 125# **BSA** 1.4 m^2 **Et Tube place** 24@ lip **Et Tube press.** 20 mm Hg
Initial V_E 5.4 L V_T 600 ml **f** 9 F_IO_2 0.3

Date/Time	6/28 / 9:00AM					
Mode	A/C					
P_{peak} (cm H_2O)	25					
$P_{plateau}$ (cm H_2O)	21					
P_{peak}-P_{Plat}(cm H_2O)	4					
Machine						
Vt deliv. (ml)	525					
F(actual)	9					
Patient						
Vt del. (ml)	Ø					
F(actual)	Ø					
V_E total (L.min)	4.73					
V_A total (L.min)	3.6					
PEEP/(CPAP) (cm H_2O)	Ø					
C_D (ml/cm H_2O)	21					
C_S (ml/cm H_2O)	25					
V_t sigh (ml)	Ø					
sigh f	Ø					
F_IO_2 (analyzed)	0.3					
PaO_2 (mmHg)	140					
SaO_2%	97					
$PaCO_2$ (mmHg)	42					
HCO_3 (mEq/L)	25					
PaO_2/PAO_2	.89					
$P(A\text{-}a)O_2$	18					
Q_s/Q_t	2%					
end-tidal CO_2 or $TcPCO_2$	5%					
V_D/V_t	.25					
VC (liters)	1.3					
MIP (cm H_2O)	-25					
Vital Signs						
HR	101					
BP	105/65					
Temp.	37.3°C					
Breath Sounds	↓ in bases					
Airway Temp.	36° C					
Pcuff	21 mm Hg					
Alarms	ON					
Hemodynamics						
PAP	Ø					
PCWP	Ø					
C.O.	Ø					
CVP	Ø					
Comments:						
(Sputum)	MOD AMT-CLEAR					
(Treatment)	NO					
(Others)						

FIG 8–1.
Ventilator flow sheet.

INITIAL PATIENT ASSESSMENT

When the patient is first connected to the ventilator, the initial step is to listen to breath sounds to confirm adequate volume delivery and proper ET tube placement. The alarms (apnea, low pressure, power failure, high pressure, etc.) are activated and vital signs are taken. An arterial blood gas sample is obtained about 15 minutes after ventilation begins to evaluate the effectiveness of ventilation and oxygenation. A chest film is taken to check tube placement if this has not already been done.

Mode

The mode of ventilation is recorded in the appropriate space. This might be recorded as control, assist, assist-control, intermittent mandatory ventilation (IMV), synchronized IMV (SIMV), pressure control (PC), pressure support (PS), CPAP, minimum minute ventilation (MMV), or T-tube. It might also be recorded based on ventilator classification, e.g., time-triggered PC, or time-cycled.

Sensitivity

If the patient is on a pressure-triggered mode such as the assist mode or SIMV where inspiration is initiated by a patient effort, the pressure needed to trigger the ventilator is checked. It should take no more than -1 or -2 cm H_2O to trigger the ventilator. If the ventilator is flow-triggered, the sensitivity may be a change of 2 to 3 L/min of flow. The response time and sensitivity of the ventilator varies from one brand to another. Some ventilators are more responsive, reliable, and consistent than others.

Auto-PEEP and Patient Triggering

If auto-PEEP is present, this will make it more difficult for the patient to trigger a breath. If the patient's accessory muscles are active and the patient appears to be laboring to breathe, the presence of auto-PEEP may be one cause. Measuring for auto-PEEP is appropriate when other causes have been ruled out (see Chapter 7). If auto-PEEP is present, it may be necessary to increase the flow rate to the patient or take other steps to reduce auto-PEEP. This might include changing modes to allow for more spontaneous breaths or reducing $\dot{V}_E$.

IMV and Patient Inspiratory Flow Demand

If the patient is on a continuous flow IMV system the manometer needle should not go more than -1 to -2 cm H_2O below the baseline during a patient's spontaneous inspiration. If it does, the flow from the IMV system is not adequate and must be increased. If the IMV is through the demand valve on the ventilator, the ventilator may need to be changed to one with a more responsive demand valve.

Minute Ventilation, Tidal Volume, and Rate

Volume parameters, V_T, respiratory frequency (f), and $\dot{V}_E$, can be measured using a hand-held volume-measuring device or respirometer, and a watch or clock with a sweep second hand. The respirometer is connected directly to the patient's endotracheal tube and to the patient wye connector (Fig 8–2), or at the exhalation valve. Gas exhaled from the lungs is measured for 1 minute. Frequency is counted at the same time. Tidal volume can be calculated ($\dot{V}_E = V_T \times f$) or measured directly. If the patient is on IMV or SIMV, the

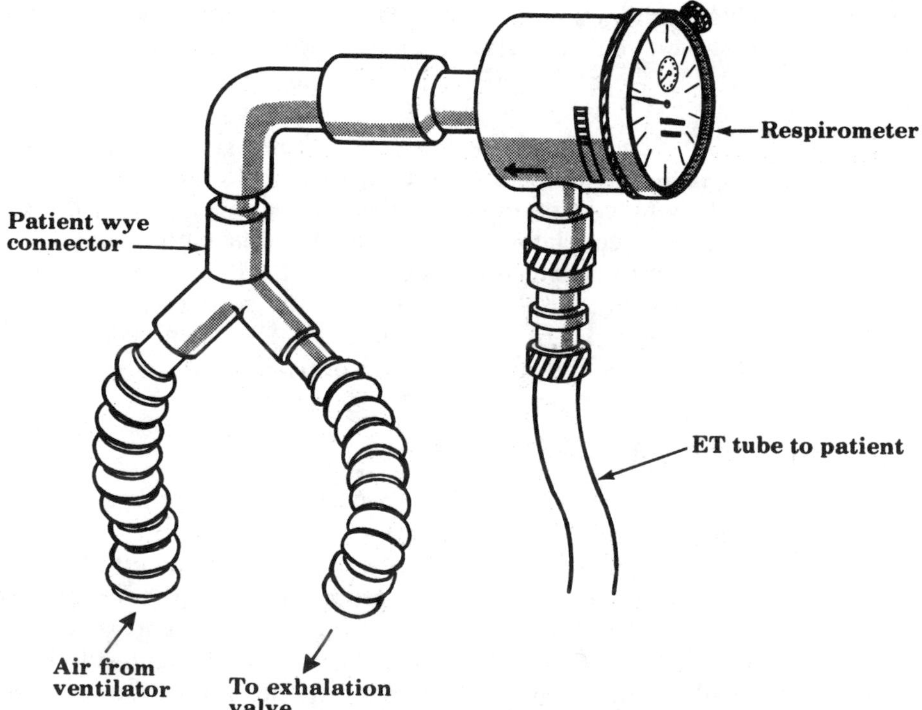

FIG 8–2.
Tidal volume measurement at the endotracheal *(ET)* tube. The respirometer is attached to the ET tube so that the patient's actual exhaled air can be measured. The respirometer can also be attached at the exhalation valve. Some respirometers read both inspiration and expiration by measuring flow in both directions.

spontaneous rate and V_T are measured and recorded separately from the machine rate and V_T.

Correcting for Tubing Compliance

If V_T is measured at the expiratory port, then the volume lost to tubing compliance (C_{Tubing}) must be subtracted from the V_T reading on the respirometer. For example, if peak inspiratory pressure (PIP) = 25 cm H_2O, V_T (at exhalation port) = 600 mL, and C_{Tubing} = 3 mL/cm H_2O, then the volume lost to the tube will be PIP × C_{Tubing}, or 25 cm H_2O × 3 mL/cm H_2O = 75 mL. The actual delivered volume to the patient's lungs will be 600 mL − 75 mL, or 525 mL.

Alveolar Ventilation

To determine $\dot{V}_A$ in patients on mechanical ventilation, three factors must be considered: anatomic dead space, normal mechanical dead space, and added mechanical dead space.

Anatomic Dead Space.—Normal anatomic dead space (V_{Dan}) is 1 mL/lb of ideal body weight (IBW). This is subtracted from actual delivered V_T to determine $\dot{V}_A$ for one breath. When the upper airway is bypassed with an ET or tracheostomy tube, V_{Dan} is decreased by about 1 mL/kg of IBW. In a 165-lb (75-kg) male, for example, V_{Dan} is 165 mL. With an ET tube in place it becomes 165 − 75 = 90 mL.

Normal Mechanical Dead Space.—Ventilator circuits have a certain amount of normal mechanical dead space (V_{Dmech}) which ranges in value from 75 to 150 mL in most patient circuits. This rebreathed volume technically increases dead space ventilation. Note that the amount of increase in dead space is nearly equal to the amount of decrease in dead space from ET intubation. Most institutions assume that these two factors balance each other when calculating $\dot{V}_A$ and ignore them.

An example of a device which increases mechanical dead space is the heat-moisture exchanger. This device acts as an artificial nose and provides warm humidified air when placed between the ET tube and the wye connector. It is sometimes used for short-term humidification in place of a cascade or pass-over–type humidifier. It contains absorbent material housed in a small plastic unit. The material collects moisture from expired air and thus provides humidity on inspiration. The material can also act as a microbial filter.

Added Mechanical Dead Space.—If V_{Dmech} is added to the patient circuit using large-bore corrugated tubing at the ET tube, this must be subtracted from the V_T when determining actual $\dot{V}_A$. For example, if the V_T is 500 mL at the

ET tube, and the added V_{Dmech} is 100 mL, then a 150-lb adult will have a $\dot{V}_A$ for one breath of $V_T - V_{Dmech} - V_{Dan}$, or $500 - 100 - 150 = 250$ mL.

Final Alveolar Ventilation.—On assist, control, or assist/control mode, the number of machine-delivered breaths are counted for 1 minute and multiplied by the V_T. Alveolar minute volume will be $(V_T - V_{Dmech} - V_{Dan}) \times f$. When a patient is on the IMV or SIMV mode, the ventilator rate and volume delivery must be calculated separately from the patient's spontaneous rate and volume delivery when determining the $\dot{V}_A$. These are added together to get total ventilation.

For example, with an SIMV rate of 5 breaths/min and machine-delivered V_T of 900 mL, $V_{Dan} = 100$ mL (corrected for ET tube), $V_{Dmech} = 50$ mL; $\dot{V}_A$ from the machine is $5 \times [900 - 100 - 50] = 3{,}750$ mL, or 3.75 L. If the patient has an additional rate of 10 breaths/min with a spontaneous volume of 350 mL; spontaneous $\dot{V}_A$ will equal $10 \times [350 - 100 - 50] = 2{,}000$ mL or 2.0 L. Total $\dot{V}_A$ will equal $3.75 + 2.0 = 5.75$ L/min.

VENTILATION AND $Paco_2$

When arterial carbon dioxide partial pressure ($Paco_2$) is increased above the patient's normal value and the pH decreases, respiratory acidosis is present. Patient $\dot{V}_A$ is not adequate. When the ventilator is volume-controlled or volume-limited, increasing the V_T up to 15 mL/kg will decrease the $Paco_2$. If the V_T is already at 15 mL/kg, then the rate can be increased. If the ventilator is pressure-cycled, the cycling pressure is increased.

When $Paco_2$ is decreased below the patient's normal value and pH reflects a respiratory alkalosis, then excessive $\dot{V}_A$ is present. To decrease ventilation in a volume-controlled or volume-limited ventilator, decrease the respiratory rate. Then, if necessary, decrease the V_T but preferably not below 10 mL/kg. If the ventilator is time-cycled, decrease the rate first if necessary. If the ventilator is pressure-cycled, decrease the rate first, and then the cycling pressure, if needed.

If the patient is in respiratory alkalosis on assisted ventilation, decreasing the machine rate setting may have no effect on the patient's rate if the patient is initiating all breaths. Decreasing V_T may be effective unless the patient just increases his or her respiratory rate and thus maintains a high $\dot{V}_A$. In this situation three alternatives are available. First, institute IMV or SIMV to allow the patient to breathe without getting a machine breath with every inspiration. Second, sedate and, if necessary, paralyze the patient to completely control breathing. This may be needed for patients with seizures or with tetanus, but otherwise is not the best choice. Third, add V_{Dmech}. The equation for adding

TABLE 8–1.

Calculation of Mechanical Dead Space Volume Needed to Increase $Paco_2$

$$V_{Dmech} = \frac{Paco_2' - Paco_2}{Paco_2' - (Paco_2 - P_{ACO_2})} \times (V_T - V_{DAN})$$

where V_{DMECH} = mechanical dead space to add

$Paco_2$ = actual $Paco_2$

$Paco_2'$ = desired $Paco_2$

P_{ACO_2} = alveolar CO_2

1. Assume that $\dot{V}/\dot{Q}$ is normal, then $Paco_2 - P_{ACO_2}$ is <10 mm Hg
   Use $Paco_2 - P_{ACO_2} = 5$ mm Hg
2. Example: $Paco_2' = 40$ mm Hg
   $Paco_2 = 30$ mm Hg
   $V_T = 900$ mL
   $V_{DAN} = 200$ ml
   $$V_{DMECH} = \frac{40 - 30}{40 - 5} \times (900 - 200)$$
   $$= \frac{10}{35} \times 700$$
   $$= 200 \text{ mL}$$
   Add 200 mL V_{DMECH} to achieve a $Paco_2 = 40$ mm Hg
3. To determine the volume of a length of large-bore corrugated tubing, fill the tubing with water and pour it into a graduated cylinder
4. Add the V_{DMECH} between the ET tube and the patient circuit wye connector
5. Increase the patient's O_2 percentage slightly to correct for the decreased F_{IO_2} brought on by using V_{DMECH}

V_{Dmech} is given in Table 8–1.[57] The dead space is added between the ET tube and the patient wye connector on the ventilator circuit. This method is not as popular as using IMV. With added V_{Dmech}, patients will often increase their respiratory rate and V_T to overcome the effects of the dead space. Another possible option is to go to other modes of ventilation such as PS.

Some patients will continue to hyperventilate when on IMV or SIMV or with V_{Dmech} in use. The cause for the hyperventilation needs to be investigated and treated. Sometimes it may be due to a central nervous system lesion involving the respiratory centers and cannot be corrected.

Many patients in acute respiratory failure have mixed respiratory and metabolic disturbances, e.g., a combined respiratory acidosis and metabolic alkalosis. The metabolic alkalosis component may be from vomiting, diuretics, nasogastric suctioning, or bicarbonate administration. The pH may actually be near normal. In this case it is inappropriate to increase $\dot{V}_E$ in order to decrease the $Paco_2$. This can rapidly precipitate into a condition of metabolic alkalosis with accompanying cardiac dysrhythmias, seizures, and other neurologic disturbances. The cause of both problems should be determined and corrected.

CORRECTING Pa_{CO_2} ABNORMALITIES

In volume-controlled ventilators a change in the V_T or frequency setting is needed to correct for respiratory alkalosis or acidosis. These changes are based on the following equation:

$$\text{Known } Pa_{CO_2} \times \text{known } \dot{V}_A = \text{desired } Pa_{CO_2} \times \text{desired } \dot{V}_A$$

Since the dead space does not change significantly from moment to moment, this equation can be modified. If it is desirable to keep the rate constant and change the V_T, then the equation becomes:

$$\text{Desired } V_T = \frac{\text{known } Pa_{CO_2} \times \text{known } V_T}{\text{desired } Pa_{CO_2}}$$

If it is appropriate to keep the V_T the same and change the rate, then the equation is written:

$$\text{Desired f} = \frac{\text{known } Pa_{CO_2} \times \text{known f}}{\text{desired } Pa_{CO_2}}$$

Clinical Examples

Example 1: Respiratory Acidosis, Increasing V_T.—Let's consider an example of a patient in respiratory acidosis on mechanical ventilatory support. The patient is 6 ft 2 in. tall and weighs 190 lb (81 kg) (V_{Dan} = 190 mL). The exhaled V_T measured at the ET tube is 600 mL. Respiratory rate is 10 breaths/min. The patient is on controlled ventilation. Pa_{CO_2} is 60 mm Hg, pH is 7.33. The patient's desired Pa_{CO_2} is 40 mm Hg. What ventilator change must be made to decrease the patient's Pa_{CO_2}? Since the V_T setting is less than 15 mL/kg, it is appropriate to hold the rate constant and change the V_T.

$$\text{Desired } V_T = \frac{\text{known } Pa_{CO_2} \times \text{known } V_T}{\text{desired } Pa_{CO_2}}$$

$$\text{Desired } V_T = \frac{60 \times 600}{40} = 900 \text{ mL}$$

The new V_T is set at 900 mL to achieve a desired Pa_{CO_2} of 40 mm Hg. The $\dot{V}_A$ has been increased appropriately to correct the respiratory acidosis.

Example 2: Respiratory Acidosis, Increasing Rate.—A 5 ft 2 in. woman on controlled ventilation has a Pa_{CO_2} of 58 mm Hg; pH is 7.28; V_T at the ET tube is

800 mL. IBW is 115 lb (52 kg); VDan is 115 mL; respiratory rate is 7 breaths/min. How can a desired $Paco_2$ of 40 mm Hg be achieved?

In this case the current VT is at 15 mL/kg (52 kg × 15 mL = 780 mL) so it is appropriate to change the rate and not the VT.

$$\text{Desired f} = \frac{\text{known f} \times \text{known } Paco_2}{\text{desired } Paco_2}$$

$$\text{Desired f} = \frac{7 \times 60}{40} = 10.5 \text{ breaths/min}$$

Increasing the frequency to 11 breaths/min should decrease the $Paco_2$ to 40 mm Hg

Example 3: Respiratory Alkalosis, Decreasing the Rate.—A patient is in respiratory alkalosis ($Paco_2$ = 20 mm Hg, pH = 7.60) on the control mode with a delivered VT of 1,000 mL; f is 15 breaths/min, and VDan is 150 mL. The desired $Paco_2$ is 40 mm Hg. IBW is 70 kg. The VT setting is 15 mL/kg. It is appropriate in this case to decrease the rate and leave the VT constant.

$$\text{Desired f} = \frac{\text{known f} \times \text{known } Paco_2}{\text{desired } Paco_2}$$

$$\text{Desired f} = \frac{15 \times 20}{40} = 7.5 \text{ breaths/min}$$

Round off to 8 breaths/min. This rate should achieve the desired $Paco_2$ of 40 mm Hg.

Example 4: Combined Respiratory Acidosis and Metabolic Alkalosis.—A patient on mechanical ventilation has a $Paco_2$ of 60 mm Hg and a pH of 7.41. The patient's normal $Paco_2$ is 40 mm Hg. The fact that the high $Paco_2$ is not reflected in the pH indicates that the patient also has a metabolic alkalosis. Before the $Paco_2$ can be corrected with ventilator manipulation (increase VT or increase f) the metabolic alkalosis must be corrected. If the $Paco_2$ were decreased to 40 mm Hg, the pH would increase and the patient would have severe alkalosis. In addition, the O_2 would fall if the $\dot{V}$E were reduced.

Example 5: Dead Space Problem.—If a pure respiratory acidosis persists even after the $\dot{V}$A has been increased, the patient may have a problem with increased dead space. This can be from a high $\dot{V}$E leading to air trapping. A slow inspiratory flow rate or an uneven distribution of ventilation due to a pathologic problem in the lungs or a high I/E ratio (e.g., 3:1) could be causing the problem.

Increasing the flow rate or decreasing the I/E ratio (to 1:1 or 1:2) in the case of air trapping might help. In patients with chronic obstructive pulmonary disease (COPD), reducing the flow or increasing the expiratory time (lower rate) may correct the situation. Sometimes repositioning the patient so the least disease-compromised lung is in the down position will help. The patency of the airways also needs to be checked and efforts made to clear secretions and reduce dead space.

Example 6: Increased Metabolism.—A burn patient on SIMV has a V_T of 1,000 mL, a respiratory rate of 10 breaths/min, a Pa_{CO_2} of 40 mm Hg, and a pH of 7.39. The patient has a spontaneous rate of 15 breaths/min and a spontaneous V_T of 800 mL. In this case the patient has a very high total $\dot{V}_E$ ($\dot{V}_E$ machine = 10 L/min + $\dot{V}_E$ patient = 12 L/min, total $\dot{V}_E$ = 22 L/min). One would expect the Pa_{CO_2} to be low and it is not. There are two possible reasons: either the V_D/V_T is increased or carbon dioxide production ($\dot{V}_{CO_2}$) is increased. Both of these could be measured and calculated to determine if one or the other or both is increased.

In the case of burn victims, multiple trauma, sepsis, and multiple surgical procedures, it is not unusual for metabolism to be high. In this case the increased $\dot{V}_{CO_2}$ was due to the increased metabolic rate. Regardless of the problem, one thing is clear: the patient's work of breathing is high. However, if the machine rate is increased to decrease the patient's work of breathing, auto-PEEP is likely to result. For this particular case it may be beneficial to add PS for the spontaneous breaths to reduce the work of breathing through the ET tube and circuit.

SIGH RATE, FREQUENCY, AND VOLUME

If a low V_T is used (i.e., 4 × IBW in lb = V_T), the sigh mode is usually used. The sigh rate may be set at 10/hr with the sigh mode then cycling a sigh every 6 minutes. Along with frequency the number of consecutive sighs is set, i.e., two or three sighs occurring every 6 minutes. The sigh volume is measured following a sigh breath. It is usually set at 1.5 to 2.0 times the V_T. All three values are then recorded on the ventilator sheet.

Sigh mode is not needed with V_T of 10 to 15 mL/kg. In fact, the need for a sigh breath has never been clinically well established. However, some ventilators still offer the option to provide a sigh breath. Some clinicians like to use a periodic deep breath with patients on spontaneous modes like CPAP or PS at low settings. If the ventilator does not provide a sigh control, the practitioner can use a low SIMV setting such as one breath every 2 minutes. This would substitute for the sigh mode in this situation.

MONITORING AIRWAY PRESSURES

All positive pressure ventilators have a pressure monitor for the continuous measuring of upper airway pressure. The pressure monitor reads most accurately when it detects pressures very near the patient's upper airway. To do this the monitor tubing, usually a small-diameter plastic tube, is connected to the wye connector (patient connector) of the patient circuit. If the tubing is not visible on the circuit, pressures are probably being detected through the main patient circuit and not at the upper airway. These measures are less accurate, but are still clinically useful. Figure 8–3 shows where pressures are monitored on several ventilators.

Pressure is continually monitored to be sure that very high pressure limits are not exceeded but that a minimal pressure is maintained (low pressure limit). Intermittent readings of peak pressure (PIP), plateau pressure ($P_{Plateau}$), transairway pressure (PIP − $P_{Plateau}$), mean airway pressure ($\bar{P}aw$), and end-expiratory pressure can give information about the patient's condition.

Peak Pressure

The peak pressure, or highest pressure observed, is recorded. It is sometimes called peak inspiratory pressure (PIP). This value is used in the calculation of

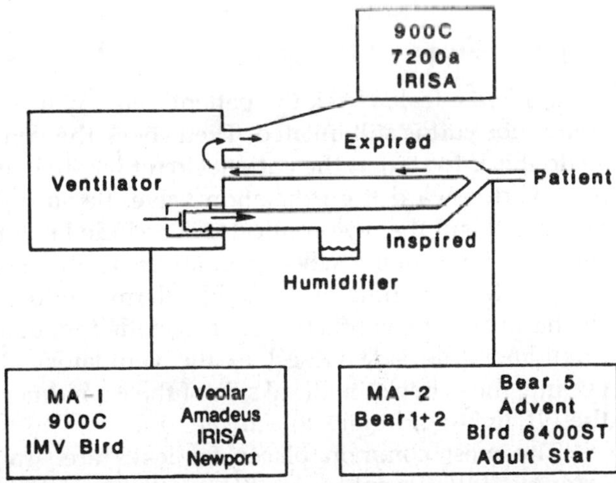

FIG 8–3.
Pressure monitoring sites of old and new ventilators. The Irisa ventilator uses measurements of pressure from the inspired and expired side in an effort to calculate proximal airway pressure. (From Branson RD: *Respir Care* 1991; 36:362–376. Used by permission.)

dynamic compliance or dynamic characteristic. When V_T is fairly constant and PIP is increasing, this might indicate a reduction in lung compliance or an increase in airway resistance (Raw). If the PIP is decreasing it might indicate the presence of a leak or an improvement in compliance or resistance.

Pressure Limit

An audible and visual alarm will be activated on most ventilators if the pressure exceeds a limit usually set at 5 to 10 cm H_2O above the PIP reading. This indication of a change in the patient's condition may signal that the airway needs to be suctioned, that Raw is increased, that lung compliance is decreasing, that the patient is coughing or biting the tube, or that water from condensation has accumulated in the circuit.

Low Pressure Alarm

Audible and visual alarms are present on many ventilators indicating that the PIP has fallen below a desired limit, usually 5 to 10 cm H_2O below ventilating pressures. This acts as an indicator that the pressure has fallen significantly, probably the result of a leak. The most common cause of a leak is disconnection of the patient from the ventilator. This is easily visible and can be rapidly corrected. If the leak is not so obvious, then the patient's ventilations need be done manually by using a resuscitation bag while the machine leak is corrected.

Checking for Leaks

To find a leak, check the patient's airway first to be sure the ET or tracheostomy tube cuff is still inflated. Then check the ventilator circuit. The easiest way to do this is to start at the patient circuit where it attaches to the ventilator outlet and work toward the exhalation valve. Be sure the patient is being manually ventilated and the wye connector is occluded before beginning the test. Squeeze the large-bore tubing where it connects to the main ventilator outlet and manually cycle the ventilator. If the PIP alarm sounds, then there is no leak between the hand and the ventilator. Then occlude the tubing on the proximal side of the humidifier (the side closest to the ventilator). Repeat the ventilator manual cycling, then check the distal side of the humidifier. The leak will be found when the PIP limit alarm fails to activate.

The most common places for leaks are around the humidifier, near an external IMV assembly, at the exhalation valve, or any place where tubing connections join. In-line thermometers, oxygen analyzers, and proximal airway pressure monitors are other potential sources for leaks. A normal leak may be present around the ET tube if the minimum leak technique is used (see below). This leak is usually insignificant and very little volume is lost.

One precaution needs to be noted. If you are using a ventilator that cycles out of inspiration based on flow, a leak in the system can prevent flow cycling. For example, the Puritan Bennett 7200ae cycles out of PS when the flow falls to 5 L/min. If there is a leak in the system that allows a flow out of the system at more than 5 L/min, the ventilator might stay in inspiration. This can cause inadvertent build-up of pressure in the patient's lungs. Fortunately, most new microprocessor ventilators also have a back-up cycling time and cycling pressure. These would end inspiration if flow did not.

False Pressure Readings or Failure of Alarms

False pressure readings can occur if the line leading to the pressure indicator, either a manometer or a digital type, is plugged with water or kinked. Pressure limit alarms will also fail to operate properly if their batteries are worn out and need replacing.

Cuff Pressure Measurement

About once or twice a shift (8-hour period) the ET or tracheostomy cuff pressure is checked to guarantee that intracuff pressures do not exceed 25 mm Hg. Tracheal wall arterial–end-capillary pressure is about 30 mm Hg. Keeping the cuff pressure below 25 mm Hg is believed to reduce the risk of tracheal necrosis associated with tube cuffs. In hypotensive patients even an intracuff pressure of only 25 mm Hg may not be safe.

There are currently cuff pressure–measuring devices that provide gauge or digital readout of cuff pressures. These devices offer an easy way of adding or removing air from the cuff. They also have very short connections so little volume is lost by connecting the cuff pilot balloon to the device.

Intracuff pressure can also be measured by using a mercury column manometer, such as those used to measure blood pressure, or an anaeroid manometer. The manometer has to be prepressurized or a significant amount of the cuff volume or pressure will be lost in the connecting tube. This can be done using a three-way or four-way stopcock between the cuff pilot balloon and the manometer. The manometer is pressurized by injecting air into it with a syringe. The amount of pressure added needs to be equal to previous pressure readings. The cuff and manometer can also be pressurized simultaneously if the cuff is being inflated or has been deflated prior to measurement (Fig 8–4).

Sometimes use of the minimum leak technique (MLT) can provide adequate cuff inflation to allow for ventilation and reduce intracuff pressure. To perform MLT, the cuff is inflated until no air leak is heard around the airway during a positive pressure inspiration. Then a small volume of air is removed from the cuff until a small leak is heard at the end of inspiration when listening over the trachea.

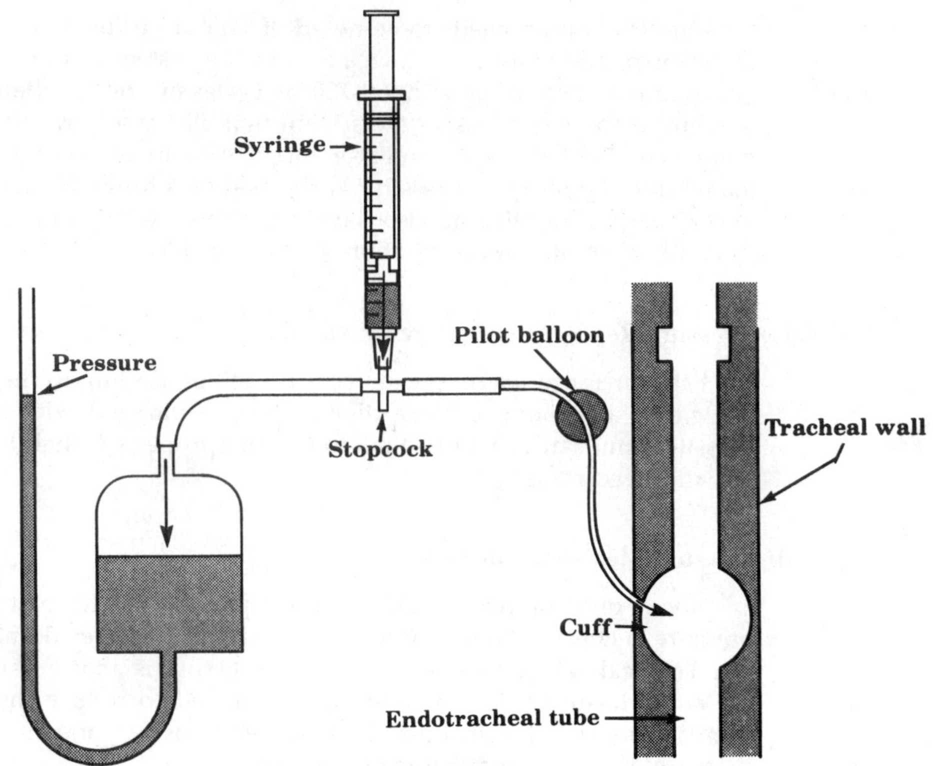

FIG 8–4.
Use of a syringe, mercury manometer, and three-way stopcock for measuring cuff pressure.

While MLT can provide low cuff pressures in some situations, it cannot do so if the cycling pressure necessary to achieve V_T delivery is too high. This occurs in patients with low lung compliance or high Raw. In this case a significant amount of volume may be lost. One solution is simply to increase the set volume on the ventilator.

In some situations it may be impossible to maintain low intracuff pressures and still provide adequate ventilation. Intracuff pressure will be high in situations where the tube size is small in relation to the size of the trachea. Again, MLT may help as can increasing the set volume to compensate for the amount of volume leaked. Better still, the tube can be replaced with a larger one.

During volume-controlled ventilation, a leak with MLT will change as PIP changes. If MLT is used when PIP is high and the PIP gradually decreases, then the volume in the cuff would eventually be larger than necessary. The leak may actually no longer exist. MLT would need to be performed again. Conversely, if

MLT is used at low PIP with volume-controlled ventilation, the leak will be too great if PIP increases.

For the collection of expired gas, as is performed in V_D/V_T, oxygen consumption ($\dot{V}O_2$), and $\dot{V}CO_2$ measurements, the cuff must be inflated enough to completely occlude the airway. Once these measurements are taken, the cuff is reinflated to MLT or its previous low pressure. Cuff leaks that are too large can actually prevent termination of PS breaths. Recall that on most ventilators PS is flow-terminated. If the leak is too large, the ventilator never reaches the minimum flow and inspiration on PS never stops (see Chapter 7).

To minimize the risk of tracheal necrosis associated with cuff overinflation, the following five-step protocol has been developed[40]:

1. Maintain MLT.
2. Establish that a "reasonable" MLT is present, i.e., only 50 to 100 mL of V_T is lost during inspiration. In a volume ventilator with a 1,000 mL V_T setting and delivery, expired V_T would be 900 to 1,000 mL.
3. The high volume–low pressure cuff should not require more than 5 mL for inflation.
4. If a minimal leak can be obtained only with a cuff volume of no more than 5 ml, ensure that: (a) intracuff pressure is less than 25 mm Hg, and (b) the cuff diameter to tracheal diameter checked on the chest radiograph is 1.5:1 or less.
5. If steps 1 through 4 cannot be achieved, follow patients for the presence of tracheal stenosis for at least 1 year.

Plateau Pressure

At the end of inhalation, before the beginning of exhalation, occlusion of the expiratory port or expiratory line can give a plateau pressure. This is also called static pressure and no gas flow is present. This measurement can be done on some ventilators by using inflation hold or inspiratory pause. After PIP is reached, the manometer needle will fall a few centimeters and remain in a plateau (static) position for a fraction of a second and then drop to zero.

Static compliance reflects the elastic recoil of the alveolar walls and thoracic cage against the volume of air in the patient's lungs. It also reflects the recoil of the patient circuit on the volume of air in the circuit. This latter component is fairly constant and not of much clinical significance.

Peak Pressure Minus Plateau Pressure

The difference between peak and plateau pressure readings (PIP − $P_{PLATEAU}$) is the amount of pressure lost to Raw, including the resistance of the

ET tube. Increased variation between PIP and $P_{PLATEAU}$ commonly means that the patient's airway needs to be suctioned, that the patient is biting on the tube, that the tube is kinked, or that the patient may need bronchodilator therapy (see Appendix G).

End-Expiratory Pressure (EEP)

Any pressure different from zero (ambient) that is present at the end of expiration is recorded. This value must be subtracted from PIP and $P_{Plateau}$ during the calculation of dynamic and static compliance, respectively. EEP is the lowest pressure measured in the expiratory phase. Common EEP maneuvers include CPAP and PEEP.

Artificially high readings (greater than zero) when CPAP or PEEP is not being used can occur if a constant flow IMV system is being used. This causes a slight PEEP to be present between machine breaths but this is not usually clinically significant.

Sometimes EEP goes undetected and is then referred to as auto-PEEP (see Chapter 7).

MONITORING COMPLIANCE AND AIRWAY RESISTANCE

Compliance Measurement

Compliance is a change in volume per unit of pressure change. The respiratory system has both a dynamic characteristic or compliance (Cdyn) and a static compliance (Cs).

Static Compliance.—In mechanically ventilated patients, the measurement of lung and chest wall compliance is called static compliance and equals about 70 to 100 mL/cm H_2O. When Cs is less than 25 mL/cm H_2O the work of breathing for the patient is very high. Static compliance is calculated by dividing volume delivery by plateau pressure minus end-expiratory pressure ($Cs = V_T/[P_{PLATEAU} - EEP]$).

The accuracy of the Cs calculation depends upon two factors: recording the actual delivered V_T, and obtaining accurate $P_{PLATEAU}$ readings. Plateau pressure reflects the pressure exerted on the volume of gas in the lung by the chest wall and alveoli and on the pressure exerted by tubing elastance on the gas volume in the patient circuit. Chest wall recoil stays fairly constant in most clinical patients as does the elastic recoil of the patient circuit. Thus, if Cs readings change over a period of time, they are usually considered a result of change in the condition of the patient's lung parenchyma (alveoli).

Causes of decreasing patient Cs include air trapping, pulmonary edema, atelectasis, consolidation, pneumonia, pneumothorax, hemothorax, pleural effusion, changes in chest wall compliance (flail chest, muscle tension), pneumomediastinum, and abdominal distention (peritonitis, ascites, herniation, abdominal bleeding). Many of these causes can be detected by evaluating breath sounds, percussion notes, palpation of the chest and abdominal wall, chest radiography, and laboratory data. Each must receive appropriate medical intervention to be corrected.

Reduced Cs implies that ventilation is less effective. In volume-cycled or volume-limited ventilation, the peak and plateau pressures will increase while delivered V_T stays fairly constant. In pressure-controlled or pressure-cycled ventilation, the PIP stays constant, plateau pressure is difficult to measure but will stay about the same, while the delivered V_T decreases (Table 8–2, examples A and B). In pressure-controlled or pressure-cycled ventilators, pressure must be increased when compliance decreases in order to maintain the V_T delivery. Reduced Cs can result in decreased Pa_{O_2} and increased Pa_{CO_2}; therefore, it is important to determine the cause and treat it.

Dynamic Compliance.—The volume delivered by the ventilator divided by the peak pressure is the *dynamic characteristic.*[7] This is often referred to as dynamic compliance or dynamic effective compliance (DEC).[22] Since it is measured during airflow it consists of both the recoil of the lungs and chest wall plus the pressure caused by Raw. Because it includes both compliance and resistance components, it is actually an impedance measurement.[7, 22] Most people still refer to it as dynamic compliance. The Cdyn includes the ventilator circuit, the compliance of the chest wall and lungs, and the resistance of the ET tube, circuit, and airways: Cdyn = V/(PIP − EEP).

Dynamic compliance decreases whenever Cs decreases or Raw increases. Distinguishing between lung and airway problems is done by monitoring changes in PIP, $P_{PLATEAU}$, and their difference. If PIP and $P_{PLATEAU}$ are both increasing with the same V_T delivery and the difference between the two (P_{TA}) is fairly constant, the Cs is decreasing (Table 8–2, example C). If PIP increases along with the difference between PIP and $P_{PLATEAU}$ (increased P_{TA}), then Raw is increasing (Table 8–2, example D). Calculation of Cdyn and Cs confirms these findings. If Cdyn is constant or decreasing and Cs is decreasing, then most likely lung compliance is decreasing. If Cdyn is decreasing and Cs is constant, the airway resistance is increasing.

Bronchoconstriction will increase airway resistance but will not affect Cs; however, if severe bronchospasm occurs, the airways will be completely occluded and Cs will decrease while airway resistance does not change.[4] The administration of bronchodilators can help to reverse bronchospasm and constriction in some patients.

With volume-controlled or volume-limited ventilation, the Cdyn decreases as PIP increases, and volume delivery stays nearly constant. In pressure-controlled or pressure-cycled ventilators, however, a decreased Cdyn will de-

TABLE 8–2.

Simplified Examples Showing Changes in Delivered Tidal Volumes and Peak and Plateau Pressure, Reflecting Compliance Changes*

Example A: Decreasing dynamic characteristic (Cdyn) on a pressure-cycled ventilator

Time	PIP	V_T	Cdyn
1	25	500	20
2	25	400	16
3	25	300	12

Constant pressures with decreasing volume

Example B: Decreasing dynamic characteristic (Cdyn) on a volume-cycled ventilator

Time	PIP	V_T	Cdyn
1	25	500	20
2	30	500	17
3	35	500	14

Constant volume with increasing pressures

Example C: Decreasing static compliance (Cs) and dynamic characteristic (Cdyn) on a volume-cycled ventilator with a constant airway resistance

Time	PIP	Cdyn	$P_{PLATEAU}$	Cs	P_{TA}	Volume
1	25	20	20	25	5	500
2	30	17	25	20	5	500
3	35	14	30	17	5	500

Increasing peak and plateau pressures; volume and pressure lost to the airways are constant; the lung, itself, is less compliant

Example D: While dynamic characteristic (Cdyn) decreases, static compliance (Cs) is the same on a volume-cycled ventilator during increased airway resistance

Time	PIP	Cdyn	$P_{PLATEAU}$	Cs	P_{TA}	Volume
1	25	20	20	25	5	500
2	30	17	20	25	10	500
3	35	14	20	25	15	500

Increasing PIP with constant volumes and plateau pressures; airway resistance (Raw) is increasing (P_{TA} = PIP − $P_{PLATEAU}$)

Example E: Increasing dynamic characteristics (Cdyn) and static compliance (Cs) on a volume-cycled ventilator

Time	PIP	Cdyn	$P_{PLATEAU}$	Cs	P_{TA}	Volume
1	25	20	23	22	2	500
2	23	22	21	24	2	500
3	20	25	18	28	2	500

Peak and plateau pressures are decreasing, delivered volume and transairway pressures are constant; the lungs are more compliant

Example F: Compliance measurements with PEEP

Time	PIP	Cdyn	$P_{PLATEAU}$	Cs	P_{TA}	PEEP	Volume
1	30	20	28	22	2	+5	500
2	35	20	33	22	2	+10	500
3	40	18	37	20	3	+12	500

$$\text{Cdyn} = \frac{\text{volume}}{\text{PIP} - \text{EEP}}$$

$$\text{Cs} = \frac{\text{volume}}{P_{\text{Plateau}} - \text{EEP}}$$

Addition of increasing PEEP results in increasing peak and plateau pressures. Delivered tidal volume and pressure lost to the airways remain constant in this example.

*PIP = peak pressure (in cm H_2O); V_T = tidal volume; P_{TA} = transairway pressure (in cm H_2O); $P_{PLATEAU}$ pressure (in cm H_2O); EEP = end-expiration pressure; volume is in liters, compliance in mL/cm H_2O.

crease the delivered V_T. The pressure setting must be increased to maintain delivered V_T. During volume-controlled ventilation, decreasing PIP with a constant delivered V_T may signal improvement in compliance or Raw (Table 8–2, example E). A drop in cycling pressure, however, might also indicate a leak. Delivered V_T needs to be checked. During pressure-controlled ventilation, an increased V_T delivery with the same pressure also indicates an improvement in compliance or a decrease in Raw, or both.

Remember that when PEEP is used it must be subtracted from plateau and PIP readings to calculate Cs and Cdyn (Table 8–2, example F).

Airway Resistance

Airway resistance increases under the following conditions: increased secretions, mucosal edema, bronchospasm, artificial airway problems, and aspiration. For Raw to be present flow must also be present. When there is no flow, there is no Raw. Total resistance is actually the sum of Raw and tissue resistance, but tissue resistance does not usually change in the clinical setting. Exceptions to this include the development of ascites and pleural effusion.

Normal Raw ranges from 0.6 to 2.4 cm H_2O/L/sec. With an ET tube in place, this can increase to 6 cm H_2O/(L/sec) or more. With emphysema or asthma, Raw increases from 3 to 18 cm H_2O/L/sec. This value can be estimated on ventilator patients by measuring P_{TA} (PIP − $P_{PLATEAU}$) and using the ventilator flow knob value as the flow in liters per minute. This is not an accurate flow measure, but used over a period of time it can give relative changes in Raw. For example, if PIP is 35 cm H_2O, $P_{PLATEAU}$ is 34 cm H_2O, and the flow is set at 30 L/min (0.5 L/sec), Raw will be:

$$\text{Raw} = P_{TA}/\text{flow (L/sec)}$$

$$\text{Raw} = (\text{PIP} - P_{PLATEAU})/\text{flow}$$

$$\text{Raw} = (35 - 34 \text{ cm } H_2O)/(0.5 \text{ L/sec})$$

$$\text{Raw} = 2 \text{ cm } H_2O/\text{L/sec}$$

Many newer microprocessor ventilators are now equipped with software programs that are capable of calculating and graphing both compliance and resistance values. Some of the values for this graphing are taken from measurements of pressure (see Fig 8–3) and expired flow and volume (Fig 8–5).

Compensation for increased Raw can be made by treating the cause, such as suctioning the airway, clearing an obstruction, or giving a bronchodilator (see Appendix G). Changing the flow rate or pattern can also change the pressure lost to Raw.

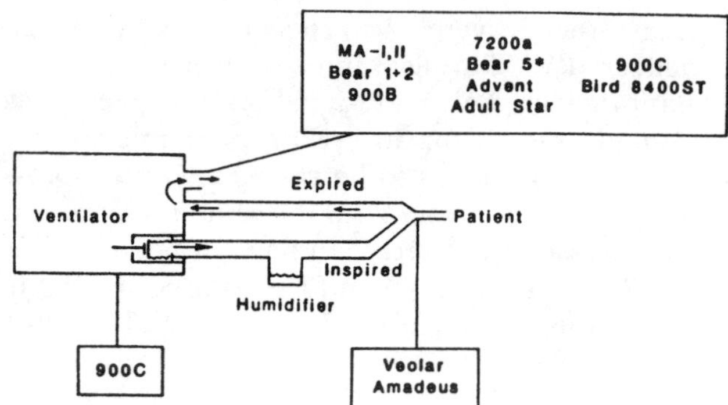

FIG 8–5.
Placement of flow-volume transducers in old and new ventilators. Although the BEAR 5, 7200a, and Advent measure flow and volume on the expired side, microprocessor compensation for compressible volume is available. (From Branson RD: *Respir Care* 1991; 36:362–376. Used by permission.)

TABLE 8–3.
Correlation of Pressure-Volume Curve Data and Clinical Findings to Evaluate Pulmonary Condition*

Diagnosis	Cs	Cdyn	Chest Radiograph	Pa_{O_2}	PCWP	Treatment
Pulmonary edema (cardiogenic)	↓	↓	↑ Vascular markings, possible; ↑ heart size	↓	↑	Diuretics, digitalis, morphine, oxygen, rotating tourniquets
ARDS	↓	↓	Diffuse infiltrate	↓	Normal	PEEP and supportive care
Pneumonia	↓	↓	Consolidation in affected area	↓	Normal	Antibiotics and supportive care
Atelectasis	↓	↓	Collapse of affected area	↓	Normal	Treat cause and give supportive care
Pneumothorax	↓	↓	No vascular markings in affected area	↓	Normal	Chest tube; chest drainage if severe
Bronchospasm	No change	↓	Possible hyperinflation	↓	Normal	Bronchodilator therapy

*Cs = static compliance; Cdyn = dynamic characteristic; Pa_{O_2} = arterial oxygen partial pressure; PCWP = pulmonary capillary wedge pressure; ARDS = adult respiratory distress syndrome; PEEP = positive end-expiratory pressure; ↓ = decreased; ↑ = increased.

Bedside Measuring of Pressure-Volume Curves

By ventilating the lung at different volumes and recording the peak and plateau pressures, you can plot the volume-pressure relationships for dynamic and static characteristics.[4,7] When this is done daily a progression of patient lung-airway changes can be monitored and evaluated. The procedure is as follows:

1. If possible, explain the procedure to the patient. The patient is normally in the supine position and relaxed.
2. Inflate the airway cuff to eliminate leaks and check the system for leaks.
3. Dial in inspiratory pause, or inflation hold, or pinch the expiratory line before the end of inspiration for each volume measurement.
4. Select a series of V_T settings. For example, 7, 10, 13, and 16 mL/kg or 500, 750, 1,000, and 1250 mL.
5. For each volume setting record: PIP, $P_{PLATEAU}$, end-expiratory pressure, and delivered V_T (subtract EEP from PIP and $P_{PLATEAU}$ before recording).

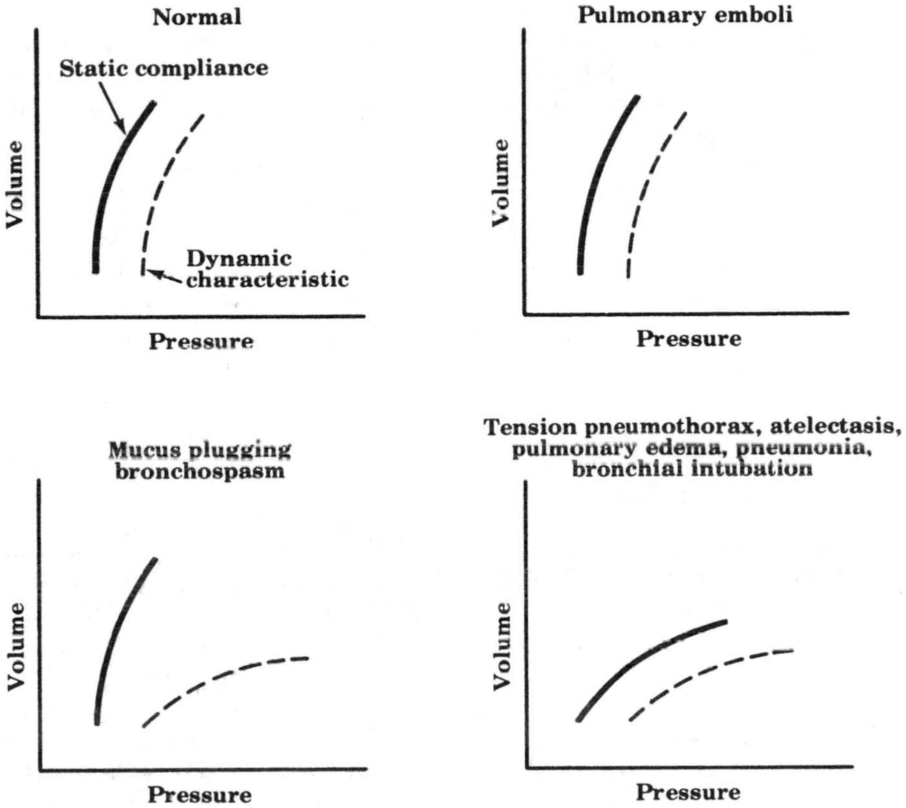

FIG 8–6.
Pressure-volume curves reflecting changes in static compliance (Cs) and dynamic characteristic (Cdyn) during mechanical ventilation. Under normal conditions the Cs and Cdyn curves will be similar. Since pulmonary emboli do not affect resistance or compliance, neither curve will change in this condition. With mucous plugging, airway resistance increases and the Cdyn curve shifts to the right and flattens (more pressure is required) while the Cs curve does not change. In conditions which reduce lung compliance both curves will shift to the right and flatten. (Redrawn from Bone RC: *Respir Care* 1983; 28:597–603.)

6. Remove inspiratory pause or inflation hold.
7. Return cuff pressures to minimum leak or initial pressure.
8. Perform a complete ventilator check.
9. Plot date (Table 8–3, Fig 8–6).
   Caution: If pressure rises rapidly and markedly, discontinue the study to avoid barotrauma.

Figure 8–6 illustrates changes in the curves that can be expected with acute respiratory distress with sudden hypoxemia caused by airway problems and pulmonary emboli.[4] It shows those conditions which affect the airway, shift the dynamic curve to the right, and flatten it. When neither curve changes but the patient develops hypoxemia, then a pulmonary embolus is suspected. Figures 2–10 and 2–13 illustrate examples of compliance curves that can be graphed by some microprocessor ventilators like the Hamilton Veolar, the BEAR 5, and the Siemens Servo 300.

With high V_T or PEEP, seeing the static curve decrease or shift to the right can signal hyperinflation of the lung.[7] In this way optimal V_T and PEEP settings can be selected which do not increase the risk of barotrauma. Combining the clinical data and the pressure-volume curve analysis can help the clinician establish the causes of changes in the patient's condition and treat them appropriately (see Table 8–3).[4]

MONITORING OXYGENATION TO PATIENTS

Delivery to Tissues

Adequate O_2 delivery to the tissues depends on several factors, including F_{IO_2}, arterial O_2 content (Ca_{O_2}), and cardiac output (CO). Methods of evaluating these parameters include measuring inspired O_2, O_2 saturation, hemoglobin, abnormal hemoglobin, arterial blood gases, O_2 content, $P(A\text{-}a)_{O_2}$, Pa_{O_2}/P_{AO_2}, shunt, CO, mixed venous oxygen saturation ($S\bar{v}_{O_2}$), and venous oxygen content ($C\bar{v}_{O_2}$). Actual O_2 delivery to the tissues is very important since it gives information about O_2 availability and potential tissue utilization of O_2. This is evaluated by measuring arteriovenous oxygen content difference [$C(a - v)_{O_2}$], $\dot{V}_{O_2}$, and $S\bar{v}_{O_2}$.

Measuring F_{IO_2} in Ventilator Patients

The F_{IO_2} is measured and recorded at least every 2 hours. It is best to keep F_{IO_2} below 0.5 to prevent the complications associated with a high F_{IO_2} while keeping the Pa_{O_2} greater than 60 mm Hg and the O_2 content near normal (20 vol %). In patients with COPD the normal Pa_{O_2} may be nearer to 50 mm Hg, and desired F_{IO_2} values are usually low (24%–28%).

A variety of O_2 analyzers are available for measuring O_2 percentage. The FIO_2 is measured on the inspiratory side of the patient circuit as close to the patient as possible during the inspiratory phase. When an analyzer is used to continually monitor FIO_2, it is done before the gas is humidified as the accumulation of moisture from high humidity can alter the readings. Some ventilators, like the Servo 900C and the 300, have built-in O_2 analyzers.

Adjusting FIO_2

Since it is desirable to keep the PaO_2 between 60 and 100 mm Hg, an arterial blood gas analysis is obtained and the results compared to the FIO_2 being delivered. A linear relationship exists between PaO_2 and FIO_2 for any patient as long as the cardiopulmonary status remains fairly constant.[36, 37] Because of this correlation, the PaO_2 and FIO_2 can be used to select the FIO_2 necessary to achieve a desired PaO_2:

$$\frac{\text{(Known) } PaO_2}{\text{(Known) } FIO_2} = \frac{\text{(desired) } PaO_2}{\text{(desired) } FIO_2}$$

The desired FIO_2 will be equal to the product of desired PaO_2 times known FIO_2 divided by the known PaO_2:

$$\text{(Desired) } FIO_2 = (PaO_2 \text{ desired} \times FIO_2 \text{ known})/PaO_2 \text{ known}$$

This equation will not be true if the cardiopulmonary status (CO or $\dot{V}A$) changes significantly. It does, however, provide a method for making an informed change in the FIO_2 which will come closer to achieving the desired PaO_2 than will a random change in FIO_2.

Some institutions use the PaO_2/PAO_2 ratio for predicting the FIO_2. The PaO_2/PAO_2 estimates what fraction or percentage of available O_2 in the lungs is actually reaching the arterial level. This ratio is also valuable as an index of oxygenation and lung function and is easier to interpret than $P(A - a)O_2$.[24, 27, 33] A patient with a PaO_2/PAO_2 of 0.60, where about 60% of PAO_2 is reaching the arteries, is far better off than one with a PaO_2/PAO_2 of 0.25, where only about 25% of available PAO_2 is reaching the arteries. The range for normal PaO_2/PAO_2 is between 0.75 and 0.95.[24] The ratio of PaO_2 to FIO_2 is also used to estimate O_2 levels, but is not as accurate as PaO_2/PAO_2.[24, 27]

Selection of PEEP

If an adequate PaO_2 cannot be maintained on FIO_2 values less than or equal to 50%, then PEEP is considered as an alternative form of therapy. High FIO_2 values not only have toxic effects but can also increase intrapulmonary shunting which further contributes to hypoxemia.[54] When Pa_{O_2} remains very low on F_{IO_2} values up to 0.5, then significant shunting is present and ventilation-perfusion ($\dot{V}/\dot{Q}$) abnormalities are severe. Either high F_{IO_2} values or PEEP or both are required for the Pa_{O_2} to be significantly affected[38] (see Chapter 10).

Tissue Hypoxia

When cellular O_2 tensions are not adequate to maintain aerobic metabolism, tissue hypoxia occurs. Hypoxia is usually caused by a decrease in Ca_{O_2}, CO, or local tissue perfusion. Hypoxia has four basic categories:

1. Histotoxic hypoxia (dysoxia) results when the cells are unable to utilize O_2. Examples are cyanide poisoning or septic shock.
2. Anemic hypoxia is present when hemoglobin concentration is lower than normal (15 g/dL) or when the hemoglobin is abnormal and unable to transport O_2 as in sickle cell anemia, carbon monoxide poisoning (carboxyhemoglobin), and methemoglobin (see Appendix H).
3. Circulatory hypoxia or stagnant hypoxia occurs when the cardiovascular system fails to transport the O_2 to the tissues, usually because of a low CO.
4. Hypoxemic hypoxia is the most common type and can be due to low inspired oxygen pressure (P_{IO_2}), hypoventilation, shunting, $\dot{V}/\dot{Q}$ mismatching, and diffusion defects.

Continuous Monitoring of Oxygenation

There is a significant time delay between the moment when an arterial blood gas sample is taken and when the results are received and analyzed. In some patients this delay is critical and undesirable. Repeated sampling of arterial blood may be undesirable in very small patients, such as newborn infants, where loss of blood is another important factor. For these and other reasons, it is important to have a method for continuously monitoring O_2 and CO_2. Techniques for continuous monitoring of gases, such as pulse oximetry and capnography, are covered in Chapter 9.

VITAL SIGNS AND PATIENT EVALUATION

Nothing replaces the presence of personnel at the patient's bedside to help prevent the occurrence of mishaps and complications. Harm to the medical-surgical patient in the intensive care unit (ICU) occurs most often when the patient is unattended.[1] Knowing that realistically we cannot always have someone at the bedside, we rely on monitors and alarms to do some observing for us (see Chapter 6). Monitoring can be done either intermittently or on a continuous basis.

Observation and recording of blood pressure (BP), heart rate (HR), temperture, and patient color every hour or two helps to evaluate possible changes in the patient's overall condition. Keep in mind that in mechanically ventilated patients, respiration and HR are constantly monitored. This may also be true with temperature and BP. Monitoring, however, only alerts one to critical changes. Moderate changes in any of these vital signs with hourly checks alerts the clinician to possible hypoxemia, impending cardiovascular collapse (decreased or increased BP and HR), or to the presence of infection (increased temperature).

Heart Rate

The use of the electrocardiogram (ECG) provides a noninvasive method of continuously monitoring HR and periodically observing rhythm. It is essential that a three-lead ECG be used constantly with any patient on ventilatory support. This device must provide both maximum and minimum alarms (audible and visual) in the event that bradycardia or tachycardia of unacceptable limits occurs. Leads are generally placed on the chest, one near each clavicle, and one near the fourth intercostal space at the left axillary line. It is important to place leads so that an easily discernible QRS complex can be electronically detected by the monitor.

The oscilloscope is viewed or scanned by a computer for changes in HR and rhythm. When an audible alarm signals, it alerts personnel that a potentially dangerous change in rate or rhythm has occurred. It may even signal that the patient has become disconnected from the ventilator resulting in severe hypoxemia or hypercarbia. Other factors which can affect HR include direct changes in the condition of the myocardium (infarction, hypoxia, drug reaction) or anxiety, pain, elevated temperature, or stress.

Temperature

A patient's skin temperature can be measured orally, in the axilla, or on any extremity. Core temperature is done by using rectal, esophageal, or pulmonary artery temperatures. Many disorders can lead to changes in temperature.[2] Hyperthermia can be caused by infection, tissue necrosis, late-stage carcinomatosis, Hodgkin's disease, leukemia, and metabolic states such as hypothyroidism. Low-grade temperature elevation can be due to accidental or surgical trauma, atelectasis, fistulas, hematomas, and foreign bodies. Hypothermia can result from metabolic diseases, central nervous system problems, drugs (phenothiazines, tricyclic antidepressants, benzodiazepines), and other substances (alcohol, heroin, carbon monoxide).[2]

Systemic Arterial Blood Pressure

The patient's BP can be monitored intermittently using either a stethoscope and sphygmomanometer, or continuously using invasive intravascular arterial catheters. Invasive arterial pressure monitoring is used for postoperative open heart surgery patients or critically ill patients. It provides a continuous, direct measurement of BP.

Arterial catheters are usually placed in small vessels such as the radial artery where collateral circulation can be demonstrated. Allen's test for collateral circulation is performed by holding the patient's hand with the palm up, occluding the radial and ulnar arteries, and having the patient open and close his hand. The hand is opened to be sure it is drained of blood (blanched) and the pressure over the ulnar artery is released. The palm will flush with blood in 15 seconds or less if collateral circulation to the hand through the ulnar artery is present. The process is repeated a second time where the pressure over the radial artery is released to demonstrate perfusion in this artery as well. Allen's test is performed whenever a radial artery puncture is done.

Arterial catheters are inserted into the artery and secured in place. The catheter is connected via patent plastic tubing to a transducer. The tubing is kept patent by the use of a pressurized intravascular bag containing a heparinized solution. The transducer is connected to a monitor that reads the pressure. These monitors can give a digital display of systolic pressure (SP), diastolic pressure (DP), and mean arterial pressure [MAP = (SP + 2 DP)/3] as well as an oscilloscope tracing of the pressure wave (see Chapter 11). The indwelling arterial line also provides an easy access route for obtaining arterial blood samples or blood for other laboratory data.

Central Venous Pressure

Indwelling venous catheters placed into the area of the superior vena cava or right atrium can be used to monitor central venous pressure (CVP), myocardial function, and fluid status in the critically ill patient (see Chapter 11). CVP measurement directly reflects right arterial pressure, right ventricular end-diastolic pressure, and right heart function. During a positive pressure breath, CVP will be elevated. Measurements of CVP during intermittent positive pressure ventilation (IPPV) is done at the end of expiration when intrapleural pressure returns to normal.

In the clinical situation where it is desirable to determine the effect of PEEP on CVP and myocardial function, CVP is measured without removing PEEP. If the CVP is to be measured without the effects of PEEP, then the patient is removed from PEEP. This procedure, however, has little clinical value and can lead to decreased functional residual capacity (FRC), increased shunting, and hypoxemia in certain patients, and is not recommended in patients on high PEEP (see Chapters 10 and 11).

Pulmonary Artery Pressure

Pulmonary artery pressure (PAP) can be monitored on a continuous basis by the use of a balloon-tipped, flow-directed, pulmonary artery catheter connected by a transducer to a monitor. Pulmonary artery catheters are used in critically ill patients who have severe cardiopulmonary complications or problems with fluid management (see Chapter 11).

A four-lumen catheter can provide information about the preload and afterload of the left and right heart, including pressures in the right atrium (CVP), pulmonary artery (PAP), and estimates of left heart filling with pulmonary capillary wedge pressure (PCWP). It can also provide access to blood samples from the right atrium and pulmonary artery. Cardiac output can be measured by thermodilution techniques.

Evaluation of mixed venous blood samples obtained from the pulmonary artery can provide valuable information about the cardiopulmonary status of the patient. Normal mixed venous oxygen pressure ($P\bar{v}O_2$) is approximately 40 mm Hg. Values lower than normal can result from arterial hypoxemia, increased metabolic rate, and a decrease in CO. Values higher than normal can occur with septic shock and cyanide poisoning or incorrect sampling technique.

Cardiac output, also measured with a four-lumen catheter, is a valuable tool for assessing the function of the heart in its delivery of O_2 to the tissues (see Chapter 11). Normal CO is about 4 to 8 L/min. Cardiac index (CI) is the CO divided by the BSA and is a better indicator of cardiac function since it takes into account body size. Normal CI is 2.5 to 4.5 L/min/m^2. A drop in CO or CI can occur with heart failure, hypovolemia, or as a result of mechanical ventilation. High CO may result from an elevation in metabolic rate as occurs with fever, seizures, shivering, and in certain stressful disease states such as sepsis, burns, and multiple trauma.

FURTHER PATIENT EVALUATION AND CARE

Airway Care

When vital signs are taken and breath sounds checked, the presence of abnormal breath sounds may indicate the need for suctioning. The removal of thick tenacious secretions can be facilitated by instilling 1 to 2 mL of sterile normal saline or half-normal saline into the airway and hyperinflating the patient with a resuscitation bag. This forces the irrigating solution into the airways and may help to thin out secretions for removal by suctioning. The amount, color, and sputum characteristics are written on the ventilator flow sheet along with the evaluation of breath sounds following suctioning.

The ET tube tape is checked to see if it is clean and still able to keep the tube in the correct position. When tube tape becomes excessively moist, it may lose its ability to perform its function and need to be changed. The position of the tube is also checked. Usually the ET tube is secured at the 23-cm marking for men and at the 21-cm marking in women.[9] Flexion and extension of the neck can result in tube movement of an average of about 2 cm downward and upward in the trachea.[12] In addition, it is important to check for the presence of bilateral breath sounds, although these are not always reliable in the case of right mainstem intubation.[9] For this reason alone, it is also advisable to get a chest film every 24 hours to ensure proper tube placement and check for any pathologic changes from the previous film.[2] For patients with tracheostomy tubes in place, the stoma and tracheostomy tube must be cleaned and cared for regularly. This procedure is outlined in Appendix G.

The temperature of the inspired air at the airway can be checked by observing the temperature indicated by the in-line thermometer. Temperatures above 37°C near the airway may lead to increased body temperature or thermal burns of the airway and must be decreased. Those below 30°C or so may not be adequate to maintain the relative humidity of the inspired air.

The humidifier water level is checked to guarantee that it is adequate. The patient circuit is checked for water present in the tubing due to rainout. This water must *not* accidently empty into the patient airway or the humidifier since it can lead to infection. It must be disposed of appropriately since all patient secretions are considered contaminated. Some hospitals empty water traps into a glove, tie off the end of the glove, and dispose of it with contaminated waste. Others use a plastic container intended for that use only and empty it with contaminated liquid wastes.

Artificial "noses" are sometimes used in mechanically ventilated patients for humidity administration. These fall into two categories: heat-moisture exchangers (HMEs) and hygroscopic condenser humidifiers (HCHs). HMEs rely on the exchange of heat and water vapor through a mesh or gauze or use a hydrophobic filter. HCHs use a hygroscopically treated insert to improve the exchange of heat and water vapor.[49]

These are both designed without a water reservoir or heating element. They basically consist of a small plastic housing containing the described material. HMEs and HCHs are placed between the wye connector of the ventilator and the ET tube. As the patient exhales, the warm, high moisture content of the exhaled air condenses on the material. The now warm, damp material gives up moisture to the dry medical gases going to the patient on inspiration.

These devices are intended for short-term use (24–48 hours) in normothermic, well-hydrated patients. They are not suggested for patients who need therapeutic humidity for retained secretions.[53] Artificial noses provide a small amount of VDmech. They also provide in-line resistance to ventilation. This can increase a patient's work of breathing during spontaneous ventilation.[49]

Sputum and Airway Infections

Patients on mechanical ventilation with artificial airways in place are at high risk for infections of the upper airway. Some of the causative agents are discussed in Chapter 7. An elevated temperature accompanied by an increased white blood cell count ($>10,000/mm^3$) may signal the presence of infection. A sputum specimen is collected and examined for color, quantity, and consistency. It is then sent to a laboratory for culture, sensitivity, and wet sputum analysis (Table 8–4).

Yellow sputum suggests the presence of pus (white blood cells) and possible infection. Green thick secretions suggest that the sputum has been in the airway for a while since the breakdown of mucopolysaccharides, one of the components of sputum, results in a green color.[55] Foul-smelling green sputum occurs with *Pseudomonas* infections. Pink-tinged sputum may indicate fresh blood or it can also occur following treatment with epinephrine, isoproterenol, racemic epinephrine, or isoetharine. Fresh blood may be present with airway trauma, pneumonia, or possibly with pulmonary infarction or emboli. Brown coloration usually means old blood. Rust-colored sputum might indicate a *Klebsiella* infec-

TABLE 8–4.
Wet Sputum Analysis for Cytology and Causative Organism or Agent*

Cytology	Evaluation
Presence of alveolar macrophages	Hallmark of bronchopulmonary secretions usually indicates patient is recovering from disease
Squamous cells present and possibly several types of bacteria	Specimen originated from or was contaminated by secretions above larynx
Heavily pigmented alveolar macrophages	Patient is a smoker
Eosinophils present	Reversible (possibly allergic) airway disease present
Polymorphonuclear leukocytes	Infectious process present (especially true with predominant infective bacteria present on the slide)
Ciliated bronchial epithelial cells with degenerative cell changes	Exacerbation of bronchial asthma or problem secondary to a viral infection if eosinophils are not present also
Lipid-ladened alveolar macrophages	May indicate lipoid pneumonia

*From Epstein: *Resp Care* 1978; 1151–1173. Used by permission.

tion. Copious pink, frothy secretions indicate the presence of pulmonary edema. The evaluation of sputum can be correlated with other clinical signs and symptoms, physical findings, and radiographic reports[50] to get a complete picture of the patient's condition.

Physical Examination of Chest

A physical examination of the chest is done on mechanically ventilated patients, ideally every shift, but minimally once a day. This examination includes inspection, palpation, percussion, and ausculation. These results are recorded in the chart and compared to the most recent previous findings. Abnormal results or significant changes must be evaluated for cause and treated appropriately.

Different conditions will produce different physical findings. For example, in a patient with severe asthma and air trapping, the percussion note is hyperresonant, breath sounds and chest excursion are diminished, use of accessory muscles is increased, and high-pitched wheezes are present. In pneumonia, the chest is dull to percussion, breath sounds are decreased, and crackles (rales) occur late in inspiration over the affected area. Pleural effusion gives a dull percussion note over the affected area, breath sounds are absent, and a pleural friction rub may be audible on ausculation. With a large pneumothorax, the tracheal position is shifted away from the affected side, percussion is hyperresonant over the area, and breath sounds are absent.

Whenever a ventilator check is performed the breath sounds are evaluated and the overall physical appearance of the patient is observed. Brief consideration of breath sounds may reveal low-pitched wheezes (rhonchi), indicating the possible need for suctioning; high-pitched wheezes, indicating the potential need for bronchodilator therapy; absence of breath sounds, indicating the possible presence of pneumothorax, complete airway obstruction, complete lung collapse, improper ET tube placement, or pleural effusion. Combining physical findings with ventilatory findings (such as increased PIPs) and the chest radiograph can confirm the cause of abnormal findings and point to appropriate treatment.

Assessment of the patient also includes evaluation of the use of the respiratory muscles. Increased use of the accessory muscles of inspiration or paradoxical breathing (retraction of the stomach during inspiration and protrusion during exhalation) indicate that the patient's work of breathing is increased and respiratory muscle fatigue is present.[2]

Abdominal distention might indicate the presence of accumulated intestinal gas postoperatively or the swallowing of air. If the patient is postoperative or a victim of trauma, the distension might be a result of bleeding. Ascites (fluid in the abdominal space) can occur for a number of reasons and can also lead to abdominal distention. Whatever the cause, this problem can impair ventilation by applying pressure upward on the diaphragm, thereby creating a restrictive breathing problem. The cause needs to be determined and corrected.

Aerosolized Medications

As in floor care, the respiratory care practitioner (RCP) is frequently asked to administer aerosolized medications to mechanically ventilated patients. The most commonly given drugs are bronchodilators. These drugs are administered in two possible ways: by metered dose inhalers (MDIs) and small volume nebulizers (SVNs).

There are several steps that need to be followed using SVNs. If a nebulizer unit is part of the ventilator, it is used in preference to an "add-on" unit. The RCP needs to be familiar with the ventilator in use to know what modes the nebulizer can be used in, and what the flow requirements are of the unit. The risks of adding a nebulizer into a patient circuit are several. First, the external nebulizer, by virtue of being powered by a continuous external gas source, will affect the ventilator's function. This is particularly true of microprocessor ventilators that rely on the monitoring of exhaled gas flows and pressures. Expiratory monitors will read differently from previous settings since they will pick up the flow rate from the added nebulizer. Second, when the expiratory valve closes to deliver a positive pressure breath, the added flow will increase volume delivery in the circuit and the patient. Third, in any assist mode, the flow added to the circuit must be overcome by the patient before he or she is able to assist-trigger the ventilator. In flow-sensitive modes or in assist modes like PS, patients with weak inspiratory efforts may be unable to trigger the machine.[3] This will not cause an alarm situation since the expiratory flow monitors will detect the flow from the external gas source.

Other problems can also arise that have not yet been reported in the literature. For this reason, when adding an external nebulizer it is advisable to put the patient in a nonassisted mode. This will guarantee ventilation during the treatment. In addition, if the expiratory gas monitors are not functioning because of the added flow, the alarms for low V_T and low $\dot{V}_E$ may be rendered nonfunctional. In addition, the medications that pass through the expiratory valve and flow-measuring devices may "clog" these devices and change their function. Using a main flow gas filter is advisable to prevent accumulation of these medications on the expiratory valves and monitors.

Placement of the SVN is also important. No adequate clinical data are available at this time to establish where the best placement is. When an SVN is placed in the circuit, it can be put at the wye connector in the inspiratory gas flow line or at the manifold about midway between the ventilator and the wye connector. Some studies suggest that delivery of the medication may be best when the nebulizer is at the manifold and when it is powered during inspiration only. However, not enough data are available at present to decide this for purposes of clinical use.[13, 27]

Administration of bronchodilators by MDI with ventilator patients is usually done with a special adaptor placed at or very near the wye connector. The unit is generally activated when the ventilator cycles into inspiration. When an aerosol-holding chamber is used, the MDI is activated at the end of exhalation, just prior to inspiration.[26]

Only a very small percentage of the medications delivered either by MDI or SVN to ventilated patients actually reaches the lungs. The ET tube obstructs much of the medication delivery. The smaller the tube, the more it obstructs the drug flow into the lungs. Since this affects medication delivery, it may change how much of the medication is needed. However, at the present time, the effectiveness of bronchodilator therapy in ventilated patients and the dosage necessary has not yet been established.

Fluid Balance

Since positive pressure ventilation can affect fluid balance and renal output, it is important to monitor fluid levels. This can be done with several measures. Basically, monitoring urinary output regularly, comparing fluid intake to output daily, and measuring body weight daily will provide the minimally essential information to alert one to a significant change in fluid balance.

Normal urine production is about 50 to 60 mL/hr or approximately 1 mL/kg/hr. Oliguria is a urinary output of less than 400 mL/day or less than 20 mL/hr. Polyuria is a urinary output of more than 2,400 mL/day or 100 mL/hr.[2] Decreases in urinary output can be due to:

1. Decreased fluid intake and low plasma volume.
2. Decreased CO from positive pressure ventilation decreasing venous return, positive pressure ventilation increasing plasma antidiuretic hormone (ADH), heart failure, relative hypovolemia (dehydration, shock, hemorrhage).
3. Decreased renal perfusion.
4. Renal malfunction.
5. Postrenal problems such as obstruction or extravasation of urinary flow from the urethra, bladder, ureters, or pelvis.

A blocked Foley catheter is one of the most common causes of sudden drops in urinary flow. This is quickly treated with irrigation of the catheter. Laboratory evaluation of acute renal failure includes tests of blood urea nitrogen (BUN), serum creatinine, the BUN/serum creatinine ratio, serum and urine electrolytes, urine creatinine, and the glomerular filtration rate.[2] A gain in body weight that is not caused by increased food intake is probably due to fluid retention. When urine production is down and body weight is up, the cause must be found and corrected or pulmonary edema can result. Other clues lie in the blood cell count. Fluid retention causes a dilution effect (hemodilution) leading to low hemoglobin, hematocrit, and cell counts. Dehydration can cause hemoconcentration and lead to false high readings of the same variables.

For a patient on positive pressure ventilation, in which the effects of $\overline{P}aw$ can lead to decreased CO and increased plasma ADH, attempts to decrease $\overline{P}aw$ need to be made. PAP monitoring is valuable in this situation. If CO increases when $\overline{P}aw$ is decreased, the fluid balance problem is due most likely to positive pressure ventilation. If not, then the answer to the fluid retention must be looked for elsewhere.

Relative hypovolemia can be due to dehydration, shock, or hemorrhage and will give low vascular pressures (low PAP, low CVP, and low PCWP). Dehydration can commonly result from inadequate fluid intake, vomiting, or diarrhea. Dehydration will often cause hemoconcentration. It can also be caused by fluid shifting out of the plasma and into the interstitial space.

Dehydration or relative hypovolemia is evaluated by giving fluid challenges. Between 50 and 200 mL of fluid are given at a time. Then the BPs, urinary output, and breath sounds are checked. The PCWP should reach about 7 mm Hg; it will be about 3 mm Hg or perhaps lower with dehydration or relative hypovolemia. If the PCWP is less than 3 mm Hg, then another volume of fluid (50–200 mL) is given. The monitoring procedures are repeated every 10 minutes until the PCWP is about 7 mm Hg. At this point hydration is believed to be adequate in an otherwise healthy patient.[55]

Shock is usually treated with fluid administration and appropriate medications such as dopamine, phenylephrine hydrochloride, mephentermine sulfate, norepinephrine, or metaraminol, any of which may help to increase BP. Close monitoring of vascular pressures is also indicated.

If CO and renal output are decreased and PCWP is increased, left heart failure is suspected. Chronic left heart failure will also increase PAP and CVP. These patients are treated with such drugs as digitalis to increase CO, morphine to decrease venous return to the heart, diuretics to unload excess fluids through the kidneys, and O_2 to improve myocardial oxygenation. Sodium nitroprusside can also be used to dilate both arterial and venous vessels. This reduces preload (venous return) and afterload (peripheral vascular resistance); however, the use of this agent must be monitored carefully (PCWP, PAP, and BP) because of its effects on pressures.

Renal failure or renal malfunction is another common cause of a decrease of urine in critically ill patients. Severe hypoxemia, sepsis, and other clinical problems can lead to renal malfunction. The urine is checked for blood cells and elevated protein and sugar levels, as well as specific gravity, color, and amount. Excessive losses of products not normally found in the urine and abnormal urine products in the blood will give clues regarding renal function.

Excessive fluid intake can also result from iatrogenic causes. An intravenous (IV) line may malfunction and run fluids in too rapidly. In addition, the fluid intake calculation must take into account the water gain due to inspired humidified air which occurs during mechanical ventilation and high-humidity therapy.

Measurement of Pulmonary Mechanics: Vital Capacity and Maximum Inspiratory Pressure

When the patient is spontaneously breathing, alert, and cooperative, assessing pulmonary mechanics by measuring VC and maximum inspiratory pressure (MIP), previously called negative inspiratory force (NIF), can help to establish if the patient is ready for weaning.

Vital capacity can be measured with a vane-type respirometer, such as a Wright or Dräger respirometer (see Fig 8–2). It is placed in the same position on the ET tube as it is for direct V_T measurement except that the patient is disconnected from the ventilator for the procedure. Some newer microprocessor ventilators allow this measurement to be done directly through the ventilator.

Vital capacity is the maximum exhaled volume following a maximum inspiratory effort. Accurate measurement requires dependable equipment, good patient instruction and cooperation, and encouragement by the person making the measurement. A VC greater than 15 mL/kg of IBW suggests that the patient may be able to maintain adequate spontaneous ventilation. Three separate readings are taken with a rest period between each effort. The best effort is then recorded on the ventilator flow sheet.

MIP also helps assess the adequacy of pulmonary mechanics and neuromuscular strength and is measured by having the patient inhale against an occluded airway. A manometer connected to the airway measures the subambient pressure generated (Fig 8–7; see also Fig 4–1 in Chapter 4). An MIP of −25 to −100 cm H_2O indicates the adequacy of respiratory reserve and muscle strength. A peak expiratory pressure (PEP) can also be measured by having the patient maximally exhale against the occluded airway. This value is less often used as a weaning criterion.

The MIP can also be measured in a comatose patient with functioning respiratory centers by occluding the airway during inspiration for 15 to 20 seconds and recording the MIP (see Chapter 4). In most cases, however, it is not advisable to wean and extubate a comatose, unconscious, and nonresponsive patient.

Neurologic and Psychological Status

Reflexes, level of consciousness, respiratory pattern, response to verbal commands, body posture, and purposeful movement can all help to establish the patient's neurologic status. If the patient regains consciousness while on venti-

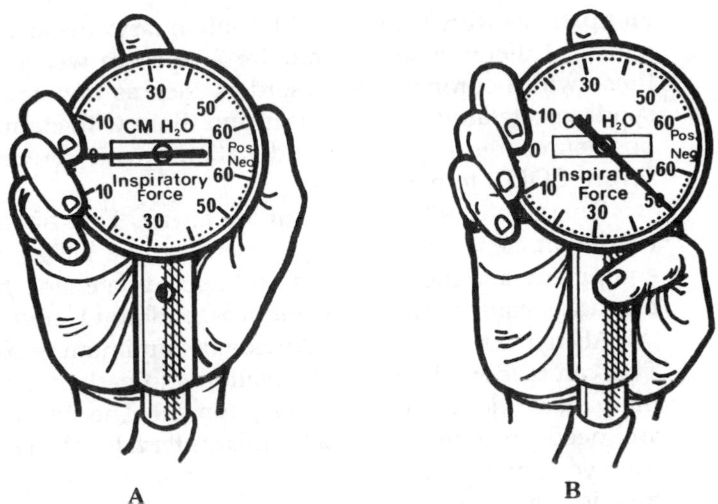

FIG 8–7.
Inspiratory force measurement. The gauge is attached to the patient's endotracheal tube **(A).** The patient is instructed to take several deep breaths while the clinician obstructs the airway by closing the open port on the gauge **(B).** The negative pressure detection, measured here as −50 cm H_2O, is the patient's inspiratory force or peak inspiratory pressure.

latory support, it is important to make the patient aware of what the ventilator and the ET tube are for, and how to communicate his or her needs. Confidence in the health care personnel is very important to the patient. Whenever possible the patient is allowed to rest and sleep undisturbed and is given as much privacy as possible. Whenever an alarm sounds, it is the patient that is checked first, not the equipment. The patient is then reassured that all is well and that he or she need not be concerned about the alarm.

Patient Comfort and Safety

A patient's physical discomfort can be caused by pain from trauma or disease, an awkward body position, distended organs, inadequate ventilation, heavy tubing, bad connections, restraints, limb boards, loss of speech, inability to communicate, inability to swallow, a cough or yawn, poor oral hygiene, and overcooling or overheating due to the environmental conditions. All efforts are made to keep the patient as comfortable as possible.

The primary reason the patient was started on ventilatory support is always kept in mind. Those on short-term mechanical ventilation include postoperative patients and those with uncomplicated drug overdose. Those patients that may require several days to a week or two of ventilation include posttrauma victims, and patients with asthma, COPD, pulmonary edema, aspiration, and pulmonary emboli. Patients who may require 2 or more weeks of ventilator support are those with neuromuscular disorders such as myasthenia gravis, Guillain-Barré syndrome, tetanus, and botulism, and those with cranial tumors or hemorrhage, postneurosurgery patients, and patients with cerebrovascular accidents, and severe COPD, to name a few.

Several pieces of equipment are always kept handy. These include intubation equipment, an emergency tracheostomy kit, a thoracentesis tray, suction equipment, an emergency cart and appropriate emergency medication, arterial blood gas equipment, patient records, and an O_2 source.

Always look for ways to provide the optimum in patient safety and comfort. This can be done by keen observation and early detection of problems in both the patient and the mechanical equipment. The system is never left unattended and needs to be monitored at regular intervals. Always anticipate problems and trust your own assessment of the situation; often, the numbers from the monitors do not accurately reflect the patient's true condition.

FIGHTING THE VENTILATOR

The expression "fighting the ventilator" is used to describe a condition in which the patient is breathing one way and the ventilator is trying to do it another way. It is a situation of "respiratory distress" in the ventilator-supported patient who prior to the event was doing well on mechanical support.[59]

Recognition of Patient Distress

Since the patient generally cannot explain the problem, it is up to the clinician to identify it. The sudden onset of dyspnea can be visually recognized by the physical signs of distress shown in Figure 8–8. These include tachypnea, nasal flaring, diaphoresis, use of accessory muscles, retraction of the suprasternal, supraclavicular, or intercostal spaces, paradoxical or abnormal movement of the thorax and abdomen, abnormal findings on auscultation, tachycardia, possibly arrhythmias, and hypotension.[59] Pulse oximetry and capnography readings may change as will peak and plateau pressures.

Causes of Distress

Table 8–5 provides several causes of the patient fighting the ventilator. One that might be added is pulmonary embolus.

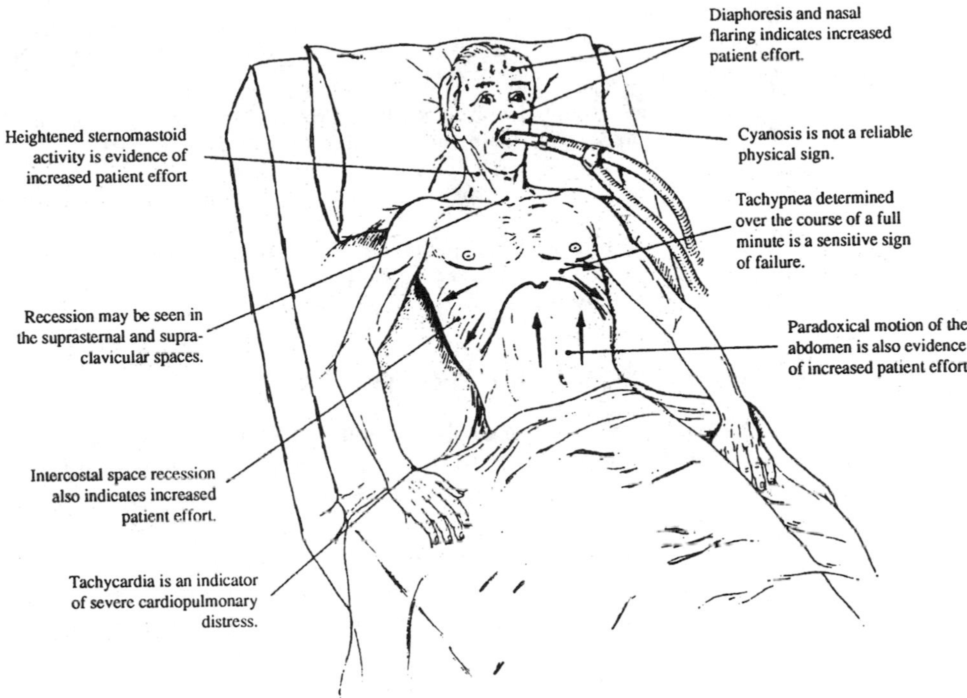
Diaphoresis and nasal flaring indicates increased patient effort.
Heightened sternomastoid activity is evidence of increased patient effort
Cyanosis is not a reliable physical sign.
Tachypnea determined over the course of a full minute is a sensitive sign of failure.
Recession may be seen in the suprasternal and supra-clavicular spaces.
Paradoxical motion of the abdomen is also evidence of increased patient effort.
Intercostal space recession also indicates increased patient effort.
Tachycardia is an indicator of severe cardiopulmonary distress.

FIG 8–8.
Physical signs of severe respiratory distress. (From Tobin MJ: *J Crit Illness* 1990; 6:819–837. Used by permission.)

TABLE 8–5.
Causes of Sudden Respiratory Distress in Patient Receiving Mechanical Ventilation*

Patient-Related Causes	Ventilator-Related Causes
Artificial airway problems	System leak
Pneumothorax	Circuit malfunction or disconnection
Bronchospasm	Inadequate F_{IO_2}
Secretions	Inadequate ventilatory support
Pulmonary edema	Inadequate trigger sensitivity
Dynamic hyperinflation	Improper inspiratory flow setting
Abnormal respiratory drive	Patient-ventilator asynchrony
Alteration in body posture	
Drug-induced problems	
Abdominal distention	
Anxiety	
Patient-ventilator asynchrony	

*From Tobin MJ: *Respir Care* 1991; 36:395–406. Used by permission.

TABLE 8–6.

Steps in the Management of Sudden Distress in a Ventilator-Supported Patient*

1. Remove the patient from the ventilator
2. Initiate manual ventilation using a self-inflating resuscitation bag containing 100% O_2
3. Perform a rapid physical examination and assess monitored indices
4. Check patency of the airway and pass a suction catheter
5. If death appears imminent, consider and treat most likely causes: pneumothorax, airway obstruction
6. Once the patient is stabilized, perform more detailed assessment and management

*From Tobin MJ: *Respir Care* 1991; 36:395–406. Used by permission.

Management of Sudden Respiratory Distress

Management of the problem begins with several specific steps listed in Table 8–6. The initial step is disconnection from the ventilator and manual ventilation of the patient. If the patient's distress is relieved immediately, the problem is in the ventilator. If the distress persists, then the problem lies with the patient. Suspect an obstructed airway or pneumothorax.

A common problem that occurs with the ventilator is inadequate ventilatory support. This might be inadequate O_2 levels, a $\dot{V}_E$ that is too low, a flow that is too low, inadequate machine sensitivity, leaks in the system, auto-PEEP, or an unexpected ventilator malfunction. Oxygen levels and $\dot{V}_E$ can be increased, as can flow. An inadequate flow rate might also be corrected with a change in flow pattern, such as using a descending ramp rather than a rectangular wave.[51] Sometimes changing the mode of ventilation can help the patient. Switching, for example, from assist to PS or to SIMV, depending on the patient's needs, can change the ventilatory pattern and relieve distress. The RCP should examine each possibility, one at a time, and then check the patient's response to the change before proceeding to the next possibility.

Machine Sensitivity.—Inadequate machine sensitivity may be due to inappropriate settings, trapping of gas in the circuit or system, a poorly responsive internal demand valve, the use of an external nebulizer which is blocking the machine's ability to sense a patient's breath, water in the inspiratory line, or the presence of auto-PEEP increasing the amount of pressure the patient must generate to begin a breath.

Auto-PEEP and Sensitivity.—Auto-PEEP is unintentional PEEP (see Chapter 7). Just briefly, increasing the flow rate or using a mode which allows more spontaneous ventilation can help reduce auto-PEEP levels. The use of extrinsic PEEP can also help in patients with early airway closing, such as those with COPD. Using PEEP in the presence of auto-PEEP in the COPD patient population may help increase machine sensitivity.[59] To trigger the ventilator, pressure only needs to drop below alveolar pressure rather than below zero. This can be explained by using a waterfall as an analogy[60] (Fig 8–9). The height of the falls represents the critical closing pressure of the airways in patients with COPD with auto-PEEP. By elevating the downstream pressure (with PEEP), outflow of gas is not blocked. The auto-PEEP level is not changed, but the closing pressure is not reached and the airways remain open. This is true when the downstream pressure is equal to the value of the critical closing pressure (Fig 8–9,B).

If machine sensitivity were set at -1 cm H_2O, without the added PEEP, a patient would have to breathe in -11 cm H_2O to get a breath started (Fig 8–9,A). With PEEP added, the patient only needs to generate the -1 cm H_2O for the machine to sense the effort. Unfortunately, if too much PEEP is added, the pressure upstream increases and the hyperinflation (the auto-PEEP) level gets even higher (Fig 8–9,C).[59]

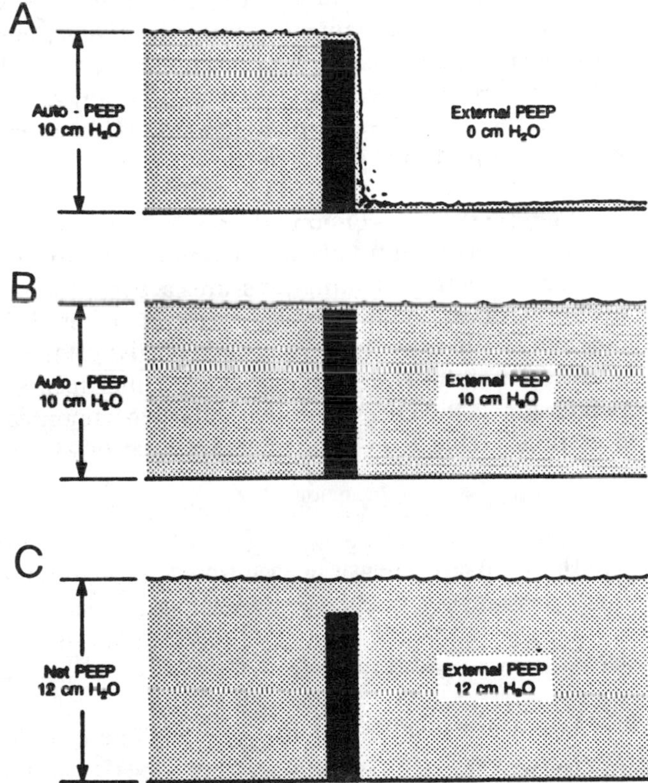

FIG 8–9.
A–C, analogy of a waterfall over a dam *(solid block)* is used to explain the effect of external PEEP (upstream pressure) during expiration. See text. (From Tobin MJ, Lodato RF: *Chest* 1989; 96:449–451.)

Ventilator Malfunction and Leaks.—Ventilator malfunction and circuit leaks can be checked while the patient is being manually ventilated. If need be, a separate ventilator can be used. Ventilator complications are described in Chapter 7.

Airway Problems.—Sudden distress related to airway malfunction might include secretions in the tube, migration of the tube into the right mainstem bronchus, and migration of the tube above the vocal cords. This can be corrected with suctioning and irrigation for secretions and repositioning of the tube for tube migration. Cuff herniation or rupture can also occur and requires a new tube. Tube kinking is not as common with polyvinylchloride ET tubes, but occasionally happens. Repositioning might help this problem. Tracheoesophageal fistula can lead to an inability to deliver a preset V_T. This usually results with protracted intubations. Innominate artery rupture usually only occurs within the first 3 weeks following a tracheotomy. Mortality is high. Immediate indications are blood spurting from the tracheotomy site. In this situation the cuff must be overinflated. Another option is to apply pressure internally with a finger inserted through the stoma. The finger is inserted as far as possible toward the carina and pulled forward. This attempts to compress the artery against the posterior aspect of the sternum.[59]

Pneumothorax.—Pneumothorax is another potential problem (see Chapter 7). Between 60% and 90% of pneumothoraces in ventilated patients are under tension.[59] When ventilating pressures are less than 60 cm H_2O, barotrauma does not often occur. When pressures exceed 70 cm H_2O, on the other hand, a 43% incidence of barotrauma has been reported.[47] Pneumothorax can be recognized as dyspnea if the patient is conscious. Other measures include auscultation and percussion of the chest, cardiovascular assessment, and evaluation of ventilating pressures (Table 8–7). If a pneumothorax is strongly suspected and death is

TABLE 8–7.
Patterns of Alteration in Thoracic Pressure-Volume Relationships*†

	Case 1		Case 2	
	1 hr ago	Now	1 hr ago	Now
Tidal volume (mL)	600	600	600	600
Plateau pressure (cm H_2O)	10	10	10	20
Peak pressure (cm H_2O)	20	40	20	40
Static compliance (mL/cm H_2O)	60	60	60	20
Dynamic characteristic (mL/cm H_2O)	30	15	30	15

*From Tobin MJ: *Respir Care* 1991; 36:395–406. Used by permission.
†In case 1, because plateau pressure is unchanged, suspect an airway problem. In case 2, because plateau pressure is increased and there is no increase in the gradient between peak and plateau pressure, suspect a pneumothorax, mainstem intubation, or atelectasis.

TABLE 8–8.
Pharmacologic Agents Used to Produce Sedation and Neuromuscular Blocking*

Diazepam	2–5 mg IV every 5 min to maximum of 20–30 mg
Morphine	2–5 mg IV every 5 min to a maximum of 20–30 mg
Succinylcholine	0.6–1.0 mg/kg (2–10 min duration)
Pancuronium	0.06–0.1 mg/kg (1–2 hr duration)

*From Tobin MJ: *Respir Care* 1991; 36:395–406. Used by permission.

imminent, a 14- or 16-gauge fluid-filled syringe is inserted into the second intercostal space at the midclavicular line.[59] If the patient is stable, there is time for a confirming chest film with later tube placement and pleural drainage as needed.

Pulmonary Embolism.—Acute pulmonary embolism is another sudden-onset problem that can lead to the patient's fighting the ventilator. The rapid onset of hypoxemia from the embolus leads to all the signs of distress previously described. Disconnection and manual ventilation does not help the condition. One possible clue occurs when a patient is monitored with a capnograph. The cause is often detected by the RCP who is caring for the patient. A fall in the end-tidal CO_2 value and elevation of the arterial–end-tidal CO_2 pressure gradient may lead to the suspicion of an embolus. An angiogram is confirmative. The patient will have an increase in HR, BP, and respiratory rate. Even with high ventilator rates and flows, the patient may still be using accessory muscles to breathe and will begin to pale. Checking airway patency, ventilating pressures, and increasing the F_{IO_2} may not alleviate a falling arterial oxygen saturation (Sa_{O_2}) showing on the pulse oximeter. This is sometimes an acute emergency that leaves the clinician feeling helpless in determining cause and treatment.

Paralyzing and Sedating Patient.—When all efforts have been made to recognize and correct the cause of the patient's distress, sometimes it becomes necessary to use medications. The use of a sedative alone or with a neuromuscular blocking agent may relax the patient and permit control of ventilation. Table 8–8 shows some agents used for sedation and neuromuscular block.[59]

Summary

Patients breathing out of synchrony with the ventilator and those in distress who are connected to mechanical breathing support are in an emergency situation. To repeat, always make every attempt at ventilating the patient. First, disconnect and manually ventilate. Check for airway patency. Make a systematic attempt to find the cause of the problem and correct it.

STUDY QUESTIONS

1. A patient on a 50% Venturi mask has a Pa_{O_2} of 45 mm Hg. The patient is to be switched to a mechanical ventilator. What F_{IO_2} would you set to achieve a Pa_{O_2} of 60 mm Hg?
   a. 0.9.
   b. 0.75.
   c. 0.67.
   d. 0.55.
   e. 1.0.
2. A patient on mechanical ventilation has a V_T ordered by the physician that is approximately 7.5 mL/kg of IBW. What other parameter or mode must be set to accommodate this patient?
   a. Inflation hold.
   b. Expiratory retard.
   c. PEEP.
   d. Sigh mode.
   e. IMV.
3. A patient has the following ventilator settings: V_T, 750 mL; f, 8 breaths/min; PIP, 25 cm H_2O; inflation hold, 0.5 second. Arterial blood gases show Pa_{CO_2} of 41 mm Hg, pH of 7.43, Pa_{O_2} of 89 mm Hg on 0.25 F_{IO_2}. Blood pressure is 80/40 mm Hg. What ventilator change would you make?
   a. None at this time.
   b. Increase the F_{IO_2}.
   c. Reduce the pressure limit.
   d. Remove the inflation hold.
   e. Increase the rate.
4. On which of the following patients would you recommend the use of either expiratory retard or *low* levels of PEEP (<5 cm H_2O)?
   a. Congestive heart failure.
   b. COPD.
   c. Adult respiratory distress syndrome (ARDS).
   d. Closed head injury.
   e. Recovery from anesthesia after surgery.
5. The patient is a 21-year-old woman. Following minor surgery, she is still under the effects of anesthesia. Her height is 62 in., her weight is 110 lb, and her BSA is 1.5 m^2. What initial ventilator settings would be appropriate for this patient?
   a. V_T = 500 mL, f = 9 breaths/min.
   b. V_T = 725 mL, f = 8 breaths/min.
   c. V_T = 850 mL, f = 6 breaths/min.
   d. V_T = 850 mL, f = 10 breaths/min.
   e. V_T = 1,000 mL, f = 8 breaths/min.

6. A constant inspiratory flow of 40 L/min is being used on a patient. The ventilator I/E ratio indicator shows inspiratory time greater than expiratory time. What change could be made to correct this problem without changing the $\dot{V}_E$?
   a. Shorten the expiratory time.
   b. Increase the rate.
   c. Lengthen the inspiratory time.
   d. Increase the flow rate setting.
   e. Reduce the V_T.

A patient with COPD is being given prednisone, theophylline, and furosemide (Lasix). Which of the following should be checked regularly?
   a. Na^+.
   b. Cl^-.
   c. K^+.
   d. HCO_3^-.
   e. Hemoglobin.

8. A patient with COPD has the following arterial blood gases: pH, 7.18; Pa_{CO_2}, 89 mm Hg; Pa_{O_2}, 55 mm Hg on 24% O_2. HCO_3^- is 38 mEq/L. The patient is 65 years old and weighs 140 lb. What mode of ventilation and initial settings would be appropriate?
   a. IMV = 8 breaths/min, V_T = 1,200 mL.
   b. Assist-control = 13 breaths/min, V_T = 1,000 mL.
   c. IMV = 8 breaths/min, V_T = 800 mL.
   d. Control mode = 12 breaths/min, V_T = 600 mL.
   e. SIMV = 14 breaths/min, V_T = 450 mL.
9. A 5 ft 4 in. man with pickwickian syndrome (weight = 340 lb) is to be placed on mechanical ventilatory support. Which of the following V_T and rate settings would be most appropriate?
   a. V_T = 875 mL, f = 11 breaths/min.
   b. V_T = 520 mL, f = 8 breaths/min.
   c. V_T = 450 mL, f = 10 breaths/min.
   d. V_T = 1,100 mL, f = 6 breaths/min.
10. The following values are obtained from a patient's ventilator flow sheet.

Time	Volume	PIP	PPLATEAU
1:00	850 mL	36 cm H_2O	33 cm H_2O
2:00	850 mL	39 cm H_2O	32 cm H_2O
3:00	850 mL	43 cm H_2O	33 cm H_2O

   Which of the following statements about these conditions is correct?
   a. Lung compliance is improving.
   b. Lung compliance is getting worse.
   c. Airway resistance is improving.
   d. Airway resistance is getting worse.
   e. There has been no change in lung characteristics.

11. A patient on mechanical ventilatory support is suctioned for large amounts of foul-smelling green sputum. The patient has a temperature of 39°C and an elevated white blood cell count. The most likely cause of this problem is:
    a. Overheated cascade humidifier.
    b. Cardiogenic pulmonary edema.
    c. Allergic reaction to acetylcysteine.
    d. Normal response to being intubated.
    e. *Pseudomonas* infection.
12. Which of the following are potential problems related to the addition of an externally powered nebulizer to a mechanical ventilator circuit?
    a. It affects ventilator function.
    b. Expiratory monitor readings will change from previous values.
    c. It may add volume to the delivered V_T.
    d. It may affect sensitivity.
    e. All of the above.
13. List five ways in which urinary output can decrease in ventilated patients.
14. The sudden onset of dyspnea can be visually recognized by the physical signs of distress. Describe these findings in a ventilated patient with respiratory distress.
15. What is the initial step to take in managing a patient in distress who is being mechanically ventilated? How can you tell if the problem is with the ventilator or the patient?

ANSWERS TO STUDY QUESTIONS

1. c.
2. d.
3. d.
4. b.
5. b.
6. d.
7. c.
8. c.
9. a.
10. d.
11. e.
12. e.
13. Decreases in urinary output can be due to: (a) decreased fluid intake and low plasma volume; (b) decreased CO from positive pressure ventilation decreasing venous return, positive pressure ventilation increasing plasma ADH, heart failure, relative hypovolemia (dehydration, shock,

hemorrhage); (c) decreased renal perfusion; (d) renal malfunction; (e) post-renal problems such as obstruction or extravasation of urinary flow from the urethra, bladder, ureters, or pelvis.

14. Tachypnea, nasal flaring, diaphoresis, use of accessory muscles, retraction of the suprasternal, supraclavicular, or intercostal spaces, paradoxical or abnormal movement of the thorax and abdomen, abnormal findings on auscultation, tachycardia, possibly arrhythmias, and hypotension.
15. The initial step is disconnection from the ventilator and manual ventilation of the patient. If the patient's distress is relieved immediately, the problem is with the ventilator. If the distress persists, then the problem lies with the patient. Suspect an obstructed airway or pneumothorax.

REFERENCES

1. Abromson NS, Wald KS, Grenvik ANA, et al: Adverse occurrences in intensive care units. *JAMA* 1980; 244:1582–1584.
2. Balk RA, Bone RC: Patient monitoring in the intensive care unit, in Burton GG, Hodgkin JE, Ward JJ (eds): *Respiratory Care: A Guide to Clinical Practice,* ed. 3. Philadelphia, JB Lippincott Co, 1991, pp 705–718.
3. Beaty CD, Ritz RH, Benson MS: Continuous in-line nebulizers complicate pressure support ventilation. *Chest* 1989; 96:1360–1363.
4. Bone RC: Diagnosis of causes for acute respiratory distress by pressure-volume curves. *Chest* 1976; 70:740–746.
5. Bone RC: Pressure-volume measurements in detection of bronchospasm and mucous plugging in acute respiratory failure. *Respir Care* 1976; 21:620–626.
6. Bone RC: Monitoring the patient and ventilator during respiratory failure. *Curr Rev Respir Ther* 1979; 1:139–143.
7. Bone RC: Monitoring ventilatory mechanics in acute respiratory failure. *Respir Care* 1983; 28:597–603
8. Branson RD: Enhanced capabilities of current ICU ventilators: Do they really benefit patients? *Respir Care* 1991; 36:362–376.
9. Brunel W, Coleman DL, Schwartz DE, et al: Assessment of routine chest roentgenograms and the physical examination to confirm endotracheal tube position. *Chest* 1989; 96:1043-1045.
10. Chatburn RL, Carlo WA, Lough MD: Clinical algorithm for pressure-limited ventilation of neonates with respiratory distress syndrome. *Respir Care* 1983;28:1579–1586.
11. Cohen A, Taeusch HW, Stanton C: Usefulness of the arterial/alveolar oxygen tension ratio in the care of infants with respiratory distress syndrome. *Respir Care* 1983; 28:169–173.
12. Conrardy PA, Goodman LR, Lainge F, et al: Alteration of endotracheal tube position: Flexion and extension of the neck. *Crit Care Med* 1976; 4:8–12.
13. Consensus Conference on Aerosol Delivery. *Respir Care* 1991; 36:913–1044.
14. Conway M, Durbin GM, Ingram D, et al: Continuous monitoring of arterial oxygen

tension using a catheter-tip polarographic electrode in infants. *Pediatrics* 1976; 57:244–250.

15. Cox PM, Schatx ME: Pressure measurements in endotracheal cuffs: A common error. *Chest* 1974; 65:84–87.
16. Craig KC, Pierson DJ: Expired gas collection for deadspace calculations: A comparison of two methods. *Respir Care* 1979; 24:435–437.
17. Cross DE: Recent developments in tracheal cuffs. *Resuscitation* 1973; 2:77–81.
18. Dimas S, Kacmerak RM: Intrapulmonary shunting. *Curr Rev Respir Ther* 1978; 1:35–39, 43–47.
19. Dixon RJ: *Assessment of the Pulmonary Patient.* Denver, Multi-Media Publishing, Inc, 1984.
20. Douglas ME, Downs JB, Dannemiller FJ: Changes in pulmonary venous admixture with varying inspired oxygen. *Anesth Analg* 1976; 55:688–693.
21. Epstein J: The sputum wet prep technique, eosinophils and reversible obstructive lung disease. *Respir Care* 1978; 23:1151–1173.
22. Fleming WH, Bowen JC, Petty C: The use of pulmonary compliance as a guide to respiratory therapy. *Surg Gynecol Obstet* 1972; 134:291–293.
23. Freeman C, Cicerchia E, Demers RR, et al: Static compliance, static effective compliance and dynamic effective compliance as indicators of elastic recoil in the presence of lung disease. *Respir Care* 1976; 21:323–326.
24. Gilbert R, Keighley JF: The arterial/alveolar oxygen tension ratio: An index of gas exchange applicable to varying inspired oxygen concentrations. *Am Rev Respir Dis* 1974; 109:142–145.
25. Goddard P, Keith I, Marcovitch H, Roberton NRC, et al: Use of continuous recording intravascular oxygen electrode in the newborn. *Arch Dis Childhood* 1974; 49:853–860.
26. Hess D: How should bronchodilators be administered to patients on ventilators? *Respir Care* 1991; 36:377–394.
27. Hess D, Maxwell C: Which is the best index of oxygenation: $P(A - a)O_2$, PaO_2/P_AO_2 or PaO_2/F_IO_2? *Respir Care* 1985; 30:961–963.
28. Holzapfel L, Robert D, Perrin F, et al: Static pressure-volume curves and effect of positive end-expiratory pressure on gas exchange in adult respiratory distress syndrome. *Crit Care Med* 1983; 11:591–597.
29. Hylkema BA, Barkmeijer-Degenhart P, van der Mark TW, et al: Central venous versus esophageal pressure changes for calculation of lung compliance during mechanical ventilation. *Crit Care Med* 1983; 11:271–275.
30. Kacmarek RM, Dimas S: Pulmonary deadspace: Concepts and clinical application. *Curr Rev Respir Ther* 1979; 1:147–151.
31. Krouskop RW, Cabatu EE, Chelliah BP, et al: Accuracy and clinical utility of an oxygen saturation catheter. *Crit Care Med* 1983; 11:744–749.
32. Martin L, Jeffreys B: Use of a mini-computer for storing, reporting, and interpreting arterial blood gases/pH and pleural fluid pH. *Respir Care* 1983; 28:301–308.
33. Maxwell C, Hess D, Shefet D: Use of the arterial/alveolar oxygen tension ratio to predict the inspired oxygen concentration needed for a desired arterial oxygen tension. *Respir Care* 1984; 29:1135–1139.
34. McPeck M: The impact of computer-age technology on respiratory therapy. *Respir Care* 1982; 27:855–865.

35. McPherson SP: *Respiratory Therapy Equipment,* ed 5. St Louis, Mosby–Year Book, Inc, 1990.
36. Mithoefer JC, Holford FD, Keighley JFH: The effect of oxygen administration on mixed venous oxygenation in chronic obstructive pulmonary disease. *Chest* 1974; 66:122–132.
37. Mithoefer JC, Keighley JF, Karetzkey MS: Response of the arterial PO_2 to oxygen administration in chronic pulmonary disease. *Ann Intern Med* 1971; 74:328–335.
38. Murray JF: Pathophysiology of acute respiratory failure. *Respir Care* 1983; 28:531–541.
39. Nahrwold ML: Rapid calculation of derived hemodynamic parameters using a programmable calculator. *Anesthesiol Rev* 1981; 8:15–19.
40. Neff TA, Clifford D: A new monitoring tool—the ratio of the tracheostomy tube cuff diameter to the tracheal air column diameter (C/T ratio). *Respir Care* 1983; 28:1287–1290.
41. Nelson EJ, Morton EA, Hunter PM: *Critical Care Respiratory Therapy.* Boston, Little, Brown & Co, 1983.
42. Nelson RD, Wilkins RL, Jacobson WK, et al: Supranormal $P\bar{v}O_2$ in the presence of tissue hypoxia: A case report. 1983; 28:191–194.
43. Off DO, Braun SR, Tompkins B, et al: Efficacy of the minimum leak technique of cuff inflation in maintaining proper intracuff pressures for patients with cuffed artificial airways. *Respir Care* 1983; 28:1115–1120.
44. Osborn JJ: Monitoring respiratory function. *Crit Care Med* 1974; 2:217–220.
45. Peris LV, Boix JH, Salom JV, et al: Clinical use of the arterial/alveolar oxygen tension ratio. *Crit Care Med* 1983; 11:888–891.
46. Peters RM, Brimm JE, Utley JR: Predicting the need for prolonged ventilatory support in adult cardiac patients. *J Thorac Cardiovasc Surg* 1979; 77:175–182.
47. Peterson GW, Baier H: Incidence of pulmonary barotrauma in medical ICU. *Crit Care Med* 1983; 11:67–68.
48. Pollitzer MJ, Soutter LP, Osmund E, et al: Continuous monitoring of arterial oxygen tension in infants: Four years of experience with an intravascular oxygen electrode. *Pediatrics* 1980; 66:31–36.
49. Polysongsang Y, Branson RD, Rashkin MC, and Hurst JM: Effect of flowrate and duration of use on the pressure drop across six artificial noses. *Respir Care* 1989; 34:902–907.
50. Rau JL, Pearce DJ: *Understanding Chest Radiographs.* Denver, Multi-Media Publishing, Inc, 1984.
51. Rau JL, Shelledy DC: The effect of varying inspiratory flow waveforms on peak and mean airway pressures with a time-cycled volume ventilator: A bench study. *Respir Care* 1991; 36:347–356.
52. Richman KA, Jobes DR, Schwalb AJ: Continuous in vivo blood gas determination in man: Reliability and safety of new device. *Anesthesiology* 1980; 52:313–317.
53. Scanlan CL, Spearman CB, Sheldon RL: *Egan's Fundamentals of Respiratory Care.* St Louis, Mosby–Year Book, Inc, 1990.
54. Shapiro BA, Cane RD, Harrison RA, et al: Changes in intrapulmonary shunting with administration of 100 percent oxygen. *Chest* 1980; 77:138–141.
55. Shapiro BA, Harrison RA, Kacmarek RM, et al: *Clinical Applications of Respiratory Care.* St Louis, Mosby–Year Book, Inc, 1985.

56. Silage DA, Maxwell C: A lung diffusion determination/interpretation program for hand-held computers. *Respir Care* 1983; 28:1587–1590.
57. Suwa K, Geffin B, Pontoppidan H, et al: A nomogram for deadspace requirement during prolonged artificial ventilation. *Anesthesiology* 1968; 29:1206–1210.
58. Tobin MJ: Respiratory parameters for successful weaning. *J Crit Illness* 1990; 6:819–837.
59. Tobin MJ: What should the clinician do when a patient "fights the ventilator?" *Respir Care* 1991; 36:395–406.
60. Tobin MJ, Lodato RF: PEEP, auto-PEEP, and waterfalls (editorial). *Chest* 1989; 96:449–451.

Chapter 9

Noninvasive Gas Monitoring and Measurement of Physiologic Dead Space and Shunt in Mechanically Ventilated Patients

On completion of this chapter the reader will be able to:

1. Name the two parameters that are measured by pulse oximetry and the two physical principles that are the basis for its operation.
2. List the Po_2 associated with each of the following saturations: 100%, 97%, 90%, 80%, 75%, and 50%.
3. Describe the basic principle of operation of the pulse oximeter.
4. Explain how pulse oximetry readings are affected by abnormal hemoglobins, such as HbCO.
5. Tell what a capnometer measures.
6. Name the two types of capnometers.
7. Discuss the normal components of a capnogram.
8. Explain the changes in end-tidal CO_2 during hyperventilation and hypoventilation.
9. Identify or describe the fast P_{ETCO_2} tracing that occurs with the following: apnea, hypoperfusion (drop in blood pressure or decreased cardiac output), mechanical dead space, obstructive airway disease, esophageal intubation.
10. Give the normal value for $P(a - ET)CO_2$ and list four disorders in which this value is greater than normal.
11. Explain the value of arterial–maximum end-expiratory P_{CO_2} measurements.
12. Give the principle of operation of the transcutaneous O_2 and CO_2 monitors.
13. Describe how heating the skin affects CO_2 and O_2 in the skin.
14. List the normal values for the Pao_2-$PtcO_2$ gradient and the $Paco_2$-$PtcCO_2$ gradient.
15. Provide the equations for calculating the V_D/V_T ratio and clinical shunt.

NONINVASIVE GAS MONITORING AND MEASUREMENT OF PHYSIOLOGIC DEAD SPACE AND SHUNT IN MECHANICALLY VENTILATED PATIENTS

Arterial blood gas results are essential in monitoring patients on mechanical ventilation. Obtaining these results requires an invasive procedure that carries risks both for the patient and the respiratory care practitioner. In the past decade noninvasive gas monitoring techniques have become available. While they do not supersede the importance of blood gas analysis, they provide alternative methods of continuous monitoring of physiologic gases that correlate well with arterial blood samples. These techniques include pulse oximetry, capnography, and transcutaneous oxygen and carbon dioxide monitoring. These methods of patient evaluation are the primary focus of this chapter. The evaluation of physiologic dead space also provides useful information for the ventilated patient and is also included.

PULSE OXIMETRY (Spo_2 AND PULSE RATE)

Accurate evaluation of arterial oxygenation is very important in the care of the critically ill patient. Oxygen therapy and ventilatory support both rely on monitoring of arterial blood gas levels as a basis for their effectiveness. More than two decades ago, refinement of arterial blood gas analyzers helped to revolutionize the field of respiratory care. Arterial blood gas sampling requires an invasive procedure of puncturing an artery. In addition, it is an occasional measurement and does not provide a method of continuously monitoring the oxygenation status.

Pulse oximetry is a continuous, noninvasive technique that can be used for evaluating oxyhemoglobin saturation (Spo_2) and pulse rate. It is done by placing a sensor over a finger or an ear lobe and measuring the absorption of selected wavelengths of light through the tissue. Oxygenated hemoglobin absorbs different wavelengths of light than does deoxygenated hemoglobin. The amount and type of absorption of light is determined and the resulting Spo_2 is read out on a meter or digital device (Fig 9–1).

Today, pulse oximeters are considered a standard of practice in the field of anesthesiology[75] and are in common use in all intensive care units (ICUs). It was declared by Severinghaus and Astrup to be "arguably the most significant technologic advance ever made in monitoring the well-being of patients during anesthesia, recovery, and critical care."[62]

History

The pulse oximeter came about because of the development of the combined technologies of oximetry, plethysmography, and microprocessor-based instrumentation.[75] Early oximeters first used a single wavelength of light. In 1935 the

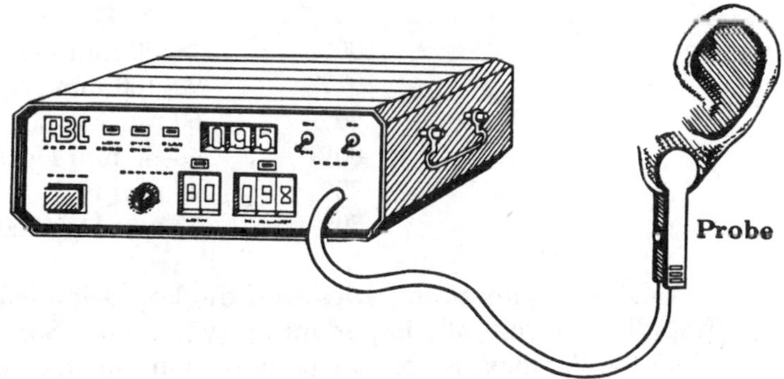

FIG 9–1.
Pulse oximeter probe placed on the ear lobe.

first dual wavelength oximeter was developed by Matthes.[62] The use of two wavelengths helped to compensate for changes in tissue thickness and blood content, among other variables, in assessing the O_2 saturation of hemoglobin. In the initial development, the oximeter required two-point calibration.

By the mid-1960s Shaw had designed an oximeter using eight wavelengths of light in an ear oximeter. By the early 1980s this device was refined, marketed, and sold by the Hewlett-Packard Corp.[62] Aoyagi, a Japanese bioengineer, devised a method using a plethysmographic signal that was sensitive to changes in O_2 saturation. He noted that the pulsatile nature of the blood flow could be detected by the absorption signal. Aoyagi found that this was due to changes in blood volume and was not affected by pigmentation, bone, or tissue.[75]

Further development of the pulse oximeter is credited to Biox (a subdivision of Ohmeda) and Nellcor. Both of these companies used microprocessor technology in improving the device. Since that time, its use has become extensive in respiratory care, pulmonary function testing, exercise testing, sleep studies laboratories, and in anesthesiology.

Oxygen Saturation and Oxygen Tension Relationships

The oximeter measures the oxygen saturation of arterial blood (Sao_2). Oxygen saturation is the percentage of hemoglobin molecules that are saturated with O_2 compared to the total number of hemoglobin molecules available.

$$Sao_2 = (Hbo_2/Hb\ total)$$

Normal Sao_2 is 97%. Below are some values for oxygen saturation (So_2) and correlating partial pressure of oxygen (Po_2) at a normal pH. These values are true for arterial or venous blood and represent important points on the oxyhemoglobin saturation curve.

So_2	Po_2
100%	≥150 mm Hg
97%	90–100 mm Hg
90%	60 mm Hg
80%	46–48 mm Hg
75%	40 mm Hg
50%	27 mm Hg (P50)

Oxygen saturation varies with the Po_2. Below 80% saturation the Po_2 falls rapidly. It is clinically important to try and keep Sao_2 about 90% to 95%. Above 90% the Po_2 may rise considerably without much change in saturation. It is not necessary to keep saturation above normal (97%) for most patients. There may be some clinical situations where full arterial saturation is desired. Examples are stroke, heart attack, and severe angina.[55]

TABLE 9–1.
Factors Affecting Affinity of Hemoglobin for Oxygen

Factors That Reduce Affinity (Right Shift of HbO_2 Dissociation Curve)	Factors That Increase Affinity (Left Shift of HbO_2 Dissociation Curve)
Increased H^+ concentration	Decreased H^+ concentration
Increase in body temperature	Decrease in body temperature
Increase in CO_2	Decrease in CO_2
Increase in 2,3-DPG*	Decrease in 2,3-DPG*
Increase in metabolism	Decrease in metabolism[55]
	Fetal hemoglobin
	Abnormal hemoglobins

*2,3-DPG (2,3 diphosphoglycerate) is produced normally in red blood cells (RBCs). Production is increased with high altitude, chronic alkalosis, and chronic hypoxia. Production is decreased in chronic acidosis, in stored (banked) blood, and as RBCs age.

Table 9–1 lists the factors that affect the affinity of hemoglobin for O_2. Abnormal hemoglobins also influence hemoglobin's affinity for O_2. Carbon monoxide is strongly attracted to the hemoglobin molecule. It has more than 200 times the affinity for hemoglobin than does oxygen. Carbon monoxide will competitively bind with hemoglobin at very low fractional concentrations of carbon monoxide in inspired gas (F_{ICO}). The result is carboxyhemoglobin (HbCO). Other abnormal hemoglobins states like sickle cell anemia, methemoglobinemia, and sulfhemoglobinemia reduce the binding of O_2. These factors must all be kept in mind when evaluating O_2 tension and saturation levels.

Function of Pulse Oximeter

Pulse oximeters use the combined principles of spectrophotometry and optical plethysmography to measure Sa_{O_2}. A plethysmograph is a device used to determine the variation in the size of an organ.[25] Optical plethysmography uses light absorption technology to determine change in volume to separate the pulsatile blood flow from other constant, nonchanging components of the tissue. Spectrophotometry uses various wavelengths of light to evaluate the light absorption of different substances.[47]

Pulse oximeters operate on the basic principle that oxygenated hemoglobin and deoxygenated hemoglobin have different light absorption characteristics. When red light (wavelength of about 660 nm) passes through oxyhemoglobin, very little light is absorbed. Conversely, when red light passes through deoxyhemoglobin, more light is absorbed. As a result, oxygenated hemoglobin has a distinct red color. When infrared light (wavelength about 920 nm) is passed through oxygenated hemoglobin it has a tendency to be absorbed. Very little infrared light is absorbed by deoxyhemoglobin (Fig 9–2).[47,75] Thus, red light passes easily through red (oxygenated) blood and is easily absorbed by blue (nonoxygenated) blood.[25]

Light emitting diodes (LEDs) transmit both the infrared and red light that is provided during pulse oximetry. Calculation of So_2 is determined by comparing, at any point, the amount of infrared light absorbed to the amount of red light absorbed. The light sources originate from a probe and are directed through a piece of tissue, such as a finger, toe, ear lobe, or nose and detected on the opposite side by a optical sensor (photodetector). Part of the light is absorbed by the pulsatile vascular tissue bed. The other part of the light is absorbed by the veins, capillaries, bones, muscles, and fat layers of the tissue, which are constant. Only the pulsing blood volume varies (Fig 9–3). The oximeter compares the constant absorption of the static tissues to the nonconstant absorption of the dynamic component. As a result, the amount of reported light absorption only represents the dynamic pulsatile portion.

Technical Limitations

Accuracy of the device seems to vary depending on the reported saturations. The accuracy is acceptable for saturations above 70%, but the accuracy below

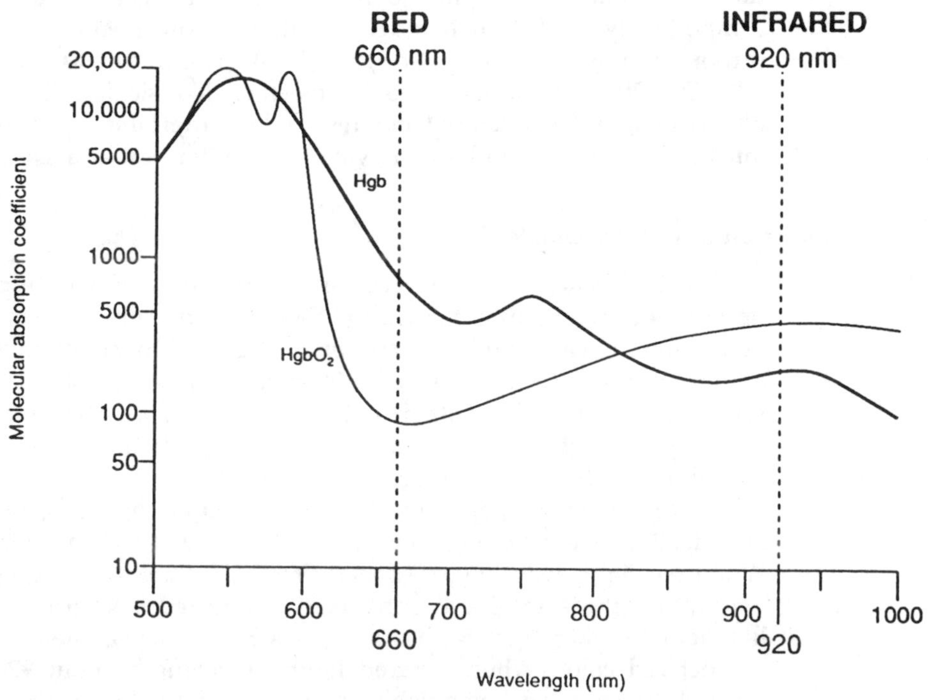

FIG 9–2.
Wavelength absorption for reduced hemoglobin *(Hgb)* and oxyhemoglobin *($HgbO^2$)*. (Courtesy of Nellcor, Inc, Hayward, Calif.)

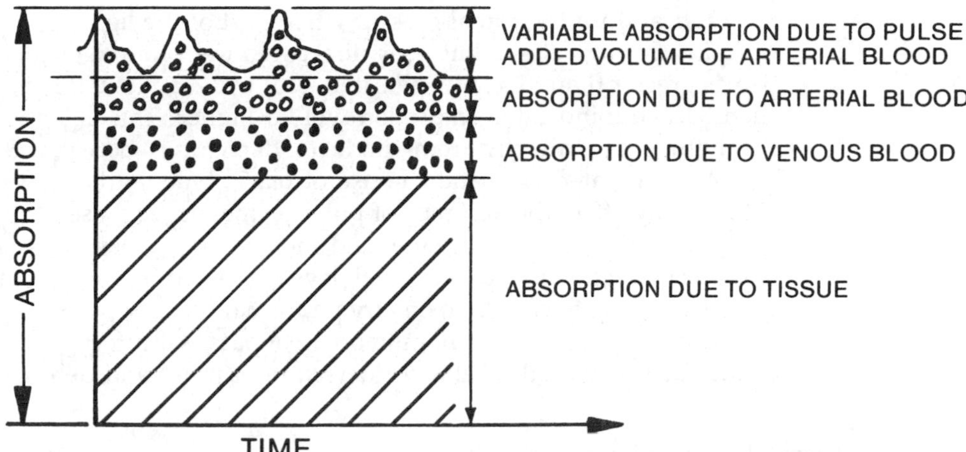

FIG 9–3.
Amount of light transmitted through a tissue is partly absorbed by each layer of the tissue. Each of the components absorbs a constant amount except the pulsing arterial portion. During systole the volume to the tissue increases. The amount of absorption varies with systole and diastole as the blood volume increases and then decreases. (Courtesy of Ohmeda, Boulder, Colo.)

70% is questionable.[75] Accuracy is also affected by such factors as abnormal hemoglobin, ambient light, low perfusion states, optical shunting, skin pigment, nail polish, and vascular dyes.

Pulse oximeters are described as evaluating only "functional" hemoglobin, i.e., the hemoglobin capable of carrying O_2.[47] "Nonfunctional" hemoglobin, such as methemoglobin and HbCO, cannot carry O_2. In other words, most pulse oximeters up to the present time (1992) do not take into account any hemoglobin that is abnormal. For example, if the oxyhemoglobin (HbO_2) content were 10 g, the HbCO 3 g, and the HHb (deoxyhemoglobin) 2 g, the total hemoglobin would be 15 g. A co-oximeter, which measures actual saturation, would see an HbO_2 saturation of 10/15, or 67%. A pulse oximeter would see 10/12 as the saturation since the HbCO is nonfunctional. Its reading would be nearer to 83%. This would give the impression of being fairly high compared to the actual low So_2. So with abnormal hemoglobin present, Spo_2 will overestimate actual saturation. For this reason, pulse oximetry is not recommended when carbon monoxide poisoning is suspected or when abnormal hemoglobins are present in significant amounts.

Bright light sources such as sunlight, bilirubin lights, infrared heat lamps, and fluorescent lights can interfere with the photodetector if they are present in significant amounts. This problem can be reduced by covering the sensor with an opaque material.[25]

Optical shunting can also occur when part of the light from the diodes does not pass through tissue but goes directly to the photodetector. If the patient's Sa_{O_2} is greater than 81%, the indicated Sp_{O_2} will read low. If the saturation is less than 85%, the indicated saturation will be higher. This is because the value of the light going directly from diode to detector is between 81% and 85%.[25] Deeply pigmented skin and the use of black, blue, and green nail polish may significantly affect the accuracy of pulse oximeters. The use of the vascular dyes methylene blue, indigo carmine, and indocyanine green can also affect its red and infrared light absorption.[75] High levels of blood bilirubin, on the other hand, do not seem to affect pulse oximetry performance. Low perfusion states, as occur during cardiac arrest or cardiopulmonary bypass, will affect pulse oximeters. They cannot be considered reliable for detection of pulse and determining Sp_{O_2}.[75]

Clinical Uses of Pulse Oximetry

Clinical uses of pulse oximetry include continuous monitoring of critically ill patients, patients with unstable oxygenation status, and patients on mechanical ventilation. These devices are also used extensively for monitoring during surgery, monitoring of infants and children, for prescribing oxygen in hospitalized patients, for prescribing long-term O_2, in emergency medicine, and for sleep studies. In addition, pulse oximetry is used in the home care setting to help evaluate the effectiveness of O_2 therapy in this environment.

CAPNOMETRY

Capnometry is the measuring of carbon dioxide in respired gases. The capnometer measures the CO_2 and gives a numeric display of the gas tension. Capnography normally contains a capnograph and a capnometer. The capnograph gives a waveform (capnogram) of the partial pressure of carbon dioxide (P_{CO_2}). There are three current methods for CO_2 measurement in gases: infrared absorption, mass spectrometry, and Raman scattering.[37] The most commonly used method is infrared. The first measuring of expired CO_2 was performed by Tyndall in 1865, but the use of infrared CO_2 gas analysis was not made possible until 1943.[25]

There is a great deal of clinical use of the CO_2 monitor, which is often referred to as P_{ETCO_2} monitoring (end-tidal CO_2), because the level of CO_2 at the end of exhalation is of greatest interest. This represents gas coming from the alveolar level. Under normal conditions, alveolar and arterial CO_2 pressures are nearly equal. As a result, monitoring of P_{ETCO_2} gives an estimate, in most cases, of arterial CO_2 changes. It provides an evaluation of ventilatory status through a noninvasive technique. This method is used not only in pulmonary function testing but for continuous monitoring in critically ill patients.

Technical Aspects

Capnography uses infrared spectrophotometry to measure and report the percentage or partial pressure of CO_2 in expired air.[36] There are two types of infrared capnometers currently in use: mainstream and sidestream. Mainstream capnometers have the sample measurement chamber placed at the endotracheal tube. Analysis is performed at the airway so there is no delay time between sampling and reporting of data. Inhaled and exhaled gas both pass directly through the chamber. Sidestream capnometers have gas from the airway extracted through a very narrow plastic tube to the sample measuring chamber. Actual analysis is performed away from the airway. There is a delay between sampling time and the time data are presented.

The disadvantage of mainstream capnometers is that they are more often handled and thus more often damaged, e.g., from dropping; also, they tend to increase dead space and add weight to the artificial airway. The disadvantage of sidestream capnometers is that they tend to plug with water or secretions, there is a delay time between aspirating and reporting of the value, and the sampling tube can be contaminated with ambient air.[29]

Carbon dioxide absorbs infrared light at a wavelength of 4.26 μm. The analyzer determines the amount of infrared absorption of the sample and thus the CO_2 level in the gas sample.[37] A schematic of a nondispersive double-beam positive-filter capnometer is illustrated in Figure 9–4. Infrared analyzers emit radiation that passes through a chopper, which is like a rotating fan blade. This permits periodic measurement of the reference and sample signal and the dark signal (neither reference nor sample signal).[29] From the chopper the beam passes

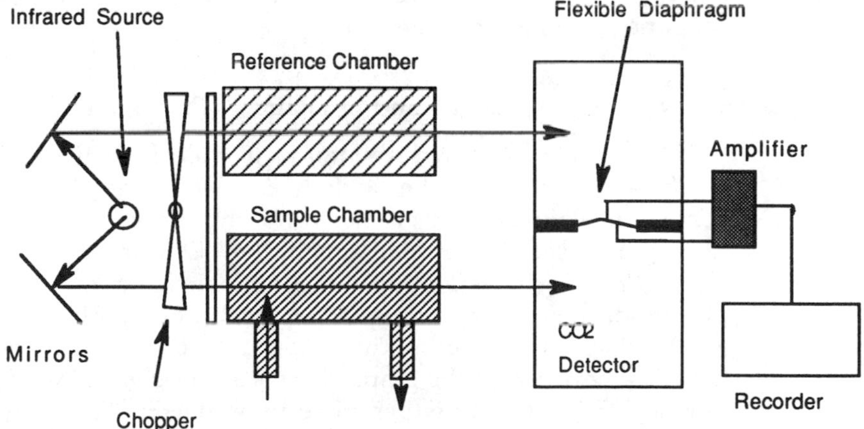

FIG 9–4.
Schematic of a nondispersive, double-beam, positive-filter capnometer. The level of CO_2 in the sample cell absorbs some of the radiation and decreases the radiation sent to the detector. A high level of radiation from the reference cell helps heat and expand the gas in the detector. This causes movement of the diaphragm. (Redrawn from references 4, 24.)

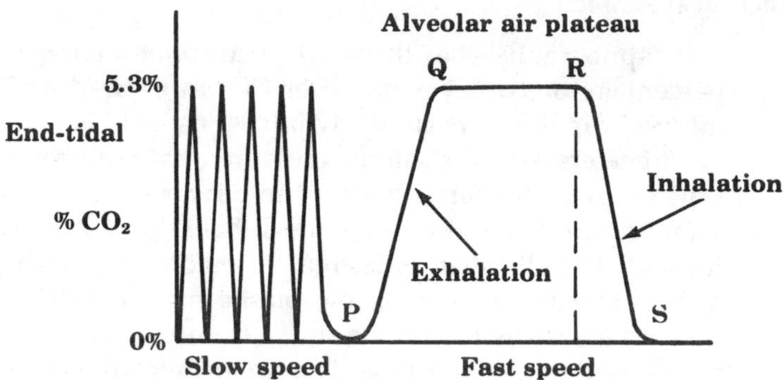

FIG 9–5.
Left, slow capnographic tracings. *Right,* fast speed, which provides the opportunity to see the different parts of the respiratory cycle.

through a filter which absorbs radiation from the nitrous oxide absorption band. This reduces interference by N_2O gas. The radiation then passes in parallel through a reference cell and a sample cell, then finally to a detector which is filled with CO_2.[25]

Radiation coming through the reference and sample cells affects the absorption of CO_2 in the detecting chamber. The CO_2 in the sample cell reduces the radiation transmitted to the detector.[29] The difference between the reference cell radiation and the sample cell radiation causes movement of a diaphragm in the detector chamber. This movement is converted to a signal which is amplified and displayed. The displayed value is either in partial pressure or concentration and is displayed over a given time. Mainstream capnometers can also be single-beam negative-filter capnometers.[29]

Physiology of CO_2 Production and Exhalation – Capnogram

Carbon dioxide is produced normally in the body tissues during metabolism. It diffuses out cells into the capillary circulation and from there passes into the venous circulation, returns to the lungs, and is excreted with exhaled gases. The capnograph records the exhalation of the CO_2 from the lungs.

Figure 9–5 shows a sample of a normal capnogram. Anatomic dead space (the conductive airways) contain low levels of CO_2. The beginning of the curve will be at zero representing the conductive airways at the beginning of exhalation. The next part of the graph rises as alveolar gas mixes with dead space gas (segment *PQ*). The curve then plateaus as alveolar air is exhaled (segment *QR*). The CO_2 at the end of the plateau (point *R*) is called end-tidal CO_2 (P_{ETCO_2}). It represents the end of the tidal breath. Normal P_{ETCO_2} varies between 4.5% and 5.5%. It is also called peak-exhaled P_{CO_2} or maximum exhaled P_{CO_2}. Inspiration is detected when the CO_2 level again falls with inhalation of ambient air (segment

RS). Besides viewing a screen, a graphic paper record, similar to an electrocardiogram (ECG) strip, can be run to provide a permanent record of the capnogram. Slow speed is used for continuous monitoring or fast speed can be selected for the evaluation of a single breath.

The alveolar level of CO_2 (P_{ACO_2}) is determined by the rate of metabolism and CO_2 production, the rate of perfusion of blood through the lungs, and the rate of ventilation of gas out of the lungs. Basically P_{ACO_2} is related to the ventilation/perfusion ($\dot{V}/\dot{Q}$) ratio. With normal $\dot{V}/\dot{Q}$ ratios, arterial carbon dioxide (Pa_{CO_2}) and P_{ACO_2} are nearly equal. In normal, healthy persons, the P_{ETCO_2} is 4 to 6 mm Hg lower than the Pa_{CO_2}.[12, 37]

If ventilation decreases, P_{ACO_2} and mixed venous carbon dioxide ($P\bar{v}_{CO_2}$) levels begin to equilibrate. P_{ACO_2} rises toward $P\bar{v}_{CO_2}$. On the other hand, with high ventilation and low perfusion (increased $\dot{V}/\dot{Q}$), the physiologic dead space increases. The P_{ACO_2} approaches inspired CO_2 in value.[29] The P_{ETCO_2} may be higher than normal when the metabolic rate increases as long as the alveolar ventilation does not increase and compensate for the change. Table 9–2 lists causes of increases in P_{ETCO_2} and it is assumed that compensation has not occurred. Table 9–3 gives examples of lower-than-normal P_{ETCO_2}, again assuming that compensation has not occurred.

In patients in whom the physiologic dead space increases, as in chronic obstructive pulmonary disease (COPD) and pulmonary embolism, the gradient between Pa_{CO_2} and P_{ETCO_2} increases and P_{ETCO_2} is less than Pa_{CO_2} (Table 9–4). In low perfusion states, such as decreased cardiac output or hypotension, the P_{ETCO_2} values will no longer parallel Pa_{CO_2}. Thus, P_{ETCO_2} cannot be used to predict Pa_{CO_2}.

TABLE 9-2.

Causes of Increased End-Tidal Carbon Dioxide Pressure*

Increased CO_2 production and delivery to lungs
Fever
Sepsis
HCO_3^- administration
Increased metabolic rate
Seizures
Decreased alveolar ventilation
Respiratory center depression
Muscular paralysis
Hypoventilation
COPD
Equipment malfunction
Rebreathing
Exhausted CO_2 absorber
Leak in ventilator circuit

*From Hess D, Maxwell C: *Respir Care* 1985; 30:961–963. Used by permission.

TABLE 9–3.
Causes of Decreased End-Tidal Carbon Dioxide*

Decreased CO_2 production and delivery to lungs
Hypothermia
Pulmonary hypoperfusion
Cardiac arrest
Pulmonary embolism
Hemorrhage
Hypotension
Increased alveolar ventilation
Hyperventilation
Equipment malfunction
Ventilator disconnection
Esophageal intubation
Complete airway obstruction
Poor sampling
Leak around endotracheal tube cuff

*From Hess D, Maxwell C: *Respir Care* 1985; 30:961–963. Used by permission.

TABLE 9–4.
Causes of Increased Difference Between Arterial and End-Tidal Carbon Dioxide Values*

Pulmonary hypoperfusion
Pulmonary embolism
Cardiac arrest
Positive pressure ventilation (especially with PEEP)
High-rate low–tidal volume ventilation

*From Hess D, Maxwell C: *Respir Care* 1985; 30:961–963. Used by permission.

Use of Slow Capnogram for Distinguishing Problems

Clinically, the slow continuous monitoring of expired CO_2 can be used to distinguish:

1. Changes in carbon dioxide production ($\dot{V}CO_2$) (as $\dot{V}CO_2$ increases, alveolar ventilation increases while expired CO_2 levels remain constant).
2. Hyperventilation (P_{ETCO_2} decreases) (Fig 9–6).
3. Hypoventilation (P_{ETCO_2} increases) (see Fig 9–6).
4. Apnea or periodic breathing (Fig 9–7).
5. CO_2 rebreathing (P_{ETCO_2} does not return to baseline) (Fig 9–8).
6. Pulmonary blood flow cessation (major pulmonary embolus or cardiac arrest or severe hypotension) (Fig 9–9).

The rapid single breath analysis can be used to detect the presence of airway obstruction and $\dot{V}/\dot{Q}$ mismatching (Fig 9–10). Here the expiratory flow curve does not rise sharply, but rises gradually. This is a result of the presence of alveoli with long time constants (empty slowly) that add CO_2-rich gas to the exhaled gas flow.[29] In patients with very slow respiratory rates (bradypnea), cardiac oscillations can sometimes be seen on the capnogram (Fig 9–11).

Clinical Applications

Capnometry has become a valuable measurement tool for spontaneous breathing in addition to its use in mechanically ventilated patients. It has gained

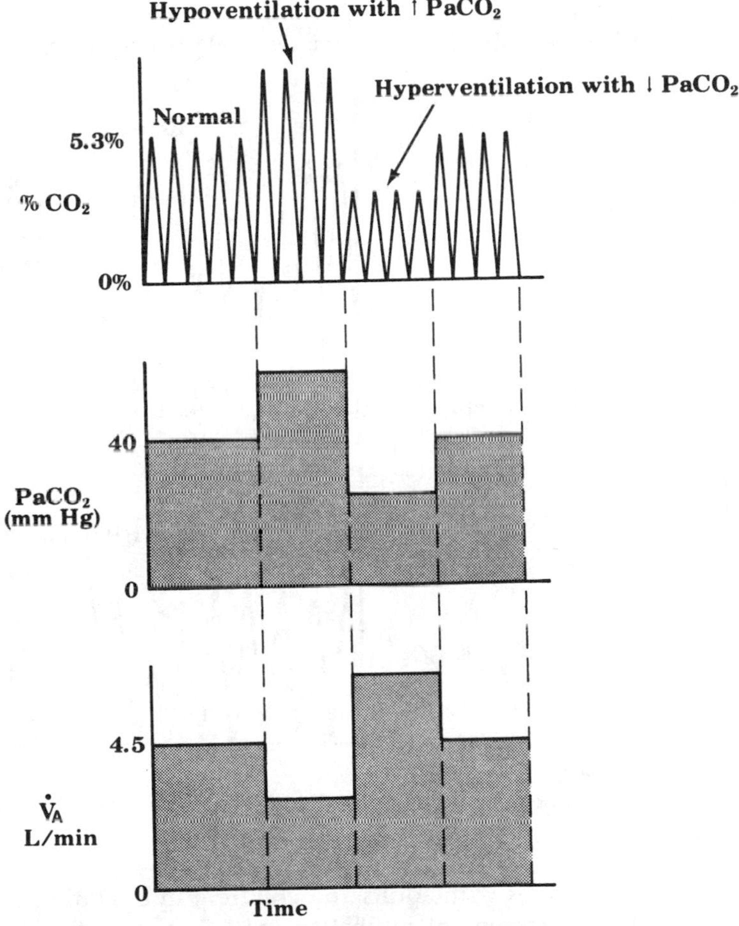

FIG 9–6.
Changes in end-tidal CO_2 (P_{ETCO_2}) with changes in ventilation. During normal alveolar ventilation ($\dot{V}_A$), Pa_{CO_2} and P_{ETCO_2} are normal. During hypoventilation, Pa_{CO_2} and P_{ETCO_2} increase. During hyperventilation, Pa_{CO_2} and P_{ETCO_2} decrease.

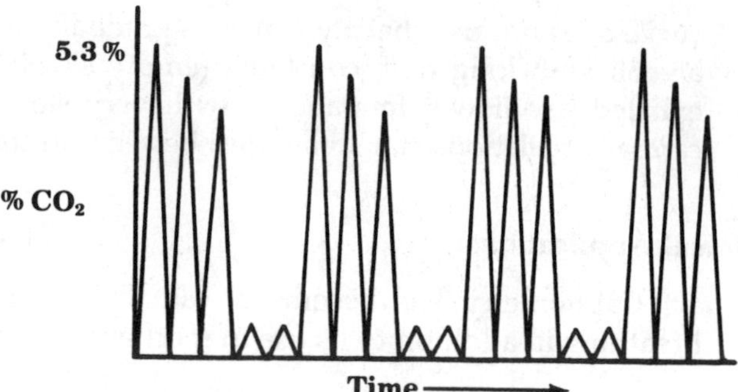

FIG 9–7.
Changes in the CO_2 curve as a result of Cheyne-Stokes respiration.

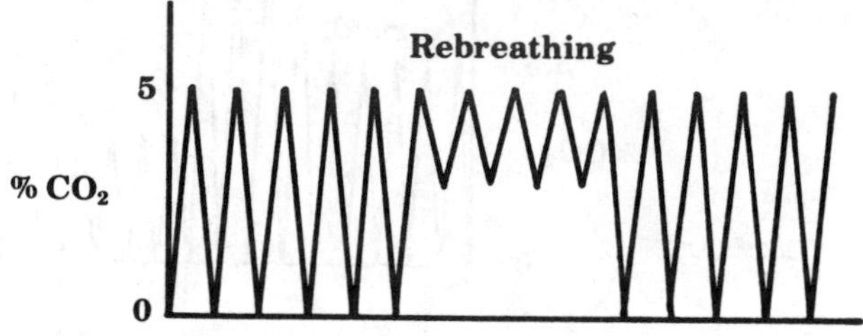

FIG 9–8.
During the rebreathing of air the CO_2 curve does not return to baseline on inhalation. This is an example of mechanical dead space.

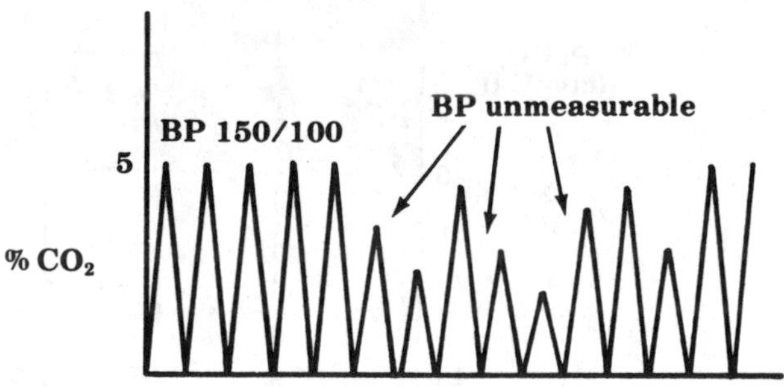

FIG 9–9.
Low blood pressure *(BP)* conditions can cause a drop in end-tidal CO_2 readings.

use in ICUs with adults and children; in operating room procedures, including the assessment of intubation; and in monitoring resuscitation efforts during cardiac arrest.[29, 37]

Artifacts.—Several artifacts can give abnormal capnographic tracings. One example is the water trap on sidestream analyzers. The trap removes moisture before the gas sample enters the CO_2 analyzer. The volume of the trap appears to be critical during ventilation at high pressures. At high airway pressures, the capnogram will falsely show a brief period of exhalation during a mechanical inspiration. The artifact can be eliminated by reducing the water trap volume from 30 to 10 mL.[72]

Capnography With IMV Ventilation.—On patients ventilated with intermittent mandatory ventilation (IMV) the capnogram will have different P_{ETCO_2} values on spontaneous breaths than with machine breaths. The P_{ETCO_2} for spontaneous breaths with moderate tidal volumes is usually higher than that for positive pressure breaths. In this situation monitoring the maximal observed P_{ETCO_2} regardless of breathing pattern is the most clinically useful indicator of Pa_{CO_2} in postcardiotomy patients.[74] These results can probably be applied to all patients.[37]

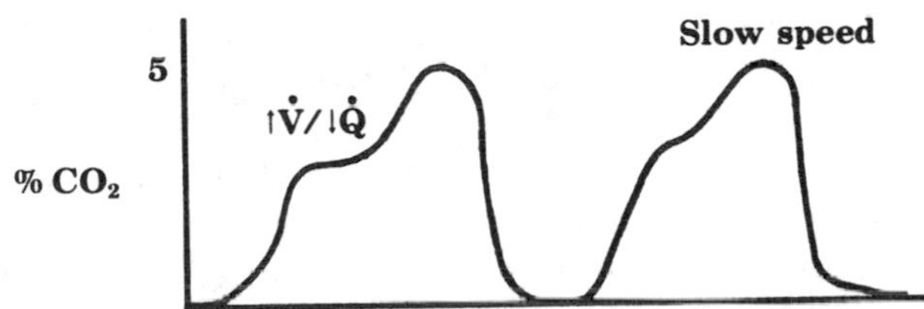

FIG 9–10.
With a slow tracing it is possible to pick up abnormalities in the CO_2 curve. Sloping expiratory curve may indicate a ventilation-perfusion ($\dot{V}/\dot{Q}$) abnormality.

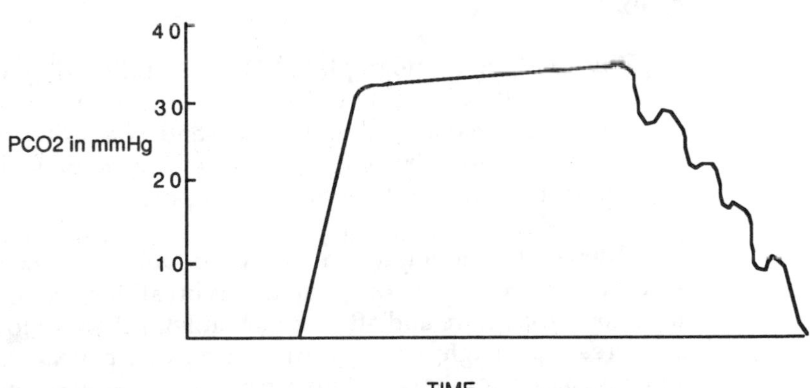

FIG 9–11.
During bradypnea, cardiac oscillations can sometimes be seen on the capnogram. (Redrawn from references 29, 68.)

Application During CPR.—During cardiac arrest, a total dead space is created if ventilation continues without perfusion. The P_{ETCO_2} will drop to near zero. Cardiopulmonary resuscitation (CPR) can restore part of the circulation but does not return $\dot{V}/\dot{Q}$ abnormalities to normal. The P_{ETCO_2} will begin to reappear as ventilation continues and circulation is partially restored, but may rise to no more than 20 mm Hg. When spontaneous cardiac contractions return circulation to near normal, the P_{ETCO_2} will begin to return to normal levels. It seems then that monitoring during CPR can be an indication of the progress and success of the event.[29, 37]

Esophageal Intubations.—Accidental intubation of the esophagus can occur during endotracheal intubation. Use of the capnograph may help in detecting this situation. If the P_{ETCO_2} values do not rise to normal levels, or if they drop significantly after several breaths, then esophageal intubation can be suspected.[29, 50] Two precautions need to be pointed out. First, there may be high levels of CO_2 in the stomach following exhaled gas ventilation or ingestion of a carbonated beverage. This is usually cleared with bag-resuscitation ventilation. Second, low circulatory states can reduce pulmonary circulation and thus exhaled CO_2 levels. The latter should not be confused with esophageal intubation.[29]

Leaks.—Endotracheal tube cuff leaks can be detected by a rise in the P_{ETCO_2} level as the delivered tidal volume decreases.[50] Gas sampling line leaks can also occur. When there is a loose connection between the sampling line and the analyzer in a sidestream analyzer, the CO_2 waveform during exhalation will show a long plateau followed by a brief peak, rather than the normal CO_2 plateau. The long plateau is due to entrainment of room air through the leaky connection. The brief CO_2 peak is caused by the next positive pressure breath which pushes undiluted end-tidal gas through the sampling line and to the analyzer.[76]

Weaning.—A capnograph can be helpful during weaning. It can show, breath by breath, a patient's ability to resume the work of breathing. It has also been suggested that a $P(a\text{-}ET)O_2$ (arterial–end-tidal CO_2 pressure gradient) of less than 8 mm Hg may be one indicator of which patients may be successfully weaned from mechanical ventilatory support.[45]

Others.—Capnography can be used during bronchoscopy and for sleep studies for the detection of spontaneous breathing and noting periods of apnea. It can be used before and after bronchodilator therapy to monitor the $\dot{V}/\dot{Q}$ ratio. A decrease in height or a return to a normal plateau rather than an upward sloping curve may show an improvement from severe obstruction. It can also be used to document the need for and effectiveness of racemic epinephrine treatments in children with severe croup.[50] Its use in infants, however, remains unclear.[29] At the present time transcutaneous CO_2 monitoring rather than P_{ETCO_2} is more frequently used in infants for evaluation of ventilatory status.

Capnographs and other CO_2 analyzers, such as the Severinghaus electrode, can also be used to measure gas samples for dead space–tidal volume (V_D/V_T) ratio calculation (see below), and for $P(a - ET)CO_2$ gradient, and arterial–end-expiratory assessments.

ARTERIAL END-TIDAL AND ARTERIAL MAXIMUM END-EXPIRATORY P_{CO_2} EVALUATION

When P_{ETCO_2} monitoring is available, there is one further maneuver that can be used in patient evaluation. After P_{ETCO_2} is recorded, the patient is asked to exhale maximally (end-expiratory) to the level of residual volume and the CO_2 value is evaluated. The difference between the arterial and maximum end-expiratory CO_2 is calculated. This gradient is normally less than 7 mm Hg. Increases in this value are indications of the presence of some abnormality.

Patients with COPD, acute pulmonary embolism, left ventricular failure, or shock have elevated arterial maximum end-expiratory P_{CO_2} gradients as well as increased $P(a - ET)CO_2$. The amount of arterial maximum end-expiratory P_{CO_2} gradient varies according to the severity of the pathologic problem (Table 9–5).

Capnography or P_{ETCO_2} alone cannot be used to predict Pa_{CO_2} in patients with COPD, pulmonary embolism, left ventricular failure, or shock. Comparison of $(Pa - ET)CO_2$ and arterial maximum end-expiratory P_{CO_2} (maximum exhalation), however, does much to shed light on patient disorders.[12, 26] By measuring P_{CO_2} at maximum exhalation the high gradients between Pa_{CO_2} and P_{ETCO_2} approach zero in patients with COPD or left ventricular failure. On the other hand, patients with severe dead space disease, such as lung embolism, have only a slight reduction in the gradient. In this way severely hypoxemic patients with large emboli can be separated from those with acute or chronic $\dot{V}/\dot{Q}$ disorders (Fig 9–12).[18, 26]

TABLE 9–5.

The Category of Problem and the Arterial Maximum End-Expiratory Carbon Dioxide Pressure*

Category	Arterial Maximum End Expiratory P_{CO_2} (mm Hg)
Normal	<7
Slightly abnormal	7–10
Moderately abnormal	11–13
Markedly abnormal	>13

*Data from references 12 and 26.

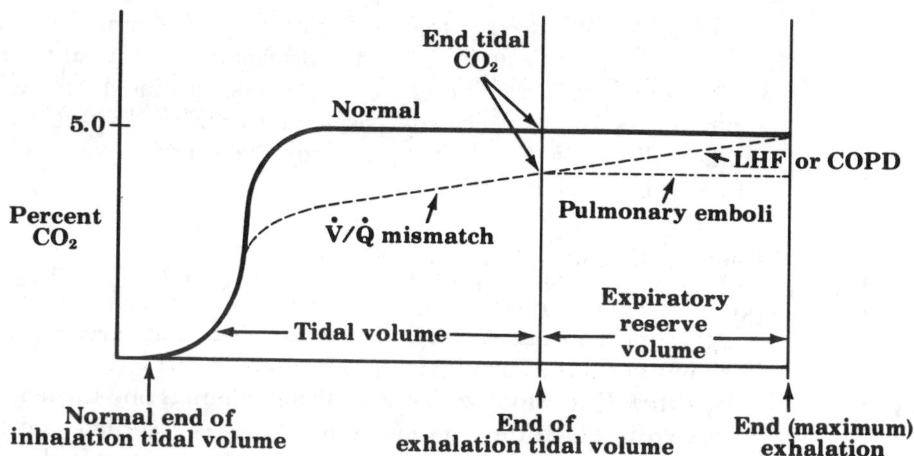

FIG 9–12.
Percent CO_2 exhaled at varying exhaled lung volumes is shown. For a normal person *(solid line)* the end-tidal CO_2 at the end of normal tidal exhalation is equal to that at maximum exhalation. With left heart failure *(LHF)* or chronic obstructive pulmonary disease *(COPD)*, the end-tidal CO_2 is less than normal at the end of a normal exhalation and may rise slightly at the end of a maximum exhalation. With pulmonary emboli present, a low end-tidal CO_2 will not rise in value at the end of a maximum exhalation. (Data from references 12, 18, 26.)

In patients with COPD, the $P(a - ET)CO_2$ is highly variable; however, the arterial–maximum end-expiratory PCO_2 gradient is relatively constant and varies directly with the severity of disease. A close approximation of $PaCO_2$ can be obtained by subtracting the initial gradient between $PaCO_2$ and $PETCO_2$ and the measured maximum end-expiratory PCO_2.[12] This can help to eliminate the need for frequent arterial blood sampling (Figs 9–12 and 9–13).

TRANSCUTANEOUS OXYGEN MONITORS

History

Gierlach in 1851 was the first to measure O_2 transport across the skin. He shellacked the shaved skin of dogs, horses, and men. When a bubble formed, he analyzed the gas content of the bubble and referred to the gases as "cutaneous respiration."[25] Gierlach also did an experiment in which he glued a horse bladder full of air to his chest for a day and measured the changes in gas concentration that took place during that time.[69]

A hundred years later, in 1951, Baumberger and Goodfriend found that O_2 diffusion through intact skin allowed for an estimation of the partial pressure of arterial oxygen (Pa_{O_2}).[3] They placed a finger in water and after a period of time measured the P_{O_2} of the water. By the early 1970s, a heated Clark electrode was being used to measure P_{O_2} of the skin.[25, 33] A commercially available transcutaneous P_{O_2} monitor ($PtcO_2$) was finally on the market by the late 1970s. Since that time, $PtcO_2$ monitors have been manufactured and sold extensively, particularly for monitoring in infants.

Physiology of Skin in Ptc_{O_2} Monitoring

The skin consists of two main layers: the epidermis and the dermis. The epidermis consists of an outer layer of dead cells that acts as a membrane and allows gas diffusion across the membrane. This layer is also called the stratum corneum. The next inner layer of the epidermis contains no blood vessels and receives its O_2 supply from the air. Carbon dioxide from the epidermis is removed by diffusion outward. It gains its nourishment from the capillaries of the underlying dermal layer. The dermis contains capillaries and a vascular supply and is considered a living tissue layer. The outward diffusion of O_2 is not possible. Normally, the skin P_{O_2} is near zero even when Pa_{CO_2} values are high. But the mechanisms that prevent this diffusion can be reversed by heating, abrasion, or chemical treatment (nicotinic acid derivatives). These reverse the lipid structure of stratum corneum and increase its gas permeability.

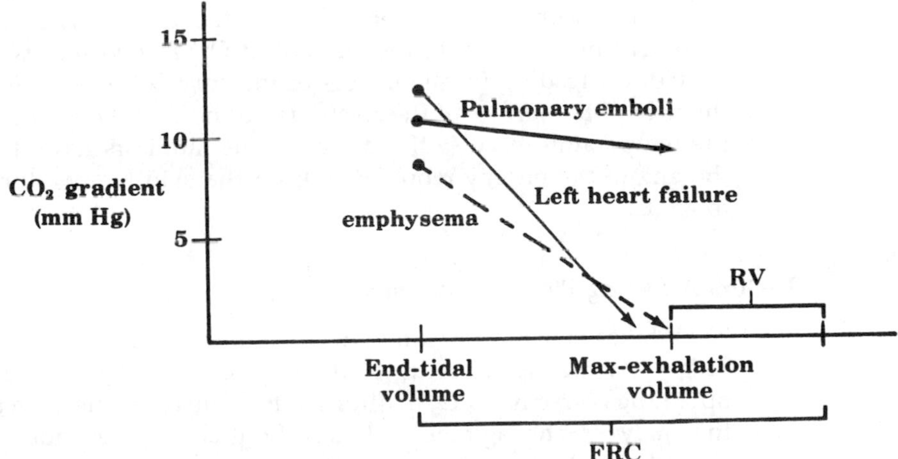

FIG 9–13.
Representation of the changes in the gradients for arterial–end-tidal CO_2 and arterial–maximum end-expiratory CO_2 with pulmonary emboli, left heart failure, and emphysema. *Dots* = arterial–end-tidal P_{CO_2} gradient; *Arrowheads* = arterial–maximum end-expiratory gradient for P_{CO_2}. (Redrawn from Hatle L, Rokseth R: *Chest* 1974; 66:352–357.)

Effects of Heating the Skin for $Ptco_2$ Monitoring

Transcutaneous O_2 monitors all require heating of the skin for the unit to function. The skin site is heated to 44 to 45° C. Heating the skin has several physiologic effects. First, it causes local vasodilation. This helps to arterialize the capillaries in the vicinity, which raises the blood Po_2. For every degree Celsius, the Po_2 increases 6% when the Po_2 is less than 100 mm Hg. For a Po_2 more than 100 mm Hg, the increase is about 6 mm Hg per degree Celsius.

Additionally, heating causes a shift to the right in the HbO_2 dissociation curve. For a specific saturation, the Po_2 will be higher. Thus, the affinity of hemoglobin for O_2 is reduced. As the O_2 diffuses outward toward the skin surface, it is consumed. Heating of the skin increases local tissue consumption and lowers the Po_2. This drop in O_2 from consumption is offset by the rise from heating. The end result is that the $Ptco_2$ is about 5 mm Hg lower than the Pao_2 in adults and nearly the same as in infants.[3, 58, 62]

Electrode Operation

The $PtcO_2$ electrode is based on the polarographic, or the Clark electrode principle.[13, 25, 69] A silver anode is usually the heated portion. Inside the electrode are one or more cathodes made of gold or platinum wires bathed in the electrolyte solution. The anode and cathodes are encased in plastic with an attached membrane (Fig 9–14). Voltage across the electrode produces a current. Oxygen from the nearby sample area diffuses across the membrane into the electrode and reacts with electrons provided by the anode. The amount of resulting current is proportional to the amount of O_2. The current is then amplified and provides a reading in millimeters of mercury. A temperature sensor measures the heat of the surface of the electrode on the skin. This sends information about the temperature back to the device. Some monitors have a display that shows the amount of energy required to keep the skin temperature at the desired 44 to 45° C.

Factors Affecting $Ptco_2$ Measurement

It takes time for the skin to heat when the sensor is first attached to the skin. This delay time is about 15 to 20 minutes. It also takes time once the device is operating correctly for O_2 to diffuse out of the capillaries and across the skin into the analyzer. The lag time for this is about 20 to 30 seconds in adults and 8 to 10 seconds in children. The amount of peripheral blood flow to the site of the sensor will also affect the $PtcO_2$ reading. For example, low cardiac output, and low perfusion states like low blood pressure, shock, and poor local perfusion, will alter the reading. In these situations, the vasodilation from the heater cannot make up for poor perfusion. The result is a low $PtcO_2$ reading. Skin metabolism and O_2 consumption vary with different skin thicknesses and age.

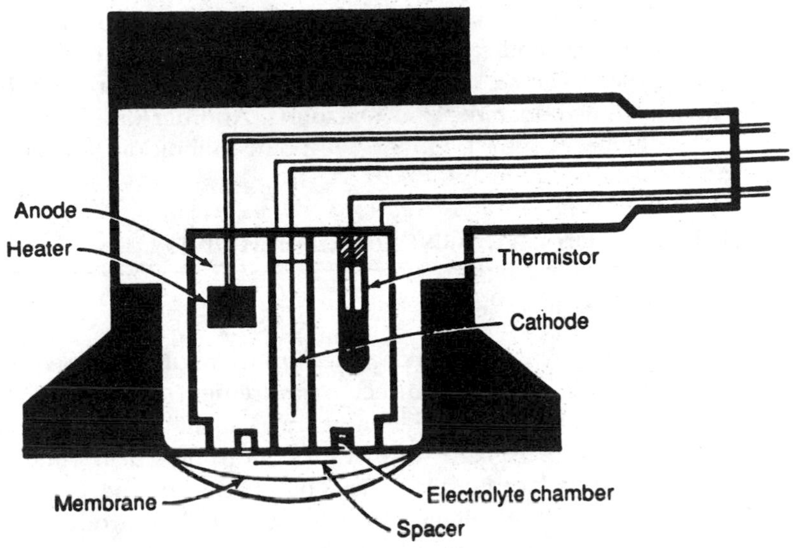

FIG 9–14.
Transcutaneous oxygen electrode. (From Deshpande VM, Pilbeam SP, Dixon RJ: *A Comprehensive Review in Respiratory Care.* Norwalk, Conn, Appleton & Lange, 1988. Used by permission.)

Correlations between Pao_2 and $PtcO_2$ are better in infants than in adults for this reason. $PtcO_2$ can, however, underestimate the Pao_2 in infants and cannot be relied upon completely for decisions on O_2 therapy. It does, however, serve as a useful reference. Other factors that affect readings include hemoglobin concentration, HbO_2 affinity, the thickness of the epidermis, capillary density, the level of epidermal hydration, and the temperature of the electrode and skin.[69]

Extensive studies have been done correlating Pao_2 and $PtcO_2$ values.[25] The advantage of the device remains its ability to provide continuous monitoring without invading the skin through blood sampling. Clinically, a decrease in $Ptco_2$ indicates hypoxemia or a loss of adequate cutaneous blood flow. A widening gradient between Pao_2 and $PtcO_2$ tells that the monitor is no longer tracking Pao_2, and indicates a reduction of skin blood flow.[69]

During mechanical ventilation, if ventilating parameters remain constant but $Ptco_2$ decreases, there is good reason to believe something has gone wrong. This might include pneumothorax, endotracheal tube displacement, worsening of the patient's cardiopulmonary condition, and so on.

Possible Hazards and Disadvantages

Because of the need to heat the skin, transcutaneous monitors can cause skin burns. For this reason the site of placement is changed every few hours. Any device that uses a heating element controlled by a thermostat runs the risk that it will fail and cause overheating. The accuracy of the device will also be affected by skin edema, deep hypothermia, sensitive skin, and drugs that affect perfusion such as dopamine and tolazoline. Another disadvantage is that transcutaneous devices require frequent two-point calibration to ensure accuracy.

TRANSCUTANEOUS CARBON DIOXIDE MONITORS

Principle of Operation

Transcutaneous P_{CO_2} ($PtcCO_2$) monitors are based on the Stow-Severinghaus principle for the indirect measurement of CO_2.[13,69] Carbon dioxide diffuses across a CO_2-permeable membrane, usually Teflon or Silastic, into the electrode. It then reacts with water to form carbonic acid which dissociates to hydrogen ions and bicarbonate ions. The change in the pH of the electrolyte causes a change in the voltage across the glass pH electrode and the silver–silver chloride reference electrode (Fig 9–15). The pH changes and the voltage change parallel the change in CO_2. Transcutaneous monitors are now available that contain elements for measuring both CO_2 and O_2. These have the obvious advantage of performing both measurements at once.

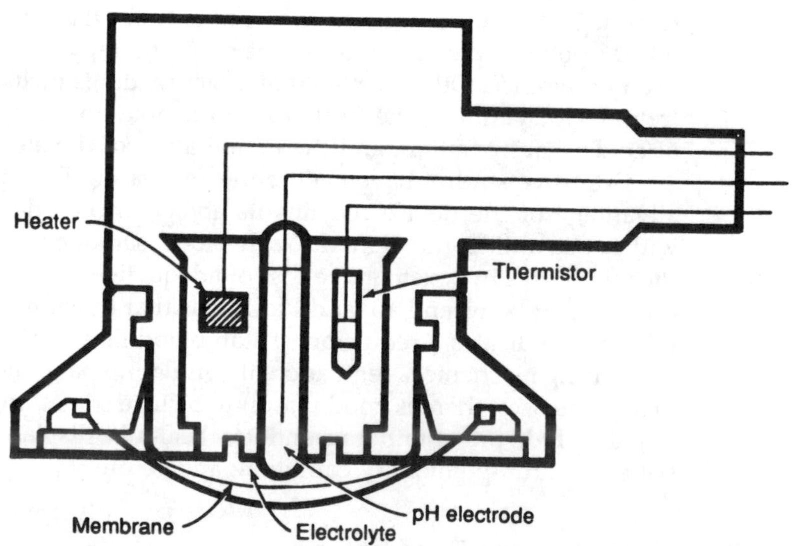

FIG 9–15.
A transcutaneous P_{CO_2} electrode. (From Deshpande VM, Pilbeam SP, Dixon RJ: *A Comprehensive Review in Respiratory Care.* Norwalk, Conn, Appleton & Lange, 1988. Used by permission.)

Skin Pco_2 and Temperature

Carbon dioxide is the only gas present in the body that can diffuse freely across the epidermis and affect pH. Since ambient CO_2 is nearly zero, levels of approximately 40 mm Hg within the skin tissue augment its outward diffusion. Likewise, measurement of $Ptcco_2$ is made at the tissue level where CO_2 is normally highest. In addition, heating the skin increases CO_2 production and elevates capillary blood Pco_2. As a result of these factors, $Ptcco_2$ overestimates $Paco_2$ by 8 to 15 mm Hg or more. But heating the electrode improves the response time of the monitor and also keeps the skin temperature constant.[61] Changes in $\dot{V}co_2$ and capillary Pco_2 are relatively constant as a result. For this reason, most $PtcCO_2$ monitors use a correction factor to compensate for these alterations in Pco_2 which allows the reading to be closer to actual $Paco_2$.[69]

Accuracy of $Ptcco_2$ Monitor

As with $PtcO_2$ monitoring, the perfusion to the area must be adequate to remove the CO_2 produced by the tissues. Carbon dioxide cannot be allowed to accumulate. When cardiac output is low and tissue perfusion down, the cells become hypoxic and accumulate lactic acid and CO_2. Administration of bicarbonate to correct for lactic acidosis actually results in an increased CO_2 level from the combining of HCO_3^- and lactic acid. $PtcCO_2$ monitoring under these conditions reflects the local tissue CO_2 and not $Paco_2$. The overall variables that affect CO_2 include $Paco_2$, blood pressure, peripheral perfusion, skin thickness, and skin temperature.[69]

Studies have been done on adults and neonates to evaluate the correlation of $PaCO_2$ and $PtcCO_2$. Correlation is good in neonates when the electrode is heated as long as perfusion is normal. Correlation is not as good in adults. Thus, $PtcCO_2$ is a valuable tool in following $Paco_2$ trends, especially in infants.[6,7]

PHYSIOLOGIC DEAD SPACE AND ITS CLINICAL MONITORING

Physiologic dead space is defined as ventilation of lung areas without perfusion and gas exchange. It is divided into anatomic dead space (V_{Dan}) which is comprised of the conductive airways down to the level of the respiratory bronchioles where gas exchange begins, and alveolar dead space (V_{DA}) where alveoli are ventilated but underperfused. In normal persons, physiologic dead space (V_D) and V_{Dan} are nearly equal. Alveolar dead space is not significant.

Anatomic dead space seldom changes in the clinical situation. It can be reduced by introducing an endotracheal tube or by doing a tracheotomy and bypassing the upper airway. It can be artificially increased by adding mechanical dead space, but even these maneuvers, once performed, do not change significantly with time.

In the hospitalized patient, VDA can change in many different situations. It can be responsible for producing hypoxemia and hypercarbia. Patients with increased VDA often have the following characteristic findings: normal lung volumes; normal lung mechanics; increased ventilation (hypoxemic response); normal distribution of ventilation in most cases; uneven distribution of capillary blood flow in the lungs; decreased diffusing capacity; hypoxemia; and normal or decreased $Paco_2$.

The classic dead space disease is pulmonary embolism which reduces the flow in the pulmonary arteries without impeding ventilation. In critically ill patients on mechanical ventilator support, changes in VDA can occur and compromise the patient's ability to receive O_2 into the arteries or eliminate CO_2. It is beneficial to monitor VD in these patients to determine if, in fact, VD is changing. If so, the patient must be treated appropriately.

It was pointed out previously that there is no significant change from the arterial–end-tidal Pco_2 to the arterial–maximum end-expiratory Pco_2 in pulmonary embolism. In addition, progressive decreases in P_{ETCO_2} may occur because of increased VDA. This alone is not conclusive evidence of increased VDA since P_{ETCO_2} will also decrease with increased alveolar ventilation ($\dot{V}_A$) and an improvement in $\dot{V}/\dot{Q}$ matching.

Another way to follow the course of VD changes in ventilated patients is to measure the dead space–tidal volume ratio (VD/VT). The normal VD/VT is 25% to 40%. This value can be calculated from the Enghoff modification of Bohr's equation.[65]

$$V_D/V_T = (Paco_2 - P\bar{E}co_2)/Paco_2$$

where $P\bar{E}co_2$ is the mixed expired partial pressure for carbon dioxide. Figure 9–16 shows a classic example of expired air collection. In this example:

$$Paco_2 = 40 \text{ mm Hg}$$
$$P\bar{E}co_2 = 20 \text{ mm Hg}$$
$$\text{Let } V_T = 500 \text{ mL}$$
$$V_D/V_T = (40 - 20)/40 = 0.50$$

Fifty percent of ventilation is wasted, i.e., unperfused. Since the VT is 500 mL, the VD will be 0.50 × 500 mL, or 250 mL.

Figure 9–17 shows an extra expiratory valve assembly for use in measuring $P\bar{E}co_2$ in mechanically ventilated patients. It eliminates the need for correcting values because of compressible volume due to tubing compliance.[1] Appendix I

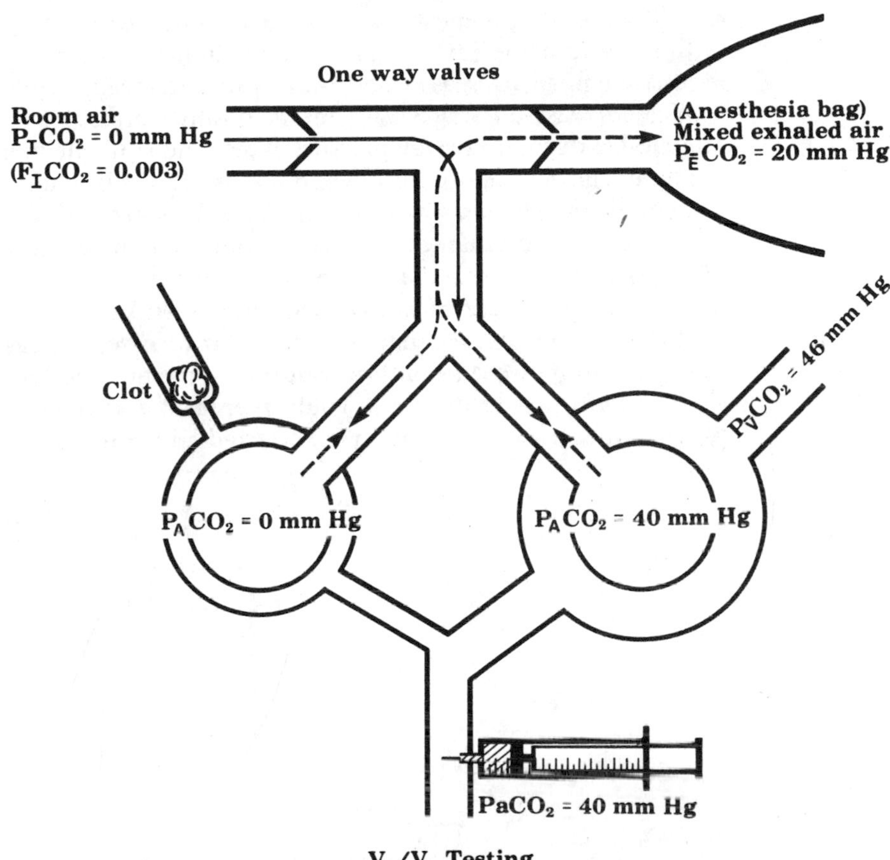

FIG 9–16.
Schematic representation of the procedure for measuring and mixing expired P_{CO_2} and Pa_{CO_2} for the calculation of the dead space–tidal volume (V_D/V_T) ratio.

describes the procedures for V_D/V_T measurement. There is also an equation for use that compenates for compressed gas if the mixed expired sample is collected at the normal expiratory valve[65]:

$$V_D/V_T \text{ corrected} = (Pa_{CO_2} - P\bar{E}_{CO_2} \text{ corrected})/Pa_{CO_2}$$

$$P\bar{E}_{CO_2} \text{ corrected} = V_T/(V_T - V_C) \times P\bar{E}_{CO_2}$$

where Vc is the volume lost due to tubing compliance.

The V_D/V_T ratio can also be estimated by using the graph illustrated in Figure 9–18. The measured minute ventilation ($\dot{V}_E$) and Pa_{CO_2} are plotted on the graph. The V_D/V_T ratio is obtained by noting the isopleth (curve) that coincides with that point. The most common cause of increased VD/VT in respiratory care is the effects of positive pressure ventilation leading to overinflation of well-ventilated areas, decreased perfusion, and decreased cardiac output.

To decrease a rising VD/VT due to positive pressure, the ventilator may be adjusted to decrease airway pressure (Paw) and slow the flow while maintaining $Paco_2$. If VD/VT does not improve, the reason may be due to causes other than the ventilator. The causes of increased VD are listed in Table 9–6.

Patients on mechanical ventilation can have increased $\dot{V}DA$ if high ventilating pressures overexpand alveoli and put pressure on adjacent capillaries reducing effective flow. Other patients with increased VD/VT include those who have COPD and those with pulmonary vascular disease. Increased $\dot{V}DA$ can also be present with increased shunting. Suppose a patient had left lower lobe atelectasis. The perfusion to that area would represent a shunt ($\dot{Q} > \dot{V}$). If this patient were on mechanical ventilation the affected lobe might not be as well ventilated

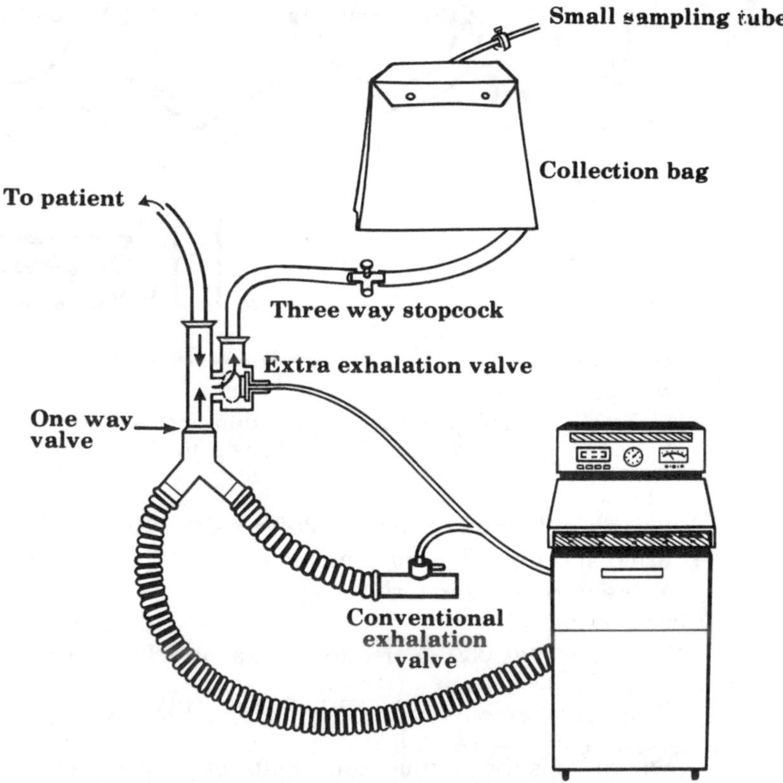

FIG 9–17.
Equipment used for collecting mixed gases from a patient on mechanical ventilation. (From Bageant RA: *Respir Care* 1977; 22:715–725. Used by permission.)

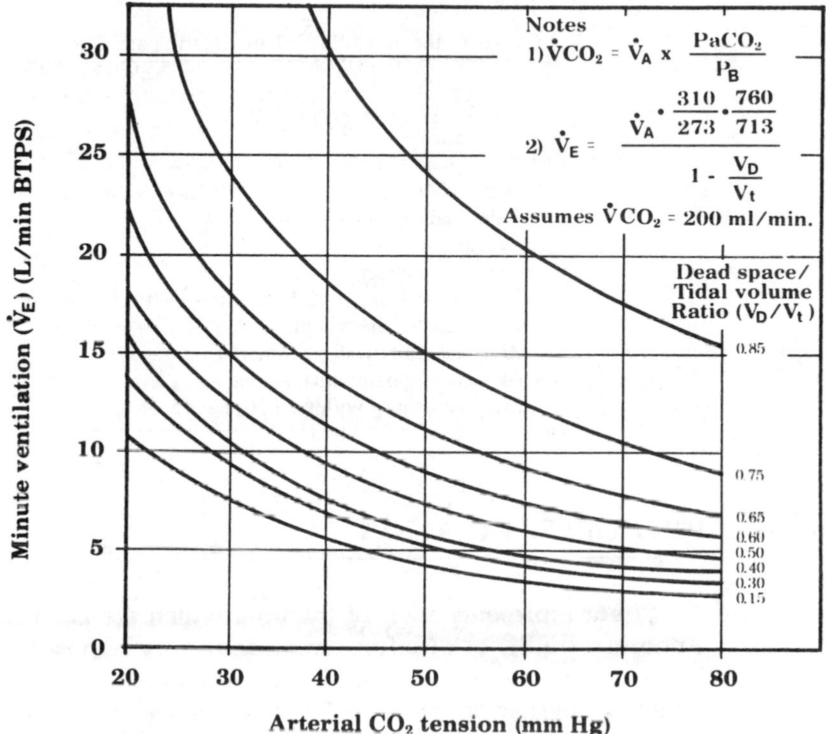

FIG 9–18.

Relationship between ventilation ($\dot{V}_E$) and arterial P_{CO_2} tension (Pa_{CO_2}) for various isopleths of the ratio of dead space to tidal volume (V_D/V_T). The notes in the *upper right hand corner* give the basic assumptions for this relationship. $\dot{V}_{CO_2}$ = CO_2 output; $\dot{V}_A$ = alveolar ventilation; P_B = barometric pressure. To obtain the V_D/V_T, measure the $\dot{V}_E$ and the Pa_{CO_2} and plot these points on the graph. The physiologic V_D/V_T ratio is obtained by noting the isopleth that coincides with this point. To obtain the $\dot{V}_E$ required to achieve a desired Pa_{CO_2}, draw a vertical line from the desired Pa_{CO_2} on the abscissa to the V_D/V_T isopleth obtained in the first step above. Draw a horizontal line from this point to the ordinate to obtain the required $\dot{V}_E$. (From Selecky PA, Wasserman K, Klein M, et al: *Am Rev Respir Dis* 1978; 117:181. Used by permission.)

as other lung areas. Pressurized gas would favor uncompromised areas, reduce their perfusion, and cause a dead space effect.

If a patient with COPD were given therapeutic O_2, it would decrease the pulmonary artery pressure by opening up pulmonary capillaries which were previously constricted due to alveolar hypoxemia. These newly opened capillaries, however, may cause blood to flow past unventilated alveoli and could shunt blood away from areas of better ventilation. The result is increased $\dot{V}_{DA}$. It is important, then, to serially monitor V_D/V_T in patients who are suspected of having dead space disorders since a variety of situations can increase V_D.

TABLE 9–6.
Causes of Increased Physiologic Dead Space (V_D)

Increased V_D
Positive pressure ventilation
Hypopnea
Tachypnea
Increased V_{DA}
Pulmonary emboli
Vascular tumors
Increased V_D effect
Positive pressure ventilation (increased intrapleural pressure)
Decreased cardiac output
Alveolar septal wall pneumonia
Atelectasis, pneumonia, edema
Increased shunt with COPD patients on O_2

CLINICAL SHUNT DETERMINATION

Shunt represents areas of the lung which are perfused but not ventilated. Abnormal shunts can lead to severe, refractory hypoxemia. For this reason it is important to monitor the shunt fraction in severely hypoxemic, critically ill patients. Physiologic shunt ($\dot{Q}s/\dot{Q}t$) (anatomic shunt plus capillary shunt) can be estimated using the clinical shunt equation:

$$\dot{Q}/\dot{Q}t = \frac{[P(A - a)O_2] \times 0.003}{[C(a - v)O_2] + ([P(A - a)O_2] \times 0.003)}$$

Using the factor $[P(A - a)O_2 \times 0.003]$ converts the reading from mm Hg to vol % (mL/100 mL), so that it becomes $C(A - a)O_2$ or the alveolar-arterial oxygen content difference.

The arteriovenous oxygen content difference $[C(a - v)O_2]$ is often given the value of 3.5 vol %, the approximate value in a critically ill patient.[14] Appendix J gives an example of a clinical shunt equation.

Acute hypoxemia accompanied by increased shunt shows that an intrapulmonary pathologic change has occurred. Sometimes mobilization of secretions or treatment with bronchodilator therapy and O_2 can help correct $\dot{V}/\dot{Q}$ mismatching, decrease shunt, and improve oxygenation. In true $\dot{V}/\dot{Q}$ inequality, increasing the F_{IO_2} will decrease the percent shunt and increase Pa_{O_2}. In true shunting, however, no matter how high the F_{IO_2}, there is never an improvement in gas exchange at the level of the shunt, and hypoxemia remains severe. Hypoxemia refractory to increases in F_{IO_2} suggests that a true shunt exists and the cause of the shunt needs to be corrected. The use of positive end-expiratory pressure (PEEP) or continuous positive airway pressure (CPAP) may be of benefit in treating hypoxemia associated with capillary shunt (see Chapter 10).

SUMMARY

This chapter has reviewed the techniques of pulse oximetry, capnometry, transcutaneous gas monitoring, and V_D/V_T, and shunt determinations. These all have value in the monitoring of certain critically ill patients and patients on mechanical ventilatory support. The type of patient population and the device indicated varies. For example, pulse oximetry is becoming very popular for monitoring a wide variety of patient populations, not just those in ICU. Capnometry has been primarily used in ICU and the operating room. Transcutaneous monitoring of CO_2 and O_2 is used mostly in newborn ICU monitoring. Calculation of V_D is seldom done at the present time, but remains an option for determining major changes in CO_2 and ventilation status. Clinical shunt is generally determined in hemodynamically unstable and in severely hypoxemic patients in the ICU, particularly those requiring PEEP or CPAP therapy.

STUDY QUESTIONS

1. Pulse oximetry is used to measure what two parameters?
2. What two physical principles are the basis for the operation of the pulse oximeter?
3. List the partial pressure of oxygen associated with each of the following saturations: 100%, 97%, 90%, 80%, 75%, and 50%.
4. Describe the basic principle of operation of the pulse oximeter.
5. How are pulse oximetry readings affected by abnormal hemoglobins, such as HbCO?
6. What does a capnometer measure?
7. What are the two types of capnometers?
8. Explain the normal components of a capnogram.
9. What changes in P_{ETCO_2} occur during hyperventilation and hypoventilation?
10. During CPR the P_{ETCO_2} monitor reads 30 mm Hg briefly and then drops to near zero and stays there. What could be the problem?
11. Give the normal value for $P(a - ET)CO_2$.
12. List four disorders in which this value is greater than normal.

13. What is the advantage for measuring arterial–maximum end-expiratory Pco_2 measurements?
14. What are the principles of operation of the $PtcO_2$ and $PtcCO_2$ monitors?
15. Describe how heating the skin affects CO_2 and O_2 in the skin.
16. What are the normal Pao_2–$PtcO_2$ and $Paco_2$–$PtcCO_2$ gradients?
17. Give the equations for calculating the VD/VT ratio and clinical shunt.

ANSWERS TO STUDY QUESTIONS

1. Spo_2 and pulse rate.
2. Oximetry and plethysmography. Microprocessor-based instrumentation is also involved.
3. The Po_2 values are: ≥150 mm Hg, 90 to 100 mm Hg, 60 mm Hg, 46 to 48 mm Hg, 40 mm Hg, and 27 mm Hg (P_{50}).
4. Pulse oximeters operate on the basic principle that HbO_2 and HHb have different light absorption characteristics. Oxyhemoglobin absorbs very little red light (wavelength 660 nm), but absorbs more infrared light (wavelength 920 nm). Deoxyhemoglobin, on the other hand, absorbs very little infrared light, but tends to absorb more red light.
5. The pulse oximeter looks only at functional hemoglobin or that able to carry O_2. It gives the Spo_2 based on the percentage of "functional" hemoglobin that is carrying O_2. For example, if there are 16 g of hemoglobin, and 5 g are HbCO, and one is HHb (reduced hemoglobin), the functional level is 11 g. If 10 g are HbO, then Spo_2 will read 91%. The actual percent saturation evaluated by a co-oximeter would be 10/16, or 63%.
6. A capnometer measures CO_2.
7. The two types of capnometers are mainstream, which is placed at the spot where CO_2 is being measured, and sidestream, which suctions off a sample of air and takes it to the capnometer to be measured.
8. At the beginning of exhalation, the VDan empties. This contains no (or very little) CO_2 so it reads zero. As exhalation progresses, the curve rises. This occurs as dead space and alveolar gas mix. The curve then plateaus. This represents alveolar air. Alveolar CO_2 is about equal to $Paco_2$. As inhalation begins, one draws in room air, which is low in CO_2, and the curve drops back to zero.
9. During hyperventilation $PETco_2$ is lower than normal, while during hypoventilation it is higher than normal.
10. This may be an esophageal intubation. Carbon dioxide may be high to begin with (exhaled gas ventilation into the stomach) but will drop to near zero and stay there afterward. The operator could disconnect the capnometer and blow into it to be sure it was still working and also recheck breath sounds to make sure they are present in the lungs.

11. The normal $P(a - ET)CO_2$ is ≤ 7 mm Hg.
12. This will be higher than normal in COPD, left heart failure, pulmonary embolism, and shock.
13. The advantage of measuring arterial–maximum end-expiratory PCO_2 is that it can help differentiate COPD, left ventricular failure, and pulmonary embolism. The last is the only one whose value will not approach zero at maximum exhalation.
14. The $PtcO_2$ monitor works on the principle of the Clark electrode. The $PtcCO_2$ monitor works on the Stow-Severinghaus principle.
15. Heating the skin increases arterialization of the capillaries, increases metabolism of local cells, and raises the partial pressures of gases. Oxygen arterialization and higher partial pressures raise its value, while a higher metabolism results in its consumption and lowers it. For CO_2, arterialization gives it a value close to $PaCO_2$. Increasing metabolism increases its level as does heating.
16. The normal PaO_2–$PtcO_2$ gradient is about 5 mm Hg in adults and less than this in infants. The $PtcCO_2$ gradient is 8 to 15 mm Hg higher than $PaCO_2$.
17. The equation for the V_D/V_T ratio is $(PaCO_2 - P\bar{E}CO_2)/PaCO_2$. The clinical shunt equation is:

$$\dot{Q}s/\dot{Q}t = \frac{[P(A - a)O_2] \times 0.003}{[C(a - v)O_2] + ([P(A - a)O_2] \times 0.003)}$$

REFERENCES

1. Bageant RA: Bedside techniques for calculating deadspace/tidal volume ratio (VD/Vt) and pulmonary shunt ($\dot{Q}s/\dot{Q}t$). *Respir Care* 1977; 22:715–725.
2. Balk RA, Bone RC: Patient monitoring in the intensive care unit, in Burton GG, Hodgkin JE, Ward JJ (eds): *Respiratory Care: A Guide to Clinical Practice,* ed 3. Philadelphia, JB Lippincott Co, 1991, pp 705–717.
3. Baumberger JD, Goodfriend RB: Determination of arterial oxygen tension in man by equilibration through intact skin. *Fed Proc* 1958; 10:10.
4. Beauchamp GG: Pulmonary function testing procedures, in Barnes T (ed): *Respiratory Care Practice.* St Louis, Mosby-Year Book, Inc, 1988, pp 32–92.
5. Burton GG, Hodgkin JE, Ward JJ: *Respiratory Care: A Guide to Clinical Practice,* ed 3. Philadelphia, JB Lippincott Co, 1991.
6. Cabal L, Cruz EB, Siassi B, et al: Skin surface PCO_2/PO_2 in preterm infants with RDS without cardiovascular compromise (abstract). *Clin Res* 1980; 28:1.
7. Cabal L, Hadgman J, Siassi B, et al: Factors affecting heated transcutaneous PO_2 and unheated transcutaneous PO_2 in preterm infants. *Crit Care Med* 1980; 9:298–304.
8. Cohen AJ, Slavin RE, Frantz ID, et al: Cutaneous carbon dioxide measurements with heated and unheated electrodes in infants (abstract). *Respir Care* 1980; 25:12.

9. Cohen A, Taeusch HW, Stanton C: Usefulness of the arterial/alveolar oxygen tension ratio in the care of infants with respiratory distress syndrome. *Respir Care* 1983; 28:169–173.
10. Conway M, Durbin GM, Ingram D, et al: Continuous monitoring of arterial oxygen tension using a catheter-tip polarographic electrode in infants. *Pediatrics* 1976; 57:244–250.
11. Craig KC, Pierson DJ: Expired gas collection for deadspace calculations: A comparison of two methods. *Respir Care* 1979; 24:435–437.
12. Darin J: Capnography. *Curr Rev Respir Ther* 1981; 3:146–150.
13. Deshpande VM, Pilbeam SP, Dixon RJ: *A Comprehensive Review in Respiratory Care.* Norwalk, Conn, Appleton & Lange, 1988.
14. Dimas S, Kacmarek RM: Intrapulmonary shunting. *Curr Rev Respir Ther* 1978; 1:35–47.
15. Dixon RJ: *Assessment of the Pulmonary Patient.* Denver, Multi-Media Publishing, Inc, 1984.
16. Douglas ME, Downs JB, Dannemiller FJ: Changes in pulmonary venous admixture with varying inspired oxygen. *Anesth Analg* 1976; 55:688–693.
17. Emrico J: Transcutaneous oxygen monitoring in neonates. *Respir Care* 1979; 24: 601–605.
18. Eriksson L, Wollmer P, Olsson CG, et al: Diagnosis of pulmonary embolism based upon alveolar dead space analysis. *Chest* 1989; 96:357–362.
19. Evans NTS, Naylor PFD: The systemic oxygen supply to the surface of human skin. *Respir Physiol* 1967; 3:21–37.
20. Fenner A, Muller R, Busse HG, et al: Transcutaneous determination of arterial oxygen tension. *Pediatrics* 1975; 55:224–232.
21. Fernandez A, de la Cal, MA, Esteban A, et al: Simplified method for measuring physiologic VD/Vt in patients on mechanical ventilation. *Crit Care Med* 1983; 11:823.
22. Gilbert R, Keighley JF: The arterial/alveolar oxygen tension ratio: An index of gas exchange applicable to varying inspired oxygen concentrations. *Am Rev Respir Dis* 1974; 109:142–145.
23. Goddard P, Keith I, Marcovitch H, et al: Use of continuous recording intravascular oxygen electrode in the newborn. *Arch Dis Child* 1974; 49:853–860.
24. Gravenstein JS, Paulus DA, Hayes TJ: *Capnography in Clinical Practice.* Boston, Butterworth Publ, 1989.
25. Harris K: Noninvasive monitoring of gas exchange. *Respir Care* 1987; 32:544–557.
26. Hatle L, Rokseth R: The arterial-to-end-expiratory carbon dioxide tension gradient in acute pulmonary embolism and other cardiopulmonary diseases. *Chest* 1974; 66:352–357.
27. Hauser CJ, Harley DP: Transcutaneous gas tension monitoring in the management of intraoperative apnea. *Crit Care Med* 1983; 11:830–831.
28. Hebrank DR, Mentelos RA: Non-invasive transcutaneous carbon dioxide monitoring. *Med Instrum* 1981; 14:203–206.
29. Hess D: Capnometry and capnography: Technical aspects, physiologic aspects and clinical applications. *Respir Care* 1990; 35:557–576.
30. Hess D, Maxwell C: Which is the best index of oxygenation – $P(A - a)O_2$, PaO_2/PAO_2 or PaO_2/FIO_2. *Respir Care* 1985; 30:961–963.

31. Huch A, Huch R: Transcutaneous, non-invasive monitoring of PO_2. *Hosp Pract* 1976; (June):43–52.
32. Huch R, Huch A, Albani M, et al: Transcutaneous PO_2 monitoring in routine management of infants and children with cardiorespiratory problems. *Pediatrics* 1976; 57:681–690.
33. Huch A, Huch R, Arner B, et al: Continuous transcutaneous oxygen tension measured with a heated electrode. *Scand J Clin Lab Invest* 1973; 31:269–275.
34. Kacmarek RM: Noninvasive monitoring techniques in the ventilated patient, in Kacmarek RM, Stoller JK (eds): *Current Respiratory Care.* Philadelphia, BC Decker, Inc, 1988, pp 182–187.
35. Kacmarek RM, Dimas S: Pulmonary deadspace: Concepts and clinical application. *Curr Rev Respir Ther* 1979; 1:147–151.
36. Kalenda Z, Kramer J: Periodic respiration. The capnographic interpretation. *Anaesthetist* 1979; 28:368–372.
37. Kirby RR, Banner MJ, Downs JB: *Clinical Applications of Ventilatory Support,* ed 2. New York, Churchill Livingstone Inc, 1990.
38. Krouskop RW, Cabatu EE, Chelliah BP, et al: Accuracy and clinical utility of an oxygen saturation catheter. *Crit Care Med* 1983; 11:744–749.
39. Levesque PR, Rosenberg H: Rapid bedside estimation of wasted ventilation (VD/Vt). *Anaesthesia* 1975; 42:98–100.
40. Litton Medical Electronics: Document #227-11-03 BA (USA)-7802. *Oxymonitor.* SM 361.
41. Malalis L, Bhat R, Vidyasagar D: Comparison of intravascular PO_2 with transcutaneous and PaO_2 values. *Crit Care Med* 1983; 11:110–113.
42. Martin L, Jeffreys B: Use of a mini-computer for storing, reporting, and interpreting arterial blood gases/pH and pleural fluid pH. *Respir Care* 1983; 28:301–308.
43. Martin RJ: Transcutaneous monitoring: Instrumentation and clinical applications. *Respir Care* 1990; 35:577–583.
44. Maxwell C, Hess D, Shefet D: Use of the arterial/alveolar oxygen tension ratio to predict the inspired oxygen concentration needed for a desired arterial oxygen tension. *Respir Care* 1984; 29:1135–1139.
45. McNabb L, Globerson T, St Clair R, et al: The arterial-end tidal PCO_2 difference in patients on ventilators (abstract). *Chest* 1981; 80:381.
46. McPeck M: The impact of computer-age technology on respiratory therapy. *Respir Care* 1982; 27:855–865.
47. Nellcor, Inc: *Principles of Pulse Oximetry,* Hayward, Calif, Clinical Education, Nellcor, Inc, 1988.
48. Nelson EJ, Morton EA, Hunter PM: *Critical Care Respiratory Therapy.* Boston, Little, Brown & Co, 1983.
49. Nelson RD, Wilkins RL, Jacobson WK, et al: Supranormal PvO_2 in the presence of tissue hypoxia: A case report. 1983; 28:191–194.
50. Nuzzo PF, Anton WR: Practical applications of capnography. *Respir Ther,* 1986, Nov/Dec, pp 12–17.
51. Osborn JJ: Monitoring respiratory function. *Crit Care Med* 1974; 2:217–220.
52. Peabody JL: The effect of tolazoline in transcutaneous PO_2 monitoring. *Pediatr Res* 1976; 10:430.
53. Peris LV, Boix JH, Salom JV, et al: Clinical use of the arterial/alveolar oxygen tension ratio. *Crit Care Med* 1983; 11:888–891.

54. Peters RM, Brimm JE, Utley JR: Predicting the need for prolonged ventilatory support in adult cardiac patients. *J Thorac Cardiovasc Surg* 1979; 77:175–182.
55. Petty TL: *Clinical Pulse Oximetry*. Louisville, Ky, Ohmeda, 1986, pp 1–9.
56. Pollitzer MJ, Soutter LP, Osmund E, et al: Continuous monitoring of arterial oxygen tension in infants: Four years of experience with an intravascular oxygen electrode. *Pediatrics* 1980; 66:31–36.
57. Richman KA, Jobes DR, Schwalb AJ: Continuous in vivo blood gas determination in man: Reliability and safety of new device. *Anesthesiology* 1980; 52:313–317.
58. Rooth G: Transcutaneous oxygen tension measurements in newborn infants. *Pediatrics* 1975; 55:232.
59. Rooth G, Hedstand U, Tyden S: The validity of the transcutaneous oxygen tension method in adults. *Crit Care Med* 1976; 4:162.
60. Selecky PA, Wasserman K, Klein M, et al: A graphic approach to asssessing interrelationships among minute ventilation, arterial carbon dioxide tension, and ratio of physiologic deadspace to tidal volume in patients on respirators. *Am Rev Respir Dis* 1984; 117:181–184.
61. Severinghaus JW: Transcutaneous blood gas analysis. *Respir Care* 1982; 27:152–159.
62. Severinghaus JW, Astrup PB: History of blood gas analysis. VI. Oximetry. *J Clin Monit* 1986; 2:270–288.
63. Shapiro BA, Cane RD, Harrison RA, et al: Changes in intrapulmonary shunting with administration of 100 percent oxygen. *Chest* 1980; 77:138–141.
64. Silage DA, Maxwell C: A lung diffusion determination/interpretation program for hand-held computers. *Respir Care* 1983; 28:1587–1590.
65. Smith ER: Measurement of physiological deadspace during mechanical ventilation. *Respir Care* 1977; 22:1341–1342.
66. Suwa K, Geffin B, Pontoppidan H, et al: A nomogram for deadspace requirement during prolonged artificial ventilation. *Anesthesiology* 1968; 29:1206–1210.
67. Swanstrom S, Elisaga VI, Cardona L, et al: Transcutaneous PO_2 measurements in seriously ill newborn infants. *Arch Dis Child* 1975; 50:913–919.
68. Swedlow DB: Capnometry and capnography: The anesthesia disaster early warning system. *Semin Anesthesia* 1986; 5:194–205.
69. Taylor W: Transcutaneous and transconjunctival blood gas monitoring. *Prob Respir Care* 1989; 2:240–254.
70. Tremper KK, Barker SJ: Pulse oximetry. *Anesthesiology* 1989; 70:98–108.
71. Tremper KK, Wakman K, Bowman R, et al: Continuous transcutaneous oxygen monitoring during respiratory failure, cardiac decompensation, cardiac arrest and CPR. *Crit Care Med* 1980; 8:377–381.
72. van Genderingen HR, Gravenstein N: Capnogram artifact during high airway pressures caused by water trap. *Anesth Analg* 1987; 66:185–187.
73. Watts CE: Carbon dioxide elimination and capnography. *Respir Ther* 1980; 10:107–113.
74. Weinger MB, Brimm JE: End-tidal carbon dioxide as a measure of arterial carbon dioxide during intermittent mandatory ventilation. *J Clin Monit* 1987; 3:73–79.
75. Welch JP, DeCesare R, Hess D: Pulse oximetry: Instrumentation and clinical applications. *Respir Care* 1990; 35:584–602.
76. Zupan J, Martin M, Benumof JL: End-tidal CO_2 excretion waveform and error with gas sampling line leak. *Anesth Analg* 1988; 67:579–581.

Chapter **10**

Improving Oxygenation: Positive End-Expiratory Pressure, Continuous Positive Airway Pressure, and Inverse Ratio Ventilation

On completion of this chapter the reader will be able to:

1. Define the following terms: PEEP, CPAP, IPAP, EPAP, CPPB, minimum PEEP, moderate PEEP, maximum PEEP.
2. List the characteristics of a patient in need of PEEP therapy.
3. Give the relative and absolute contraindications for PEEP or CPAP.
4. Describe the pathophysiology of the disease process called ARDS.
5. Explain the effects of PEEP on FRC, pleural pressure, vascular pressures, and lung water.
6. Given data from a PEEP study, select the optimal PEEP level.
7. List the parameters measured during a PEEP study.
8. Describe the effect of PEEP or CPAP on the measurement of pulmonary vascular pressures.
9. Discuss the use of positive pressure in congestive heart failure.

10. List and describe the effects of PEEP or CPAP on cardiac function.
11. Name four methods of applying PEEP or CPAP to the upper airway.
12. Compare the function of a flow resistor with that of a threshold resistor.
13. Give three examples of gravity-dependent PEEP valves and three examples of nongravity-dependent PEEP valves.
14. Draw a graph showing the difference in airway pressure waveforms with CPAP and with sPEEP and explain the effect of each on work of breathing.
15. From a drawing, identify a freestanding CPAP system and a freestanding demand flow sPEEP system.
16. Describe the use of PEEP with assisted ventilation, IMV, SIMV, PC, and PS.
17. Explain the procedure for weaning from PEEP or CPAP.
18. Compare the effects of mean airway pressure and flow patterns on tissue oxygenation.
19. Define PCIRV and VCIRV.
20. Describe three methods of obtaining IRV on a conventional volume-controlled ventilator.

IMPROVING OXYGENATION: PEEP, CPAP AND IRV

One of the major problems associated with ventilation of patients with adult respiratory distress syndrome (ARDS) and similar lung problems is oxygenation. One method for treating this is increasing the fractional concentration of oxygen of inspired gas (F_{IO_2}). But this has the associated problems of oxygen toxicity at high levels of administration. A commonly and widely used alternative is positive end-expiratory pressure (PEEP) or continuous positive airway pressure (CPAP) therapy. Recent evidence shows that this increases the risk of lung injury (see Chapter 7). An alternative strategy is to use inverse ratio ventilation (IRV). This approach is still experimental and requires more extensive research for proof of its superiority.

In this chapter the acceptable practice of using PEEP or CPAP therapy is discussed, including indications for its use, methods of administration, and associated complications. A brief section includes the more recently applied method of IRV using both pressure-controlled and volume-controlled ventilation.

HISTORY OF PEEP AND CPAP

While the history of PEEP and CPAP goes as far back as the 1870s, use of this form of therapy did not become popular until the mid-20th century. During the early 1970s investigators began extensive use of PEEP.[51, 57, 60, 99] It was found to improve oxygenation in patients with severe refractory hypoxemia, increased intrapulmonary shunt, decreased functional residual capacity (FRC), and reduced lung compliance. This mode of therapy was also applied to patients who were breathing spontaneously without the aid of mechanical positive pressure breaths. This was referred to as CPAP.

The extensive use of positive airway pressure during the past two decades and the unique way in which this mode of therapy alone affects physiologic response in the body in comparison to mechanical ventilatory support warrants some discussion. Included in this discussion is a definition of related terms; the technical aspects of their application; the indications, complications, and contraindications; finding optimal PEEP levels; weaning from PEEP and CPAP; and prophylactic PEEP.

GOAL OF PEEP OR CPAP THERAPY

The goal of PEEP and CPAP therapy is to enhance tissue oxygenation and maintain an arterial oxygen partial pressure (Pa_{O_2}) above 60 mm Hg, where saturation is 90% at normal pH, using less than 40% inspired oxygen while sustaining cardiovascular function. The availability of O_2 to the tissues can be expressed by the term *oxygen transport* which is the product of cardiac output (CO) and arterial oxygen content (Ca_{O_2}).

TERMINOLOGY

When one becomes familiar with trends in ventilatory support, one is faced with a profusion of abbreviations used to describe positive airway pressure therapy: CPPB, CPPV, CPAP, PEEP, IPAP, EPAP.[101] These are a few of the terms related to a method of supporting the respiratory system by applying positive airway pressure, or PEEP, in order to maintain pressure above ambient at the end of exhalation either during spontaneous breathing or during mechanically supported ventilation. Whether the patient is breathing spontaneously or not, a key concept to remember is that PEEP only describes the pressure on exhalation. During inhalation the pressure can be either positive, zero, or negative (Fig 10–1). CPAP is pressure above ambient maintained during spontaneous ventilation. This means that expiratory positive airway pressure (EPAP) and inspiratory positive airway pressure (IPAP) are both present with IPAP being a little less than EPAP.[33] IPAP and EPAP levels can be varied independently on some mechanical devices. It is now popular to use these in the home care of patients (see Chapter 14). CPAP and PEEP have replaced the terms CPPB and CPPV in the respiratory care vernacular. In the literature, CPAP and CPPB are often used interchangeably.

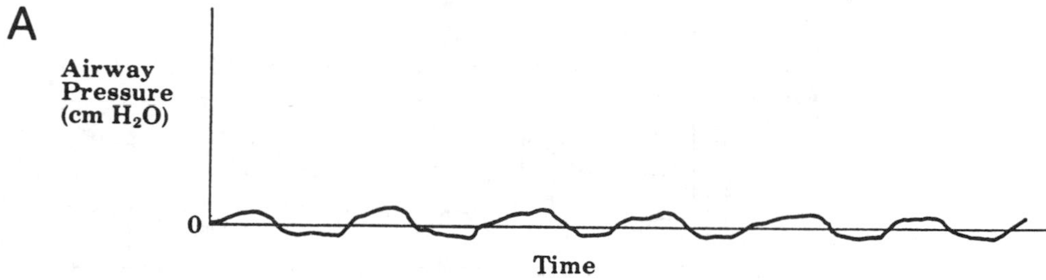

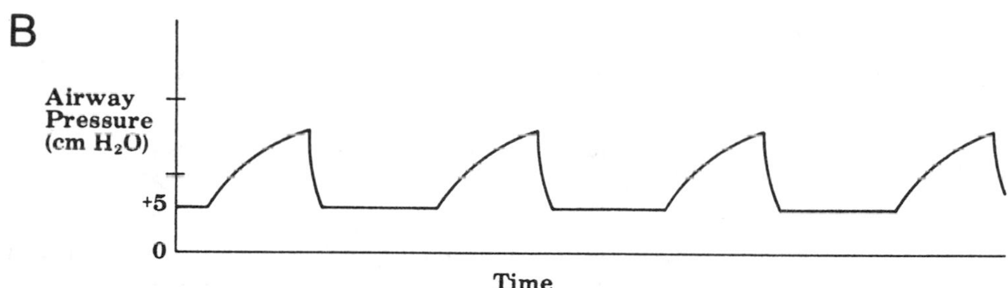

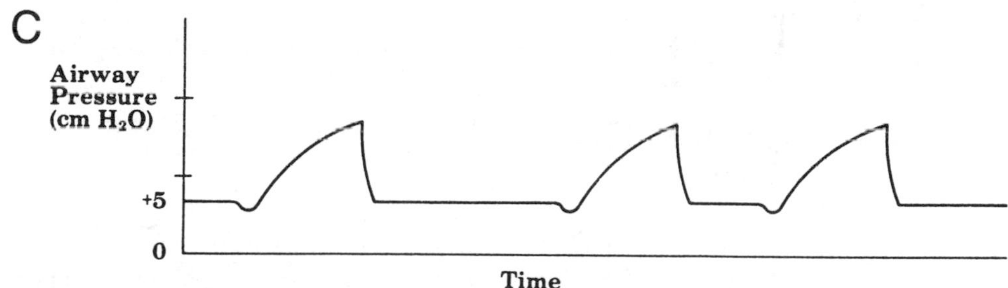

FIG 10–1.
Curves represent airway pressure in centimeters of water graphed against time. **A,** patient is breathing spontaneously against ambient pressures. The curve dips low during inspiration and rises during expiration. **B,** curve shows the pattern that occurs during controlled ventilation (IPPV) with PEEP. The patient makes no spontaneous efforts to breathe. The pressure remains above zero at all times. The pressures rise during a mechanically delivered breath. This mode is also called CPPV and IPAP plus EPAP. **C,** assisted ventilation with PEEP is shown in this curve. When the patient makes an inspiratory effort, indicated by a slight downward deflection of the curve, the ventilator detects the pressure change and delivers a positive pressure machine breath. Pressures remain above ambient. This can also be termed IPAP plus EPAP. (*Continued.*)

D

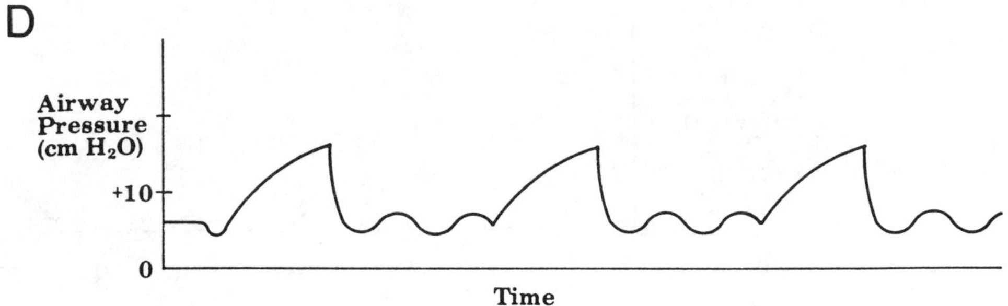

E

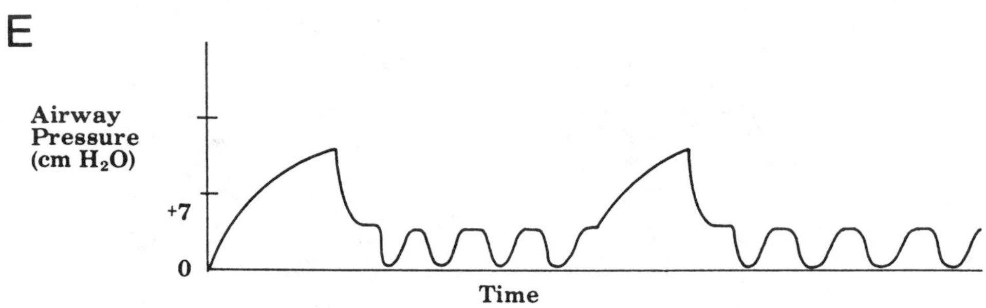

F

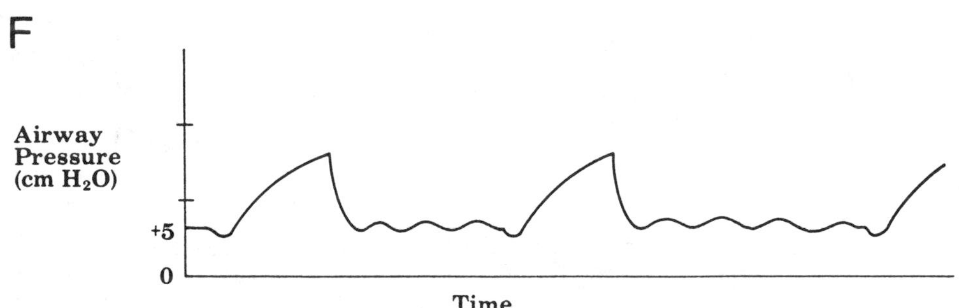

FIG 10–1 (cont.).
D, curve shows IMV used with PEEP. The patient breathes spontaneously between machine breaths at pressures that are above zero. The machine-delivered breath occurs at fixed time intervals. This is also referred to as IMV with CPAP. **E,** in this graph IMV is used with PEEP; however, during spontaneous inspiration the flow of gas to the patient is reduced and the airway pressures drop to zero or slightly below zero. This increases the work of breathing. The end of exhalation is above baseline (EPAP) and machine-delivered breaths are positive. **F,** curve shows the airway pressures that occur with SIMV and PEEP. During spontaneous breathing pressures are above zero. The machine-delivered breath occurs when the patient makes an inspiratory effort after a certain amount of time has elapsed. This is sometimes called SIMV with CPAP. (*Continued.*)

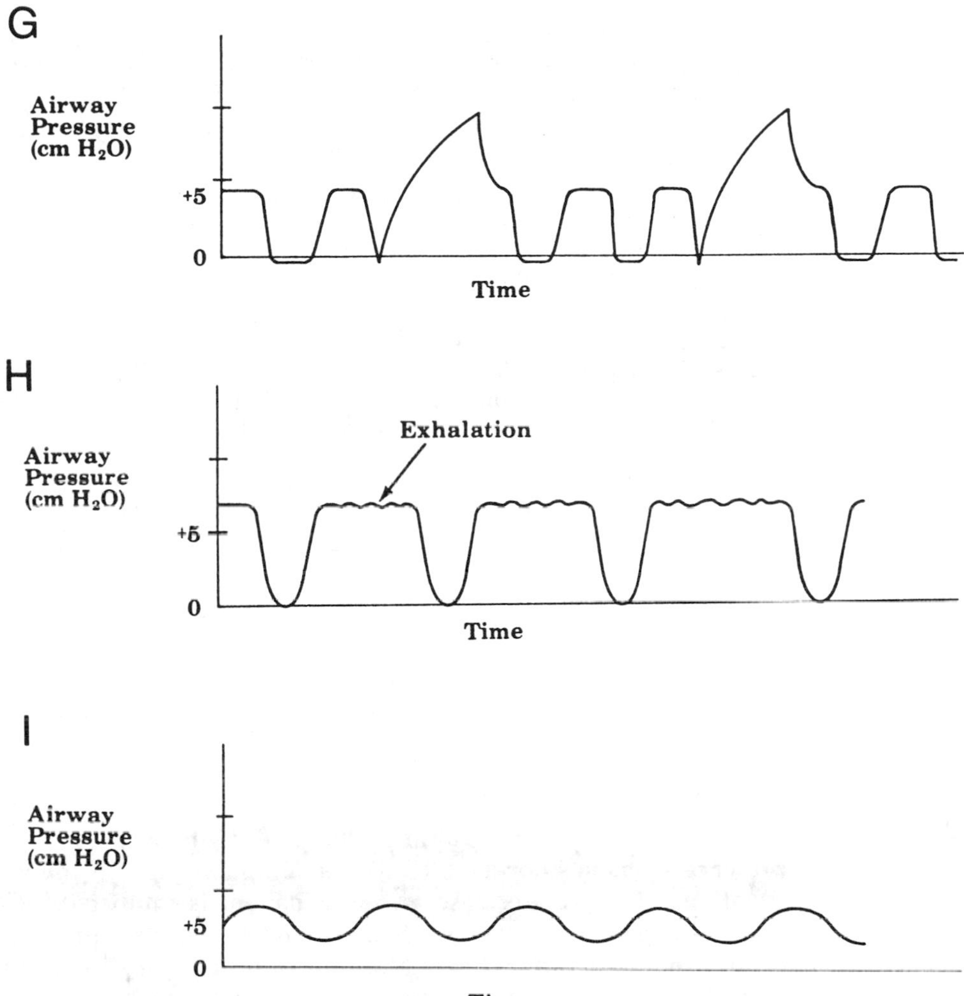

FIG 10–1 (cont.).
G, SIMV with PEEP or EPAP is shown here. During spontaneous breathing the patient inspires to ambient pressures or slightly less. During spontaneous exhalation the pressures rise to the set PEEP value. When it is time for a machine-delivered breath, the ventilator waits until a spontaneous effort detects the pressure change and delivers a positive pressure machine breath. This mode increases the work of breathing. **H,** curve here is similar to CPAP **(I).** The patient is spontaneously breathing and receives no machine breaths. During inspiration pressures drop to ambient or below. During exhalation, pressures rise to the set PEEP value. This is referred to as spontaneous PEEP (sPEEP) or EPAP. **I,** during CPAP the pressure remains above ambient at all times as the patient breathes spontaneously. This requires less work of breathing than that shown in **H.** This is also referred to as CPPB or EPAP plus IPAP. *(Continued.)*

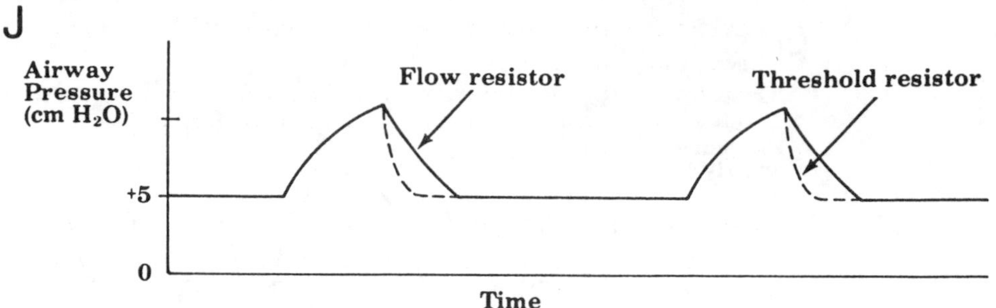

FIG 10–1 (cont.).
J, curve demonstrates IPPV plus PEEP with two different expiratory flow curves following the machine breath. When a flow resistor–type of PEEP device is used, the positive pressures remain in the lung longer. When a threshold resistor–type PEEP device is used, pressure leaves the lung more rapidly (*dashed line*).

RANGES OF PEEP

There are three levels or ranges of PEEP that are clinically employed: minimum or low PEEP, moderate PEEP, and high or maximum PEEP.[35, 96]

Minimum PEEP

It is believed that a normal glottic response is present which helps to preserve a person's normal FRC. This assumption explains the fact that, in most situations, the FRC decreases when a patient is intubated.[96] Clinically, some patients appear to do better when minimum PEEP is employed than when it is not used at all and end-expiratory pressures are zero.[55] For example, patients with chronic obstructive pulmonary disease (COPD) often use pursed lips breathing to prevent early airway closure and air trapping. When an endotracheal tube is inserted in these patients, they can no longer use this technique. Use of low levels of PEEP, 1 to 5 cm H_2O, seems to improve their clinical picture, particularly during weaning from mechanical ventilatory support.[55] For this reason, minimum PEEP is sometimes called "physiologic" PEEP.

Grunting is often observed in infants who have hyaline membrane disease. When these infants are intubated, they can no longer perform the grunting maneuver. Minimum PEEP seems to benefit these infants.

Minimum PEEP can be selected for either spontaneously breathing patients or those on mechanical ventilation in the following circumstances[96, 97]:

1. For those with a drop in PaO_2 attributed to the removal of low levels of PEEP (<5 cm H_2O).
2. For those adults on mechanical ventilatory support with low intermittent mandatory ventilation (IMV) rates (<4 breaths/min).
3. For those with significant COPD.

Since minimum PEEP is of a low level, it is not considered a problem in terms of inducing cardiopulmonary complications that can sometimes be associated with positive pressure breathing; however, this low PEEP level is not necessary for all patients.

When a patient is ready for weaning and extubation from mechanical ventilation, but becomes hypoxemic and clinically deteriorates whenever PEEP is removed, then it may be appropriate to consider use of low levels of CPAP. Another alternative is extubation of the patient. The use of mask CPAP can still provide the end-expiratory pressures if it becomes necessary. Often, CPAP is not necessary and the patient simply needs to have the endotracheal tube removed.

Moderate PEEP

Moderate PEEP is in the range of 5 to 20 cm H_2O. It is used in the treatment of refractory hypoxemia caused by increased intrapulmonary shunting that is accompanied by a decreased FRC and decreased compliance. It is the most common range of PEEP used.[17, 35]

Maximum PEEP

Values greater than 20 cm H_2O are considered "high" PEEP. This range of PEEP is beneficial in a small percentage of patients who require PEEP.

Optimal PEEP

In 1975 Suter and his coauthors[108] coined the term "best" PEEP. Since then, other authors have used the terms "optimum" PEEP[17] and "therapeutic" PEEP. Optimal PEEP is the level at which the maximum beneficial effects of PEEP occur, i.e., increased O_2 transport, increased FRC, increased compliance, and decreased shunt. This level of PEEP is optimal without producing profound cardiopulmonary side effects: decreased venous return, decreased CO, decreased blood pressure, increased shunting, increased dead space–tidal volume ratio (V_D/V_T), and barotrauma. It is considered optimal when done at safe levels of inspired O_2 (FIO_2 <0.40). It is important to note that optimal PEEP correlates with criteria other than PaO_2 alone.[35] Determining when optimal PEEP has been achieved is discussed later in this chapter.

INDICATIONS FOR PEEP OR CPAP

Some patients with acute respiratory insufficiency have severe refractory hypoxemia. Often they can maintain ventilation well enough to have a normal or even a low partial pressure of arterial carbon dioxide ($Paco_2$). The hypocarbia is attributed in this situation to hyperventilation caused by hypoxemia. These patients often have severe systemic injury such as multiple trauma, severe burns, sepsis, or aspiration, alone or in combination. The severe systemic injury results in alveolar edema, alveolar collapse, interstitial pulmonary edema, decreased FRC, reduced lung compliance, increased intrapulmonary shunting, and, consequently, severe refractory hypoxemia.

This multiple lung problem does not seem to benefit from mechanical ventilatory support alone. While the collapsed alveoli may reopen during positive pressure inspiration, the expiratory phase allows the unstable alveoli and airways to recollapse. Since about two thirds of the respiratory cycle is spent in expiration, blood passes areas of alveoli that are collapsed during this time.

PEEP maintains pressures above ambient during the expiratory phase of ventilation and helps prevent the collapse of the small airways and alveoli. The edema-filled alveoli may have their volumes partially air-filled with this technique as well. The FRC is increased both by recruitment of collapsed alveoli and by maintenance of higher lung volumes. This enhances lung compliance and gas distribution, reduces the shunt effect of the venous admixture, and helps improve oxygenation. Table 10–1 identifies the characteristics of a patient in need of PEEP therapy.

CPAP has indications similar to PEEP. The primary difference between the two is that CPAP requires that the patient provide the work of breathing at all times. If the patient is able to breathe spontaneously without much difficulty and is able to maintain a near-normal $Paco_2$, then CPAP can be applied.

The use of PEEP or CPAP allows for the reduction of Fio_2 as PEEP or CPAP improves oxygenation and helps to avoid the complications associated with

TABLE 10–1.
Indications for PEEP Therapy

P_AO_2 < 60 mm Hg on Fio_2 of 0.8*
$P(A - a)O_2$ > 300 on Fio_2 of 1.0
Refractory hypoxemia: Pao_2 increases < 10 mm Hg with Fio_2 increase of 0.2
A shunt of > 30%
Recurrent atelectasis with low FRC
Reduced compliance of the lung

*Data from Kirk B: *Respir Med* 1980; 2:38–42.

excess O_2 administration. Specific clinical indications for the use of PEEP or CPAP may include[109]:

1. ARDS.
2. Hyaline membrane disease.
3. Cardiogenic pulmonary edema in adults and children.
4. Postoperative uses, as in the treatment of postoperative atelectasis.
5. Bilateral, diffuse pneumonia.

In addition, use of CPAP by nasal mask is gaining wide acceptance in the home care of patients with sleep disorders. Home uses of varying levels of IPAP and EPAP are becoming common as a method of home mechanical ventilation (see Chapter 14).

CONTRAINDICATIONS TO PEEP OR CPAP

A relative contraindication for PEEP or CPAP is hypovolemia. If a patient is hypovolemic as a result of hemorrhage or dehydration, or relatively hypovolemic because of neurogenic or drug-induced causes, then PEEP can be detrimental as it can reduce CO and compromise circulation. In some instances of hypovolemia, the patient can be treated with volume expanders or inotropic agents, or both, to enhance blood volume and CO.

The absolute contraindication to PEEP or CPAP is an untreated significant pneumothorax or tension pneumothorax. The positive pressure might further increase the air present in the intrapleural space and cause increased mortality or morbidity. PEEP must be used with care in patients with bronchopleural fistulas or in patients with other types of barotrauma for the same reason.[28] In patients who have recently had lung surgery, PEEP can be used, but cautiously, so that a pneumothorax does not develop.

In patients with elevated intracranial pressures (ICP), PEEP or CPAP may cause further elevation by increasing central venous pressure. This does not prevent the use of PEEP in this patient group, especially if patients are severely hypoxemic. The hypoxemia is likely to be fatal if not treated; however, ICP monitoring should be employed with these patients and elevated levels appropriately treated. Sometimes mechanical hyperventilation and deliberate reduction of arterial carbon dioxide partial pressure ($Paco_2$) will help lower ICP.

In patients with hypoxemia, pulmonary hyperinflation, and increased FRC where compliance is either normal or high, PEEP therapy is *not* appropriate. An example is a patient with emphysema. The beneficial effects of PEEP occur when it is used to increase FRC in collapsed or edematous alveoli. This same effect would not occur in preexisting hyperinflation. Areas of the lung which are already hyperinflated may be further distended. This can lead to compression of adjacent capillaries and the rerouting of blood to areas which are not as well ventilated resulting in an increase in shunting, venous admixture, and further hypoxemia. The use of low PEEP may be beneficial to this type of patient if it compensates for the reduced FRC resulting from intubation. Otherwise, use of PEEP in these patients will not usually be beneficial.

When lung pathologic changes are not homogeneous, as in unilateral lung disease, PEEP may have unexpected and undesirable side effects on the distribution of blood flow and ventilation in the lungs. For this reason, unilateral lung disorders may represent a relative contraindication to the use of PEEP or CPAP.

ADULT RESPIRATORY DISTRESS SYNDROME AND PEEP

One of the clinical situations which frequently requires the use of PEEP or CPAP is ARDS. This disorder is best described as a homogeneous acute metabolic malfunction of the lung parenchyma due to a variety of severe physiologic stresses to either the lung or to some other organ system.[71] ARDS is affiliated with such events as aspiration of gastric contents, inhalation of noxious gases or chemicals, sepsis, and multiple trauma (Table 10–2). This suggests that many severe physiologic stresses might result in the development of ARDS.

The common pulmonary complications associated with ARDS include reduced FRC associated with early airway closure and alveolar collapse, reduced lung compliance, increased pulmonary vascular resistance (PVR), and ventilation-perfusion ($\dot{V}/\dot{Q}$) inequalities.[71, 96, 97, 112] Areas of atelectasis can form adjacent to pulmonary vessels which are still being perfused. A shunt effect is created, and there is perfusion without ventilation. The result is severe hypoxemia which does not respond to O_2 therapy.

TABLE 10–2.
Physiological Stress Situations Frequently Associated With Subsequent Development of ARDS

Aspiration of gastric contents
Smoke inhalation or chemical-induced lung injury
Thoracic and nonthoracic trauma
Near-drowning
Drug ingestion
Oxygen toxicity
Pancreatitis
Sepsis
Interstitial viral pneumonitis
Massive blood transfusion
Prolonged cardiopulmonary bypass

Despite the widespread areas of tissue injury and the diffuse infiltrates that are seen on chest radiographs, there does not seem to be a homogeneous distribution of gas exchange abnormalities and mechanical changes. A portion of the lung appears to have normal $\dot{V}/\dot{Q}$ ratios despite marked increases in shunt and dead space.[69] These areas of normal function are scattered throughout areas of significantly abnormal lung.

Patients with ARDS are usually treated with CPAP or PEEP. The use of positive pressure at the end of exhalation maintained at the airway may provide enough pressure against collapsed airways and alveoli to reach their critical opening pressure and expand these areas with air. This can reduce shunt and allow for the lowering of F_{IO_2} to safer levels (< 0.4 F_{IO_2}) while still maintaining O_2 transport to the tissues. If patients are able to maintain their Pa_{CO_2} within normal limits without excessive work of breathing, then CPAP alone may be enough and mechanical ventilatory support with PEEP may not be necessary.

PULMONARY EFFECTS OF PEEP

The use of PEEP or CPAP increases FRC. The amount of change in FRC brought on by the use of PEEP will vary with the compliance of the lung and the amount of PEEP. The volume distribution in the lung depends on both FRC and alveolar distending pressure. The lower the lung compliance, the greater the pressure required to increase alveolar volume. With ARDS the dependent areas of the lung tend to be less compliant than the apices. In ARDS with PEEP or CPAP, it appears that more of the pressure is dissipated into the dependent spaces and a greater portion of the change in FRC per unit of lung is distributed to these areas. This is an advantage since the perfusion is better here and this helps to reduce the amount of shunting and increases the Pa_{O_2}. However, PEEP may overdistend normal functional units as well. This must be watched for when using PEEP.

Figure 10–2 shows a pressure-volume (compliance) curve which describes the changes that occur from normal compliance to reduced compliance with ARDS. When PEEP is applied to the injured lung and increases the lung volume and compliance, the pressure-volume curve moves up and to the right, toward more normal conditions. With patients on CPAP this makes the work of breathing lower, i.e., less pressure change is required to move the same volume.[54]

The recruitment of collapsed alveoli by reaching and maintaining the critical opening pressure appears to be the primary mechanism by which PEEP aids in reducing shunting and improving oxygenation in conditions such as ARDS. Table 10–3 shows the data in a patient in whom increasing increments of PEEP showed no significant effect until 15 cm H_2O was used, at which time the Pa_{O_2} improved markedly.[8] This represents the point at which alveolar recruitment has probably occurred.

When alveoli are edematous (fluid-filled), PEEP might increase the volume of the alveoli so that the fluid no longer completely or significantly fills that alveolar volume. The other possibility is that PEEP redistributes lung water to other areas of the lung.[69] This may explain the apparent clearing that is seen on a chest radiograph.[105] Or it may redistribute the lung water to other areas. Where respiratory bronchioles are collapsed or obstructed, PEEP might overcome the closure and increase the airway diameter allowing the gas to then move more easily into the alveoli. All of these factors would theoretically contribute to improved $\dot{V}/\dot{Q}$ matching, reduced intrapulmonary shunting, and increased lung compliance and volumes.

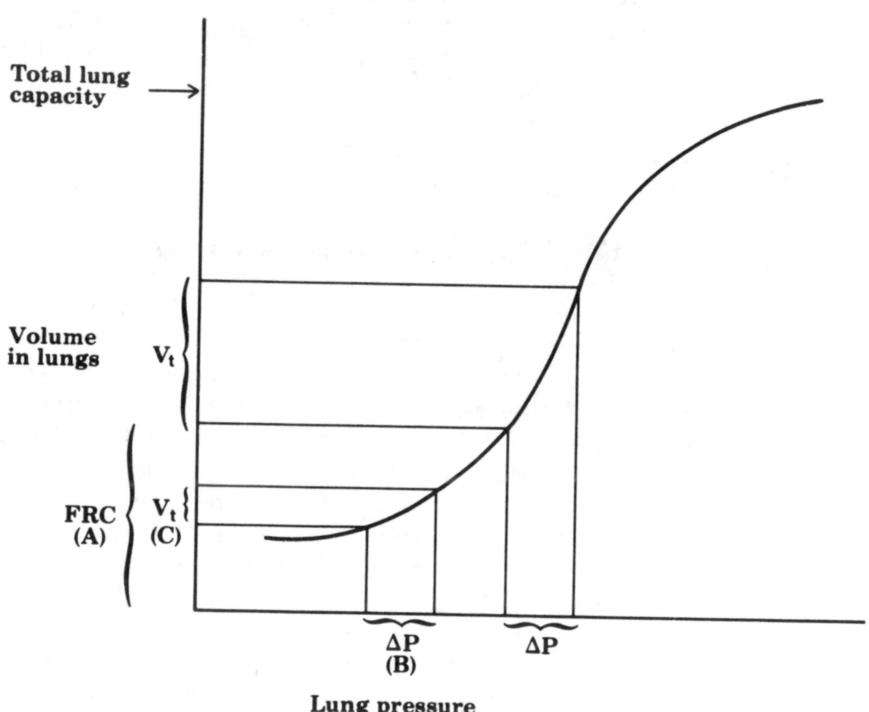

FIG 10–2.
Curve represents the pressure-volume (compliance) relationships in the lung. As pressure to the lung increases, the volume in the lung increases. At normal lung volumes *(FRC)*, very little pressure change *(ΔP)* results in a good tidal volume *(Vt)* at the steepest part of the curve. This represents a condition of normal compliance. In lungs with low compliance, at the bottom left-hand part of the curve, the FRC is low. Here an equal pressure change *(ΔP) (B)* produces only a small tidal volume *(Vt) (C)*. Theoretically, by placing a patient with stiff lungs on PEEP therapy, the compliance becomes improved toward normal, that is toward the steeper portion of the curve at the same time that the FRC is increasing from low to normal.

TABLE 10–3.
Data from a Patient With ARDS on Mechanical Ventilation 24 Hours After Admission*†

PEEP (cm H_2O)	BP (mm Hg)	HR (beats/ min)	PCWP (mm Hg)	CO (L/ min)	Cs (cm H_2O)	V_T (mL)	f (breaths/ min)	$\dot{V}_E$ (L/ min)	Ppeak (cm H_2O)	Pa_{O_2} (mm Hg)	$P\bar{v}_{O_2}$ (mm Hg)	F_{IO_2}	Pa_{CO_2} (mm Hg)	pH
0	130/65	130	16	4.8	28	1,100	6	6.6	50	40	27	0.8	38	7.41
5	120/55	135	13	4.2	31	1,100	6	6.6	58	45	37	0.8	40	7.40
10	135/65	125	18	5.8	33	1,100	6	6.6	60	50	35	0.8	41	7.42
15	130/70	120	19	5.9	36	1,100	6	6.6	55	115	37	0.8	45	7.42
20	110/50	130	25	4.1	27	1,100	6	6.6	63	150	29	0.8	41	7.40

*Data from Bone RC: *Respir Care* 1982; 27:482–407.
†PEEP = positive end-expiratory pressure; BP = blood pressure; HR = heart rate; PCWP = pulmonary capillary wedge pressure; CO = cardiac output; Cs = static compliance; V_T = tidal volume; f = respiratory rate; $\dot{V}_E$ = minute ventilation; Ppeak = peak pressure; Pa_{O_2} = partial pressure of arterial oxygen; Pv_{O_2} = mixed venous oxygen partial pressure; F_{IO_2} = fractional concentration of oxygen in expired gas; Pa_{CO_2} = partial pressure of arterial carbon dioxide.

TRANSMISSION OF AIRWAY PRESSURE TO PLEURAL SPACE

With the addition of positive pressure to the thorax, the risk of transmitting this pressure to the intrapleural space, the mediastium, and the thoracic vessels is present. If the pulmonary injury is uniform, then this is not too great a problem. When chest wall compliance is normal and lung compliance is low, less of the airway pressure (Paw) is transmitted to the pleural space; however, if lung compliance is near normal and chest wall compliance is low, then more of the pressure would be transmitted to the pleural space.[97]

Static compliance measured during mechanical ventilation estimates both lung and chest wall compliance. Chest wall compliance remains fairly constant when patients are comatose or paralyzed on controlled ventilation; however, during the use of IMV when the patient is breathing spontaneously or whenever a patient is fighting the ventilator, the chest wall compliance can vary. This is important to remember when monitoring patients on PEEP. If the pulmonary pathologic changes are not evenly distributed throughout the lung, the use of PEEP can lead to increased $\dot{V}/\dot{Q}$ mismatching. The following case presented by Kanarek and Shannon[53] illustrates such a situation:

> A 12-year-old boy was admitted and treated in the hospital following an accident in which the right femur was fractured and a closed head injury (concussion) was sustained. Two days after admission the chest radiograph showed right upper and middle lobe infiltrates. *Streptococcus pneumoniae* and *Staphylococcus aureus* were cultured. In spite of antibiotic therapy, the infection finally involved the entire right lung with only moderate involvement of the left lung. The patient remained hypoxemic although 100% O_2 was being administered.

TABLE 10–4.

Cardiopulmonary Measurements at Differing Levels of Positive End-Expiratory Pressure (PEEP)*†

	PEEP (cm H_2O)		
	15	5	0
Pa_{O_2}	35	51	71
Pa_{CO_2} (mm Hg)	51	46	54
pH	7.49	7.50	7.49
CI L/min/m^2	2.62		2.46
PAP (mm Hg)	37/20		36/20
P_{Peak} (cm H_2O)	46	35	30
LL%	33	44	59
RL %	67	56	41

*From Kanarek DJ, Shannon DC: *Am Rev Respir Dis* 1975; 112:458.
†LL% = percent distribution of total perfusion to the left lung; RL% = percent distribution of total perfusion to the right lung. For other abbreviations, see text.

To treat the hypoxemia, PEEP was instituted with mechanical ventilation. During a PEEP study, an xenon 133 pulmonary perfusion scan was done to assess pulmonary blood flow. The scan showed a shift of perfusion to the severely involved right lung with increasing PEEP. The Pa_{O_2} decreased at high PEEP levels (Table 10–4). The results of the scan imply that ventilation was distributed predominantly to the unaffected left lung. It was possible that the exudate present in the right lung provided a buffer to high PEEP and less of the pressure was exerted in the right intrapleural space. The left lung capillaries were not similarly protected and left PVR increased. It was also speculated that the positive pressures favored distribution to the left lung because of the high relative compliance in the left lung capillaries and shifted the perfusion to the right lung. Removal of PEEP allowed a redistribution of blood flow.

PEEP AND LUNG WATER

The use of PEEP in patients with diffuse lung injury (ARDS) and pulmonary edema was once believed to be of benefit because it reduced the amount of edema present. The theory held that positive pressure in the alveoli was transmitted to the interstitial space. As a result, the pressure gradient between the pulmonary capillary and the interstitial space was decreased and there was less of a tendency for edema to form in the interstitial space or the alveolus. Other studies do not support this hypothesis, however, but suggest the lung water either remains unchanged or increases.

The two primary forces responsible for fluid movement in the normal lung are hydrostatic pressure and osmotic pressure. These forces are balanced between the interstitial (extravascular) space and the intravascular space. Most of the time the net fluid movement is from the vascular space to the interstitium with removal of the interstitial fluid through lymphatic drainage. This helps to keep the alveoli and interstitial spaces free of water or fluids that interfere with normal gas exchange.

When PEEP is added to normal ventilating pressures the intravascular hydrostatic pressure in the alveolar vessels increases as does the pressure surrounding the interstitial space. The net pressure gradient across the perialveolar vessels theoretically does not change; however, the interstitial pressure surrounding the vessels in the lungs not adjacent to alveoli (extraalveolar vessels, such as pre- and postcapillary vessels and larger vessels) decreases as the PEEP is increased. Radial tension on these vessels produced by an expanding lung structure may cause them to enlarge. As a result the resistance to blood flow is lower.[41] Assuming the CO does not change, the hydrostatic pressure in these vessels stays the same or may increase with PEEP.[101] Since the internal pressure is constant and the external (interstitial) pressure is decreasing in the extraalveolar vessels, there is a tendency for fluid to move out of these vessels; thus, lung edema formation is increased as is total lung water to the extraalveolar perivascular and peribronchial interstitial space.[59, 81, 89, 112]

The apparent improvement in the appearance of the chest radiograph that often follows the use of PEEP with ARDS most likely reflects increased air in the alveolar spaces so that the ratio of air in the lung to the lung water is increasing even though actual lung water may be rising. PEEP appears to improve gas exchange by increasing alveolar ventilation which allows ventilation to occur despite increased lung water.[109] Firm answers to these theories are not yet available.[63, 83]

Clinical observations of patients with cardiogenic pulmonary edema, on the other hand, seem to give evidence to the contrary. Positive pressure ventilation appears to reduce the appearance of the thin, pink, frothy secretions that are produced in copious amounts in this type of pulmonary edema. Intermittent positive pressure ventilation (IPPV) has been seen to improve the cardiovascular status of these patients.[38] In the clinical setting, PEEP is usually used for pulmonary edema when there is an increased pulmonary capillary permeability rather than when pulmonary edema is a result of increased hydrostatic pressure (cardiogenic pulmonary edema).

In patients with congestive heart failure (CHF), CO and systemic blood pressure may rise with the increased intrathoracic pressures. This occurs especially where venous engorgement is sufficient to prevent great vessel collapsing with increased intrapleural pressures. The pooling of the blood outside the thorax and the decreased right ventricular filling permit the heart to work in a more efficient and effective manner.[19] Thus, IPPV may improve patients with CHF by decreasing preload and reducing afterload.

Clinicians often treat CHF with diuretics to decrease the preload to the heart; however, overzealous use of diuretics can place the patient at risk for hypovolemia when IPPV is applied.

SELECTING APPROPRIATE PEEP OR CPAP LEVEL (OPTIMAL PEEP)

The goal of PEEP therapy is to improve oxygenation to the tissues by reducing the shunt effect and increasing FRC and lung compliance. Because of the potential cardiovascular and pulmonary complications related to PEEP and CPAP therapy, therapy must also be aimed at minimizing all potential side effects (Figs 10–3 and 10–4). The medical literature describes several ways of determining when this goal has been reached. The consensus of these different approaches is:

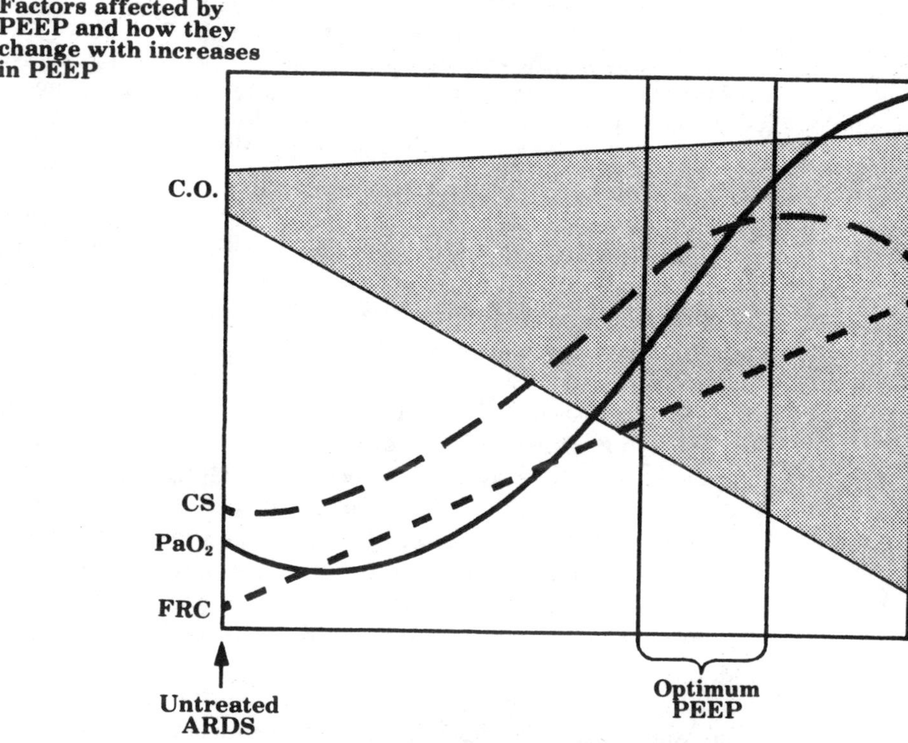

FIG 10–3.
Curves represent the physiologic factors that change during the application of PEEP or CPAP. As the PEEP level is increased, Pa_{O_2}, FRC, and static compliance *(Cs)* normally increase. Cardiac output *(C.O.)*, represented by the *shaded area*, can increase slightly, stay the same, or decrease. The optimal PEEP level can be expected to occur where Pa_{O_2}, FRC, and Cs are high. Cardiac output should be maintained near normal so that O_2 transport to the tissues remains high.

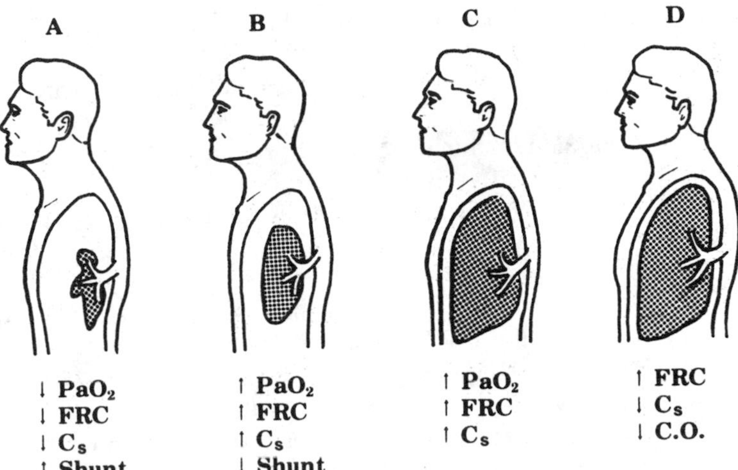

FIG 10–4.
A, stiff lungs and increased shunt result in a drop in FRC and Pa_{O_2}. **B** and **C,** as PEEP is increased, compliance (Cs) and Pa_{O_2} improve as FRC increases, resulting in a lowering of the shunt effect. **D,** too much PEEP has been used and Cs and cardiac output (CO) decrease as FRC is increased above the optimal level.

1. PEEP should be increased in increments of 3 to 5 cm H_2O per step.
2. An optimal oxygenation point should be achieved which allows adequate tissue oxygenation (optimal oxygen transport) at a safe F_{IO_2}.
3. Cardiovascular status should be monitored and maintained at an adequate level.

The clinical data used in assessing these objectives consist of several different measurements. While some authors try to select one specific datum, such as shunt or optimal compliance, it is better to look at several factors together in deciding when the optimal PEEP level has been reached with a patient.

In general, mild forms of acute lung injury require lower levels of PEEP (5–15 cm H_2O). More severe forms require higher PEEP (10–30 cm H_2O). On rare occasions (approximately 20% of patients) more than 20 cm H_2O of PEEP is needed. About 5% of the time, more than 30 cm H_2O is needed.[97] This figure may be on the decline since some clinicians are turning to other modes of ventilation, such as IRV, to avoid the tissue damage associated with high ventilating pressures. Performing an optimal PEEP study is a function most often reserved for patients requiring 10 cm H_2O or more of PEEP. When a PEEP or CPAP study is performed it requires monitoring of:

1. Ventilatory data: tidal volume (V_T), frequency (f), minute ventilation ($\dot{V}_E$), peak pressure (P_{PEAK}), plateau pressure ($P_{Plateau}$), PEEP, static compliance

(Cs), breath sounds, arterial blood gases (Pa_{O_2}, Ca_{O_2}, pH, Pa_{CO_2}), alveolar-arterial oxygen difference [$P(A-a)O_2$] or Pa_{O_2}/F_{IO_2} ratio, shunt (calculated clinical shunt, $\dot{Q}s/\dot{Q}t$), and arterial–end-tidal carbon dioxide gradient [$P(a-ET)CO_2$].

2. Hemodynamic data: blood pressure, CO (by thermodilution), arteriovenous oxygen difference $C(a-v)O_2$, mixed venous oxygen tension and saturation ($P\bar{v}_{O_2}$, $S\bar{v}_{O_2}$), pulmonary artery pressure (PAP), pulmonary capillary wedge pressure (PCWP), and oxygen transport (CO $\times$ Ca_{O_2}).

These data are used to assess the total cardiopulmonary response of the patient to the PEEP challenge and to establish the desired end point or optimal PEEP level (see Fig 10–3).

Obviously, this list is so daunting it is no wonder clinicians seek one quantitative determination to use as the indication for PEEP therapy. Whenever this has been attempted, however, an exception to the use of that determination has always appeared. Many determinations are evaluated to assess the patient's response to the PEEP challenge. These may include any of the following, depending on the individual patient's clinical picture:

1. A Pa_{O_2} of 60 to 100 mm Hg. This represents an arterial oxygen saturation (Sa_{O_2}) of 90% to 97% at a normal pH on an F_{IO_2} of less than or equal to 0.4.
2. A point at which O_2 transport is optimal. Normal O_2 transport is about 1,000 mL/min (5 L/min $\times$ 20 vol %).
3. A shunt of less than 15%.[30, 111]
4. A minimal amount of cardiovascular embarrassment. This includes adequate systemic blood pressure, CO (decrease of $\leq$20%), and pulmonary vascular pressure.
5. Improving lung compliance.[108]
6. A Pa_{O_2}/F_{IO_2} ratio of more than 300.
7. The point of minimal arterial–end-tidal P_{CO_2} gradient [$P(a-ET)CO_2$].[76, 80]
8. Optimal mixed venous oxygen values.[25, 77]

INITIATING PEEP THERAPY

If a patient's clinical condition suggests that PEEP or CPAP therapy is necessary, then it should be started as soon as possible. The patient will undoubtedly have been treated with O_2 in an attempt to relieve the hypoxemia. Oxygen concentrations greater than 50% for more than 24 to 48 hours can lead to O_2 toxicity. Positive pressure therapy along with F_{IO_2} values of 0.5 or more may damage pulmonary cells in even less than 24 hours; therefore, the patient must be started on PEEP and CPAP early to avoid lung damage from O_2. When

PEEP has achieved good O_2 transport, then the F_{IO_2} can be reduced, maintaining the alveolar oxygen tension (P_{AO_2}) between 60 and 100 mm Hg. When the F_{IO_2} is 0.40 or less, a satisfactory level of PEEP and oxygenation has been achieved for most clinical situations.

CPAP is appropriate for patients with good V_T, vital capacity, inspiratory force, reasonable respiratory rate, low-to-normal Pa_{CO_2}s, and pH in the normal range. These parameters indicate that the patient is able to maintain the work of breathing and can do well on CPAP alone. This has fewer complications associated with it than does IPPV plus PEEP. If the patient does not meet these criteria or has an increased work of breathing, then mechanical ventilatory support needs to be instituted along with PEEP.

Performing Optimal PEEP Study

Figure 10–5 presents a flow sheet that can be used for monitoring patients receiving PEEP or CPAP therapy. Once the baseline data are obtained (an initial measurement and calculation of all parameters), then 5 cm H_2O of PEEP or CPAP is instituted. Figure 10–6 shows the effects of PEEP on pressure readings.

Blood Pressure.—The patient's blood pressure is checked within the first few minutes of receiving PEEP or CPAP to be sure it is not significantly decreasing, i.e., decreasing by more than 20 mm Hg systolic.[22] If it does decrease, the patient may be hypovolemic or have obtunded neurologic reflexes that prevent the adequate maintenance of blood pressure.

Breath Sounds.—A brief examination of the chest (auscultation, palpation, and percussion) can give an early indication of any barotrauma that may have occurred or any other changes in the patient's lung condition.

Patient Appearance.—The patient's appearance—color, level of consciousness, signs of anxiety or pain—is checked frequently. A sudden deterioration in the patient's condition may signal cardiovascular collapse or the sudden development of pneumothorax. Approximately 15 to 30 minutes following the increase in PEEP, all of the ventilatory and hemodynamic parameters are measured and calculated.

Peak and Plateau Pressures.—Measurements of P_{Peak} and $P_{Plateau}$ can be used to evaluate the compliance and airway resistance changes. If airway resistance increases significantly during a PEEP trial, then the cause must be investigated and treated. As PEEP is increased, the peak pressure will also rise.

Respiratory Rate, Tidal Volume, Minute Ventilation.—Measuring V_T and $\dot{V}_E$ is best accomplished by measuring exhaled volumes at the endotracheal tube.

If this is not possible because of the use of continuous flow systems, then other methods of measurement are available. They are described in greater detail elsewhere.[45, 51, 72] Normally one does not expect $\dot{V}_E$ to change as a direct result of using CPAP or PEEP; consequently, the Pa_{CO_2} is not directly affected. If a patient has been hyperventilating (low Pa_{CO_2}) due to hypoxemia prior to the use of

	0	5	10	15	20	25	30
Minutes/time	15	30	45	60	75	90	105
Blood Pressure (mm Hg)	117/80	120/85	120/80	110/70	115/75	115/75	90/65
P_{Peak} (cm H_2O)	33	39	43	51	51	53	60
P_{PL} (cm H_2O) (plateau)	28	33	37	48	45	47	58
$V_{t\ spontantous}/V_{t\ ventilator}$	200/1000	200/1000	250/1000	250/1000	250/1000	250/1000	250/1000
$f_{spontaneous}/f_{ventilator}$	4/10	4/10	3/10	4/10	3/10	5/10	6/10
$\dot{V}_E$ Total (l/min)	10.8	10.8	10.8	11.0	10.8	11.3	11.5
C_s (ml/cm H_2O)	36	36	37	35	40	45	36
PaO_2 (F_IO_2 = 1.0)	43	59	65	73	103	152	167
CaO_2 (vol %)	15.3	17.8	18.3	18.9	19.2	19.4	19.6
$PaCO_2$ (mm Hg)	37	37	38	37	39	37	38
pH	7.41	7.42	7.42	7.42	7.40	7.41	7.41
$P(A\text{-}a)O_2$ (mm Hg)	607	591	585	577	547	498	483
$PaCO_2 - P_{ET}CO_2$ (mm Hg)	16	15	13	10	9	8	15
$P\bar{v}O_2$ (or $S\bar{v}O_2$) (mm Hg or %)	27	37	38	38	39	40	34
C.O. L/min	4.1	4.2	4.0	4.5	4.4	4.4	3.3
$C(A\text{-}\bar{V})O_2$ (vol %)	5.3	5.2	5.4	5.0	4.9	4.9	6.7
PCWP (mm Hg)	3	5	8	11	12	13	18
PAP (mm Hg)	37/21	39/25	41/24	43/25	40/21	38/24	45/30
C.O. x CaO_2 Oxygen transport	627	748	732	851	845	854	647

Comments: Bilateral scattered crackles present in both lungs.

FIG 10–5.

Example of a PEEP study flow sheet including ventilation, oxygenation, and hemodynamic data. Key points to observe when first reviewing a PEEP study are: (1) blood pressure, (2) mixed venous oxygen ($P\bar{v}O_2$), and (3) O_2 transport. Note that these three values decline at a PEEP of 30 cm H_2O. Blood pressure drops to 90/65, $P\bar{v}O_2$ drops to 34 mm Hg, and O_2 transport drops to 647 mL/min. An optimal PEEP level is +25 cm H_2O where these parameters and others indicate that O_2 transport is improving without significant cardiovascular side effects.

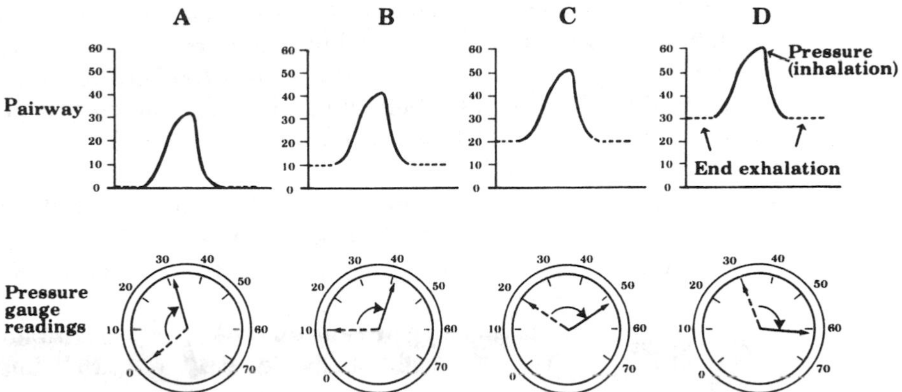

FIG 10–6.
High PEEP levels can be expected to give rises in peak and plateau pressure readings on the ventilator manometer. The baseline reading rises above zero and reflects the increase in FRC.

CPAP or PEEP, then relief of the hypoxemia with PEEP (or CPAP) can be expected to be accompanied by a fall in $\dot{V}_E$ and a rise in $Paco_2$ toward the patient's normal levels.[54] High levels of PEEP expand the conductive airways. This may be due in part to dilation of terminal and respiratory bronchioles. This increases dead space and can increase $Paco_2$.[69]

Compliance.—The measurement of Cs in the patient on PEEP therapy is considered a good indicator of the effects of low-to-moderate PEEP on the lung. As PEEP progressively improves lung volumes, compliance can be expected to increase. When PEEP reaches a point where it overdistends alveoli, then compliance can be expected to fall.

The calculation of Cs requires a $P_{Plateau}$, end-expiratory pressure, and V_T measurements. If V_T is measured at the exhalation valve, then correction must be made for the changes in tubing compliance during a ventilated breath with PEEP (Appendix K). If auto-PEEP is suspected, it is measured and considered part of the end-expiratory pressure (see Chapter 7).

In patients with chest wall injury or with hypovolemic conditions, the use of Cs alone will not be a good indicator of optimal PEEP or cardiovascular changes with PEEP even at low levels of PEEP. More invasive monitoring techniques are recommended. If PEEPs above 15 cm H_2O are used, compliance is not a good evaluator of cardiovascular function and pulmonary artery catheter monitoring is indicated.

Pao_2, Fio_2, and Pao_2/Fio_2.—The usual approach to the management of Fio_2 and PEEP is to start with high Fio_2 and incrementally decrease the Fio_2 as PEEP or CPAP improves oxygenation. A Pa_{O_2} of 60 mm Hg with a normal pH represents 90% saturation of hemoglobin and represents a good acceptable end point.

The Pa_{O_2}/F_{IO_2} ratio reflects the relationship between available O_2 and actual arterial O_2, i.e., venous admixture and shunt. Values over 300 (e.g., Pa_{O_2} = 100 on an F_{IO_2} of 0.33) indicate a good ratio.

Pa_{CO_2} and pH.—Adequacy of ventilation can be determined by regular evaluation of Pa_{CO_2} and pH as PEEP is increased. If values are not being maintained near the patient's normal, then appropriate adjustment should be made.

Alveolar-Arterial Oxygen Tension [$P(A-a)O_2$].—With incremental increases in PEEP the $P(A-a)O_2$ will usually decrease, reflecting improvement in $\dot{V}/\dot{Q}$. This can also be assessed by calculating Pa_{O_2}/P_{AO_2} or Pa_{O_2}/F_{IO_2} ratios.

Arterial End-Tidal Carbon Dioxide Tension Gradient [$P(a-ET)CO_2$].—($P(a-ET)CO_2$) will be lowest when gas exchange units are maximally recruited without being overdistended by PEEP. In other words, an increase in PEEP which increases the $P(a-ET)CO_2$ gradient past its minimum represents a PEEP which can be expected to produce a drop in CO and an increase in V_D/V_T. It has been suggested that this value may be a more sensitive indicator of excessive PEEP than shunt and Pa_{O_2}. It is especially useful if a pulmonary artery catheter is not in use.[76]

The normal $P(a-ET)CO_2$ gradient is 4.5 ± 2.5 mm Hg during both mechanical and spontaneous ventilation. It usually increases with ARDS as the physiologic dead space increases. The data in Table 10–5 were extrapolated from a study by Murray and his colleagues[76] on oleic acid–treated dogs and gives an example of changes that might be expected in $P(a-ET)CO_2$ with increased PEEP. The findings of Murray et al. have not been confirmed by others.[44]

TABLE 10–5.

A PEEP Study to Evaluate Use of $P(a-ET)CO_2$ Gradient for Assessing PEEP in Dogs Injected With Oleic Acid*

	PEEP					
	0	5	10†	15	20	25
$P(a-ET)CO_2$	17	13	8	8	10	14
$\dot{Q}s/\dot{Q}t$ (%)	14	3	2	2	2	2
Cs (mL/cm H_2O)	18	20	16	12	7	9
Pa_{O_2} (on F_{IO_2} = 0.5)	95	180	>200	>200	>200	>200
O_2 delivery (mL/min)	250	200	300	280	220	180

*Data from Murray JF, Modell JH, Gallagher TJ, et al: *Chest* 1984; 85:100–104.

†10 cm H_2O represents a PEEP level where all parameters are optimal. With greater increases in PEEP, the $P(a-ET)CO_2$ rises and the O_2 delivery and Cs fall. Note that shunt ($\dot{Q}s/\dot{Q}t$) and Pa_{O_2} remain high.

Hemodynamic Data

In addition to the measurement of blood pressure, hemodynamic monitoring also includes evaluation of mixed venous oxygen ($P\bar{v}O_2$ or $S\bar{v}O_2$), CO, $C(a-v)o_2$, pulmonary vascular pressures (PAP, PCWP), and O_2 transport. All of these values require invasive monitoring (pulmonary artery catheterization).

Mixed Venous Oxygen Tension and Saturation.—Normal $P\bar{v}o_2$ ranges between 35 and 40 mm Hg which represents a saturation of about 75%. A $P\bar{v}o_2$ of 28 mm Hg is probably the minimal acceptable level and this represents an $S\bar{v}O_2$ of about 50%.[25] Some patients needing PEEP therapy will have a low $P\bar{v}o_2$, usually due to arterial hypoxemia. As PEEP is increased it often leads to an increase in Pao_2 and $P\bar{v}o_2$ with no net change in $P(a-v)o_2$. This indicates that O_2 transport is improving since there is no apparent change in CO. There is also a net decrease in intrapulmonary shunt fraction.

PEEP may increase PaO_2 and $P\bar{v}o_2$ with a net decrease in $C(a-v)o_2$ and improvement in O_2 delivery. If oxygen consumption ($\dot{V}o_2$) is constant, this suggests a rise in CO. In patients in whom $P\bar{v}o_2$ decreases with PEEP and $C(a-v)o_2$ increases, CO may be decreased and O_2 delivery is reduced; however, if $P\bar{v}o_2$ was high to start with, no deleterious effects may result. If $P\bar{v}o_2$ does not change as PEEP is increased, a rising Pao_2 may reflect an improvement in lung function with a reduction in O_2 delivery; however, this reduced delivery may not be clinically significant.[78]

Cardiac Output.—Thermodilution measurement of CO provides key information about the body's response to increased PEEP. As PEEP improves the $\dot{V}/\dot{Q}$ relationship, myocardial oxygenation also improves. This may enhance cardiac performance. As intrapleural pressures increase or as the gas exchange units become overdistended, however, venous return decreases and cardiac function is altered. Cardiac output then declines (Table 10–6). The drop in CO with increased PEEP is sometimes referred to as "circulatory preload depression"[112] or relative hypovolemia associated with increased PEEP.

Some clinicians augment vascular volumes with fluid administration (fluid challenge) and give inotropic agents to maintain cardiac function as PEEP is increased until they are satisfied that O_2 transport or delivery is sufficient to provide the tissues with O_2. Steps in performing a fluid (volume) challenge have been described by Shapiro[97] and are given in Appendix L.

Arteriovenous Oxygen Difference.—$C(a-v)o_2$ is normally about 5 vol %. It reflects the utilization of O_2 by the tissues. An increase in $C(a-v)o_2$ with an increase in PEEP may indicate hypovolemia, cardiac malfunction, decreased venous return to the heart, and a decreased CO from PEEP, or an increase in $\dot{V}o_2$. A decrease in $C(a-v)o_2$ with an increase in PEEP might be caused by a rise in CO due to improved or augmented cardiac function and volume, and reduced O_2 extraction by the tissues from reduced metabolic rate or histotoxic hypoxia.

Use of Pulmonary Vascular Pressures With PEEP

When moderate-to-high levels of PEEP are used (>15 cm H_2O) it becomes increasingly important to closely evaluate the hemodynamic changes that occur by using a pulmonary artery catheter. PCWP is especially important to watch when establishing optimal PEEP because it reflects left heart filling and can also be used to indicate overinflation of the lungs during PEEP therapy. Values for PCWP rise very high with an increase in PEEP (see Chapter 11).

The pressures in the thoracic vessels normally rise with the use of PEEP. The data in Table 10–7 show changes in PCWP with PEEP.[107] This does not mean that the actual transmural pressure (Ptm) in the vessels may be unaffected. Noncompliant lungs help to protect the vessels from being "squeezed" by the

TABLE 10-6.

Effects of Increased PEEP on $P\bar{v}O_2$ and Related Parameters

	PEEP (cm H_2O)				
	0	5	10*	15	20
$P\bar{v}O_2$ (mm Hg)	35	37	39	37	35
$C(a - \bar{v})O_2$ (mL/100 mL)	3.7	3.7	3.6	3.8	4.1
CO (L/min) (O_2 transport)	7.0	7.0	7.5	6.7	6.5
CO × CaO_2(mL/min)	850	875	950	850	825

*10 cm H_2O of PEEP represents a point where $P\bar{v}O_2$ is nearest normal, and cardiac output (CO) and O_2 transport are at their highest. Note that as PEEP continues to increase, the $C(a - \bar{v})O_2$ continues to rise and $P\bar{v}O_2$ falls. The CO falls reflecting a slower perfusion rate and more time for O_2 extraction at the tissues.

TABLE 10–7.

Effects of Increased PEEP on Wedge Pressure (PCWP) and Pulmonary Vascular Resistance (PVR)*†

	PEEP (cm H_2O)			
	0	5	10	15
PaO_2 (mm Hg) (FIO_2 = 1.0)	90	150	300	500
PAP (mm Hg)	39/15	42/17	45/20	47/21
PCWP (mm Hg)	8	12	15	18
CVP (cm H_2O)	9	13	14	16
CO (L/min)	4.3	4.8	4.4	4.7

*Data from Sugerman HJ, Rogers RM, Miller LD: *Chest* 1972; 62(suppl):865–945.

†PaO_2 increases substantially. Central venous pressure (CVP) increases slightly. Cardiac output (CO) did not change significantly. The increase in PCWP is matched by an increase in pulmonary artery pressure (PAP). Data indicate that in patients with decreased compliance and decreased FRC and no hypovolemia, minimal changes occur in systemic and pulmonary vascular pressures or in CO.

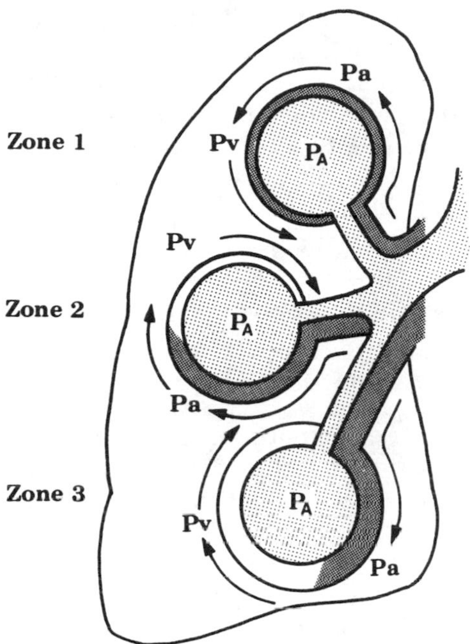

FIG 10–7.
In the normal lung the greatest amount of perfusion and ventilation are to the dependent (lower) lung zones. The *Zone 3* regions represent areas of lung where pulmonary artery pressure (PAP) exceeds pulmonary venous pressure (PvP) which exceeds pulmonary alveolar pressure (*PA*). In *Zone 2* lung areas (normally the middle region) PAP > PA > PvP. In *Zone 1* lung areas (normally the upper regions) PA > PAP > PvP. Pulmonary vascular pressure monitoring is most accurate if the catheter is in a zone 3 region. *Pa* = pulmonary artery blood (deoxygenated); *Pv* = pulmonary venous blood (oxygenated).

rising lung volumes (increased FRC) up to a point. These falsely elevated vascular pressures do not give an accurate picture of the true filling of the left heart. This can best be determined by calculating the transmural PCWP which more truly reflects left heart pressures and filling (see Chapter 11 and Appendix M).

Rises and falls in the pulmonary vascular pressure readings monitored by an oscilloscope will occur during the respiratory cycle. Because of this, pressures are read during exhalation only regardless of whether the patient is spontaneously breathing on CPAP or is on mechanical ventilation with PEEP. If the patient is receiving very high PEEP, PEEP need not be removed to measure PCWP, PAP, or central venous pressure (CVP) readings. This might precipitate severe hypoxemia which is difficult to reverse.[24, ,98, 111] PCWP may reflect alveolar pressure (PA) or Paw and not left heart pressures if the pulmonary artery catheter is located in a nondependent area of the lung (Fig 10–7).[7]

At high levels of PEEP there can be a divergence of wedge and left arterial pressures because of overinflation of alveoli and redistribution of pulmonary blood flow.[109] Thus, during an optimal PEEP study when PEEP is increased and PCWP rises markedly, the lungs may be overinflated and the PEEP may need to be reduced (Fig 10–8).

PCWP and left atrial pressure (LAP) may be markedly decreased when pulmonary blood flow is reduced as a result of significantly decreased venous return to the right heart due to PEEP therapy. This occurrence is a PEEP-induced relative hypovolemia, and requires a reduction in the amount of PEEP being used or intravenous (IV) fluid administration.[105]

Oxygen Transport

The use of O_2 transport as a tool for evaluating the effect of PEEP is very important since it reflects both cardiac and pulmonary function as well as the carrying capacity of the blood. The normal value for O_2 transport is approximately 1,000 mL/min. If CO is low, it may be enhanced by slightly reducing the PEEP level or by the use of volume-loading (IV fluids) or inotropic agents or both. A low Ca_{O_2} may be improved by increasing PEEP, increasing F_{IO_2}, or by increasing hemoglobin levels (giving blood) if the patient is anemic.

An example of the effect of PEEP on cardiovascular responses is shown in Table 10–7.[107] It provides the hemodynamic data on a patient with diffuse interstitial edema. The Pa_{O_2} increased substantially with PEEP. After achieving +15 cm H_2O, it was possible to lower the F_{IO_2} of the patient to 0.4 and maintain an adequate Pa_{O_2}. The CVP increased slightly. Cardiac output and PVR did not change significantly. The increase in PCWP was matched by increases in PAP. In patients with decreased compliance and FRC and no hypovolemia, there is minimal change in cardiovascular values.[107]

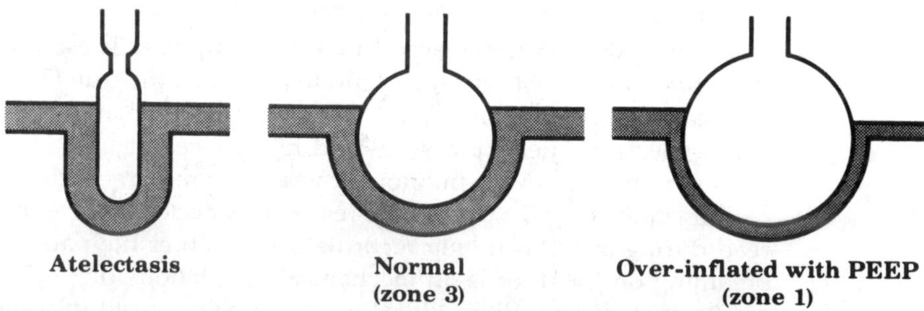

FIG 10–8.
ARDS creates many lung regions with atelectasis *(left)*. With PEEP these atelectatic areas can be reexpanded creating more zone 3 areas of lung *(center)*; however, overexpansion with PEEP can reduce perfusion to ventilated alveoli and create zone 1 areas of lung *(right)*.

PEEP AND CONGESTIVE HEART FAILURE

Patients in CHF often have reduced CO and impaired cardiac function. They progressively develop pulmonary edema (cardiogenic pulmonary edema) that differs from edema associated with ARDS. The permeability characteristics of the pulmonary vessels and alveoli remain normal, but the pulmonary hydrostatic pressures rise due to the back-up of blood in the pulmonary circulation from the left heart. As the edema develops in the lungs, the patient becomes progressively more hypoxemic. PVR increases and eventually the right heart work increases. Over a long period of time the patient will develop peripheral edema.

When patients in CHF are admitted to the hospital they usually present with pink frothy secretions and bilateral crackles (rales) indicative of the presence of pulmonary edema. These patients often benefit from positive pressure therapy. The positive pressure may help to reduce the venous return to the heart and the amount of blood the heart must pump. This reduces the work of the heart. Increased F_{IO_2} values and positive pressure also help improve oxygenation. This may increase myocardial oxygenation and function. In some instances, PEEP or IPPV is beneficial to patients with CHF. This effect, however, is not predictable. In patients with aortic or mitral valve replacement, PEEP has been associated with changes in V_D/V_T and decreased cardiac index (CI).

HAZARDS OR COMPLICATIONS OF PEEP

The hazards associated with the use of PEEP include altered cardiovascular function, high pressure physical lung injury (barotrauma), reduced renal function, and increased ICP. In general, the use of CPAP, as opposed to mechanical ventilation with PEEP, has fewer complications. The effects of PEEP on normal heart function are greater than with IPPV alone. PEEP with IPPV decreases CO more than PEEP with IMV or CPAP alone.[8]

Thoracic Vessel Pressure and Pulmonary Vascular Effects

PEEP increases the pressure measured in all thoracic vessels.[47,48] The vascular pressures generally increase in the same amounts as the pleural pressure.[114] PEEP also increases intracardiac pressures.[47,48] The effect of PEEP on the pulmonary vasculature varies. High levels of PEEP can stretch alveoli and the vessels adjacent to their corners. This can compress these vessels and cause an increase in PVR. PEEP can also reduce overall pulmonary blood flow by two to three times normal, redistribute pulmonary blood flow so that there is less flow to the nondependent lung zones, and shift the flow outward toward the periphery of the lung as if the lung had been exposed to a centrifugal force. PEEP also reduces bronchial blood flow to all lobes and causes bronchial veins to return their flow to the left atrium at low levels and to the right atrium at levels greater than 10 cm H_2O.

Altered Cardiovascular Function

Transmission of positive airway pressures to the vessels in the pleural space can result in reduced venous return to the heart, decreased CO, decreased blood pressure, altered right and left ventricular function, and increased PVR.

With diffuse lung disease, which reduces lung compliance, the effects of PEEP tend to be minimal. As PEEP is increased, lung compliance also increases to a point and then generally decreases. As long as compliance is increasing with PEEP, PVR tends to decrease. This is attributed to both alveolar recruitment and an increase in FRC to a higher point in the compliance curve. Once compliance becomes lower with an increase in PEEP, one would expect PVR to increase.

In order to maintain venous return with PEEP, venous pressure must rise. In patients with good vascular reflexes the rising intrathoracic pressures are usually accompanied by increasing peripheral vasoconstriction, and venous return is maintained. If the normal vascular reflexes are impaired or if hypovolemia is present, then venous return and CO cannot be maintained. In normovolemic patients it is unusual to get a reduction in CO with 5 to 10 cm H_2O of PEEP. Most decreases in CO occur when more than 15 cm H_2O is applied.[37] Major cardiac effects of PEEP include the following:

1. Transmural pressure changes in the heart.
2. Altered right ventricular function.
3. Interventricular septal shifting.
4. Decreased CO (not due to decreased venous return but to other causes).
5. Altered left ventricular function.
6. Endocardial blood flow changes.
7. Neural and humoral effects on the heart.

Transmural Pressure Changes.—The effective filling of the heart is determined by the pressure difference between the inside of the heart and the intrathoracic pressures. This is called the cardiac *transmural pressure.* The more positive this value, the greater the filling of the heart; the less positive this value, the lower the filling of the heart. Because intrathoracic pressure changes during each part of the respiratory cycle (inspiration plus expiration), COs change during the respiratory cycle. PEEP may decrease CO by reducing transmural filling pressures in the heart.[86] Transfusing fluids can restore CO and increase filling pressures.[86]

Right Ventricular Function.—The use of PEEP may be beneficial when used appropriately and may lead to reexpansion of formerly atelectatic (underexpanded) areas of the lung. If excessive levels of PEEP are employed so that overdistention results, then PVR may increase as a result of the stretching and narrowing of the pulmonary capillaries. In this situation, the work of the right heart must increase to pump blood through the lungs. This is called an increased afterload. Increased afterload can potentially lead to increased right atrial and right ventricular end-diastolic (filling) pressures.[83] Apparently this does not affect the ability of the right heart to pump blood but only increases the amount of work it must perform. Still, less blood volume is moved since venous return (preload) is down.

Interventricular Septal Shifting.—With PEEP the increased right ventricular afterload from increased PVR may induce a shift of the interventricular septum to the left. This may not alter right ventricular function, but potentially could decrease left ventricular compliance, volume, and left ventricular diastolic (filling) pressure.[40, 63, 83, 109]

Decreased Cardiac Output.—PEEP increases FRC and lung volume, as well as intrapleural pressure. When pleural pressures are kept from increasing by using open chest animal preparations, increasing PEEP still results in decreased CO. This decrease occurs when the pleural pressure is not increased but lung volume is increasing.[109] This is related to alteration in left ventricular function. Controversy still exists over the interpretation of these findings.[70]

Left Ventricular Function.—There are several reasons why left ventricular function might be altered with PEEP:

1. Changes in coronary blood flow as the heart is compressed by the increased lung volume.
2. Increases in right ventricular afterload from increased PVR reducing the preload to the left heart.
3. Reflex change in the contractility of the left ventricle.
4. Humoral-mediated response.
5. Change in the contour of the heart and its chambers. Leftward displacement of the interventricular septum may occur with PEEP leading to a possible reduction in left ventricular volume and function.[15, 109]

Endocardial Blood Flow Changes.—The flow in the coronary vessels depends upon a pressure gradient. The pressure gradient responsible for the flow to the left ventricular myocardium is the difference between systemic diastolic pressure and left ventricular end-diastolic pressure (coronary perfusion pressure). The pressure gradient to the right ventricle is estimated by the difference between aortic systolic pressure and pulmonary artery systolic pressure.[63]

Because of the effect of several other factors on myocardial blood flow, e.g., left ventricular diastolic pressure, intrathoracic pressure, and humoral and neural reflex mechanisms, it is difficult to study endocardial blood flow in response to PEEP. It is speculated that the effects of PEEP on coronary blood flow may be responsible for some of the changes in cardiac function seen with PEEP. Ischemia of the myocardium due to decreased coronary perfusion may contribute to myocardial dysfunction.

Neural and Humoral Effects.—In studies using dogs, it has been demonstrated that a neural reflex arc may be present in the lungs. It is comprised of sensory vagal afferent nerves going from the lung to the central nervous system that inhibit vasal motor tone through autonomic system efferent nerve fibers. This vagosympathetic neural reflex arc may be responsible for arterial vasodilation and depression of left ventricular function which has been reported with the use of PEEP.[83] There is also evidence from animal studies that a humoral-mediated depression of CO may occur with PEEP. Lung expansion may cause the release of humoral substances such as prostaglandins or perhaps some unidentified substance which depresses left ventricular function. The importance of these phenomena in humans is uncertain at present.[64, 83, 109]

Barotrauma

Alveolar damage, subcutaneous emphysema, pneumothorax, pneumomediastinum, and pneumopericardium are examples of the barotrauma or extraalveolar gas that is known to occur with PEEP. As much as a 14% incidence of barotrauma has been reported, much of which is the result of using high PEEP with mechanical ventilation (PEEP >25 cm H_2O). Barotrauma is also more apt to occur when only patchy lung involvement is present, resulting in regional changes in compliance and resistance predisposing certain areas of the lung to rupture.[78] Various underlying lung disorders may actually predispose patients to alveolar rupture during mechanical ventilation and PEEP.

It is not the high peak pressures that result in alveolar rupture, but high P_A and high lung volume changes. Ways of reducing the likelihood of alveolar rupture during mechanical ventilation or PEEP therapy are: (1) use small V_T settings in patients with COPD or similar causes of hyperinflation; (2) decrease V_T as the PEEP level is raised; (3) monitor compliance during PEEP studies as an index of increased chance of alveolar rupture; (4) avoid right mainstem intubation; (5) do not use end-inspiratory hold (pause); (6) do not use sigh breaths with high volumes; (7) monitor for auto-PEEP in cases where it is likely to occur and correct for auto-PEEP when present; and (8) use PEEP cautiously in patients prediposed to alveolar rupture (unilateral, patchy, or cavitary lung disease; nosocomial pneumonias; sepsis; late-stage ARDS; COPD; asthma).[92]

Reduced Renal Output

A decrease in urine production is associated with PEEP and is attributed to reduced or altered renal perfusion and changes in circulating antidiuretic hormone (ADH) levels. PEEP may also decrease the levels of atrial natriuretic peptide (ANP). This substance is normally produced in the atria. PEEP may reduce its levels by mechanical compression of the atria or by decreasing right atrial stretching by affecting the venous return. It may also reduce sodium excretion from the kidneys by (1) increasing glomerular filtration, (2) changing the distribution of blood flow in the kidneys, (3) inhibiting aldosterone production, or (4) altering ADH release.

Increased Intracranial Pressure

A reduction in venous return to the heart caused by elevated intrapleural pressures can cause an elevation of ICP. This is especially hazardous to patients with closed head injury or cranial tumors and occurs postoperatively in some neurosurgical patients and patients who are already at risk for elevated ICP. In the presence of severe, refractory hypoxemia, PEEP would not be contraindicated in the presence of increased ICP.

TECHNIQUES FOR SETTING UP PEEP OR CPAP

CPAP or sPEEP (spontaneous PEEP) can be achieved through the use of a freestanding setup (one without a mechanical ventilator) or with the use of a mechanical ventilator in which the rate is turned to zero or the mode to sPEEP or CPAP. The various methods for achieving CPAP or PEEP include CPAP or EPAP by a continuous flow (closed) system (freestanding), EPAP (sPEEP) by demand flow (open) system (freestanding), PEEP with controlled ventilation, PEEP with assisted ventilation, and PEEP with IMV or synchronized IMV (SIMV). Each of the components necessary for establishing these forms of CPAP and PEEP will be considered. In addition, the application of the pressure to the airway by various methods and the achievement of positive expiratory pressure through resistance devices is discussed. CPAP used in home care is covered in Chapter 14.

Application of CPAP or PEEP Device to Patient Airway

The positive pressures employed with CPAP or PEEP can be applied to the airway by means of a head box, face mask, nasal prongs (nasal cannula) and masks, or endotracheal tube.

Head Box.—A clear plastic chamber holds the patient's head (infant or adult) and an adjustable neck iris provides a seal around the neck. Humidified gas flows into the chamber at 10 to 30 L/min. High flows provide the desired pressure and compensate for leaks in the system. Excess gas exits the system by means of an outlet tube or valve that allows adjustment of outward flow and controls the CPAP level.[51, 65, 107]

The head box may help to prevent the need for intubation, but it also makes some patient care procedures difficult. Ulceration of the neck and high noise levels are two additional difficulties. The use of head chambers requires that the patient perform the work of breathing, protect the lower airway, and maintain a normal $Paco_2$. This system is not commonly used for administering PEEP or CPAP.

Face Mask.—CPAP or PEEP administered with a soft silicon plastic mask also elimiantes the need for endotracheal intubation in select patient groups. A variety of tight-fitting masks can be applied to the face, with the pressure adjusted up to as much as 15 cm H_2O. Leaking around the mask, however, may create a problem at higher levels of CPAP or PEEP. Patients receiving mask CPAP or PEEP are usually alert, awake, and oriented. They should be able to protect their lower airway, support the work of breathing, and maintain a normal $Paco_2$ without excessive ventilatory effort. They should have a Pao_2/Fio_2 ratio of more than 300 mm Hg with a stable cardiovascular system. The hazards of mask CPAP include vomiting and aspiration, CO_2 retention and increased work of breathing, skin necrosis and discomfort from the mask, and cerebral hemorrhage at high CPAP levels (infants).

Nasal Prongs (Nasal Cannula) and Masks.—By taking advantage of the fact that neonates are obligate nose breathers, plastic or Silastic nasal prongs can be fitted into an infant's nares and pressures up to about 15 cm H_2O of CPAP or PEEP can be administered. Loss of pressure from the system can occur through the mouth at high pressure levels ($>$15 cm H_2O) or when an infant cries. Problems of nasal CPAP or PEEP include gastric distention, pressure necrosis, swelling of nasal mucosa, and abrasion of the posterior pharynx.

Nasal masks and nasal "pillows" are now used in adult care in the home setting. Masks come prefabricated or can be molded to patient use. Nasal pillows resemble the nasal prongs used with infants, and provide a cushioning pillow for comfort (see Chapter 14).

Endotracheal Tube.—In patients who do not meet the criteria for mask CPAP, endotracheal intubation may be necessary to provide an airway for the patient and administration of CPAP or PEEP.

Resistance Devices Used on Exhalation Line to Provide CPAP or PEEP

During inspiration with PEEP therapy, the pressure may vary above, at, or below ambient. With CPAP, inspiratory pressure always remains above zero. The force or pressure the patient must generate to obtain inspiratory air flow depends on the use of either high gas flow systems, pressurized reservoirs, demand valves, or demand flow systems. Expiratory pressure, on the other hand, is kept above ambient with CPAP or PEEP and can employ a variety of resistance devices which are either flow resistors or threshold resistors.

Flow Resistors.—A flow resistor achieves expiratory pressure by creating a resistance to gas flow through an orifice. As the diameter of the orifice increases in size, the pressure level decreases. As the orifice decreases in size the pressure level on exhalation increases. Changes in expiratory gas flow rates also vary the expiratory pressure applied with a flow resistor. The higher the expired gas flow, the higher the expiratory pressure generated, and vice versa.[4] An ideal flow resistor is one in which pressure would increase linearly as the flow increases.[4] A flow resistor is technically an expiratory retard device. If the expiratory period were prolonged, the expiratory pressure could actually reach ambient (zero) at the end of exhalation.[35] An example of a flow resistor is a variable orifice screw clamp. Other examples are the Siemens Servo 900B PEEP valve and the Baby Bird overflow valve.

Threshold Resistors.—Ideally, a threshold resistor is a device that provides a constant pressure throughout the expiratory phase regardless of the rate of gas flow or the rate of ventilation.[4] When a threshold resistor is used in the exhalation line of a nonrebreathing system, the flow of exhaled air proceeds unimpeded until the pressure falls to the preset "threshold" value. At that time the exhaled gas flow stops and the system pressure is maintained.

In theory a threshold resistor allows unimpeded exhalation, and therefore does not give an expiratory retard[4, 97] (Fig 10–1,J). In fact, many threshold resistors also impede expiratory gas flow. There may be some resistance to flow depending on the diameter or opening through which exhaled gas must flow. Examples of threshold resistors are underwater column or "bucket" PEEP devices. Any expiratory resistance in this device depends on the diameter of the tube through which exhaled gas flows. Other examples are the Emerson water column PEEP valve and the Bird Demand CPAP system. A variety of threshold resistors are available. The two major types are gravity-dependent resistors and nongravity-dependent resistors[51]:

1. Examples of *gravity-dependent threshold resistors* include the water bottle (Fig 10–9), the water column (Fig 10–10), and the weighted ball (Fig 10–11).[51, 113]

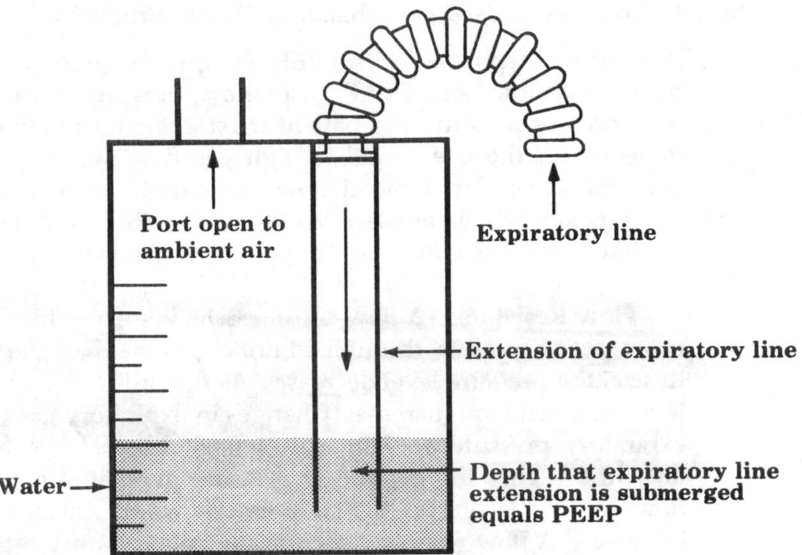

FIG 10–9.
Water bottle threshold resistor. The expiratory tube of the ventilatory device (mechanical ventilator or freestanding CPAP system) is submerged in a bottle of water. The amount of pressure exerted on exhalation is directly related to the height of the water in the submerged tube. This is true as long as the cross-sectional area of the submerged tube is the same as the cross-sectional area of the exhalation line. Coughing or forced expiration with flows greater than 20 to 30 L/min will increase the PEEP level transiently.

2. *Nongravity-dependent devices* include the spring-loaded valves (Fig 10–12), balloon-type expiratory valves (Fig 10–13), opposing gas flow systems[51] (Fig 10–14), magnetic PEEP valves, and electromechanical valves.[101]

In magnetic valves a disc of ferromagnetic metal is held against a valve seat by a magnet. The distance between the magnet and the disc is adjustable. This controls the level of PEEP. The closer the magnet to the disc, the higher the PEEP required to separate them. Flow resistance in these devices depends on how large an area the gas flow can pass through.[90] Ventilators which control their PEEP valves electromechanically include the Hamilton Veolar, which uses an electromagnetic pin to dynamically position a diaphragm over the exhalation port.[101, 102] As exhaled gas flow increases, the valve is controlled to open further. This helps keep pressures from rising above the desired PEEP level. This threshold resistor actually controls its flow resistance characteristics. The Servo 900C also has an electronically controlled valve, commonly called a scissor valve. If pressure measured during exhalation rises above the set PEEP, the valve opens wider to allow easier expiratory flow. When the expired pressure reaches the preset PEEP level, the valve closes. A disadvantage of this valve is that the diameter for exhaled gas is fairly narrow. For this reason it has flow-resistive properties.[4, 101]

Circuitry for Spontaneous CPAP or EPAP with Freestanding Systems and Mechanical Ventilators

Either CPAP or EPAP (sPEEP) can be provided by a freestanding system without using a ventilator. CPAP or sPEEP can also be provided through some mechanical ventilators by simply eliminating the mechanical breath. If the patient has been on mechanical ventilation and requires only CPAP at some point in the weaning process, then it is easier to use the ventilator than to assemble a separate freestanding CPAP system. For example, on the Puritan Bennett 7200, CPAP can be administered by changing the ventilator's mode selector to the CPAP mode and then adjusting the PEEP level until the desired pressure is recorded on the indicator. On the IMV Emerson, CPAP can be achieved by

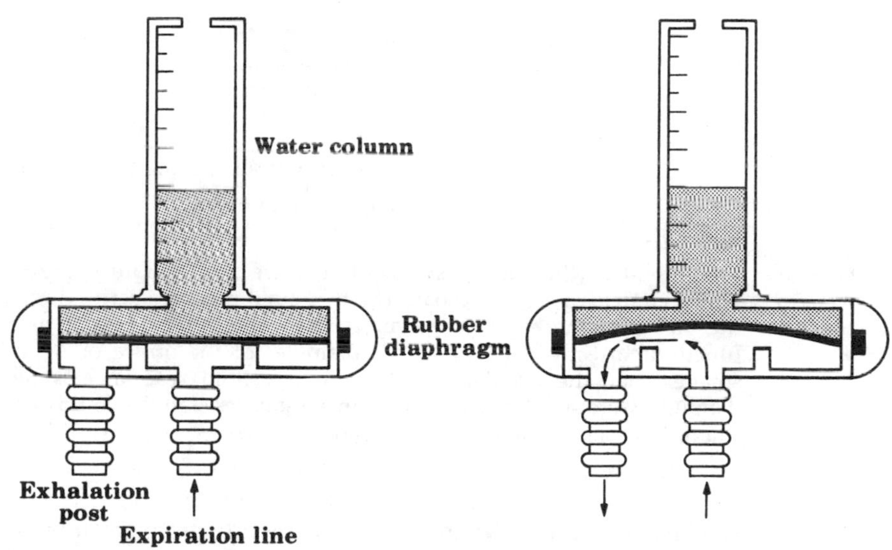

FIG 10–10.
Water column threshold resistor. In this device the expiratory line is connected to a specially designed expiratory valve in which a column of water sits on top of a flexible rubber expiratory diaphragm. The PEEP level is a function of the weight of the column of water and the surface area of the diaphragm. This is a true threshold resistor which is not significantly affected by expiratory flow changes. Flows must reach about 200 L/min for increased resistance to occur.[101] One example is the Emerson PEEP valve.

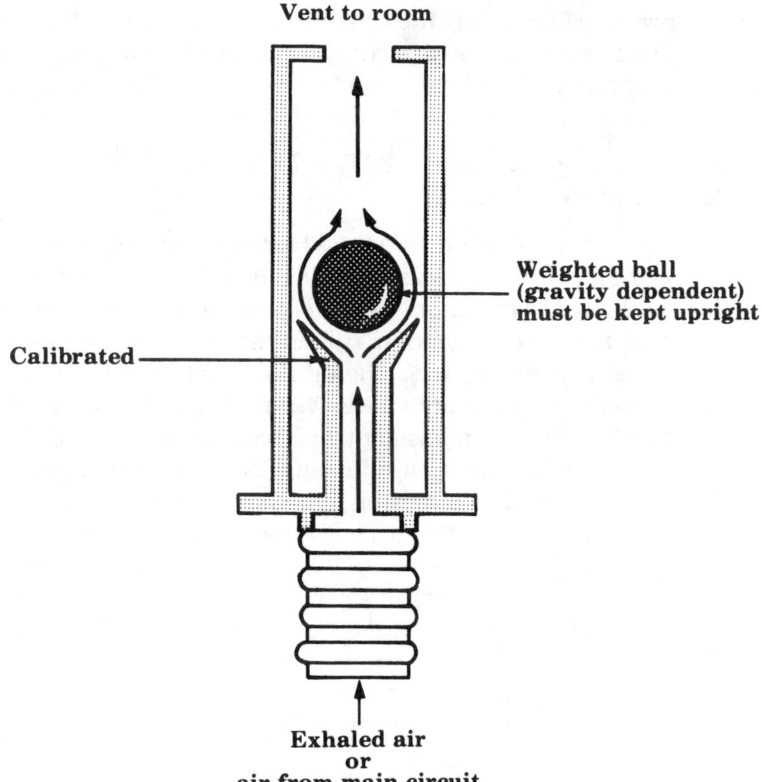

FIG 10–11.
Weighted-ball (threshold resistor) PEEP valve. An expiratory line is connected to a valve which contains a weighted ball. The threshold pressure varies directly with the weight of the ball over the expiratory orifice. The valve must be kept in a vertical position to function correctly. As long as the diameter of the orifice on which the ball sits is not smaller than the exhalation tube, the threshold resistance is nearly constant. If the diameter were smaller, orifice resistance (flow resistance) would affect the PEEP level. An example of this is the Boehringer valve.

turning the pump switch off, providing adequate gas flow to the IMV bag, and adding the desired amount of water to the water column until the desired CPAP is reached.

There are two types of freestanding or stand-alone CPAP or EPAP systems: continuous flow CPAP, which is a closed system, and demand flow spontaneous PEEP, which is an open system. Both systems mandate that the patient not require mechanical support, but still need support for a reduced FRC and hypoxemia. The patient must be able to comfortably maintain a near-normal $Paco_2$.

Continuous Flow CPAP.—In a continuous flow CPAP system, gas flows from a blended source of air and O_2 at the desired F_{IO_2} into a reservoir bag (anesthesia bag) and then to a heated humidifier. The air passes from the humidifier to a main flow inspiratory tube through a one-way valve and then into the patient (Fig 10–15). Exhaled air passes through a main expiratory line. This may also have a one-way valve in it, toward the expiratory resistor (PEEP device) which provides the desired positive expiratory or baseline pressure. The flow through the system must be adequate to provide the desired system pressure, meet the patient's flow demand, provide the desired O_2 concentration, and prevent CO_2 build-up. The one-way valve in the expiratory line can help to do this by making sure flow is unidirectional and by preventing the rebreathing of exhaled air.

A pressure relief valve, usually located close to the pressurized reservoir, provides a safety pop-off (pressure limiting) mechanism in the event the expiratory resistor becomes obstructed or fails to operate. The pop-off pressure is usually +5 cm H_2O above the desired threshold pressure. A pressure manometer connected close to the patient connector gives a reading of upper airway pressure and serves to monitor system pressure. Also near the patient's upper airway is a safety pop-in valve. This valve connects room air to the system. If the gas source fails the patient can open this one-way valve and breathe room air. Because of the risk of apnea or source gas failure, some systems also add a high and low pressure alarm. A temperature monitor and control device provide a

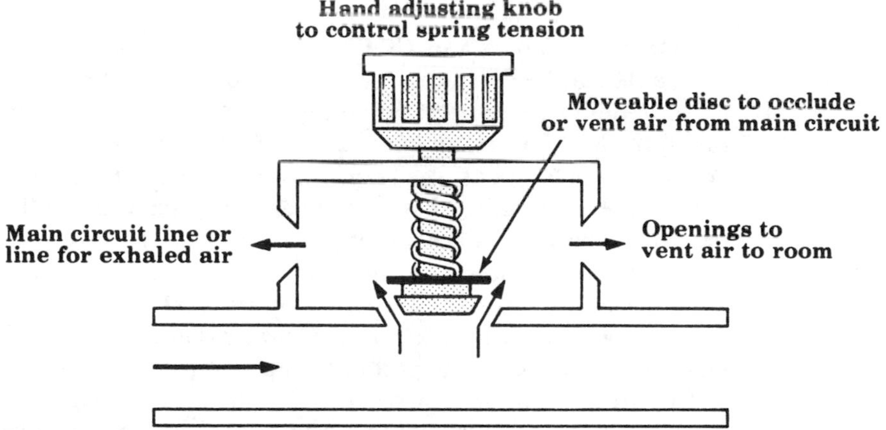

FIG 10–12.
Spring-type PEEP valve. A manually adjusted spring with a valve housing can be attached to an expiratory line to provide PEEP. The amount of pressure required to open the valve and allow flow out of the system is related to the tension (elastic recoil) present in the spring. In this device, if the diameter of the expiratory line decreases or the patient's expiratory gas flow increases, PEEP will increase.

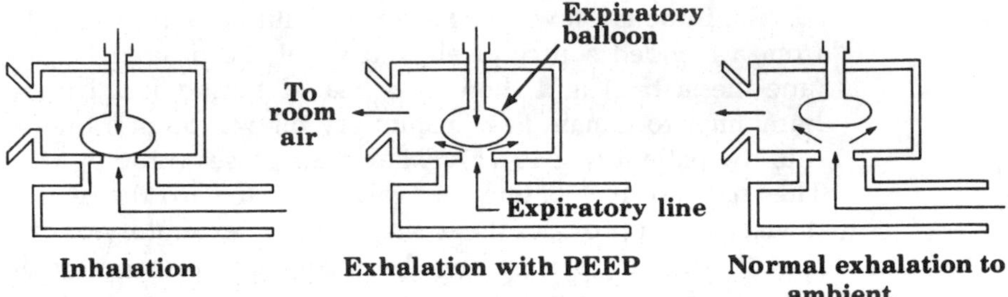

FIG 10–13.
Balloon-type PEEP valve. A partially inflated balloon present in the exhalation valve assembly creates a threshold resistor. As the volume within the balloon increases it creates pressure over the outlet orifice and its surface. When expiratory flow varies, PEEP also varies. During normal inhalation with IPPV the balloon occludes the expiratory orifice and air goes into the patient's lungs. During exhalation with PEEP the balloon volume partially occludes the exhalation orifice. During normal unimpeded exhalation to ambient pressure, the balloon completely deflates and does not affect the expired gas flow (no PEEP). Examples of this device include the Puritan Bennett: MA-1 and MA 2 + 2, and the BEAR 2.

method for assessing the appropriateness of the temperature level and a way of correcting very high or very low temperatures. It is a good idea to have a water trap in the inspiratory line for catching and removing condensation. This is not mandatory, but does help to avoid the necessity of removing the patient from the system in order to empty the tubing.

Demand Valves and CPAP.—Another type of CPAP device provides gas from a demand valve rather than from a pressurized reservoir bag. The demand valve is designed to open when a patient's inspiratory effort drops the system pressure by a few centimeters of water pressure below the baseline pressure. When the valve opens, gas flows into the system and to the patient to meet the demand. As the patient begins to exhale, the expired gas flow raises the system pressure slightly over the preset pressure level. The flow from the demand valve stops. Exhaled air is vented through the threshold resistor.[4] The demand valve system is a CPAP system since inspiratory pressures do not fall below zero. One of the problems with demand valve systems is that many of them require some work of breathing on the part of the patient to open the system. This may cause a transient drop in pressure (-4.5 to -9.0 cm H_2O below baseline). The demand valve may actually provide a positive pressure boost later in the inspiratory phase. This has been evaluated in mechanical ventilators which allow for CPAP through a demand valve (BEAR-1, Monaghan 225/SIMA, Puritan Bennett MA-2 and MA-2+2, Servo ventilators 900B and 900C).[36, 80]

A comparison between a continuous flow CPAP (Emerson IMV or CPAP ventilation) and a demand valve CPAP (MA-2) indicated that demand valve

CPAPs may require increased $\dot{V}O_2$ and may produce increased carbon dioxide production ($\dot{V}CO_2$) compared with the continuous flow systems.[42] Newer ventilator systems with improved demand valves cause only a slight increase in work of breathing which can basically be eliminated by using low levels (+10 cm H_2O) of pressure support.

Demand Flow EPAP (sPEEP).—Demand flow EPAP systems are not the same as demand valve systems. Demand flow systems require that the patient open a one-way valve to a gas reservoir which is at ambient pressures, and contains gas at the desired F_{IO_2}. Pressures on inspiration drop below zero. Blended gases flow through a heated humidifier and into a large-bore tube that acts as an unpressurized reservoir (Fig 10–16). When the patient breathes in, reservoir gas flows to the patient. When the patient breathes out, exhaled air is directed down the main expiratory tube toward the expiratory resistor (PEEP

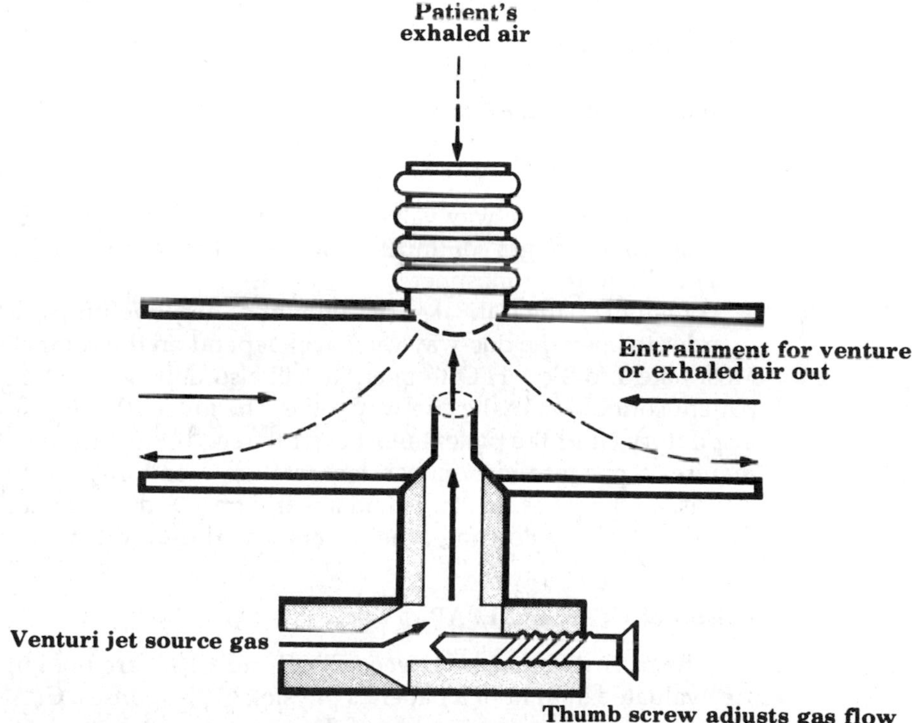

FIG 10–14.
Opposing gas flow system for PEEP. An opposing flow system is basically a Venturi device which exerts pressure against the patient's exhaled air. This maintains a positive pressure and creates PEEP or CPAP. An example is present on the Bourns BP200 ventilator.

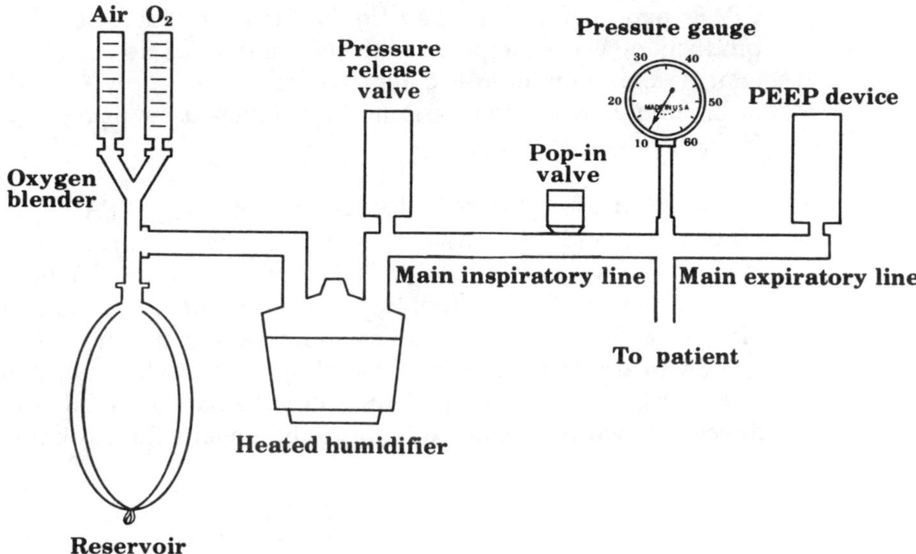

FIG 10–15.
Continuous flow CPAP circuit.

valve) through a one-way valve. This valve prevents rebreathing of air. During exhalation, source gas continues to flow into the reservoir tubing and the excess is vented into the atmosphere.

When the patient inhales, the amount of negative pressure that is generated in order to open the one-way valve will depend on the competency of the valve. Most take 1 to 2 cm H_2O to open. It will also depend on the distance from the patient connection to the one-way valve. The longer the distance, the greater the inspiratory effort the patient must exert to receive the inspired gas.[51] This system requires a pressure manometer, temperature monitoring and regulation, apnea alarms, a high pressure alarm, and a water trap. A disadvantage of the system is that if inspiratory flow fails, the patient can end up breathing only ambient air.

Comparison of CPAP and EPAP

The basic differences between EPAP and CPAP are not important until they are evaluated in light of a patient's physiologic responses. CPAP systems require a high pressure reservoir and gas flow source and a closed circuit system that can provide the needed positive pressure during both inspiration and expiration. The flow of gas from the reservoir must meet or exceed the patient's peak inspiratory flow rate. This can generally be provided with a flow rate four times the patient's measured $\dot{V}_E$. An EPAP system does not use a pressurized reservoir as long as it is required that the inspiratory phase be below ambient and not positive. The expiratory resistance on either system needs to be kept to a minimum by using a low resistance exhalation valve.

To further illustrate the difference between the two, look at the pressure curves that are generated as the inspiratory flow rate is changed (Fig 10–17). When CPAP is operated at high flows, the work of breathing is low. The work of breathing is the integral of the pressure difference which must be generated to move a volume of gas[56] ($W = \int PV$) where W is work, P is pressure, and V is volume.[32] Figure 10–17 shows hypothetical pressure curves that are generated during spontaneous ventilation on a circuit with expiratory pressures at 15 cm H_2O and at constant flow rates of 60 L/min *(I)*, 45 L/min *(II)*, 30 L/min *(III)*, 15 L/min *(IV)*, and 5 L/min *(V)* on inspiration. Curves *I*, *II*, *III*, and *IV* all represent CPAP. Curve *V* represents EPAP. Note that the difference between curve *IV* and curve *V* is small. In both of these curves the patient must overcome a large pressure difference to receive an inspiratory flow of gas. Thus, the work of breathing with CPAP can, on occasion, be nearly as high as it is with EPAP. Gas flows through a system which can provide inspiratory flows and pressures similar to curve *I* require minimal patient respiratory effort. To achieve this curve, gas flows through the system must be kept high (3 to 4 × $\dot{V}_E$). The volume can be inspired from the pressurized reservoir without a significant change in the system pressure.

Physiologically, the patient has two basic responses to these two systems. (1) With EPAP the work of breathing is increased, but the mean airway pressure

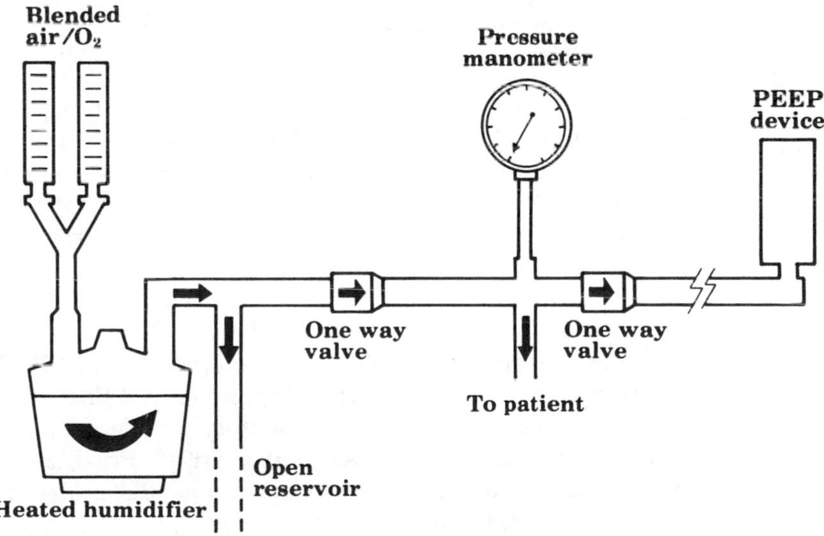

FIG 10–16.
Demand flow spontaneous PEEP circuit (open system).

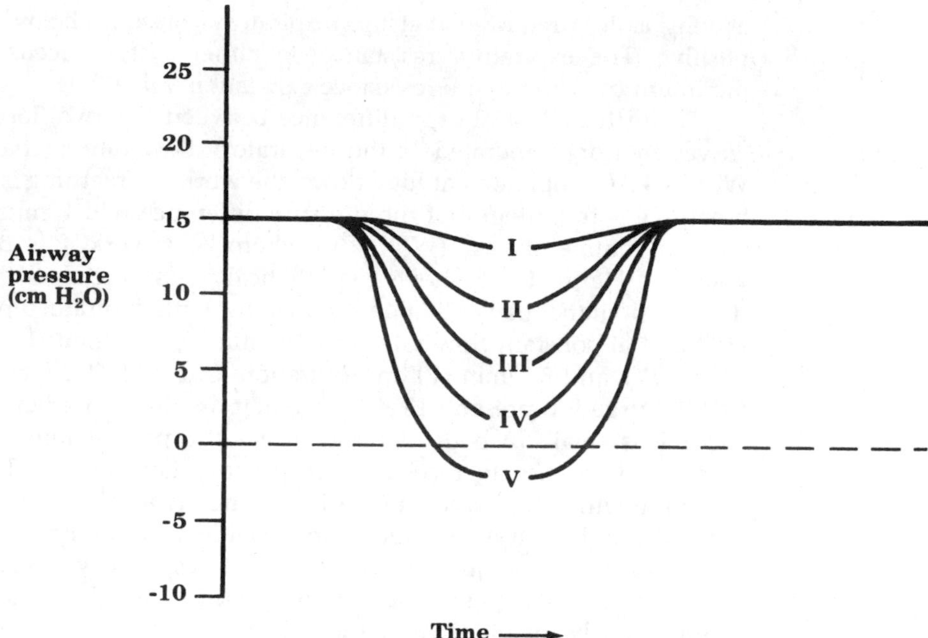

FIG 10–17.
Airway pressure changes vary during inspiration when a patient is on a continuous flow CPAP system, depending on the amount of inspiratory flow provided. The inspiratory flow rate varies as follows: *I* = 60 L/min, *II* = 45 L/min, *III* = 30 L/min, *IV* = 15 L/min, *V* = 5 L/min. The lower the flow rate, the greater the change in pressure between exhalation and inhalation. (Data from references 32 and 56.)

($\overline{P}aw$) is lower. With lower positive pressure, the intrapleural pressure is lower, venous return to the heart is improved, and one would anticipate CO to be improved. (2) With the CPAP system, the work of breathing is low but intrapleural pressures are higher and venous return and CO can be lower compared with EPAP.[30, 51]

It would appear that EPAP has fewer effects on the cardiovascular system than CPAP, but this is not always the case. The afterload on the heart may be less during inspiration with CPAP, compared with EPAP, due to a lowering of the transmural aortic pressure. Opponents of EPAP cite the increased work of breathing and the potential circulatory problems, such as increased venous return in the face of increased left heart afterload, as reasons why CPAP is a better method of supporting a patient's FRC and oxygenation. In terms of increasing lung volume delivery and FRC, CPAP appears to be more effective than identical levels of EPAP. Patients on EPAP have been seen to have an end-expiratory thoracic squeeze similar to a Valsalva maneuver and they show clinical deterioration.[56, 57] The effective FRC may be reduced in these patients and may explain their worsening clinical picture. Given all the possibilities, CPAP is preferable to EPAP.

PEEP WITH CONTROLLED VENTILATION

Most conventional mechanical ventilators provide a method for administering PEEP at the end of exhalation between controlled mechanical ventilator breaths. When they do not, PEEP can be administered by adding a threshold resistor, such as a water bottle or water column, at the expiratory valve on the ventilator. It is important that the tubing from the valve be the same diameter as the threshold resistor or PEEP valve, or the expiratory pressures may not be what is desired. The exhaled air must all pass through the PEEP valve or the desired PEEP may not be maintained. Upper airway pressure tracings similar to Figure 10–1,B are produced with continuous ventilation plus PEEP. Desired PEEP levels may be obtained by dialing in the appropriate PEEP on the ventilator until the manometer registers the desired PEEP, or by adjusting the water level in the water column or bottle until the manometer reads appropriately.

Continuous ventilation with PEEP has a disadvantage in that it usually results in a higher $\overline{P}aw$ than other forms of ventilation and a higher incidence of cardiovascular complications and pulmonary barotrauma. For example, with comparable peak pressures and PEEP, IMV with PEEP appears to have fewer problems associated with it than control or assist-control ventilation with PEEP.

PEEP WITH ASSISTED VENTILATION

With assisted ventilation, the ventilator delivers a positive pressure breath to the patient when the patient makes an inspiratory effort and triggers the mechanism. Sensitivity is adjusted with assisted ventilation so that a pressure change of 1 or 2 cm H_2O below zero triggers the machine breath. Assisted ventilation can also be used with PEEP. With this mode of ventilation, the inspiratory phase consists of a machine-delivered breath and the expiratory phase is against resistance so the baseline is above ambient (Fig 10–1,C). As with normal assisted ventilation (baseline of zero), it is desirable for a small change in sensitivity to trigger a machine breath with a patient on assisted ventilation with PEEP. Otherwise the patient must inhale all the way to zero pressure or less. This would increase the work of breathing.

Suppose the patient is on a PEEP of +7 cm H_2O. It would be desirable for the machine to give a breath when the pressure was about 5 to 6 cm H_2O. Some ventilators have an automatic sensitivity adjustor so that when PEEP is dialed in, the preset sensitivity is adjusted to that level. Examples of this include the BEAR 2, 3, and 5, the Puritan Bennett 7200ae, the Servo 900C and 300, and the Veolar.

If the sensitivity is set at -2 cm H_2O for assisted ventilation, then the same or less effort is required to cycle the machine regardless of the level of PEEP.

Other ventilators need to have the sensitivity readjusted. The MA-1 is an example. Sensitivity can be readjusted by occluding the patient wye connector, dialing in the desired PEEP, turning the machine sensitivity up until the ventilator automatically cycles (rapidly), and decreasing the sensitivity until the spontaneous cycling stops. The patient can then be connected to the ventilator at the new PEEP level.[27]

PEEP WITH IMV

There are two techniques of applying positive expiratory pressure with IMV. With one technique the patient must open a one-way valve to receive air during spontaneous breathing. This is an open demand flow system IMV which returns spontaneous inspiratory pressures to below zero (Fig 10–1,E). By adding a PEEP valve to the expiratory line this becomes an IMV with EPAP. The other type of IMV with PEEP uses a reservoir bag which is inflated with enough pressure to keep the one-way valve open into the system from the reservoir between machine-delivered breaths. A continuous flow of gas passes through the patient circuit. When flows are adequate, the patient's inspiratory effort results in pressures remaining above ambient. Thus, baseline airway pressures stay above zero. This is best described as IMV with CPAP (Fig 10–1,D). The addition of a threshold resistor to the expiratory line in the setting provides a continuous flow IMV with CPAP.

Continuous Flow IMV vs. Demand Flow IMV

The use of demand flow IMV with EPAP, as opposed to continuous flow IMV with CPAP, has been debated. In the demand flow system the patient must open a one-way valve. This increases the work of breathing for the patient. Supporters of demand flow IMV with EPAP suggest that the reduction in $\overline{P}aw$ has cardiovascular advantages. The difference between the work of breathing with IMV and EPAP vs. IMV with CPAP parallel the differences seen with CPAP vs. EPAP.

SIMV With CPAP

With SIMV the ventilator is sensitive to patient effort when a machine breath is due to be delivered. Between these assisted machine breaths the patient can breathe spontaneously at ambient pressures. Current ventilators offer the feature of CPAP with SIMV. Between machine breaths the patient can breathe spontaneously at pressures above ambient. This is achieved by the use of demand valves or a bellows which activates when a patient makes a spontaneous inspiratory effort. They then provide gas flow to meet the demand of the patient's inspiratory effort and gas flow to meet the inspiratory flow demands without actually giving a positive pressure machine breath. The spontaneous inspiratory breathing pressure stays above zero. During exhalation, the demand valve closes. The exhaled air then passes to the threshold resistor which is set at the desired end-expiratory pressure (EPAP). Since pressures at the airway always keep a positive baseline, this mode of ventilation is most appropriately called SIMV with CPAP (see Fig 10–1,F). Ventilators which provide this feature include the 7200ae, the BEAR 5, the Servo 900C, and the Veolar.

The work of breathing may increase with SIMV and CPAP compared with regular IMV with CPAP. This is demonstrated by an increase in $\dot{V}O_2$ and $\dot{V}CO_2$.[42] Further evaluation is needed to support these findings.

PEEP WITH PRESSURE SUPPORT AND PRESSURE CONTROL

Microprocessor or third-generation ventilators can provide pressure support (PS) and pressure control (PC) modes of ventilation. These ventilators also give the option of PEEP with these additional modes. In PS, the baseline value is above zero during this assist mode of ventilation. With PC, PEEP can also be dialed in. When PC is used with IRV, air trapping and the resulting auto-PEEP are not uncommon (see Chapter 7). Adding external or extrinsic PEEP can cause significant hemodynamic effects. For this reason, it must be used with caution.

USES OF PEEP FOR OTHER THAN ACUTE LUNG INJURY

Mask CPAP in Postoperative Atelectasis and Hypoxemia

Some attention has been given to the use of CPAP by mask as a way to prevent postoperative pulmonary complications, such as atelectasis, and help speed the return of the lungs to their preoperative volume. Use of mask CPAP has been shown to return baseline lung volumes in patients that had received upper abdominal surgery more rapidly than when treated with frequent coughing and deep breathing alone. It also appears to help reduce the incidence of atelectasis in postoperative patients and to improve oxygenation. Levels of CPAP in these studies varied from about 5 to 15 cm H_2O. These were applied over various intervals ranging from hourly administration of 25 to 35 breaths to continuous use for up to 6 to 10 hours. The exact levels needed to accomplish the desired results still need to be determined.

Sleep Apnea

Nasal CPAP (NCPAP) has become an option for the management of obstructive sleep apnea (see Chapter 14). Levels of 5 to 15 cm H_2O may help prevent pharyngeal obstruction by causing a pneumatic splint. Another way in which it may work is by increasing FRC which results in an increase in the pharyngeal cross-sectional area.

Neonatal Apnea

One of the common respiratory problems of low-birth-weight infants is apnea. The use of CPAP in these neonates may reduce obstructive apnea. The possible mechanism of this benefit of CPAP may be that it improves airway patency.

Cystic Fibrosis

One of the common forms of treatment for cystic fibrosis is chest physiotherapy. Some physicians in Denmark have experimented with the use of EPAP in this patient group. They apply EPAP by mask using a one-way inspiratory valve and a one-way expiratory flow resistor. This is commonly referred to as a positive expiratory pressure (PEP) mask. The flow resistor is designed to prevent end-expiratory pressures from falling back to zero. The device obtains expiratory pressures of 10 to 20 cm H_2O at midexhalation. It is used for 15- to 20-minute periods, three to four times a day. This procedure may help improve the expectoration of secretions, reduce residual volume (less hyperinflation), and improve airway stability.

Chronic Obstructive Pulmonary Disease

Some research has looked at the use of CPAP in patients with asthma and bronchiolitis. Findings suggest that PEEP or CPAP may produce mechanical dilation of the airways and reduce the load on the inspiratory muscles induced by asthma. These findings need more clinical evaluation to establish their safe role in these patient groups. While PEEP or CPAP is not commonly used in COPD, low levels may help prevent small airway closure.

AIRWAY SUCTIONING WITH PEEP

There are some patients whose clinical picture deteriorates rapidly when PEEP is discontinued for the purpose of suctioning. For this type of patient it is appropriate to use manual ventilation using a resuscitation bag adapted with

PEEP or to suction through a specially adapted endotracheal-ventilator connector.[11,51] This allows suctioning without disconnecting the patient from the ventilator and helps in maintaining PEEP. A closed continuous tracheal suction is also available which provides a system for using a suction catheter without disconnecting the patient from the ventilator. The most common example of this is the Ballard suction catheter.

WEANING FROM PEEP

The exact length of time that PEEP is needed before the alveoli are stable in patients with ARDS is not known.[22] Premature weaning from PEEP is not without problems. In patients whose Pa_{O_2} drops to 65 mm Hg or lower with a reduction in PEEP of 5 cm H_2O, as long as 24 hours is required to return their Pa_{O_2} values to baseline when PEEP is reinstituted. These patients may also require higher PEEP and may develop complications like pneumothorax, hypotension, or reductions in $S\bar{v}_{O_2}$ within 2 hours following the resumption of PEEP.[22]

It takes from 3 to 8 minutes to reach the lowest immediate Pa_{O_2} drop after PEEP is discontinued. The greatest drop occurs in the first minute[22] (Fig 10–18). The highest incidence of failure to wean from PEEP occurs in patients who are on PEEP for only short periods. This may be linked to inappropriate clinical judgment as to the readiness of the alveoli to maintain function and stability.[19]

There are a few criteria which may be useful in indicating that the patient is ready for a trial reduction in PEEP. These are guided by an acceptable Pa_{O_2} on an F_{IO_2} of less than 0.40. The patient must be hemodynamically stable and nonseptic. If the lung compliance is improved (Cs >25 mL/cm H_2O) and the Pa_{O_2}/F_{IO_2} ratio is high (>300), then the chances of successful lowering of PEEP are about 80%.[110] A recommended procedure for weaning from PEEP is as follows:

1. Obtain baseline arterial blood gases and determine that the criteria have been met.
2. Reduce PEEP by +5 cm H_2O.
3. Obtain an arterial blood gas analysis to determine the effect of the reduction in PEEP. It may be advisable to return the PEEP level to where it was (at step 1) until the blood gas results are obtained.
4. If the patient's Pa_{O_2} falls by less than 20% of the previous PEEP level for Pa_{O_2}, then the patient is ready to tolerate the lower PEEP level.
5. If the patient has more than a 20% reduction in Pa_{O_2} along with an increase in shunt, then the patient is not ready to have the PEEP reduced and it should be returned to its previous level.

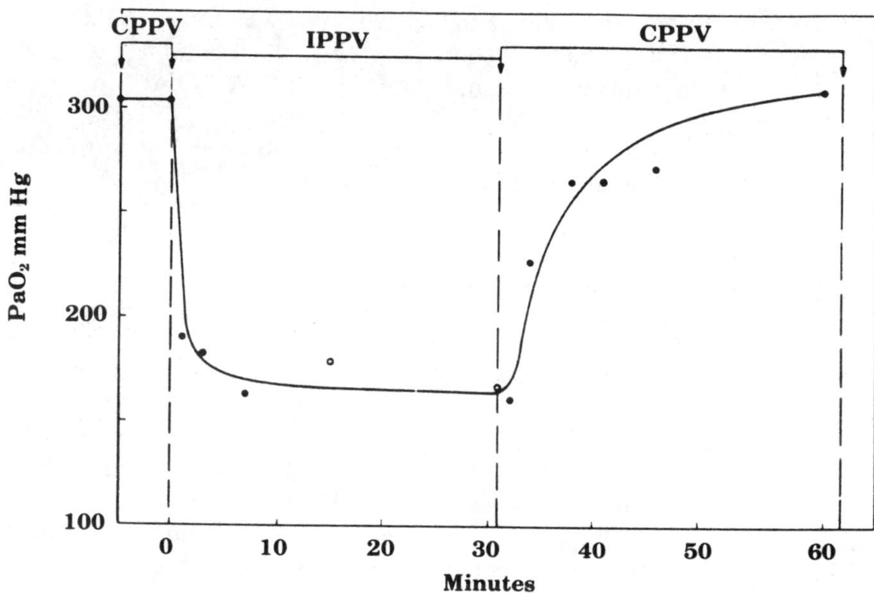

FIG 10–18.
Time sequence of Pa_{O_2} change with alteration of ventilation pattern in eight patients. The mean Pa_{O_2} with CPPV was 304 mm Hg. After a change to IPPV it fell by 129 mm Hg within 1 minute, and a further fall of 32 mm Hg occurred over the next 3 minutes. *Open circles* represent mean values of only six patients (in one patient a large fall in Pa_{O_2} required reapplication of CPPV after 6 minutes; a second value was not available owing to clotting of the blood sample). On reapplication of CPPV, the Pa_{O_2} rose gradually to its initial value. (From Kumar A, Falke KJ, Geffin B, et al: *N Engl J Med* 1970; 283:1433. Used by permission.)

6. Wait between reductions in PEEP and reevaluate the initial criteria. If the patient is stable, then reduce the PEEP by another 5 cm H_2O. This might take only 1 hour or may require as long as 6 hours.
7. When the patient is at +5 cm H_2O and needs only to be turned to zero, then an additional evaluation is involved. If reducing the PEEP to zero results in a worsening of the patient's condition, then it may be appropriate to leave the patient at +5 cm H_2O until it is time to extubate. It may be necessary to place the patient on 5 cm H_2O of CPAP by mask after extubation.[35]

More than likely, however, patients will do fine once they are extubated. The complete removal of PEEP prior to extubation may not be necessary and may be detrimental to patients with compromised lung-thorax mechanisms leading to a deterioration of FRC and Pa_{O_2}.

INVERSE RATIO VENTILATION FOR IMPROVING OXYGENATION

In addition to PEEP or CPAP for the treatment of severe hypoxemia, current reviews suggest that IRV may provide another method for improving oxygenation. This improvement seems to be related to $\overline{P}aw$ and the flow rates and patterns by which the pressures are administered.

Importance of Mean Airway Pressure

Mean airway pressure is the pressure measured at the airway opening during one respiratory cycle (inspiration plus expiration) (see Chapter 7). It represents the average pressure applied by the ventilator. $\overline{P}aw$ is affected by $\dot{V}_E$, PEEP, and different flow patterns. In patients that are passively ventilated (control support), $\overline{P}aw$ is a major determinant in oxygenation because it changes P_A and alveolar recruitment.[69]

Flow patterns alone can affect gas exchange independent of $\overline{P}aw$. Improvement in gas exchange and decreases in intrapulmonary shunting have been shown to occur with ventilatory patterns that keep end-expiratory pressure above zero even when $\overline{P}aw$ and V_T are constant.[69] This pressure at end-exhalation may help prevent alveolar and airway collapse. Keeping alveoli open may reduce dead space and help mixing of gases at the alveolar level by improving collateral ventilation. Thus, end-expiratory pressures as well as $\overline{P}aw$ can improve oxygenation.

One way to ventilate patients with ARDS and avoid the risk of barotrauma and alveolar damage might be to adjust flow patterns to improve $\overline{P}aw$ but keep peak pressure and P_A at a minimum. Using IRV may provide such an approach. There are two basic ways of providing IRV: (1) pressure-controlled ventilation in which pressure is preset and inspiration is time-triggered and time-cycled (see Chapter 6); (2) volume-controlled ventilation in which inspiration is made longer by using slow inspiratory flows, inspiratory pause, or descending flow patterns with long inspiratory times. The first is called pressure-controlled inverse ratio ventilation (PCIRV). The second is called volume-controlled inverse ratio ventilation (VCIRV). IRV by either method provides a way to increase $\overline{P}aw$ independent of PEEP.

Methods of Providing Inverse Ratio Ventilation

Pressure-controlled ventilation is available in some of the microprocessor ventilators. In this mode the operator presets the ventilating pressure, rate, and inspiratory time. Inspiration can be longer than expiration (IRV). Pressure delivery is constant and the inspiratory waveform is descending. It is possible that the descending flow pattern may provide better gas distribution than the constant

TABLE 10-8.
Comparison of Volume-Controlled (VCIRV) and Pressure-Controlled (PCIRV) Inverse Ratio Ventilation*

VCIRV	PCIRV
Advantages Available on all ventilators Guaranteed minute ventilation Precise control of flow pattern Familiar mode to most clinicans Peak inspiratory flow lower than PCIRV Disadvantages Peak alveolar pressures can vary; pressures must be monitored carefully Deep sedation usually necessary to prevent dyssynchronous breathing	Advantages Peak distending pressures precisely controlled Some patients may tolerate without deep sedation Larger experience published in the literature Disadvantages Tidal volume varies with changing respiratory mechanics; minute ventilation must be monitored carefully Not available on all ventilators Not a familiar mode to many clinicians ? Greater shear forces

*From Marcy TW, Marini JJ: *Chest* 1991; 100:494–504. Used by permission.

flow pattern generally used with volume-cycled ventilation.[2, 69, 74] During PCIRV, P_A values will equalize with the preset pressure. Volume delivery varies with compliance and resistance. For this reason, it is important in this mode to monitor exhaled V_T and $\dot{V}_E$. Auto-PEEP is generated as inspiration exceeds expiration (see Chapter 7).

Volume control with IRV is an attractive alternative to PCIRV and may not have some of the problems associated with PCIRV (see Chapters 6 and 7). Almost any volume ventilator can be adjusted to provide IRV. Since VCIRV uses a volume ventilator, V_T is assured. Using a constant or a descending waveform, very slow inspiratory flows will produce IRV. Also, an inspiratory pause can achieve the same effect of IRV. Using inspiratory pause tends to increase $\bar{P}aw$ more than a slow flow rate. But slow flow rates with descending or constant patterns produce lower peak pressures. With this mode, the pressure limit must always be set at a safe level. This is usually considered to be 10 cm H_2O above the peak pressure for a normal ventilator breath. The problem is that as hyperinflation increases with IRV, the peak airway pressure and P_A rise and may increase the risk of barotrauma. The advantages and disadvantages of VCIRV and PCIRV are shown in Table 10–8.

RISKS OF INVERSE RATIO VENTILATION

Regardless of the way in which it is applied, IRV has several risks associated with it. These include the risk of barotrauma such as pneumothoraces due to hyperinflation of the lung. Cardiac output may decrease with hyperinflation (auto-PEEP). The inverse ratio may be uncomfortable for the patient and require sedation and paralysis. This is especially true if the machine is in an assist mode as the patient can trigger the ventilator which can lead to dyssynchronous breathing.[69] In addition, since the PA rises (35–40 cm H_2O) and the end-expiratory pressure is above 10 cm H_2O, the delivered VT may be very small. Increasing respiratory rate in PCIRV can actually reduce alveolar ventilation as air trapping (auto-PEEP) rises. With VCIRV, increasing the rate may increase Ppeak and $\overline{P}aw$ to dangerous levels.

IMPLEMENTING INVERSE RATIO VENTILATION

IRV is being used in the management of ARDS, but clinical research has not demonstrated that IRV is equal to or better than conventional ventilation with PEEP. At present there are no physiologic guidelines for its safe use. Marcy and Marini[69] have described their method for using IRV which has shown to be safe and effective in their practice. It will be reviewed here.

Regular Ventilator Management With ARDS

Adults with ARDS are managed with volume-cycled ventilation, using assist-control at a VT of 7 to 10 mL/kg and a PEEP of 7 to 10 cm H_2O to compensate for the decrease in lung volume associated with the supine position.[69] Additional PEEP is used to reduce F_{IO_2} needs and to maintain Sa_{O_2} at greater than 85%. At PEEP levels greater than 10 cm H_2O a pulmonary artery catheter is inserted to monitor CO data. Patients are frequently repositioned, if possible, to maximize volume recruitment and avoid alveolar collapse. They are carefully monitored and worked with to help avoid respiratory infections and to clear secretions.

The VT is maintained to keep PA below 35 cm H_2O to avoid lung injury. Sometimes, a low VT (6–8 mL/kg) with a respiratory rate that avoids high ventilation is used to maintain pH at 7.35, with bicarbonate infusion when necessary to balance any rise in CO_2.

Increasing Inspiratory Time

When excessive levels of PEEP, high levels of inspired O_2, or high peak distending pressures are unavoidable, Marcy and Marini[69] consider using inverse inspiratory-expiratory (I/E) ratios. High I/E ratios are apparently more effective early in the disease process when some normal, recruitable alveoli are still present. They consider IRV as a method to raise $\overline{P}aw$ to a "minimum" effective level.

For this procedure the following parameters are monitored: gas exchange, pulse oximetry, hemodynamic data, $\dot{V}_E$ and Paw, including end-expiratory pressures (extrinsic PEEP plus auto-PEEP). The patient is sedated and paralyzed if these agents have not already been instituted. This helps prevent assynchronous breathing, fosters patient comfort, and allows $\overline{P}aw$ to reflect relaxed lung expansion without active expiratory or inspiratory efforts.

Constant and descending flow patterns are available as is inspiratory pause on most volume-controlled ventilators for increasing I/E. Since most ventilators have a flow rate control, there seems to be better control over $\overline{P}aw$ by changing flow rate than by employing an inspiratory pause maneuver. In addition, peak airway pressure tends to be lower with a descending flow pattern than with a constant flow. For this reason, Marcy and Marini[69] favor the use of a descending flow pattern over a constant flow or an inspiratory hold. When initiating VCIRV with a descending ramp flow pattern, the authors begin by switching flow waveforms without changing PEEP or peak flow rate. This helps to maintain a lower airway pressure while increasing inspiratory time and $\overline{P}aw$. The peak flow setting must be at least four times the $\dot{V}_E$ setting to avoid

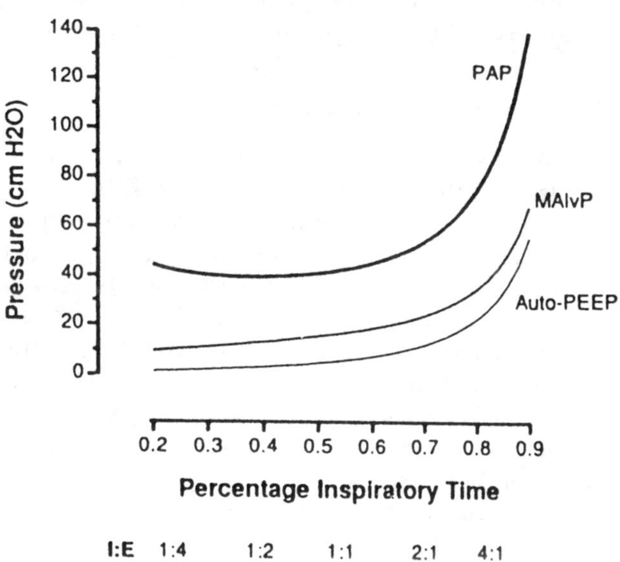

FIG 10–19.
Graph of the predicted peak airway pressure *(PAP),* mean alveolar pressure *(MAlvP),* and auto-PEEP as the I/E ratio (or inspiratory time percentage) is increased during volume-controlled ventilation. Predictions were made using a model of constant flow, volume-controlled ventilation in a respiratory system with low compliance (0.04 L/cm H_2O), expiratory resistance greater than inspiratory resistance (20 vs. 10 cm H_2O/[L/sec]), and ventilator settings of 1 L V_T at a respiratory frequency of 20 breaths/min. At I/E ratios exceeding 2:1, the airway and alveolar pressures rise hyperbolically. (From Marcy TW, Marini JJ: *Chest* 1991; 100:494–504. Used by permission.)

overdistention at the beginning. They then decrease flow rate slowly while observing its effects. The pressure limit is set at 10 cm H_2O over the normal V_T inflation pressure. Tidal volume, respiratory rate, and PEEP are adjusted as needed to maintain an end-inspiratory P_A of 35 to 40 cm H_2O. Total end-expiratory pressure is between 10 and 15 cm H_2O and is adjusted by altering extrinsic (external) PEEP.

On ventilators which do not have a descending ramp waveform, a constant flow pattern is used. With constant flow, $\overline{P}aw$ is varied by increasing the length of inspiratory pause rather than by changing the flow rate. The initial flow rate, again, must be at least four times $\dot{V}_E$. Pressure limit is set the same as with a descending ramp waveform. Pause length is gradually increased when a constant flow is used until O_2 saturation is adequate or until the I/E ratio is 2:1. Values higher than this may have significant effects on CO and hemodynamic conditions. This also helps keep P_A values from becoming too high and causing tissue damage (Fig 10–19). It must be emphasized that an inverse ratio may not be necessary in maintaining adequate oxygenation.

Once the patient's condition has improved and O_2 exchange is better, then inspiratory time can be shortened with faster flow rates with the descending ramp waveform, or inspiratory pause is shortened if a constant waveform was used.

SUMMARY

The primary focus of this chapter has been on PEEP and CPAP therapy. It is a common and widely used method for improving oxygenation in severely hypoxemic patients who are refractory to O_2 therapy. Its use will undoubtedly continue for many years to come. A newer method for improving oxygenation, IRV, is becoming more frequently used in the critical care setting although clinical trials have not yet demonstrated its advantages over more conventional PEEP or CPAP modes. The next few years will, perhaps, provide more insight into this technique.

STUDY QUESTIONS

1. Which of the following are potential complications of PEEP therapy?
   I. Reduced cardiac output.
   II. Altered cardiac function.
   III. Barotrauma.
   IV. Increased ICP.

V. Reduced urinary output.
a. I only.
b. I and III.
c. II, III, and V.
d. I, II, III, and IV.
e. I, II, III, IV, and V.

2. sPEEP is most nearly the same as:
a. auto-PEEP.
b. EPAP.
c. IPAP.
d. CPAP.
e. IRV.
3. Patients with COPD can benefit significantly from PEEP levels higher than 10 cm H_2O. True or false?
4. A primary goal of PEEP therapy is to improve O_2 transport. True or false?
5. A PEEP study is being done on a patient. When the PEEP is increased from +10 to +15 cm H_2O the CO goes from 4 to 2 L/min. What would be the next most appropriate step?
a. Decrease the F_{IO_2}.
b. Increase PEEP to +20 cm H_2O.
c. Decrease PEEP to +10 cm H_2O.
d. Measure the blood pressure.
e. Make no changes at this time.
6. A patient is on +13 cm H_2O of CPAP on a freestanding, continuous flow system. During inspiration the manometer shows a pressure of +3 cm H_2O. During expiration the pressure is +13 cm H_2O. This indicates:

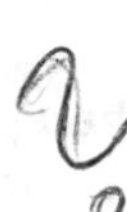

a. The patient needs ventilatory support.
b. The gas flow rate is inadequate.
c. The patient is ready to be weaned.
d. Work of breathing is low.
e. The CPAP level is too low.
7. During mechanical ventilation with IMV plus PEEP, the PEEP level is +10 cm H_2O and peak pressure is 44 cm H_2O. The PEEP is increased to +15 cm H_2O and the peak pressure rises to 50 cm H_2O. The rise in peak pressure indicates:
a. A normal occurrence with an increase in PEEP.
b. Bronchospasm.
c. Presence of a pneumothorax.
d. FRC had decreased.
e. Compliance had changed.
8. PEEP therapy is commonly used in which of the following conditions?
I. ARDS.
II. IRDS.

III. Right-sided pneumonia.
IV. Cerebrovascular accidents.
  a. I only.
  b. I and II.
  c. III and IV.
  d. I, II, and IV.
  e. I, II, III, and IV.

9. A 38-year-old patient who has ARDS is being mechanically ventilated. The results of an arterial blood gas analysis are: pH = 7.38, $Paco_2$ = 42 mm Hg, Pao_2 = 55 mm Hg. The ventilator settings are: Fio_2 = 0.9, f = 10 breaths/min, VT = 850 mL, PEEP = 5 cm H_2O. Based on this information, which of the following might be changed to improve the patient's oxygenation status?
  a. VT.
  b. Respiratory rate.
  c. O_2.
  d. PEEP.
  e. Sigh.
10. In what way does PEEP usually affect $Paco_2$ and Pao_2 levels?
  a. Increases Pao_2 and $Paco_2$.
  b. Increases Pao_2 and decreases $Paco_2$.
  c. Both are decreased.
  d. $Paco_2$ is usually unaffected but Pao_2 increases.
  e. Pao_2 remains the same and hypocapnea results.
11. A patient is being given ventilatory support with a CPAP system at +10 cm H_2O. The respiratory care practitioner finds the patient in acute ventilatory distress, using accessory muscles to breathe, and looking frantic. The manometer needle on the system is showing progressive increases in pressure from 10 to 12 to 15 to 17 cm H_2O and so on. The most likely cause of the problem is:
  a. A large leak in the circuit.
  b. Inadequate flow of gas to the reservoir.
  c. Malfunction or obstruction of the PEEP or CPAP valve.
  d. The patient is going into respiratory failure.
  e. The manometer is malfunctioning.
12. Assessment for optimal PEEP is being determined in a mechanically ventilated patient. PEEP is increased progressively from +5 to +10 to +15 cm H_2O. Volume delivery remains constant at 750 mL. Pao_2 increases progressively from 55 to 63 to 78 mm Hg. Blood pressure remains fairly constant. $P\bar{v}o_2$ goes from 27 to 36 and finally to 30 mm Hg at +15 cm H_2O of PEEP. Based on these findings the most appropriate action is:
  a. Use a PEEP of +5 cm H_2O only.
  b. Use a PEEP of +10 cm H_2O.

c. Use a PEEP of +15 cm H_2O.
d. Increase the PEEP to +20 cm H_2O and repeat the study.
e. Do nothing at this time.

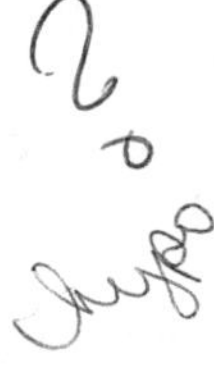

13. A 70-kg man on IMV ventilation has a VT of 650 mL, a rate of 12 breaths/min with no spontaneous breaths, 40% O_2, +5 cm H_2O of PEEP, and the following blood gases on these settings: pH = 7.48, $Paco_2$ = 30 mm Hg, Pao_2 = 78 mm Hg. Which of the following is appropriate?
    a. Increase the PEEP to + 10 cm H_2O.
    b. Increase the Fio_2 to 0.5.
    c. Increase the VT.
    d. Decrease the respiratory rate.
    e. Decrease the VT.
14. A patient in the intensive care unit is being mechanically ventilated on a volume ventilator, SIMV at a rate of 4 breaths/min. The patient's oxygenation and lung compliance are within acceptable limits. Work of breathing seems slightly increased since the patient is using some accessory muscles to breathe. How much PEEP would you suggest for this patient?
    a. 5–10 cm H_2O.
    b. 10–15 cm H_2O.
    c. 2–5 cm H_2O.
    d. 15–20 cm H_2O.
    e. No PEEP is indicated.
15. The first measurement following administration of PEEP is:
    a. Heart rate.
    b. Blood pressure.
    c. PCWP.
    d. PAP.
    e. FRC.
16. A patient on CPAP of +10 cm H_2O has a respiratory rate of 36 breaths/min. The pH is 7.33, $Paco_2$ is 48 mm Hg, Pao_2 is 75 mm Hg (Fio_2 = 0.5). The most appropriate action is:
    a. Increase CPAP to +15 cm H_2O.
    b. Increase the Fio_2.
    c. Begin mechanical ventilation.
    d. Decrease CPAP to +5 cm H_2O.
    e. Make no change.
17. Based on the following table, what is the optimal PEEP setting?

PEEP (cm H_2O)	Pao_2 (mm Hg)	CO (L/min)	$P\bar{v}o_2$ (mm Hg)	Cs (mL/cm H_2O)
+5	50	3.5	27	25
+10	75	4.0	30	30
+15	90	4.5	35	37
+20	95	4.3	32	35
+25	105	4.0	30	33

a. +5 cm H_2O.
b. +10 cm H_2O.
c. +15 cm H_2O.
d. +20 cm H_2O.
e. +25 cm H_2O.

18. Which of the following indicate that a patient is ready to be weaned from PEEP or CPAP?
    a. $Pa{O_2}$ is 80 mm Hg on 30% O_2.
    b. Patient is stable and has no active infections.
    c. Lung compliance is 37 mL/cm H_2O.
    d. $Pa{O_2}/F{I}{O_2}$ ratio is 500.
    e. All of the above.
19. Which of the following methods can be used to produce IRV on a conventional volume ventilator?
    I. Use of slow inspiratory times.
    II. Use of slow expiratory times.
    III. Increasing V_T.
    IV. Increasing pause time.
        a. I only.
        b. II and III.
        c. I and IV.
        d. II, III, and IV.
        e. IV only.
20. Peak airway pressures are more important in increasing oxygenation than Paw. True or false?

ANSWERS TO STUDY QUESTIONS

1. e.
2. b.
3. false.
4. true.
5. c.
6. b.
7. a.
8. b.
9. d.
10. d.
11. c.
12. b.
13. d.
14. c.
15. b.
16. c.
17. c.
18. e.
19. c.
20. False.

REFERENCES

1. Albert RK: Non-respiratory effects of positive end expiratory pressure. *Resp Care* 1988; 33:464–471.

2. Al-Saady N, Bennett E: Decelerating inspiratory flow waveform improves lung mechanics and gas exchange in patients on intermittent positive-pressure ventilation. *Intensive Care Med* 1985; 11:68–75.
3. Ashbaugh DG, Petty TL, Bigelow DB, et al: Continuous positive pressure breathing (CPPB) in adult respiratory distress syndrome. *J Thorac Cardiovasc Surg* 1969; 57:31–41.
4. Banner JM: Expiratory positive pressure valves: Flow resistance and work of breathing. *Respir Care* 1987; 32:431–439.
5. Banner MJ, Gallagher TJ, DeHaven CB: PEEP/CPAP Part II: Application and techniques in clinical practice. *Curr Rev Resp Ther* 1978; 1:11–15.
6. Bartlett RH: Respiratory therapy to prevent pulmonary complications of surgery. *Respir Care* 1984; 29:667–669.
7. Berryhill RE, Benumof JL: PEEP-induced discrepancy between pulmonary artery wedge pressure and left atrial pressure: The effects of controlled versus spontaneous ventilation and compliant versus non-compliant lungs in dogs. *Anesthesiology* 1979; 51:303–308.
8. Bone RC: Complications of mechanical ventilation and positive end-expiratory pressure. *Resp Care* 1982; 27:402–407.
9. Branson RD: PEEP without endotracheal intubation. *Respir Care* 1988; 33:598–612.
10. Branson RD, Hurst JM, DeHaven CB: Mark CPAP: State of the art. *Resp Care* 1985; 30:846–857.
11. Bumstead D: A modification of the Laerdal infant resuscitator for the simple and safe delivery of CPAP and PEEP. *Respir Care* 1984; 29:270–272.
12. Bunnell S: The use of nitrous oxide and oxygen to maintain anesthesia and positive pressure for thoracic surgery. *JAMA* 1912; 58:835.
13. Cassidy SS, Eschenbacher WL, Robertson CH, et al: Cardiovascular effects of positive pressure ventilation in normal subjects. *J Appl Physiol* 1979; 47:453–461.
14. Cassidy SS, Gaffney FA, Johnson RL: A perspective on PEEP (editorial). *N Engl J Med* 1981; 304:421–422.
15. Cassidy SS, Robertson CH, Pierce AK, et al: Cardiovascular effects of positive end-expiratory pressure in dogs. *J Appl Physiol* 1978; 44:743–750.
16. Cherniack V, Vidyasagar D: Continuous negative chest wall pressure in hyaline membrane disease: One year experience. *Pediatrics* 1972; 49:753–760.
17. Civetta JM, Barnes TA, Smith LO: Optimal PEEP and intermittent mandatory ventilation in the treatment of acute respiratory failure. *Respir Care* 1975; 20:550–557.
18. Civetta JM, Brons R, Gabel JC: A simple and effective method of employing spontaneous positive pressure ventilation. *J Thorac Cardiovasc Surg* 1972; 62:312–317.
19. Conway CM: Hemodynamic effects of pulmonary ventilation. *Br J Anaesth* 1975; 47:761–766.
20. Coiurnard A, Motley HL, Werko L, et al: Physiological studies of the effects of intermittent positive pressure breathing on cardiac output in man. *Am J Physiol* 1948; 152:162–174.
21. Craig KC: Weaning from positive end-expiratory pressure, in Zschoche D (ed): *Comprehensive Review of Critical Care.* St Louis, Mosby–Year Book, Inc, 1985, pp 318–322.
22. Craig KC, Peirson DJ, Carrico JC: The clinical application of PEEP in ARDS. *Respir Care* 1985; 30:184–201.

23. Crawford CA, Downs JB: Chest tube pressurization for bronchopleural fistula: A case report. *Respir Care* 1979; 24:932–935.
24. Davidson R, Parker M, Harison RA: The validity of determinations of pulmonary wedge pressure during mechanical ventilation. *Chest* 1978; 73:352–355.
25. Demers RR, Irwin RS, Braman SS: Criteria for optimum PEEP. *Respir Care* 1977; 22:596–601.
26. Demers RR, Pratter MR, Irwin RS: Use of the concept of ventilator compliance in the determination of static total compliance. *Respir Care* 1981; 26:644–648.
27. Demers RR, Saklad M: Assisted PEEP-assisted mechanical ventilation with positive end-expiratory pressure. *Respir Care* 1974; 19:435–441.
28. Feeley RW: Mechanical ventilatory support: Current techniques and recent advances. Chicago, Annual Refresher Course Lectures, *American Society of Anesthesiology*, 202, 1983, pp 1–7.
29. Fuleihan S, Wilson R, Pontoppidan H: Effect of mechanical ventilation with end-inspiratory pause on blood-gas exchange. *Anesth Analg* 1976; 55:122–130.
30. Gallagher RB: Acute respiratory failure: Rationale of therapy. *Respir Care* 1982; 27:1527–1529.
31. Gherini M, Peters RM, Virgilio RW: Mechanical work on the lungs and work of breathing with positive end-expiratory pressure and continuous positive airway pressure. *Chest* 1979; 76:251–256.
32. Graybar GB, Smith RA: Apparatus and techniques for intermittent mandatory ventilation, in Kirby RR, Graybar GB (eds): *Intermittent Mandatory Ventilation.* Boston, Little, Brown & Co, 1980, pp 53–80.
33. Greenbaum DM, Millen JE, Eross B, et al: Continuous positive airway pressure without tracheal intubation in spontaneously breathing patients. *Chest* 1976; 69:615–620.
34. Gregory GA. Comment on continuous positive airway pressure device claims (letter). *Pediatrics* 1976; 58:467.
35. Grenvik A, Eross B, Powner D: Historical survey of mechanical ventilation, in Kirby RR, Graybar GB (eds): *Intermittent Mandatory Ventilation.* Boston, Little, Brown & Co, 1980, pp 1–10.
36. Grenvik A, Oslick T, Mobel JJ: Volume controlled ventilators: Part 2. *Technol Respir Ther* 1983; 3:1–2.
37. Griebel JA, Piantadosi CA: Hemodynamic effects and complications of mechanical ventilation, in Fulkerson WJ, MacIntyre NR (eds): *Problems in Respiratory Care. Complications of Mechanical Ventilation.* Philadelphia, JB Lippincott Co, 1991, pp 25–35.
38. Guyatt GH: Positive pressure ventilation as a mechanism of reduction of left ventricular afterload. *Can Med Assoc J* 1982; 126:1310–1312.
39. Halvey A, Sirik Z, Adam YG, et al: Long-term evaluation of patients following the adult respiratory distress syndrome. *Respir Care* 1984; 29:132–137.
40. Haynes JB, Carson SD, Whitney WP, et al: Positive end-expiratory pressure shifts left ventricular diastolic pressure-area curves. *J Appl Physiol* 1980; 48:670–676.
41. Helmholz HF: Static total compliance and "best PEEP." *Respir Care* 1981; 26:637–638.
42. Henry WC, West GA, Wilson RS: A comparison of the oxygen cost of breathing between a continuous-flow CPAP system and a demand-flow CPAP system. *Respir Care* 1983; 28:1273–1281.

43. Hess D: The use of PEEP in clinical settings other than acute lung injury. *Respir Care* 1988; 33:581–597.
44. Hess D: Capnometry and capnography: Technical aspects, physiologic aspects and clinical applications. *Respir Care* 1990; 35:557–576.
45. Hess D, Kacmarek RM (eds): Noninvasive monitoring in respiratory care. Parts I and II. *Respir Care* 1990; 35:482–556, 660–746.
46. Hirsch C, Kacmarek RM, Stanek D: Work of breathing during CPAP and PSV imposed by the new generation mechanical ventilators: A lung model study. *Respir Care* 1991; 36:815–828.
47. Hudson LD: Cardiovascular complications in acute respiratory failure. *Respir Care* 1983; 28:627–633.
48. Hudson LD: Evaluation of the patient with acute respiratory failure. *Respir Care* 1983; 28:542–552.
49. Hudson LD, Weaver LJ, Haisch CE, et al: Positive end-expiratory pressure: Reduction and withdrawal. *Respir Care* 1988; 33:613–619.
50. Jardin F, Farcot JC, Boisante L, et al: Influence of positive end-expiratory pressure on left ventricular performance. *N Engl J Med* 1981; 304:387–390.
51. Kacmarek RM, Dimas S, Reynolds J, et al: Technical aspects of positive end-expiratory pressure (PEEP): Parts I, II and III. *Respir Care* 1982; 27:1478–1517.
52. Kacmarek RM, Petty TL: Historical development of positive end expiratory pressure (PEEP). *Respir Care* 1988; 33:422–433.
53. Kanarek DJ, Shannon DC: Adverse effects of positive end-expiratory pressure on pulmonary perfusion and arterial oxygenation. *Am Rev Respir Dis* 1975; 112:457–459.
54. Katz JA: PEEP and CPAP in perioperative respiratory care. *Respir Care* 1984; 29:614–629.
55. Khan FA, Mukherji R, Chitkara R, et al: Positive airway pressure in patients receiving intermittent mandatory ventilation at zero rate. The role in weaning in chronic obstructive pulmonary disease. *Chest* 1983; 84:436–438.
56. Kirby RR: *PEEP, CPAP, and IMV Revisited. Convention Lecture Series, AART*. Tempe, Ariz, Biosystems Institute, 1982, pp 81–92.
57. Kirby RR: The use of PEEP, in *Refresher Course Notes, American Society of Anesthesiology* (abst 203). Chicago, 1982, pp 1–7.
58. Kirby RR: Best PEEP: Issues and choices in the selection and monitoring of PEEP levels. *Respir Care* 1988; 88:569–580.
59. Kirby RR, Banner MJ, Downs JB: *Clinical Applications of Ventilatory Support*, ed 2. New York: Churchill Livingstone Inc, 1990.
60. Kirby RR, Downs JB, Civetts JM, et al: High levels of positive end-expiratory pressure (PEEP) in acute respiratory insufficiency. *Chest* 1975; 67:156–163.
61. Kirk B: Early diagnosis and management of hypoxemic respiratory failure. *Semin Respir Med* 1980; 2:38–42.
62. Kumar A, Konrad JF, Gerrin B, et al: Continuous positive pressure ventilation in acute respiratory failure. Effects on hemodynamics and lung function. *N Engl J Med* 1970; 283:1430–1431.
63. Laver MB: Hemodynamic adjustment to mechanical ventilation: The role of coronary artery diseases, in *33rd Annual Refresher Course Lectures, American Society of Anesthesiology* (abst 209), Chicago, 1982, pp 1–7.

64. Liebman PR, Patten MT, Manny J, et al: The mechanism of depressed cardiac output on positive end-expiratory pressure (PEEP). *Surgery* 1978; 83:594–598.
65. Loveland SR, Campbell RL, Comer PB, et al: A noninvasive device for ventilatory assistance. *Respir Care* 1979; 24:612–619.
66. Lutch JS, Murray JF: Continuous positive pressure ventilation: Effects on systemic oxygen transport and tissue oxygenation, *Ann Intern Med* 1972; 76:193–202.
67. Manny J, Grindlinger G, Mathe AA, et al: Positive end-expiratory pressure, lung stretch and decreased myocardial contractility. *Surgery* 1978; 84:127–133.
68. Manny J, Patten MT, Liebman PR, et al: The association of lung distention, PEEP and biventricular failure. *Ann Surg* 1978; 187:151–157.
69. Marcy TW, Marini JJ: Inverse ratio ventilation in ARDS: Rationale and implementation. *Chest* 1991; 100:494–504.
70. Marini JJ, Culver BH, Butler J: Mechanical effects of lung distention with positive pressure on ventricular function. *Am Rev Respir Dis* 1981; 124:382–386.
71. Maunder RJ: *Update: Prophylactic PEEP. Convention Lecture Series, AART.* Phoenix, Ariz, Biomed Systems and American Hospital Supply, 1983, pp 69–74.
72. Maxwell C, Goodrich CC: A modification of the Bennett MA-1 ventilator to permit on-demand flow and exhaled volume monitoring during continuous flow IMV with PEEP. *Respir Care* 1980; 25:941–942.
73. Miller CR, Smith ER, Lytle S, et al: Experience with a chamber for continuous negative pressure treatment of infants with respiratory distress. *Respir Care* 1977; 22:931–934.
74. Modell H, Cheney F: Effects of inspiratory flow pattern on gas exchange in normal and abnormal lungs. *J Appl Physiol* 1979; 46:1103–1107.
75. Murray JF: Pathophysiology of acute respiratory failure. *Respir Care* 1983; 28:531–541.
76. Murray JF, Modell JH, Gallagher TJ, et al: Titration of PEEP by the arterial minus end-tidal carbon dioxide gradient. *Chest* 1984; 85:100–104.
77. Nelson RD, Wilkins RL, Jacobsen WK, et al: Supranormal Pvo_2 in the presence of tissue hypoxia: A case report. *Respir Care* 1983; 28:191–194.
78. Nicotra MB, Stevens PM, Viroslav J, et al: Physiologic evaluation of positive end expiratory pressure ventilation. *Chest* 1973; 64:10–15.
79. Op't Holt TB: Work of breathing and other aspects of patient interaction with PEEP devices and systems. *Respir Care* 1988; 33:444–453.
80. Op't Holt TB, Hall MW, Bass JB, et al: Comparison of changes in airway pressure during continuous positive airway pressure (CPAP) between demand valve and continuous flow devices. *Respir Care* 1982; 27:1200–1209.
81. Pare PD, Warriner B, Baile EM, et al: Redistribution of pulmonary extravascular water with positive end-expiratory pressure in canine pulmonary edema. *Am Rev Respir Dis* 1983; 127:590–593.
82. Patten MT, Liebman PR, Manny J, et al: Humorally mediated alterations in cardiac performance as a consequence of positive end-expiratory pressure. *Surgery* 1978; 84:201–205.
83. Pick RA, Handler JB, Friedman AS: The cardiovascular effects of positive end-expiratory pressure. *Chest* 1982; 82:345–350.
84. Pierson DJ: Alveolar rupture during mechanical ventilation: Role of PEEP, peak airway pressure, and distending volume. *Respir Care* 1988; 33:472–486.

85. Quan SF, Falltrick RT, Schlobohm RM: Extubation from ambient or expiratory positive airway pressure in adults. *Anesthesiology* 1981; 55:53–56.
86. Qvist J, Pontoppidan H, Wilson RS, et al: Hemodynamic responses to mechanical ventilation with PEEP. *Anesthesiology* 1975; 42:45–55.
87. Ralph DD, Robertson HT, Weaver LJ, et al: Effects of positive end-expiratory pressure on ventilation-perfusion distribution in patients with adult respiratory distress syndrome (abstract). *Am Rev Respir Dis* 1980; 121:180.
88. Riedinger MS, Shellock RG, Swan HJC: Reading pulmonary artery and pulmonary capillary wedge pressure waveforms with respiratory variations. *Heart Lung* 1981; 10:657–658.
89. Rizk NW, Murray JF: PEEP and pulmonary edema. *Am J Med* 1982; 72:381–383.
90. Sanyal SK, Avery TL, Hughes WT, et al: Management of severe respiratory insufficiency due to *Pneumocystis carinii* pneumonitis in immunosuppressed hosts: The role of continuous negative-pressure ventilation. *Am Rev Respir Dis* 1977; 116:223.
91. Sanyal SK, Turner S, Ossi M, et al: Continuous negative chest-wall pressure therapy in management of severe hypoxemia due to aspiration pneumonitis: A case report. *Respir Care* 1979; 24:1022–1025.
92. Scanlan CL, Spearman CB, Sheldon RL: *Egan's Fundamentals of Respiratory Care*, ed 5. St Louis, Mosby–Year Book, Inc, 1990.
93. Scharf SM, Caldini P, Ingram RH: Cardiovascular effects of increasing airway pressure in the dog. *Am J Physiol* 1977; 232:H35–H43.
94. Scharf SM, Ingram RH: Influence of abdominal pressure and sympathetic vasoconstriction on the cardiovascular response to positive end-expiratory pressure. *Am Rev Respir Dis* 1977; 116:661–670.
95. Schmidt GB, O'Neill WW, Kotb D, et al: Continuous positive airway pressure in the prophylaxis of the adult respiratory distress syndrome. *Surg Gynecol Obstet* 1978; 143:613–618.
96. Shapiro BA: *PEEP: Why- When- How Much? 33rd Annual Refresher Course Lectures, American Society of Anesthesiology* (abst 215). Chicago, 1982, pp 1–7.
97. Shapiro BA, Harrison RA, Kacmarek RM, et al: *Clinical Application of Respiratory Care.* St Louis, Mosby–Year Book, Inc, 1985.
98. Shasby DM, Dauber IM, Pfister S, et al: Swan-Ganz catheter location and left arterial pressure determine the accuracy of the wedge pressure when positive end-expiratory pressure is used. *Chest* 1981; 80:666–670.
99. Smith RA: PEEP/CPAP, Part I—Historical and theoretical consideration. *Curr Rev Respir Ther* 1978; 1:3–8.
100. Smith RA: Physiologic PEEP. *Respir Care* 1988; 33:620–629.
101. Spearman CB: Positive end-expiratory pressure: Terminology and technical aspects of PEEP devices and systems. *Respir Care* 1988; 33:434–443.
102. Spearman CB, Sanders HG: The new generation of mechanical ventilators. *Respir Care* 1987; 32:403–418.
103. Spearman CB, Sheldon RL, Egan DF: *Egan's Fundamental of Respiratory Therapy.* St Louis, Mosby–Year Book, Inc, 1982.
104. Springer RR, Stevens PM: The influence of PEEP on survival of patients in respiratory failure. *Am J Med* 1979; 66:196–200.
105. Stevens PM: Positive end-expiratory pressure breathing, in *Basics of Respiratory Disease*, vol 5. New York, American Thoracic Society, 1977, pp 1–6.

106. Stoller JK: Respiratory effects of positive end expiratory pressure. *Respir Care* 1988; 33:454–463.
107. Sugerman HJ, Rogers RM, Miller LD: Positive end-expiratory pressure (PEEP): Indications and physiologic considerations. *Chest* 1972; 62(suppl):86S–94S.
108. Suter PM, Fairley HB, Isenberg MD: Optimum end-expiratory airway pressure in patients with acute pulmonary failure. *N Engl J Med* 1975; 292:284–289.
109. Tyler DC: Positive end-expiratory pressure: A review. *Crit Care Med* 1983; 11:300–307.
110. Weaver LJ, Haisch CE, Hudson LD, et al: Prospective analysis of PEEP reduction (abstract). *Am Rev Respir Dis* 1979; 119:182–187.
111. Weisman IM, Rinaldo JE, Rogers RM: Positive end-expiratory pressure in adult respiratory failure. *N Engl J Med* 1982; 307:1381–1384.
112. Wilson RS: *Management of Respiratory Failure. Annual Meeting Refresher Course Lectures. American Society of Anesthesiology* (abst 102). Chicago, 1983, pp 1–5.
113. Woods R, Rogers RM, Sugerman HJ, et al: An inexpensive continuous positive end-expiratory pressure (PEEP) adaptor for positive pressure respirators. *Chest* 1972; 61:376–378.
114. Zarins CK, Virgilio RW, Smith DE, et al: The effect of vascular volume on positive end-expiratory pressure–induced cardiac output depression and wedge–left atrial pressure discrepancy. *J Surg Res* 1977; 23:348.
115. Zwillich CW, Pierson DJ, Creagh CE, et al: Complications of assisted ventilation. *Am J Med* 1974; 57:161–169.

Chapter **11**

Hemodynamic Monitoring of the Ventilated Patient

With Thomas D. Baxter, B.S., R.R.T.

On completion of this chapter the reader will be able to:

1. Discuss the phases of the normal cardiac cycle.
2. Define terms specific to cardiac function including heart rate, pulse pressure, stroke volume, cardiac output, cardiac index, preload, afterload, and contractility.
3. Describe the components of hemodynamic monitoring systems.
4. Explain how dynamic pressure element and static pressure head affect hemodynamic measurements.
5. Discuss arterial catheter insertion, maintenance, and complications.
6. Discuss central venous pressure monitoring.
7. List and explain the function of the various lumina in a pulmonary artery catheter.
8. Describe the insertion of a pulmonary artery catheter and identify the waveforms produced by the anatomic structures through which it floats.
9. List the normal values for parameters measured using a pulmonary artery catheter.
10. Explain how PCWP reflects left ventricular function.
11. Describe mixed venous sampling using the pulmonary artery catheter.
12. Identify complications associated with the pulmonary artery catheter.
13. Discuss the effect mechanical ventilation has on hemodynamic monitoring.
14. Discuss which phase of the ventilatory cycle hemodynamic measurements should be taken to obtain a more accurate reading.
15. Calculate PWCPtm.

In today's intensive care unit (ICU), hemodynamic monitoring has become a common tool in the management of critically ill patients. The data obtained from hemodynamic monitoring is used by nurses, physicians, and respiratory care practitioners in the care of these patients.

Hemodynamic monitoring of critically ill patients can be either noninvasive or invasive. Noninvasive monitoring includes vital signs, and physical assessment of the patient (see Chapter 8). Invasive monitoring includes evaluation of data obtained from arterial lines, central venous lines, and pulmonary artery catheters. This chapter reviews invasive vascular monitoring and focuses on the effects of mechanical ventilation on data from hemodynamic monitoring.

BASIC CARDIOVASCULAR CONCEPTS

A few essential concepts of cardiovascular physiology related to hemodynamic monitoring are reviewed in this section to help the reader prepare for an understanding of invasive monitoring.

Cardiac Cycle

The cardiac cycle has two distinctive phases: systole and diastole. Systole is the period of contraction of the heart. During systole blood is forced into the pulmonary artery and aorta from the right and left ventricles, respectively. Diastole is the relaxation phase of the cardiac cycle. During this phase the cardiac muscles relax and the ventricles fill with blood. The cardiac cycle is the occurrence of mechanical events of both the atria and ventricles that are stimulated by electrical events. We measure the mechanical events during invasive monitoring. We measure the electrical events with the electrocardiogram (ECG). The mechanical events can be separated into several phases. These include atrial systole, isovolumetric contraction, ejection, isovolumetric relaxation, rapid ventricular filling, and reduced ventricular filling.

Atrial Systole.—Normally, following the firing of the sinoatrial (SA) node (P wave on the ECG), the atria contract. The a wave on an atrial pressure tracing represents atrial contraction. This sends blood from the atria into the ventricles. Pressure in the right atrium is 3 to 6 mm Hg, and in the left, 3 to 8 mm Hg. The cuspid valves (tricuspid in the right ventricle; bicuspid or mitral in the left ventricle) are open at this time. The semilunar valves (pulmonic and aortic) are closed (Fig 11–1,A). Atrial systole accounts for about 20% to 40% of ventricular filling. The rest occurs by venous return to the heart and blood going directly into the ventricles.

Isovolumetric Contraction of Ventricles.—As ventricular systole begins, the pressure inside the ventricles rises. When ventricular pressure exceeds pressure in the atria (the atria are relaxed at this time), the cuspid valves close. This produces the c wave on the atrial pressure tracing. The pressure in the ventricles continues to rise as the ventricles continue to contract. The pressure is still below the pressure in the respective arteries (right ventricle—pulmonary artery; left ventricle—aorta). All the valves are closed during this period. The volume of blood in the heart does not change, but pressure builds. Thus, it is called an isovolumetric contraction and it is the time when myocardial oxygen consumption is greatest.

Ejection.—When intraventricular pressure exceeds arterial pressure the semilunar valves, pulmonic and aortic, open. This occurs when ventricular pressures finally exceed arterial diastolic pressures. Pulmonary artery diastolic pressure is about 5 to 15 mm Hg. Aortic diastolic pressure is about 60 to 90 mm Hg.

Blood is ejected from the ventricles into the arteries. Ventricular and arterial systolic pressures eventually are equal. Pulmonary artery and right ventricular pressures increase to about 15 to 25 mm Hg. Aortic and left ventricular pressures increase to about 90 to 140 mm Hg (Fig 11–1,B). The important feature of this phase of the cardiac cycle is the rapid ejection of blood from the heart and into the arteries during the early part of this phase. A total of about 70 to 80 mL of

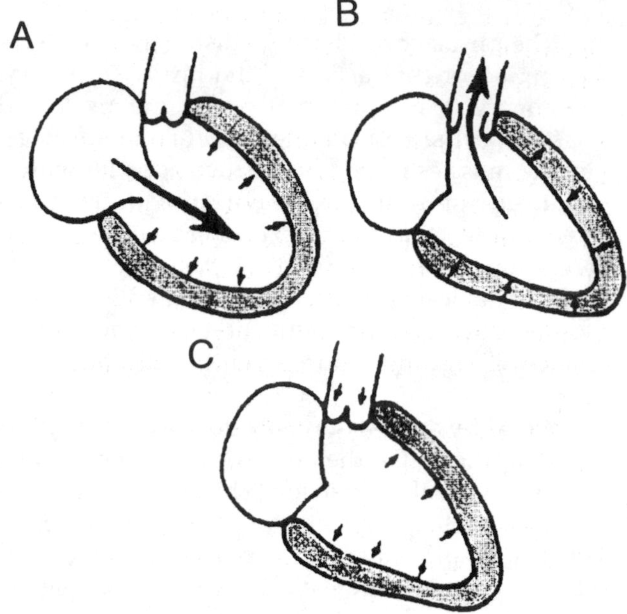

FIG 11–1.
A, atrial systole. Blood is ejected into the ventricle and as blood volume increases myocardial muscle fibers stretch and pressure increases within the ventricle. **B,** ventricular systole. Ventricular myocardial muscle fibers contract and blood is ejected into the pulmonary or aortic artery. **C,** isovolumetric relaxation. The pressure within the blood vessels is now greater than in the empty ventricle and the valves (pulmonic and aortic semilunar) close.

blood leave each ventricle (stroke volume). As the ventricular volume decreases, the pressures also decrease and finally plateau. The amount of blood remaining in the ventricle is called the end-systolic volume (ESV). Normally, it is about 70 to 75 mL. This blood, in the ventricles, still exerts a certain amount of pressure. This is called the ventricular end-systolic pressure.

Isovolumetric Relaxation.—After systole is ended, the ventricle begins to relax. This represents the beginning of diastole. As the heart relaxes, the pressure in the ventricles falls as the internal volume of the ventricle increases. Pressure in the arteries is slightly higher than in the ventricles for a brief period of time. Some blood actually starts to fall back toward the ventricles from the arteries. This blood catches in the leaflets of the pulmonic and aortic valves. The valves then snap shut. As they shut a small pulse of pressure is generated as blood hits the valve. This creates a slight upward deflection of the pressure tracing of the heart called the dicrotic notch. Following this event, when all of the valves in the heart are again closed (Fig 11–1,C), the heart continues to relax. Blood volume in the heart does not change. Thus, it is called the isovolumetric relaxation phase.

Rapid Ventricular Filling.—While the ventricles were in systole, blood was still returning to the heart from the veins. This blood was entering and filling the atria while these other events were taking place. This rise in blood volume in the atria is marked by the v wave on the atrial pressure tracing. Eventually, the pressure from this build-up of atrial blood exceeds the pressure in the now "relaxed" ventricles. This results in the opening of the cuspid valves and blood falls from the atria into the ventricles. This marks a period of rapid filling of the ventricles. This accounts for 60% to 80% of the blood volume in the ventricles.

Reduced Ventricular Filling.—As diastole continues, blood continues to return to the heart and pass through the atria and into the ventricles.

Summary.—These events occur in the right and left heart simultaneously. The pressure waveforms from these phases are identical in both the right and left atria, the right and left ventricles, and the pulmonary artery and aorta. The only difference is in the amount of pressure generated in the right heart compared to the left heart (Table 11–1).

Terms Specific to Cardiac Function

There are several terms used frequently during hemodynamic monitoring. These include: heart rate, pulse pressure, stroke volume, cardiac output, cardiac index, preload, contractility, afterload, and vascular resistance. These are briefly reviewed below.

TABLE 11–1.
Normal Pressures in the Right and Left Heart

Site	Pressure (mm Hg)
Right atrial pressure	3–6
Right ventricular diastolic pressure	0–6
Right ventricular systolic pressure	15–25
Pulmonary artery pressure	Diastolic 10–15 Systolic 15–25
Left atrial pressure	3–8
Left ventricular diastolic pressure	0–8
Left ventricular systolic pressure	90–140
Systemic arterial pressure	Diastolic 60–90 Systolic 90–140

Heart Rate, Pulse Pressure, Stroke Volume, Cardiac Output, Cardiac Index.—The heart rate is simply the number of beats (ventricular systolic events) per minute. The actual pulse pressure that is created by the heart can be detected by feeling the pulse over an artery. The term *pulse pressure* is actually defined as the systolic pressure minus the diastolic pressure. Normal pulse pressure is about 40 mm Hg (120 − 80 mm Hg). A low pulse pressure may indicate that the output of the heart (stroke volume) is down and vice versa. The pulse gives proof of a mechanical event: contraction of the heart and output of blood. On the other hand, when you look at an ECG monitor, the QRS complex shows the electrical event that occurs before ventricular systole. It does not prove that the mechanical event occurred. For this reason, when a pulse is not felt even if the ECG tracing shows electrical activity, we believe that little or no blood is coming from the heart. In this circumstance we assume that the patient is in cardiac arrest. This is referred to as electrical-mechanical dissociation (EMD).

Cardiac output (CO or $\dot{Q}_T$) is the volume of blood pumped from the heart in 1 minute. It can be calculated in two ways. One is to multiply the heart rate (HR) times the stroke volume (SV) (stroke volume is the volume of blood ejected from a ventricle during each systole).

$$CO = HR \times SV$$

Normal HR is about 72 beats/min (range 60–100). Normal SV is about 70 mL/beat. Thus CO = 72 × 70, or 4.9 L/min. Normal CO is about 5 to 8 L/min.

The second method for calculating the CO is called the Fick equation:

$$CO = (\dot{V}O_2)/C(a - v)O_2$$

where $\dot{V}O_2$ is oxygen consumption, and $C(a-v)O_2$ is the arteriovenous oxygen content difference. Normal $\dot{V}O_2$ is about 250 mL/min. Normal $C(a-v)O_2$ is 5 vol % (mL/100 mL of blood). Thus normal CO is 5,000 mL/min, or 5 L/min.

Cardiac output is affected by such things as the circulating blood volume, myocardial contractility, valve function, metabolic rate, pericardial function, and vascular resistance. It can be measured indirectly by thermodilution techniques using a pulmonary artery catheter, dye dilution techniques, or by the Fick equation.

Cardiac output is more accurately expressed as cardiac index (CI). This is CO divided by body surface area (BSA): CO/BSA = CI. This eliminates body size as a variable. Normal CI is 2.5 to 4.5 L/min/m^2. The CI increases with increases in metabolism, septic shock, and exercise. The CI decreases during shock, hypovolemia, cardiac failure, obstructive shock (pulmonary embolus), and low metabolic rates.

Preload.—The volume of blood present in the ventricles at the end of diastole is called the ventricular end-diastolic volume (VEDV). It is also referred to as preload. In actuality, preload refers to the amount of stretch of the myocardial fibers. This volume, pushing on the sides of the ventricles, causes fiber stretching and exerts a pressure that can be measured by the pulmonary artery catheter. Preload of the left side of the heart is estimated by measuring the pulmonary capillary wedge pressure (PCWP). This is a close approximation of the left ventricular filling pressure (LVEDP). The catheter can be used to estimate the preload of the right heart by measuring right atrial pressure (RAP), which is equivalent, in most conditions, to central venous pressure (CVP).

In its simplest terms, preload can be thought of as the volume of blood that returns to the heart. Actual preload is influenced by the total circulating blood volume, the amount of venous return to the heart, the strength of atrial contraction, and the compliance of the ventricle. Preload has a profound effect on myocardial muscle performance. As preload increases, myocardial performance increases.[9]

Afterload.—Afterload refers to the amount of resistance or impedance against which the heart must work in order to move blood from the ventricle into the artery (pulmonary or aorta). The higher the vascular resistance, the harder the heart has to pump in order to move the blood. One way to think of afterload is to compare it to a man opening a door on a windy day. The harder the wind blows, the harder the man has to push on the door to get it open. If the valve between the ventricle and the artery is the door, the more pressure (vascular resistance) that is in the artery, the harder the ventricle has to contract to pump the blood out.

Blood viscosity also affects afterload. The thicker the blood, the harder it is to pump. Of course, the function of the heart valves can also affect afterload. If they are narrow (stenosis), they can increase afterload.

Contractility.—The force of myocardial contraction is called its contractility. It is dependent on the ability of myocardial muscle fibers to stretch and shorten in response to the blood volume in the ventricles. The strength of a contraction depends on how filled it is with blood, how stretched the fibers are prior to contraction, and how much work it must do to pump the blood out. These all affect the stroke volume that is pumped from the heart. Figure 11–2 shows ventricular performance response to various levels of VEDV.

Resistance.—Vascular resistance is the factor which opposes or impedes blood flow through conductive vessels. It is very similar to airway resistance in breathing. Resistance is present whenever there is flow through a tube or vessel. The resistance is a result of the fluid or blood sliding against vessel walls, passing through branches of vessels, and sliding over itself. Vascular resistance can be calculated using a similar equation to the one for airway resistance. $R = \Delta P/\text{flow}$. More specifically, systemic vascular resistance (SVR) is:

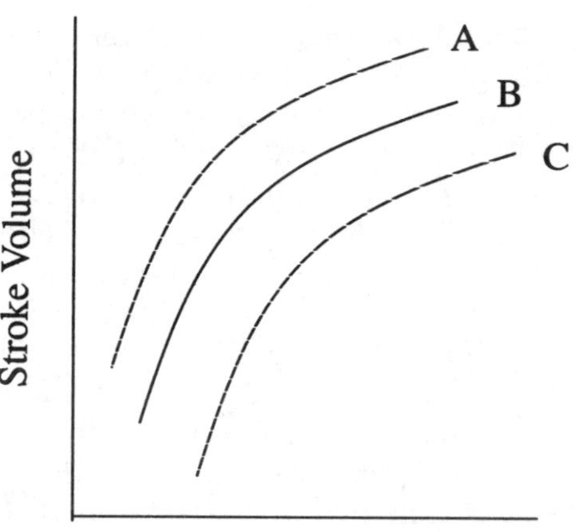

FIG 11–2.
Ventricular function curve. Normally *(curve B)* as end-diastolic pressure (volume) increases there is an increase in stroke volume to a point (the curve plateaus and may decrease). For a given preload (end-diastolic pressure) stroke volume will increase in response to an increased strength of contraction (positive inotropic effect) *(curve A)*. A decreased strength of contraction, for a given preload, will cause a decreased stroke volume *(curve C)*.

$$\text{SVR} = (\text{MAP} - \text{CVP})/\text{CO}$$

where MAP is mean arterial blood pressure; (MAP = [systolic + 2(diastolic)]/3), CVP is central venous pressure, and CO is cardiac output. Normal SVR is 900 to 1,400 dynes $\times$ cm $\times$ sec^{-5}.

Pulmonary vascular resistance (PVR) is:

$$\text{PVR} = (\overline{\text{PAP}} - \text{PCWP})/\text{CO}$$

where $\overline{\text{PAP}}$ is mean pulmonary artery pressure [systolic + 2(diastolic)]/3, PCWP is pulmonary capillary wedge pressure, and CO is cardiac output. Normal PVR is about 150 to 250 dynes $\times$ cm $\times$ sec^{-5}.

Increases in PVR increase the afterload of the right heart. This can occur in conditions which impede the blood flow through the pulmonary capillary bed, such as chronic obstructive pulmonary disease (COPD), pulmonary edema, and hypoxemia (pulmonary vasoconstriction). Increases in SVR increase the afterload of the left heart. This can be caused by events which impede blood flow through the systemic circulation such as narrowing or obstruction of vessels.

HEMODYNAMIC MONITORING SYSTEMS

Hemodynamic monitoring systems consist of equipment used to detect a small physiologic signal (vascular pressure changes), change this to an electrical impulse, amplify this signal, and record this amplified signal on a recorder or monitor. Invasive vascular monitoring systems commonly include monitors for arterial catheters, central venous catheters, and pulmonary artery catheters.

A typical invasive vascular monitoring system consists of the catheter, located inside a vessel, which is connected by hollow plastic tubing filled with a heparinized solution of saline. This solution is connected to a pressurized bag to maintain a positive pressure of fluid inside the tubing. This special pressure tubing is connected to a transducer which converts the fluid pressure to an electrical signal. The transducer is connected by wire or cable to an amplifier which is finally connected to a recorder or monitor or to both (Fig 11–3).

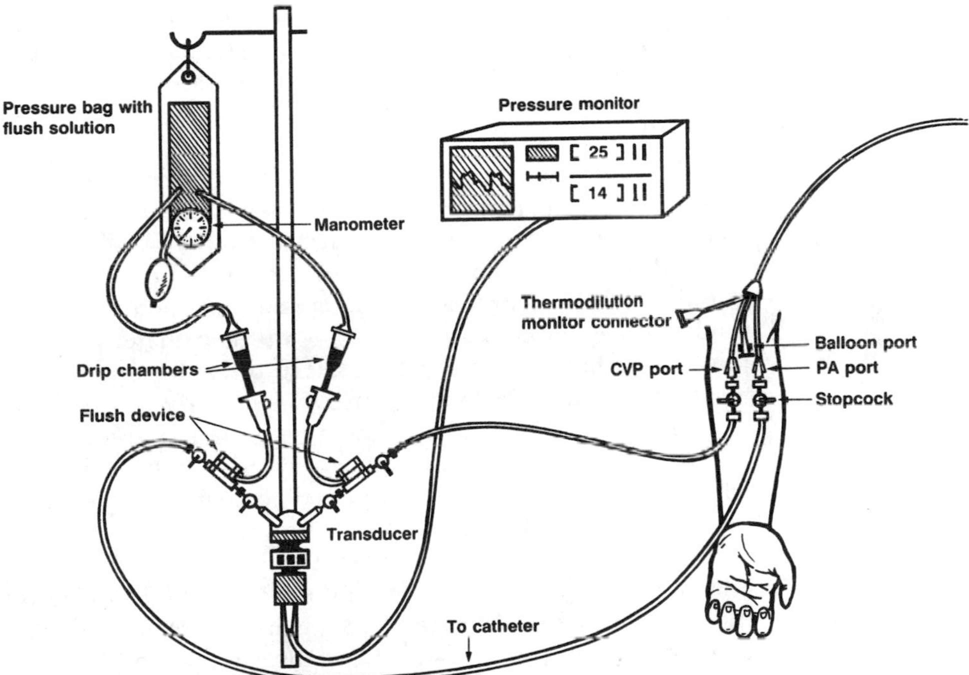

FIG 11–3.
Invasive vascular monitoring system showing the catheter connected from the vessel to a transducer and pressurized IV bag containing heparinized saline. The transducer is connected to an amplifier and recording device and monitor. (The transducer pictured is an old-style type used for easier visualization. Newer transducers are smaller and made out of plastic.)

Transducers are devices used to convert fluid pressure to an electrical signal. The transducer shown in Figure 11–3 is one of the larger styles and is used here for easier visibility. Newer transducers are small, wafer-shaped devices and are disposable. The more common type of transducer used in hemodynamic monitoring is a strain gauge which employs a Wheatstone bridge and a metal diaphragm.

Fluid enters the dome portion of the transducer by way of the fluid-filled plastic line. A diaphragm separates the fluid from the electronic portion of the transducer. Changes in pressure in the fluid result in movement of the diaphragm. This causes an increase or decrease in the length of the wires of the Wheatstone bridge. This in turn causes an imbalance or change in resistance in the current running through the Wheatstone bridge. A voltage signal change results. This signal is sent to an amplifier. Since biological signals are so small, amplifiers are necessary to enhance this signal received from the transducer. The amplifier receives the current from the Wheatstone bridge and sends the amplified signal to a monitor and recorder. One example of a monitor is a cathode ray tube (CRT). The amplified signal can be received and converted to a waveform pattern on the CRT screen. In this way, changes in waveform can be viewed.

Fluid Pressures

Fluid can exert pressure while it is in motion (hydrodynamic pressure) or while at rest (hydrostatic pressure). These pressures play integral roles when using hemodynamic monitoring systems. There are two factors which affect fluid-filled systems, the dynamic pressure element and the static pressure head.[9] The dynamic pressure element is pressure applied to fluid inside a system by fluid outside a system. It has to do with the catheter position in relation to the flow of the blood within the vessel. In order for an arterial line to accurately measure pressures that are the direct result of the work of the left heart, it must be placed with the end of the catheter facing the direction of blood flow ("looking" upstream). A pulmonary artery catheter, which measures pressures within a vessel or chamber, is placed so that the tip of the catheter is facing downstream and therefore with the flow of blood.

Static pressure head refers to the pressure placed on the transducer as related to the tip of the catheter. If the catheter tip is higher than the transducer, the monitor will read higher than the actual pressure owing to the fluid going downstream (due to gravity) from the catheter tip to the transducer. If the catheter tip is placed lower than the transducer, the fluid will flow away from the transducer toward the catheter tip and produce a reading lower than the actual pressure. The degree of error, according to Darovic,[9] is 1.86 mm Hg for each centimeter of distance from the reference point (e.g., if the transducer is 5 cm above the reference point, then the corrected measurement should be 9.3 mm Hg [$5 \times 1.86 = 9.3$]).[9] This can be avoided by leveling the transducer with the midthoracic line of the patient—the epistatic line. This is about 5 cm behind the sternal angle (the angle of Lewis). Once the epistatic line has been determined, it is important to zero-balance the transducer to this reference point. Zero-balancing the transducer references the transducer to atmospheric pressure, which is usually read as zero.

Arterial Catheters

Arterial catheters are invasive catheters placed into a systemic artery for monitoring blood pressure on a continuous basis and providing easy access to arterial blood for sampling. Peripheral artery catheterization is used in hemodynamically unstable patients.

The most common insertion sites are the radial, brachial, femoral, and dorsalis pedis arteries. The radial artery is the most common site because good collateral circulation is available through the ulnar artery. This can be demonstrated with Allen's test. It is also easily accessible. The insertion procedure is summarized in Table 11–2. An arterial pressure pattern is shown in Figure 11–4. Normal systemic arterial pressures are 90 to 140 mm Hg systolic and 60 to 80 mm Hg diastolic.

The most common complications of artery catheters are infection and ischemia of tissue distal to the catheter.[11, 19] Factors which may lead to the development of infection are: (1) insertion by cutdown rather than percutaneously, (2) use of the catheter for more than 4 days and (3) inflammation at the insertion site.[19] Ischemia can be the result of either thrombosis or distal embolization.

TABLE 11–2.
Insertion and Maintenance of Arterial Catheters

Aseptically assemble, flush, and test tubing and catheter
Perform Allen's test to assure ulnar artery refill time of 5–15 sec
Prepare and drape area of insertion (sterile technique necessary)
If necessary, infiltrate skin around insertion site with 1% lidocaine
Insert the catheter percutaneously at approximately a 30-degree angle (if pulse is weak or otherwise inaccessible, surgical cutdown may be necessary)
Advance the catheter into the artery while holding the needle secure
Remove the needle and secure the catheter
Attach tubing for drip solution and observe monitor for proper waveform
Frequently monitor:
- Insertion site for signs of infection
- Extremity distal to insertion site for adequate circulation

Catheter should be removed if:
- There is clot formation as evidenced by difficulty with blood sampling or a persistently dampened waveform
- Extremity distal to insertion site becomes ischemic
- Insertion site infection

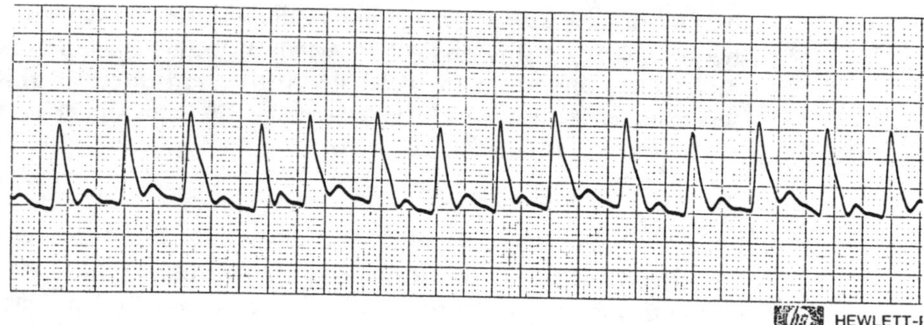

FIG 11–4.
Typical arterial waveform pattern.

Occasionally necrosis will result, but incidence of necrosis is rare.[19] The risk of emboli can be reduced by using heparinized normal saline or heparinized Ringer's lactate (1,000 units/100 mL).[20] A constant heparin flush of 2 to 3 mL/hr is maintained to help avoid clot formation (0.9% NaCl with 100–200 units heparin/100 mL).[11, 20] Risk factors for the development of acute distal ischemia include hypotension, severe peripheral vascular disease, and the use of vasopressor drugs.[19] Bleeding can occur if the line becomes disconnected or is incorrectly handled.

In the future, arterial catheters may come equipped with miniaturized gas analyzers for the continuous monitoring of partial pressure of arterial oxygen (Pa_{O_2}), pH, and partial pressure of arterial carbon dioxide (Pa_{CO_2}). This provides a method for continuous arterial blood gas (ABG) monitoring.

Central Venous Catheters

Catheters placed in the vena cava or right atrial area are referred to as central venous lines. These are most commonly used for the administration of fluid, drugs, and nutritional solutions. RAP or CVP is the pressure of blood as it returns and fills the right heart. During systole, when the tricuspid valve is closed, the catheter shows RAPs. At end-atrial diastole, when the tricuspid valve is open, it shows right ventricular filling and estimates right ventricular end-diastolic pressure (RVEDP) or preload to the right heart.

CVP catheters are usually inserted percutaneously into a large central vein such as the internal jugular or peripherally through the medial basilic or lateral cephalic vein.[11] Measurement is usually done during exhalation and with the patient supine. The transducer is zeroed at the level of the right atrium. Complications include infection, thrombosis, embolization, vessel damage, bleeding, shearing or cutting of the catheter, and pneumothorax or hemothorax when a large central vein is used.

Low CVP values suggest a hypovolemic state such as shock, dehydration, or hemorrhage. High CVP values may indicate problems in the right heart, pulmonary circulation, or left heart. A pulmonary artery catheter is best used to distinguish among these.

Pulmonary Artery Catheter

A pulmonary artery catheter is a vascular line inserted into a large vein, floated back to the heart through the right heart, and finally positioned with its tip in the pulmonary artery. It has a balloon at its tip that is used to help float it through the heart chambers and "wedge" it into a pulmonary vessel. It was originally developed in the 1970s by Swan and Ganz for the continuous monitoring of pulmonary artery pressure to help differentiate right heart, pulmonary vascular, and left heart problems. The pulmonary artery catheter is restricted to use in patients who are hemodynamically unstable and difficult to manage. Indications for its use are listed in Table 11–3.

Characteristics of the Catheter.—The balloon-tipped pulmonary artery catheter is 110 cm long with markers every 10 cm (Fig 11–5). These markers identify the distance from the tip of the catheter to the outside of the patient or connector end of the catheter. The catheter comes with two to five lumina depending on the functions needed by a particular patient situation. One of the more commonly used is the four-lumen catheter which will be described here. One lumen, the distal lumen, goes the entire length of the catheter. Its tip lodges in the pulmonary artery. It is used for measuring pulmonary artery pressure (PAP), PCWP, and for sampling mixed venous blood from the pulmonary artery. A second lumen, the inflation lumen, is used to inflate a small balloon located near the tip of the catheter just behind the distal port. The balloon is inflated with a maximum of 1.5 mL of air during insertion to help float the catheter through the heart. Once in position, the balloon is allowed to deflate. It is periodically reinflated to measure PCWP. A third lumen, the thermistor lumen, contains a conductive wire that attaches to a thermistor located about 5 cm from the tip,

TABLE 11–3.
Indications for Use of Pulmonary Artery Catheter

Shock
Congestive heart failure and myocardial infarction, to help with evaluation and treatment of preload and afterload problems
Severe burn injury for fluid management
Diagnosis and monitoring of pulmonary hypertension
Differentiation of cardiogenic vs. noncardiogenic pulmonary edema
Evaluation of high PEEP levels (>10–15 mm Hg) and volume loading in patients with ARDS

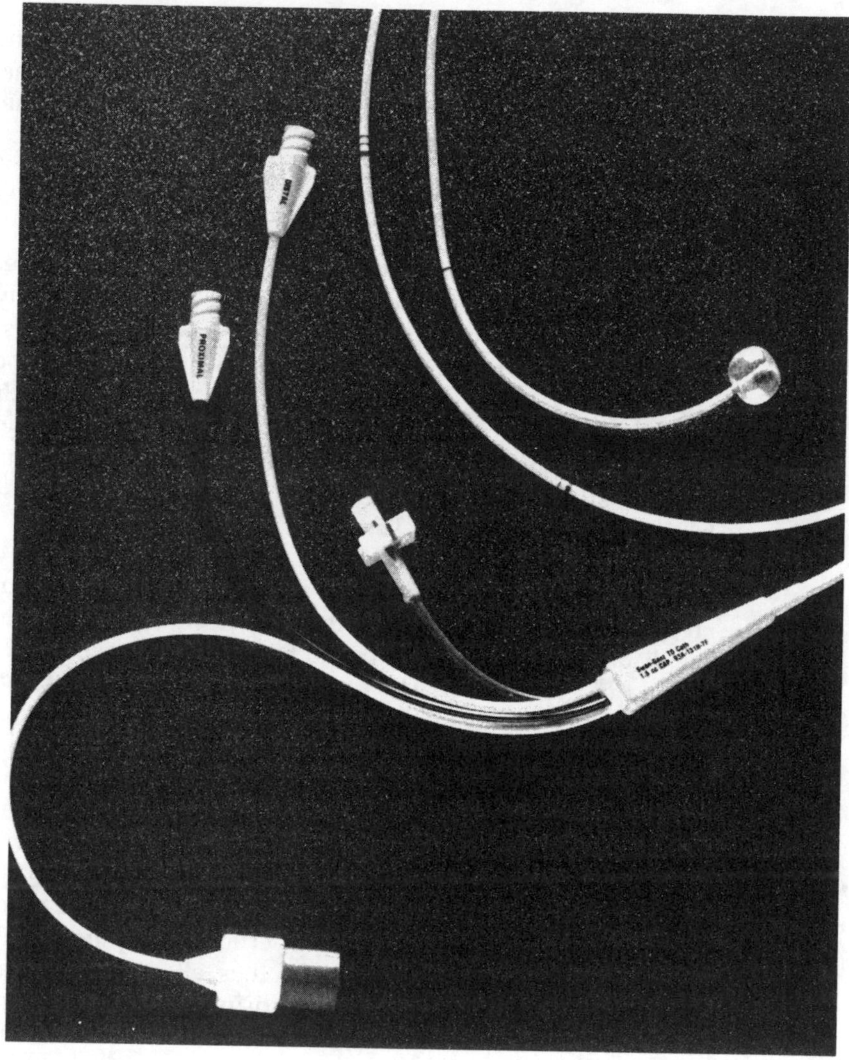

FIG 11–5.
Pulmonary artery catheter. (Courtesy of Baxter Healthcare Corp., Irvine, Calif.)

just behind the balloon. It is used for measuring temperature changes during thermodilution CO measurements.

A fourth lumen, the proximal lumen, has a port (opening) about 30 cm (third marker) from the distal tip. This proximal port is usually located in the right atrium or vena cava and is used for the measurement of RAP or CVP. (Remember, there are no valves between the vena cava and right atrium, so pressure generated in the right atrium *normally* will equal pressure in the vena cava.) It can also be used for sampling of blood in the right atrium, administration of medications, and is the site for injection of a cold bolus of fluid when a thermodilution CO measurement is performed. The distal and proximal lumina are filled with a heparinized fliud solution (Fig 11–6), connected to a transducer dome and therefore are influenced by the forces (dynamic pressure element and static pressure head) discussed earlier. The thermistor lumen contains a wire and the inflation lumen contains only air.

Insertion.—The catheter is inserted into a vein either percutaneously or by way of a cutdown, depending on the site chosen. Common sites and their relative complications are listed in Table 11–4. Complications of pulmonary artery catheters include dampening of the waveform (Fig 11–7), and catheter whip or fling (Fig 11–8), in addition to those found in other catheters: infection, thrombosis, embolization, and bleeding. Other complications are listed in Table 11–5.

After selection of the site and prior to insertion, the catheter is checked to be sure that the proximal and distal lumina are patent. This is done by instilling

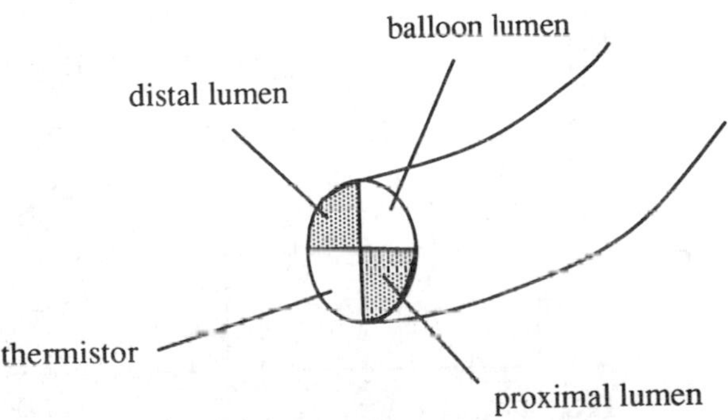

FIG 11–6.
Cross section of Swan-Ganz catheter. The *shaded areas,* the distal and proximal lumina, represent fluid-filled lumina. The balloon lumen contains only air and the thermistor lumen contains a wire which will couple to a cardiac output computer.

TABLE 11–4.
Sites of Pulmonary Artery Catheter Insertion and Their Associated Problems

Site	Associated Problems
Internal jugular	Pneumothorax, hemothorax
Subclavian	Severe thrombocytopenia (difficult to control bleeding); pneumothorax more frequent than with internal jugular; hemothorax
Antecubital	Phlebitis; movement of arm may cause the catheter tip to migrate; difficult site for catheter advancement
Femoral	Phlebitis; movement of leg may cause the catheter tip to migrate; most direct access to the pulmonary artery[20]

sterile solution in one end of the lumen and observing its outflow at the other end. The balloon is tested for leaks and symmetry. It is inflated, visualized, and submerged in a sterile solution to be sure there are no bubbles, indicating air leaks from the balloon. The catheter is then ready for insertion.

An advantage of the pulmonary artery catheter is that the pressure waveforms can be monitored during insertion. As a result, the procedure does not usually need to be done under fluoroscopy. Once the catheter is inside the vein and hooked to the transducer and monitor, the physician can watch the progression of the catheter on the monitoring screen.

When the catheter is in the vena cava, the physician inflates the balloon to help float the catheter through the heart past the tricuspid valve, through the right ventricle, out the pulmonic valve, and into the pulmonary artery. The catheter insertion is continued until the wedge position is achieved. That is, the balloon wedges against the walls of a pulmonary artery. Figure 11–9 shows the waveforms generated during insertion of the catheter into a large vein through to a wedged position.

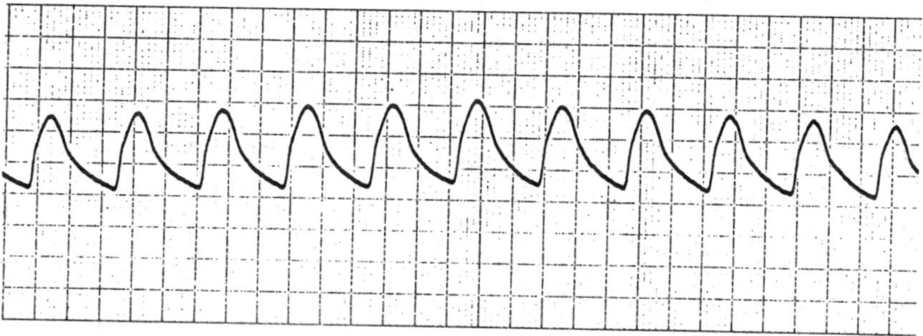

FIG 11–7.
Dampened waveform.

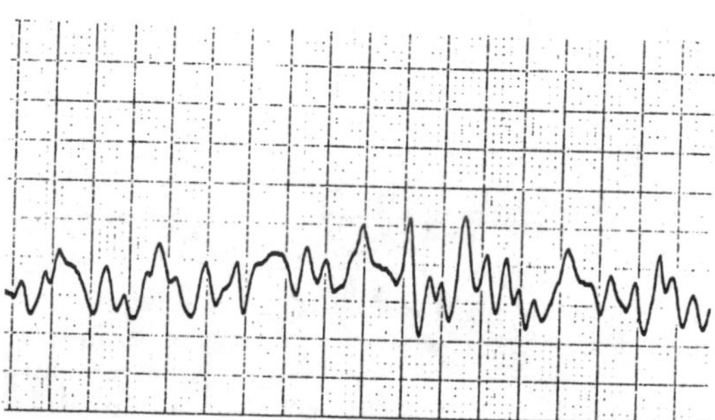

FIG 11–8.
Example of catheter whip or fling.

TABLE 11–5.
Complications Associated with Pulmonary Artery (PA) Catheterization

Complications*	Cause
Cardiac arrhythmias	Heart valve or endocardium irritation by the catheter
PVCs	
Ventricular tachycardia	
Ventricular fibrillation	
PACs	
Atrial flutter	
Atrial fibrillation	
Insertion procedure or insertion site	
Infection	Nonsterile technique or irritation of the wound
Pneumothorax	Air entering pleural space during insertion
Air embolism	Air entering vessel during insertion
Access vessel thrombosis or phlebitis	Irritation of vessel by catheter or nonsterile insertion technique
Pulmonary circulation	
PA rupture or perforation	Overinflation of balloon
Pulmonary infarction	Overinflation of balloon, prolonged wedging, clots formed in or near the catheter, or catheter advancement into a smaller artery
PA catheter	
Balloon rupture (air embolism)	Loss of balloon elasticity or overinflation
Catheter knotting	Excessive catheter movement
Dampened waveform (see Fig 11–7)	Air in line, clot in the system, kinks in line, catheter tip against vessel wall, overwedging or blood on the transducer
Catheter whip or fling (see Fig 11–8)	High cardiac output, or abnormal vessel diameter

*PVCs = premature ventricular contractions; PAC = premature atrial contractions.

PRESSURE MONITORING WITH PULMONARY ARTERY CATHETER

One of the advantages of monitoring with a three- or four-lumen pulmonary artery catheter is that it allows monitoring of preload of both the right and left sides of the heart separately (RAP and PCWP, respectively). This monitoring also helps in distinguishing problems that are fluid volume, left heart, right heart, or pulmonary in origin. The differentiation of origin will become clearer as monitoring of the various pressures is reviewed.

Right Atrial Pressure

Right atrial pressure, measured from the proximal lumen of the pulmonary artery catheter, produces a fluctuating waveform (Fig 11–9,A). These fluctuations in the waveform are small (pressures 3–6 mm Hg) unless there is some patho-

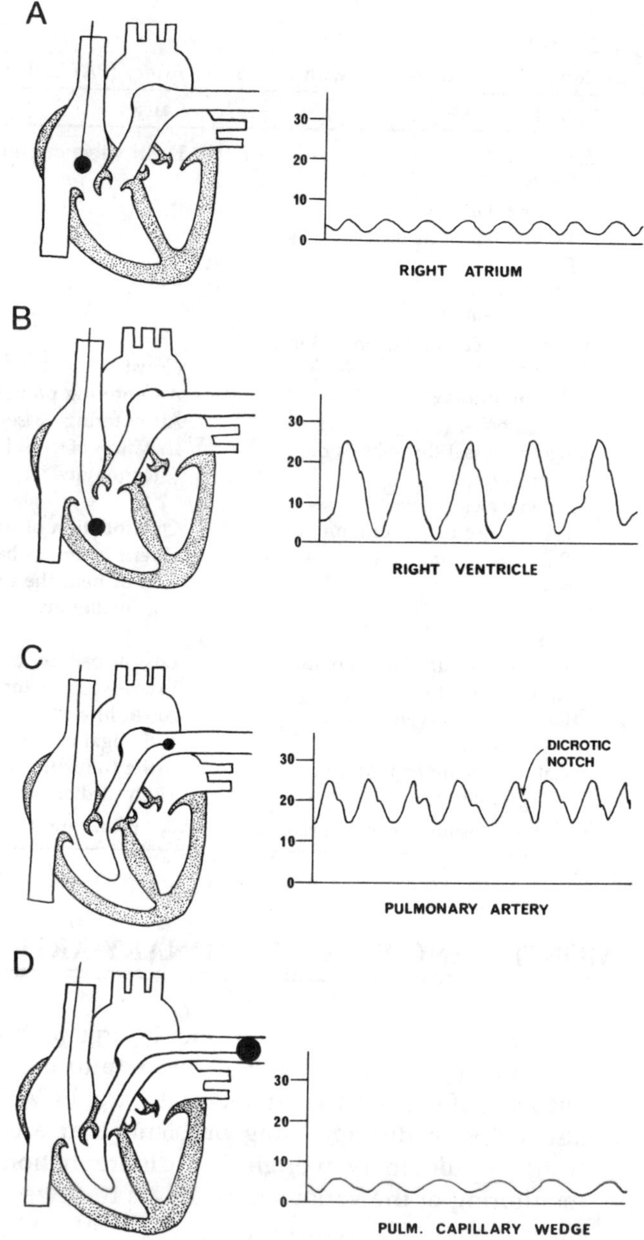

FIG 11–9.
Waveforms seen during the advancement of the catheter from the right atrium to the wedged position. **A,** central venous or right atrial pressure. **B,** pressures in the right ventricle. **C,** pulmonary artery pressures. Note the presence of the dicrotic notch. **D,** the wedged position, a reflection of left heart pressures. (From Deshpande VM, Pilbeam SP, Dixon RJ: *A Comprehensive Review in Respiratory Care.* Norwalk, Conn, Appleton & Lange, 1988, p 363–364. Used by permission.)

logic condition present (e.g., tricuspid stenosis) which would then cause an elevation in one limb of the waveform. Because of these normal fluctuations, RAP is usually measured as a *mean* value. In addition to the small waveform variations, the entire baseline is seen to rise and fall as the patient breathes.

Right Ventricular Pressure

Right ventricular pressure (RVP) is normally only seen during catheter insertion, as the catheter floats through the right ventricle (Fig 11–9,B). If during continuous monitoring the RVP waveform is identified, this indicates that the catheter has slipped from the pulmonary artery back into the right ventricle. In this circumstance, the catheter needs to be advanced back into the pulmonary artery. This is done by inflating the balloon and allowing the blood flow to carry the catheter back into the pulmonary artery.

Pulmonary Artery Pressure

Pulmonary artery pressure waveforms are continuously measured once the catheter is in place. The PAP can be distinguished by its systolic pressure of 15 to 25 mm Hg and the pulmonary artery diastolic pressure of 10 to 15 mm Hg. The normal calculated mean PAP is 10 to 15 mm Hg. The pressure waveform of the pulmonary artery (Fig 11–9,C) shows a rapid rise to peak during right ventricular systole, a gradual tapering down to the dicrotic notch (which reflects closure of the pulmonic semilunar valve), and a fall to end-diastolic level.

The baseline of the PAP waveform, as with other intrathoracic vessels, fluctuates with respirations such that the wave pattern appears to travel up- and downhill (Fig 11–10). This movement is the result of ventilation and changes in intrapleural pressure. During spontaneous ventilation, as intrapleural pressure decreases on inspiration, the wave pattern descends. During expiration it rises (Fig 11–11,A). This is the appropriate time to take a measurement. During a positive pressure breath, the curve rises as intrapleural pressures become positive and falls during the expiratory phase (Fig 11–11,B). Recall that normal intrapleural pressures are the same following either a spontaneous or a positive pressure breath (see Chapter 2). That is the reason why readings are always taken at this time.

Pulmonary Capillary Wedge Pressure

Pulmonary capillary wedge pressure (also called pulmonary artery wedge, pulmonary artery occlusion pressure, or pulmonary wedge pressure) is measured by inflating the balloon until it occludes the vessel and wedges into place (Fig. 11–12). The inflated balloon blocks blood flow past the catheter tip and the

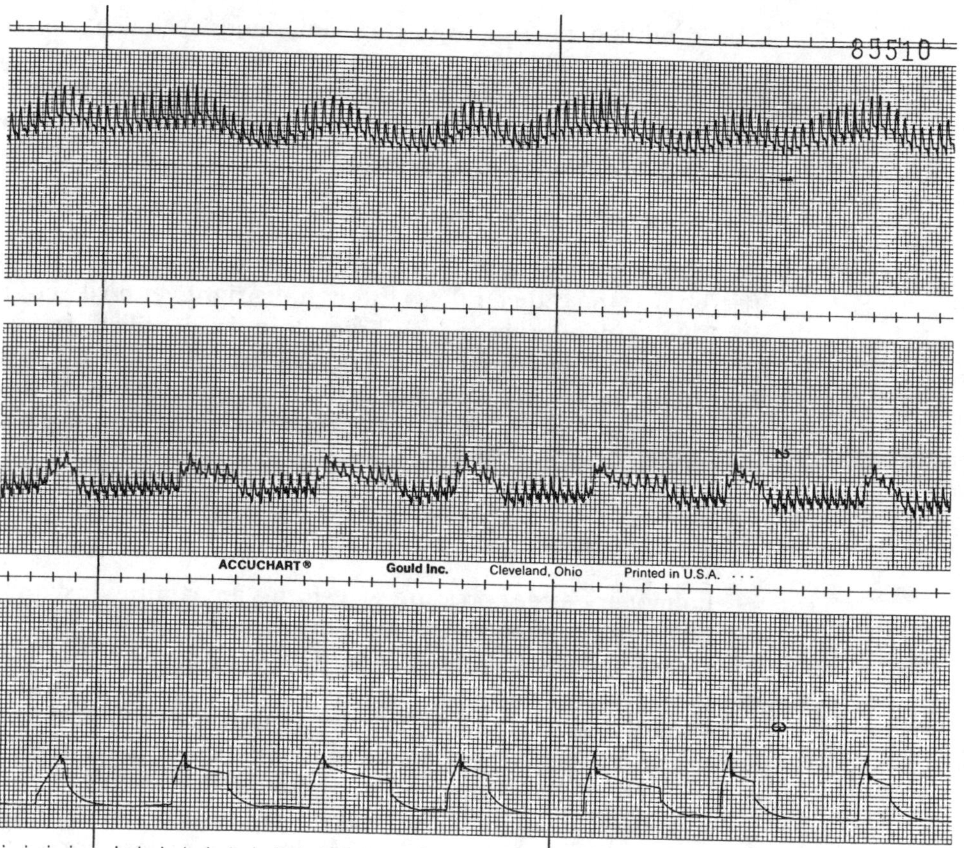

FIG 11–10.
Fluctuations in the baseline of pulmonary artery pressure (PAP) measurement during ventilation. Panel *1* is arterial pressure; panel 2 is PAP, and panel *3* is airway pressure during mechanical ventilation. Note that as the inspiratory pause increases, the effect on the PAPs lasts longer. In order to obtain an accurate measurement, pressure readings should be taken at end-exhalation[20]. (Courtesy of Jon Nilsestuen, Ph.D., RRT, University of Texas at Houston.)

pressure reading is the pressure that is in front of the catheter. This pressure is actually a retrograde pressure produced by events downstream from the catheter tip.

During ventricular diastole, with the mitral valve open, the wedged catheter views filling of the left ventricle and reads LVEDP, preload of the left heart. During ventricular systole, the mitral valve closes and the catheter views the filling of the left atrium (left atrial pressure, LAP). In this position the waveform is very similar to a right atrial tracing (Fig 11–9,D).

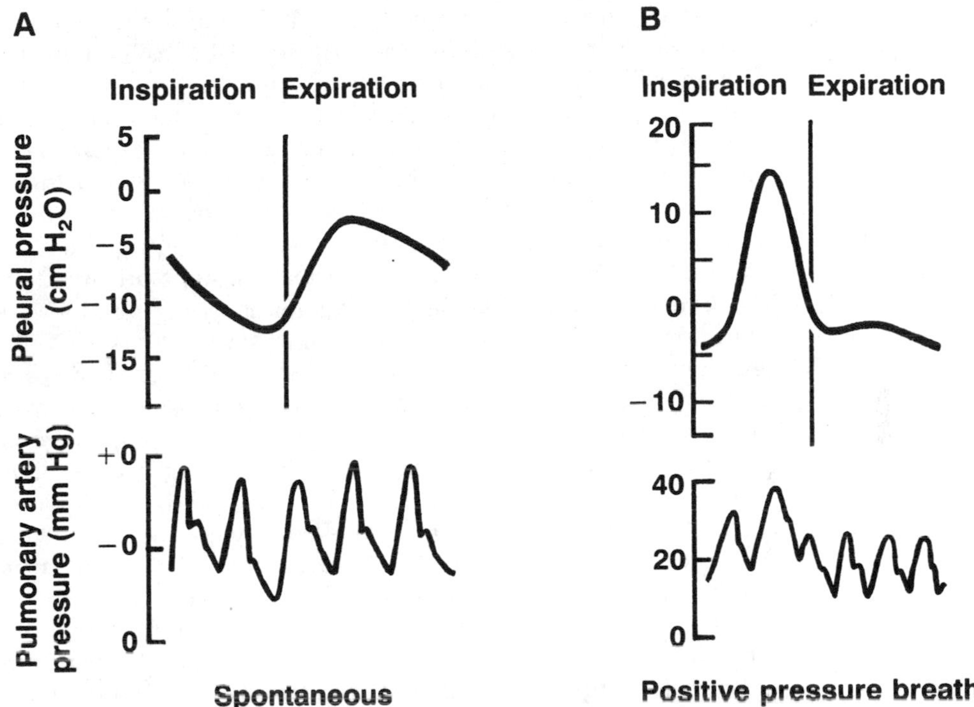

FIG 11–11.
Pulmonary artery response to ventilation. **A,** the pulmonary artery response to spontaneous ventilation. The pulmonary artery pressure (PAP) falls on inspiration and rises during expiration. **B,** the PAP in response to mechanical ventilation, rising during inspiration and falling during expiration.

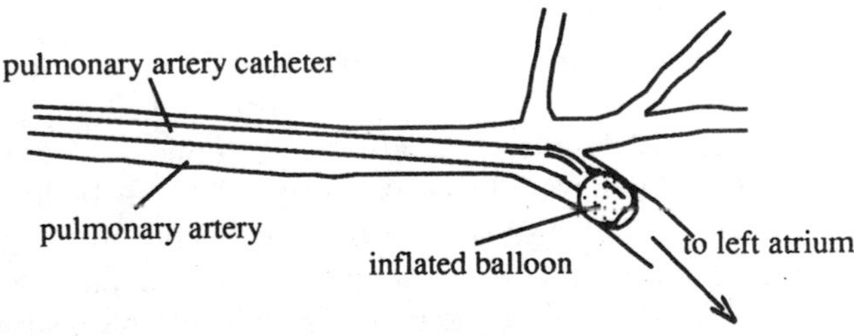

FIG 11–12.
Wedged pulmonary artery catheter.

PCWP values normally range from 5 to 12 mm Hg. PCWP is influenced by intrapleural pressures, just as all vascular pressure measurements made in the thorax are affected. Consequently, PCWP should always be measured at end-exhalation. Once the PCWP is measured, the balloon is deflated. The PAP tracing will reappear immediately if the catheter is correctly positioned and functioning. A chest film is obtained after insertion to ensure that the tip of the catheter is in the main pulmonary artery. PCWP is normally less than or equal to the pulmonary artery diastolic pressure and lower than the $\overline{PAP}$. This makes sense, since if it were higher, blood would flow backward through the pulmonary capillaries. Sometimes with severe mitral valve regurgitation, the PCWP will be transiently higher than pulmonary artery diastolic pressure.

One of the main uses of PCWP is for assessing pulmonary capillary hydrostatic pressure in the formation of pulmonary edema. PCWP can help distinguish cardiogenic pulmonary edema (increased hydrostatic pressure) from non-cardiogenic edema such as adult respiratory distress syndrome (ARDS) (normal hydrostatic pressure). PCWP greater than 18 mm Hg suggests that interstitial edema is forming. PCWP greater than 25 mm Hg usually occurs with alveolar edema from cardiac failure. On the other hand, pulmonary edema may be clinically present (bilateral infiltrates on radiograph, and bilateral crackles and wheezes on auscultation) without heart failure. If PCWP is normal and edema is clinically evident, then noncardiogenic pulmonary edema is suspect.

Between the catheter tip in the wedge position (balloon inflated) and the left atrium lies the pulmonary capillary bed. As long as this bed is unobstructed and smooth-flowing, PCWP reflects events in left heart filling. When it becomes obstructed, e.g., due to emboli, vascular damage, overinflation of alveoli (air trapping or high positive end-expiratory pressure [PEEP]), vasoconstriction from drugs or hypoxemia, then it no longer reads accurately. For this reason, in situations that change the PVR, PCWP may actually read normal in the presence of hydrostatic edema.[19]

Mixed Venous Oxygen Values

The use of a pulmonary artery catheter allows the sampling of blood from the distal tip of the catheter. This is called "mixed venous" because it is a mixture of blood from all the systemic veins before it enters the pulmonary capillary bed. Blood is sampled with the balloon in the deflated position by slowly aspirating a sample (rate of <3 mL/min).[19] If the sample is withdrawn too rapidly, it might be contaminated with pulmonary capillary blood. This would result in partial pressure of oxygen (Po_2) values higher than normal, especially if the patient is on oxygen therapy or ventilatory support.

Normal mixed venous oxygen values (pressure, saturation, content) are: $P\bar{v}o_2$, 36 to 42 mm Hg; $S\bar{v}o_2$, 75%; and $C\bar{v}o_2$, 15 vol %. Results of this sample are used to assess how much oxygen is being supplied to the tissues (arterial oxygen content [Cao_2]) in relation to demand ($\dot{V}o_2$). Mixed venous oxygen values can be expected to be lower than normal with low CO, low arterial oxygenation, and thus low oxygen transport (CO × Cao_2). Low values may also occur with a rise in metabolic rate (increased $\dot{V}o_2$). They may be higher than normal with poor sampling technique, with cyanide poisoning or other forms of histotoxic hypoxia, and also with sepsis. In sepsis, oxygenated systemic arterial blood is shunted past tissue beds. Oxygen can remain unextracted because of the peripheral vascular problems associated with sepsis.

In ARDS, mixed venous samples may appear to show variation of $\dot{V}o_2$ with oxygen delivery, even with rises and falls in CO. The reason for this is unknown. This might not reflect important changes in $\dot{V}o_2$, CO, and oxygen delivery.[19] For this reason, a mixed venous sample alone will not always be reliable.

Five-lumen cardiac catheters containing fiberoptic reflectance oximetry are now available. Optical fibers are able to read oxygen saturations inside the pulmonary artery. This may be beneficial for continuous monitoring in the event of a sudden change in patient status. Otherwise, it is expensive and similar data are available from the distal lumen of any catheter.

CATHETER COMPLICATIONS

During Insertion

During insertion, if multiple ectopic beats occur, the balloon is deflated and the catheter is pulled back.[20] Otherwise it is advanced into the pulmonary artery. The risk of perforation of the right ventricle exists if the catheter is advanced with the balloon deflated. This can result in cardiac tamponade. During insertion the catheter often forms a loop in the right ventricle. At body temperature the catheter softens and this loop unravels. This leads to migration of the catheter further distally into the pulmonary circulation. This can be detected from the monitor which will show a dampened or wedged waveform. Two possibilities exist when this condition is found. The balloon may still be inflated. Deflation of the balloon should return the PAP tracing to the screen. If it does not, then the catheter may be wedged. In this case the catheter needs to be withdrawn until only 1.5 mL is needed to inflate the balloon and reobtain the wedge reading. Failure to correct this problem can result in infarction of lung tissue.

Patient and Catheter Movement

Sometimes patient movement can result in movement of the catheter. If it moves distally, it may wedge. If it moves proximally, it may prevent wedging. Discovery of this movement can occur when the balloon is inflated to obtain a wedge reading and the waveform does not change, but continues to read PAP.

There are two possible causes of this. First, the balloon may have ruptured. You cannot add more air to test it since this creates air emboli. The second possibility is that the catheter has moved proximally, back toward the heart. To evaluate the problem, the catheter is advanced until a wedge reading is obtained. The balloon is then allowed to deflate. If the PAP waveform returns, then the catheter has migrated. If it does not return, then the balloon has ruptured and the catheter needs to be replaced.

Dampening

Air bubbles in the fluid line of the catheter can result in a dampened waveform. A dampened waveform usually is seen as a decrease in amplitude in the waveform (see Fig 11–7). Most commonly, the systolic pressure drops and the diastolic pressure rises. Dampening can also be caused by clotting at the tip of the catheter, loose connections, excessive or asymmetric balloon inflation, or the catheter tip impinging on a vessel wall.[11, 20]

EFFECTS OF MECHANICAL VENTILATION ON HEMODYNAMIC MONITORING

Intrathoracic pressure changes due to ventilation (spontaneous or mechanical) directly affect hemodynamic pressures and waveforms, i.e., thoracic intravascular measurements parallel changes in intrapleural pressure. In the spontaneously breathing patient, a decrease in intrapleural pressure during inspiration causes a corresponding decrease in PAPs (see Fig 11–11,A). During expiration, intrapleural pressure is less negative and the waveform rises. The positive intrapleural pressure applied during a mechanical ventilation breath will cause an increase in PAP during inspiration (Fig 11–11,B). During expiration, when intrapleural pressures return to normal, the waveform falls.

Figure 11–13 shows the effect of a mechanical ventilation breath on a pulmonary artery waveform and the results of doubling the tidal volume (V_T) on the same waveform. When the baseline is allowed to return to its original starting point, this change in pulmonary pressure is only realized during inspiration. With a properly maintained inspiratory-expiratory (I/E) ratio, i.e., 1:2, 1:3, or less, there is adequate time for pressure measurements to be taken at end-exhalation.[19]

The above relationship of spontaneous ventilation patterns and PAPs is true if the catheter tip is located in lung zone 3 which is where it is normally located.[20] Table 11–6 reviews the lung zones and pressure relationships in each zone.

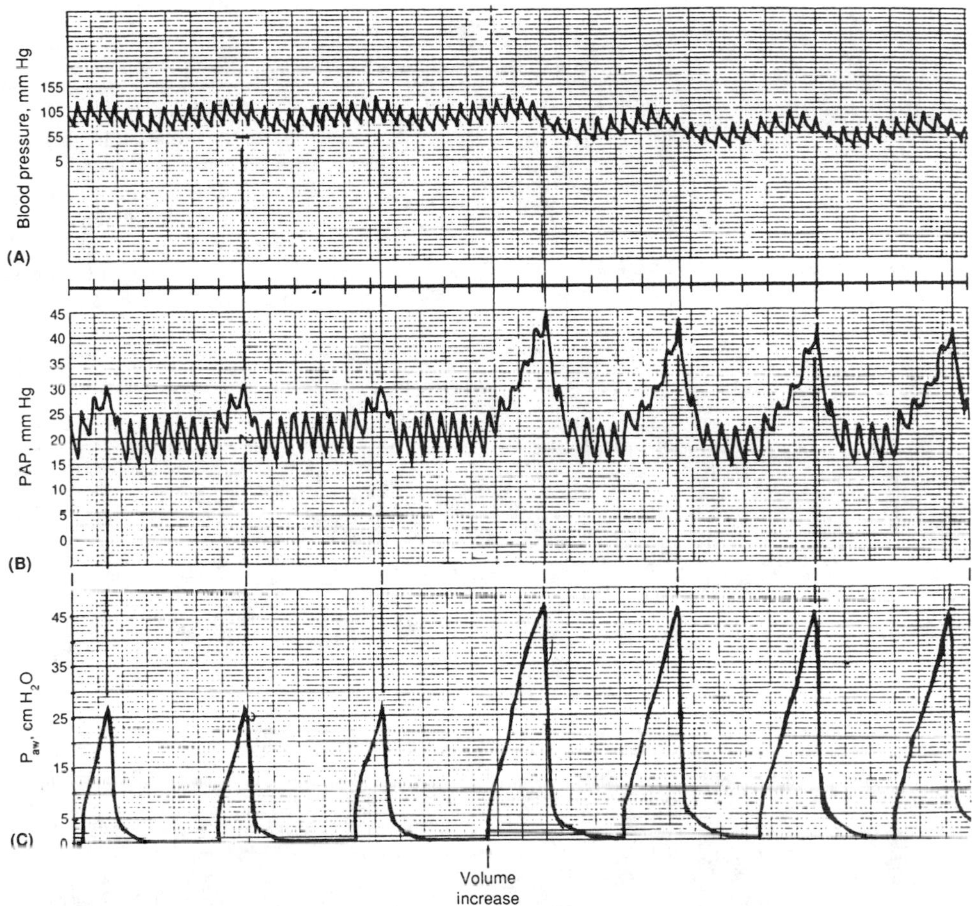

FIG 11–13.
Panel *(A)* represents arterial blood pressure, *(B)* pulmonary artery pressure (PAP), and *(C)* airway pressure (Paw) generated during mechanical ventilation. Note that PAP rises during a positive pressure breath and that blood pressure falls. (From Deshpande VM, Pilbeam SP, Dixon RJ: *A Comprehensive Review in Respiratory Care.* Norwalk, Conn, Appleton & Lange, 1988, p 372. Used by permission.)

These characteristics and pressure relationships are true in the upright lung. If the patient is supine, zone 2 conditions are dominant.[16] In zone 2, alveolar pressures have a significant effect on PAPs and the need for timely pressure measurements at end-exhalation is great. Mechanical ventilation increases zones 1 and 2 while decreasing zone 3 and care must be taken to determine the level of the transducer in relation to the catheter tip at the time of the pressure

TABLE 11–6.
Lung Zones and Pressure Relationships

Lung Zone	Pressure Relationships*	Explanation
Zone 1	$P_A > Pa > Pv$	Basically functions as alveolar dead space—ventilation in excess of perfusion
Zone 2	$Pa > P_A > Pv$	Blood flow is due to pressure difference between pulmonary artery and alveolar pressures
Zone 3	$Pa > Pv > P_A$	Blood flow is due to arterio-venous pressure differences

*Pa = arterial pressure; Pv = venous pressure; P_A = alveolar pressure.

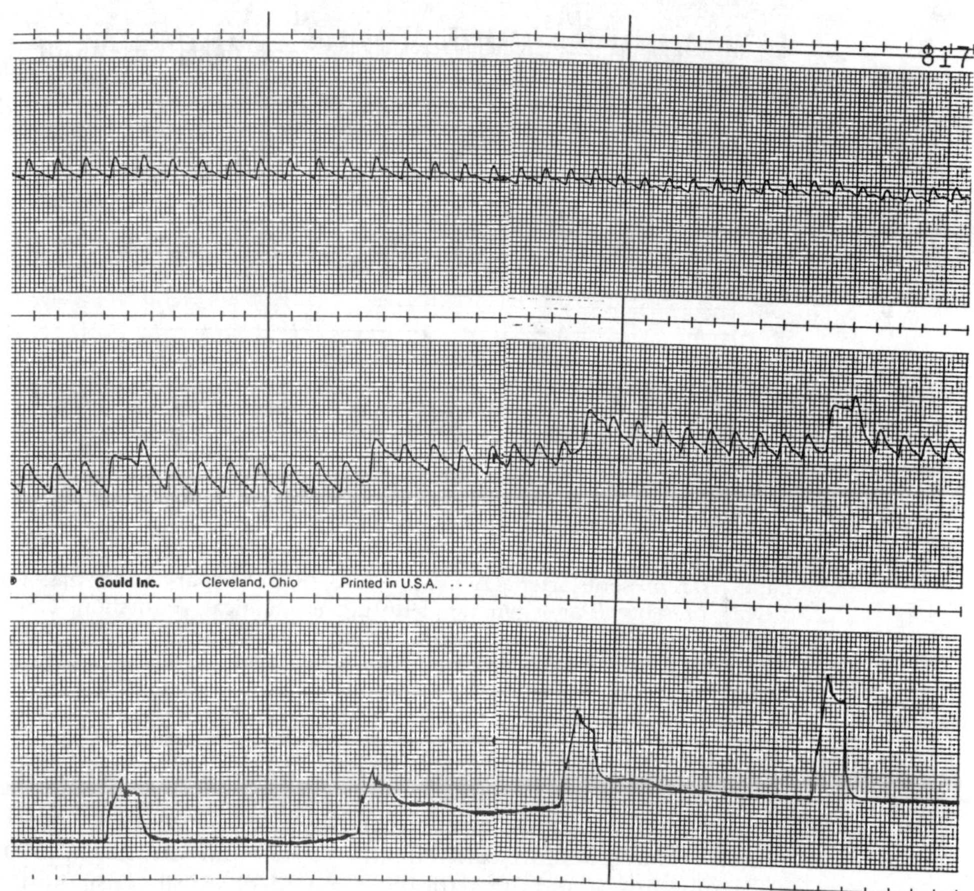

FIG 11–14.
Effects on pressures at various positive end-expiratory pressure (PEEP) levels. As PEEP is raised from 5 to 10 to 15 cm H_2O *(bottom panel)* note the corresponding rise in pulmonary artery pressures *(middle panel)* and fall in systemic artery pressure *(top panel)*. (Courtesy of Jon Nilsestuen, Ph.D., RRT, University of Texas at Houston.)

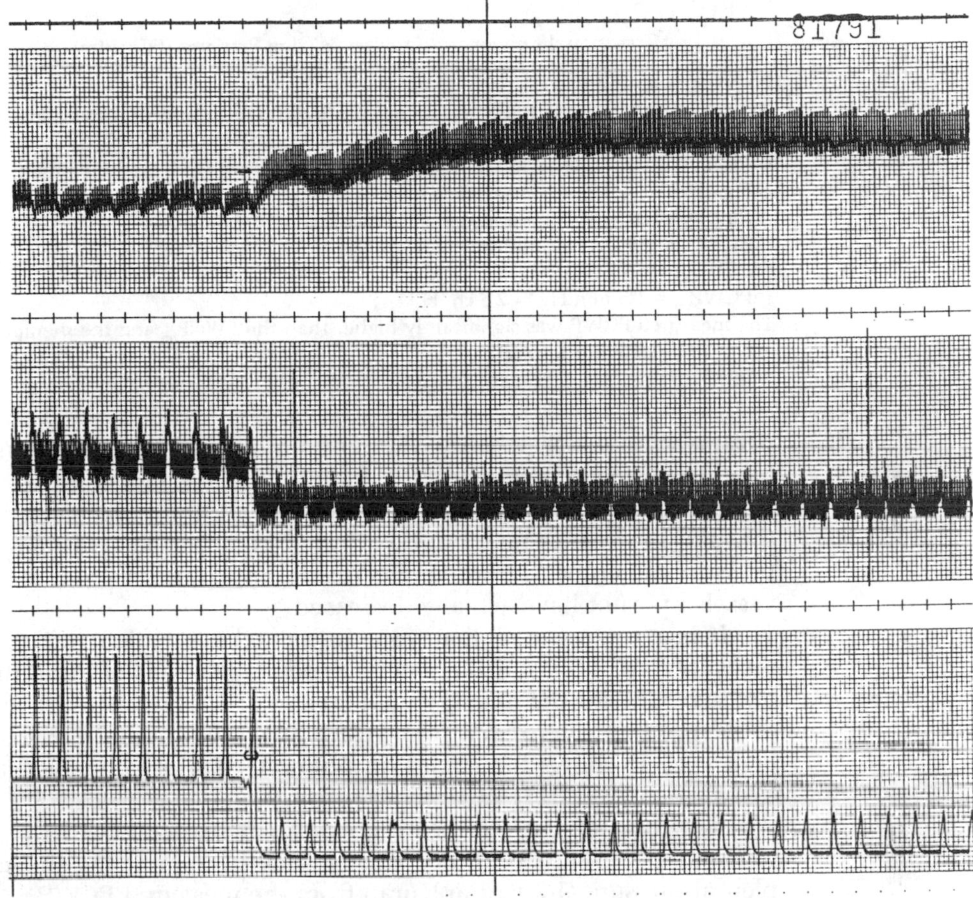

FIG 11–15.
Effects on pressures when positive end-expiratory pressure (PEEP) is removed. As PEEP is discontinued from 15 cm H_2O to zero *(bottom panel),* note the fall in pulmonary artery pressures *(middle panel),* and rise in systemic artery pressures *(top panel).* (Courtesy of Jon Nilsestuen, Ph.D., RRT, University of Texas at Houston.)

measurements. Releveling and zeroing the transducer with patients in other than "normal" positions can alleviate some of the errors in measurement.[16]

PEEP, either deliberate or inadvertent (e.g., auto-PEEP), at levels greater than 15 cm H_2O, will prolong the changes in lung zones and can produce erroneously elevated pressure readings.[20] The pressures in the thoracic circulation will rise when using PEEP therapy owing to the "squeeze" put on the vessels by the increased lung volumes (increased functional residual capacity) (Fig 11–14). PCWP, which reflects preload of the left heart, is an excellent

TABLE 11–7.

Calculating Transmural Pulmonary Capillary Wedge Pressure (PCWPtm)

PCWPtm with PEEP

Approximately ½ of the PEEP will be transmitted to the intrapleural space in a patient with stiff lungs

If PEEP = 20 cm H_2O or 15 mm Hg (1 mm Hg = 1.36 cm H_2O), and measured PCWP = 15 mm Hg, then:

Pintrapleural ≈ ½ × 15 mm Hg = 7.5 mm Hg

PCWPtm = PCWP − Pintrapleural

$PCWP_{tm}$ = 15 − 7.5

$PCWP_{tm}$ = 7.5 mm Hg = 7.5 cm H_2O

The measured PCWP was significantly higher than the $PWCP_{tm}$ and the therapeutic intervention would be different for each

parameter to watch when performing an optimal PEEP study (see Chapter 10 for a discussion on optimal PEEP studies). If PCWP increases significantly during the study, it could indicate overinflation of the alveoli. Actual blood flow through the vessels may not be affected because the transmural pressure (the pressure difference between the inside and outside of a vessel) within the vessels may not have actually decreased.

It is recommended that you do *not* take a patient off the ventilator to measure PWCP.[19, 20, 34] If the patient needs high levels of PEEP therapy, discontinuing PEEP for the time it would take to accurately measure wedge pressures could produce hypoxemia from which the patient would recover very slowly. Figure 11–15 shows the effects on pulmonary artery and systemic blood pressures when PEEP is removed.

A picture of the left heart preload can be estimated by calculating the transmural PCWP (PWCPtm). This is done by subtracting the estimated intrapleural pressure (1/2 Pıntrapleural) from the measured PCWP.

$$PCWPtm = PCWP - 1/2\ Pintrapleural\ (in\ mm\ Hg)$$

Table 11–7 shows an example of this calculation. The procedure for measuring PCWPtm is also outlined in Appendix M. The reliability of this method cannot be assured because the effects of PEEP and lung compliance differ from patient to patient. Thus, the PCWPtm calculated using this method should be used only as an estimate.

CASE STUDIES

Case 1

A 63-year-old white man is status post aortobirenal artery graft. He has a 40+-year history of tobacco use and was diagnosed with hypertension at the age of 50. He is currently in ICU suffering from acute renal failure and ARDS. The patient is 68 in. tall and weighs 68 kg (BSA 1.81 m^2). He is on a volume ventilator with a V_T of 1,000 mL, synchronized intermittent ventilation (SIMV) rate of 8 breaths/min (spontaneous respiratory rate of 4 breaths/min with a V_T of approximately 150 mL), and fractional concentration of oxygen in inspired gas (F_{IO_2}) of 0.60, and PEEP of 12 cm H_2O. The waveforms recorded while the ventilator was on the above settings are shown in Figure 11–16. Table 11–8 shows the patient's hemodynamic data and calculations during this time. See Tables 11–9 and 11–10 for definititions, values, and formulas used to obtain these data.

Interpretation.—These data are interpreted as noncardiogenic pulmonary edema due to ARDS based on the elevated PAP (52/18), CVP (12 mm Hg), normal PCWP (13 mm Hg), and normal CI (4.41 L/min/m^2). PEEP therapy is increased to treat the refractory hypoxemia. To evaluate any adverse cardiovascular effects of PEEP, blood pressure (BP), CO, CI, and urinary output are monitored.

Case 2

A 68-year-old man is being ventilated with a Puritan Bennett 7200ae following open heart surgery for a triple coronary artery bypass operation. Vital signs are stable

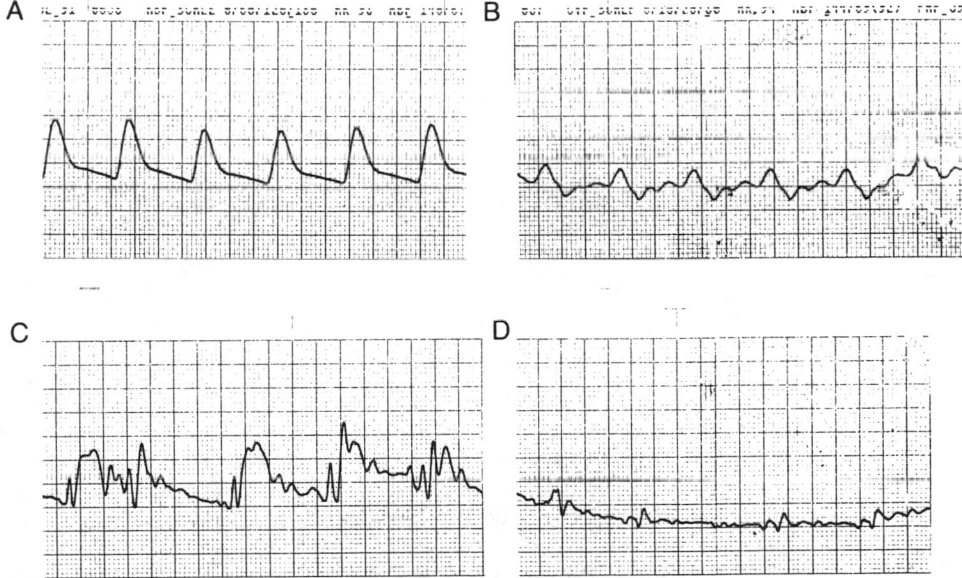

FIG 11–16.
Case 1 waveforms. **A,** arterial waveform. Absence of an identifiable dicrotic notch (representing closure of the aortic semilunar valves) is due to the catheter's position in the femoral artery. **B,** right atrial pressure. **C,** pulmonary artery pressure. **D,** wedge pressure.

TABLE 11–8.
Hemodynamic Data for Case 1

	Value
CO	7.98 L/min
CI	4.41 L/min/m^2
HR	81 beats/min
BP	159/64 mm Hg
BP, mean	92 mm Hg
PAP	52/18 mm Hg
PAP, mean	33 mm Hg
PCWP	13 mm Hg
CVP	12 mm Hg
SV	98.5 mL
SI	54.4 mL/m^2
SVR	802 dynes × cm × sec^{-5}
PVR	201 dynes × cm × sec^{-5}
Hb	14.g/dL
Temperature	37° C
Arterial blood gases	
pH	7.362
Po_2	80 mm Hg
Pco_2	46.2 mm Hg
HCO_3^-	26.5 mEq/L
Sao_2	95.2%
Mixed venous blood gases	
pH	7.339
Po_2	40 mm Hg
Pco_2	50.3 mm Hg
HCO_3^-	27.4 mEq/L
$S\bar{v}o_2$	71.2%
Cao_2	18.5 vol%
Cvo_2	13.8 vol%
$C(a-v)o_2$	4.7 vol%
O_2 transport	1,476 mL/min
$\dot{V}o_2$	375 mL/min

with a heart rate of 95 beats/min, a temperature of 37.6°C, and a BP of 130/75 mm Hg. Breath sounds are normal. The V_T is 500 mL on SIMV with no spontaneous breaths. The patient has an ideal body weight of 68 kg. The respiratory rate is 12 breaths/min. Peak pressures are 27 cm H_2O on the ventilator manometer and compliance is 20 mL/cm H_2O. PAP at end-exhalation is 25/15 mm Hg and the CO is 6.2 L/min. PCWP is 10 mm Hg. The patient is considered stable and in very good condition following his surgery.

Figure 11–13 shows the arterial blood pressure curve *(A)*, the PAP curve *(B)*, and the pressure measured at the patient's upper airway *(C)* during ventilation. As the ventilator cycles, the PAP rises and the systemic BP drops after a slight delay.

As the V_T is increased to 1,000 mL, airway pressures rise from 27 to 46 cm H_2O, arterial BP drops to 80/35 mm Hg following every positive pressure breath and does not rise to more than 100/55 mm Hg (see Fig 11–13). The drop in BP is accompanied by a decrease in CO to 4.9 L/min. The peak PAP that occurs at the peak ventilating pressure has risen to 45 mm Hg, while the end-expiratory PAP has stayed the same at 25/15 mm Hg.

Interpretation.—This patient shows the effect positive pressure can have on PAP and CO. Positive pressure ventilation can cause a decrease in systemic blood pressure, a decrease in CO, and an increase in PAP. After the VT was reduced to its previous setting (500 mL) the patient returned to his previous stable condition.[11]

Case 3

A 72-year-old man is admitted to the ICU, after stabilization in the emergency room (ER) and is being administered oxygen via nasal cannula at 2 L/min. ABGs drawn in the ER revealed pH of 7.47, $Paco_2$ of 30 mm Hg, and Pao_2 of 31 mm Hg. The patient was

TABLE 11–9.
Hemodynamic Values That Can Be Directly Measured*

	Unit	Normal value	How measured	Use
Heart rate (HR)	beats/min	60–90	Watch	Early index of tachycardia and bradycardia
Blood pressure (BP) (systemic)	mm Hg	Systolic: 90–140 Diastolic: 60–90	Blood pressure cuff or arterial line	Early index of hypertension or hypotension
Central venous pressure (CVP)	mm Hg	1–6	From CVP catheter or pulmonary artery 3- or 4-lumen catheter	Estimates right ventricular preload; also for drug and fluid administration
Pulmonary artery pressure (PAP)	mm Hg	Systolic: 15–25 Diastolic: 5–15	From pulmonary artery catheter	Measures pulmonary vascular resistance (PVR)
Pulmonary capillary wedge pressure (PCWP)	mm Hg	5–12	From pulmonary artery catheter in occluded position (balloon inflated)	Estimates left ventricular filling and preload
Cardiac output (CO)	L/min	5–8	By thermodilution or dye dilution	An important determinant of hemodynamic function
Mixed venous partial pressure of oxygen ($P\bar{v}o_2$)	mm Hg	40	From distal tip of pulmonary artery catheter	Overall assessment of cardiopulmonary function
Arterial partial pressure of oxygen (Pao_2)	mm hg	80–100	From a systemic artery	For assessing level of arterial oxygenation

*Modified with permission from Deshpande VM, Pilbeam SP, Dixon RJ: *A Comprehensive Review in Respiratory Care.* Norwalk, Conn, Appleton & Lange, 1988, p. 358.

TABLE 11–10.
Hemodynamic Values That Can Be Calculated*

	Unit	Normal Value	Formula†	Use/Comments
Mean arterial blood pressure (MAP)	mm Hg	80–100	$\frac{\text{systolic} + 2\ \text{diastolic}}{3}$	To calculate SVR; used in monitoring when giving vasoactive drugs
Pulse pressure (systemic)	mm Hg	40	Systolic − diastolic	
Stroke volume (SV)	mL	60–100	CO/HR	Gives information about cardiac performance
Cardiac index (CI)	L/min/M^2	3.5–4.5	CO/BSA	An important determinant of cardiac performance (removes body size as a variable)
Systemic vascular resistance (SVR)	dynes × cm × sec^{-5}	900–1,400	$\frac{\text{MAP} - \text{CVP}}{\text{CO}} \times 80$	Useful in diagnosis of vascular problems
Mean pulmonary artery pressure (PAP)	mm Hg	15–20	$\frac{\text{Systolic PAP} + 2\ \text{diastolic PAP}}{3}$	To calculate vascular resistance
Pulmonary vascular resistance (PVR)	dynes × cm × sec^{-5}	150–250	$\frac{\overline{\text{PAP}} - \text{PCWP}}{\text{CO}} \times 80$	
Oxygen content of arterial blood (Cao_2)	vol %	20	%sat × Hb × 1.34	
Oxygen content of mixed venous blood ($C\bar{v}o_2$)	vol %	15	%sat × Hb × 1.34	
Arteriovenous oxygen content difference [$C(a\text{-}v)o_2$]	mL/100 mL or vol %	3.5–5.0	From arteriovenous blood	An index of tissue oxygenation
Oxygen transport	mL/min	1,000‡	CO × Cao_2	An indicator of the amount of O_2 delivered to the tissues
Oxygen consumption ($\dot{V}o_2$)	mL/min	200–300	CO × $C(a-v)o_2$	Indicates metabolic rate or amount of O_2 used by the body; can be measured directly by noninvasive means, but this is very difficult

*Modified with permission from Deshande VM, Pilbeam SP, Dixon RJ: *A Comprehensive Review in Respiratory Care.* Norwalk, Conn, Appleton & Lange, 1988, p. 359.

†CO = cardiac output; HR = heart rate; BSA = body surface area; CVP = central venous pressure; PCWP = pulmonary capillary wedge pressure; % sat = percent saturation.

‡CO × Cao_2 = 5,000 mL/min × 20 mL/100 mL = 1,000 mL/min.

TABLE 11–11.
Hemodynamic Data for Case 3*

	Value
HR	127 beats/min
BP	187/59 mm Hg
CVP	5 mm Hg
PAP	59/25 mm Hg
$\overline{PAP}$	36 mm Hg
PCWP	12 mm Hg
CO	6.7 L/min
CI	3.56 L/min/m^2
SV	66 mL
SVR	1098 dynes × cm × sec^{-5}
PVR	310 dynes × cm × sec^{-5}
pH	7.33
$Paco_2$	52 mm Hg
Pao_2	42 mm Hg

*For abbreviations, see Tables 11–9 and 11–10.

TABLE 11–12.
Effects of Cardiopulmonary Disorders on Hemodynamic Values*

Condition	PAP	CVP	PCWP	CO	BP	$S\bar{v}o_2$
Pulmonary hypertension	↑	→↑	→	→↓	→↓	↓
COPD						
Pulmonary embolism (massive)						
ARDS						
Air trapping						
Fibrosis						
Congestive heart failure (cardiogenic shock)	↑	→↑	↑	↓	↓	↓
Hypovolemia	↓	↓	↓	↓	↓	↓
Dehydration						
Hemorrhage						
Septic shock						↑↓
Anaphylactic shock						
Neurogenic shock						
Hypervolemia (fluid overload)	→↑	→↑	→↑	→↑	→↑	→↑

* ↑ = increase; ↓ = decrease; → = no change.

immediately placed on a nonrebreathing mask and ABGs and vital signs were assessed with the following results: pH = 7.48; Pa_{O_2} = 56 mm Hg; HR = 116 beats/min; Pa_{CO_2} = 32 mm Hg; respiratory rate = 34 breaths/min; BP = 175/58 mm Hg.

The patient was placed on mechanical ventilation support on the following settings: V_T = 850 mL; assist-control rate = 10 breaths/min; F_{IO_2} = 0.5; PEEP = +10 cm H_2O.

Hemodynamic monitoring, following successful insertion of a pulmonary artery catheter in the subclavian vein, revealed the data contained in Table 11–11. The patient was found to have a pulmonary embolism.

Interpretation.—This patient's pulmonary embolism resulted by the presence of refractory hypoxemia. The fact that the PAP is elevated with a normal PCWP is representative of a pulmonary condition as opposed to left heart failure. The CVP is within normal limits indicating the condition is acute since the right side of the heart has not yet been affected by the elevated PAPs.[5, 8, 9]

Table 11–12 summarizes the effects some cardiovascular diseases have on various hemodynamic values. Pulmonary hypertension, congestive heart failure, and hypervolemia can present with similar hemodynamic profiles. Other clinical observations, medical history, and additional laboratory values are necessary to differentiate the type of disease. Hypovolemia will present with a unique hemodynamic profile that is easily identifiable because all hemodynamic values are decreased (with the exception of $S\bar{v}_{O_2}$, which will be elevated in septic shock).

SUMMARY

Data obtained from hemodynamic monitoring are used in the management of critically ill patients. Mechanical ventilation can have a profound effect on these data. Knowledge of the influence mechanical ventilation can have on hemodynamic data will better prepare the practitioner to make proper therapeutic interventions in the patient's care.

STUDY QUESTIONS

1. What parameters are used to estimate right and left heart preloads?
2. What can cause an abnormally high PVR?
3. If a patient is on PEEP of 18 cm H_2O and has a measured PCWP of 22 mm Hg, what is his PCWPtm?

4. What does the dicrotic notch on the pulmonary artery waveform represent?
5. How will mechanical ventilation affect PAP, PCWP, and CVP?
6. During the measurement of a patient's CVP (RAP), you note that the transducer is 6 cm above the level of the right atrium. At this position the CVP reading is 0 cm H_2O. What is the patient's approximate actual CVP?
   a. 0 cm H_2O.
   b. 7.86 cm H_2O.
   c. 11.16 cm H_2O.
   d. 15 cm H_2O.
   e. 17.16 cm H_2O.
7. You expect to see the right ventricular waveform in which of the following situations?
   I. During catheter insertion.
   II. During a normal "wedge" maneuver.
   III. When the catheter is properly placed in the pulmonary artery.
   IV. If the catheter slips back into the right ventricle.
      a. I only.
      b. III and IV only.
      c. II and III only.
      d. I and IV only.
      e. I, II, III, and IV.
8. If the Swan-Ganz catheter is properly placed, the proximal lumen is located in the:
   a. Pulmonary artery.
   b. Right ventricle.
   c. Right atrium.
   d. Wedged position.
   e. Subclavian vein.
9. Myocardial $\dot{V}O_2$ is greatest during which phase of the normal cardiac cycle?
   a. Phase 1: atrial filling.
   b. Phase II: atrial systole.
   c. Phase III: isovolumetric contraction.
   d. Phase IV: ventricular ejection.
10. A term referring to the volume of blood present in the ventricle just before systole is:
   a. Preload.
   b. Afterload.
   c. Contractility.
   d. Static pressure.
   e. Ejection fraction.

11. In the presence of vasoconstriction due to hypoxemia, the PCWP:
    a. Will read lower than actual pressure present.
    b. May read normal in the presence of hydrostatic edema.
    c. May read higher than LVEDP.
    d. May not be able to be determined.
    e. Is not affected by pulmonary vascular vasoconstriction.
12. If a patient has a CO of 6.4 L/min and a BSA of 1.8 m^2, what is this patient's CI?
    a. 2.84 L/min/m^2.
    b. 3.56 L/min/m^2.
    c. 4.60 L/min/m^2.
    d. 8.20 L/min/m^2.
    e. 11.52 L/min/m^2.
13. Which of the following corrects or minimizes the effects of fluid (blood) pressure on measurements made by a fluid-filled system?
    I. Zeroing and calibration of the equipment.
    II. Catheter orientation (positioning).
    III. Elimination of static pressure head.
    IV. Type of fluid used in the system.
    a. I, II, and III only.
    b. I and IV only.
    c. II and III only.
    d. II, III, and IV only.
    e. I, II, III, and IV.
14. The function of the transducer dome in a fluid-filled system is to:
    a. Convert a pressure signal into an electrical signal.
    b. Convert an electrical signal into a pressure signal.
    c. Act as a filter to the transducer.
    d. Respond to pressure changes in the fluid column.
    e. Act as a one-way valve for fluids going into the pulmonary artery catheter.
15. Mr. B is admitted to the ICU following abdominal surgery. He is receiving an IV infusion at 40 mL/hr and his urinary output is 15 mL/hr. A pulmonary artery catheter is successfully placed and the following data are obtained: BP = 88/68 mm Hg; CVP = 2 mm Hg; PAP = 16/6 mm Hg; CO = 3.2 L/min; pulse = 112 beats/min; PCWP = 4 mm Hg; CI = 1.18 L/min/m^2. Mr. B is most probably suffering from:
    a. Myocardial infarction.
    b. Hypovolemia.
    c. Pulmonary embolism.
    d. Cardiac tamponade.
    e. Hypoxemia.

ANSWERS TO STUDY QUESTIONS

1. CVP on the right and PCWP on the left.
2. Pulmonary hypertension, hypoxemia, COPD, or mechanical ventilation with PEEP.
3. 18 ÷ 1.36 = 13.23
   Pintrapleural = 24/2 = 12
   PCWPtm = PCWP − Pintrapleural
   PCWPtm = 22 − 12
   PCWPtm = 10 mm Hg
4. Closure of the pulmonic semilunar valve.
5. Each of the pressures will be elevated during inspiration.
6. c.
7. d.
8. c.
9. c.
10. a.
11. c.
12. b.
13. a.
14. d.
15. b.

REFERENCES

1. Assman R, Heidelmeyer CF, Trampisch HJ, et al: Right ventricular function assessed by thermodilution technique during apnea and mechanical ventilation. *Crit Care Med* 1991; 19:810.
2. Berryhill RE, Benumof JL: PEEP-induced discrepancy between pulmonary arterial wedge pressure and left atrial pressure: The effects of controlled versus spontaneous ventilation and compliant versus noncompliant lungs in the dog. *Anesthesiology* 1979; 51:303–308.
3. Bone RC: Monitoring patients in acute respiratory failure. *Respir Care* 1982; 27:700.
4. Boysen PG, McGough E: Pressure-control and pressure-support ventilation: Flow patterns, inspiratory time, and gas distribution. *Respir Care* 1988; 33:126.
5. Bustin D: *Hemodynamic Monitoring for Critical Care.* Norwalk, Conn, Appleton-Century-Crofts, 1986.
6. Civetti JM: Cardiovascular monitoring—principles and practice. *Curr Rev Respir Ther* 1979; 12:91–95.
7. Cordy DJ: Monitoring central venous pressure during mechanical ventilation. *Respir Care* 1979; 24:241–243.

8. Dailey EK, Shroeder JS: *Techniques in Bedside Hemodynamic Monitoring,* ed 2. St. Louis, Mosby–Year Book, Inc, 1981.
9. Darovic GO: *Hemodynamic Monitoring—Invasive and Noninvasive Clinical Application.* Philadelphia, WB Saunders Co, 1987.
10. Davison R, Parker M, Harrison RA: The validity of determination of pulmonary wedge pressure during mechanical ventilation. *Chest* 1978; 33:352–355.
11. Deshpande VM, Pilbeam SP, Dixon RJ: *A Comprehensive Review in Respiratory Care,* Norwalk, Conn, Appleton & Lange, 1988.
12. Downs JB, Douglas ME: Assessment of cardiac filling pressure occurring in continuous positive pressure ventilation. *Crit Care Med* 1980; 8:285.
13. Fassoulaki A, Eforakopaulou M: Cardiovascular, respiratory, and metabolic changes produced by pressure-supported ventilation in intensive care unit patients. *Crit Care Med* 1989;17:527.
14. Gengiz M, Crapo RO, Gardner RM: The effect of ventilation on the accuracy of pulmonary artery and wedge pressure measurements. *Crit Care Med* 1983; 11:502–507.
15. Gore JM, et al: *Handbook of Hemodynamic Monitoring.* Boston, Little, Brown & Co, 1985.
16. Groom L, Frisch SR, Elliott M et al: Reproducibility and accuracy of pulmonary artery measurement in supine and lateral positions. *Heart Lung* 1990; 19:147.
17. Hudson LD: Ventilatory management of patients with adult respiratory distress syndrome. *Semin Respir Med* 1981; 2:128.
18. Jastremski MS: Hemodynamic monitoring concepts every clinician should know. *Consultant* September 1982, pp 96–111.
19. Kacmerek RM, Stoller JK: *Current Respiratory Care* Philadelphia, BC Decker, Inc, 1988, pp 170–176.
20. Kirby RR, Banner MJ, Downs JB: *Clinical Application of Ventilatory Support.* New York, Churchill Livingstone Inc, 1990.
21. Marini JJ: Obtaining meaningful data from the Swan-Ganz catheter. *Respir Care* 1985; 30:572–584.
22. Matthay RA: Cardiovascular function in the intensive care unit: Invasive and noninvasive monitoring. *Respir Care* 1985; 30:432–453.
23. Osgood CF, Watson MH, Slaughter MS, et al: Hemodynamic monitoring in respiratory care. *Respir Care* 1984; 29:25–32.
24. Rajacich S, Burchard KW, Hasan FM, et al: Central venous pressure and pulmonary capillary wedge pressure as estimates of left atrial pressure: Effects of positive end-expiratory pressure and catheter tip malposition. *Crit Care Med* 1989; 17:7–11.
25. Rao TLK: Cardiac monitoring for the noncardiac surgical patient. *Semin Anesthesia* 1983; 2.
26. Reidinger MS, Shellock FG, Swan HJC: Reading pulmonary artery and pulmonary capillary wedge pressure waveforms with respiratory variations. *Heart Lung* 1981; 10:675–678.
27. Shasby DM, Dauber IM, Pfister S, et al: Swan-Ganz catheter location and left atrial pressure determine the accuracy of the wedge pressure when positive end-expiratory pressure is used. *Chest* 1981; 80:666–670.

28. Shin JA, Woods SL, Huseby JS: Effect of intermittent positive pressure ventilation upon pulmonary artery and pulmonary capillary wedge pressures in acutely ill patients. *Heart Lung* 1979; 8:322–327.
29. Sprung CL: *The Pulmonary Artery Catheter.* Rockville, Md, Aspen System Corp, 1983.
30. Tidwell SL, Ryan WJ, Osguthorpe SG, et al: Effects of position changes on mixed venous oxygen saturation in patients after coronary revascularization. *Heart Lung* 1990; 19:574.
31. *Understanding Hemodynamic Measurements Made With the Swan-Ganz Catheter.* Santa Ana, Calif, American Edwards Laboratories, 1982.
32. West JB: *Respiratory Physiology: The Essentials,* ed 2. Baltimore, Williams & Wilkins Co, 1979.
33. Wild LR, Woods SL: Comparison of three methods for interpreting pulmonary wedge pressure waveforms with respiratory variation. *Heart Lung* 1985; 14:308.
34. Wilkins RL, Sheldon RL, Krider SJ: *Clinical Assessment in Respiratory Care,* ed 2. St Louis, Mosby–Year Book, Inc, 1990.
35. Woods SL, Mansfield LW: Effect of body position upon pulmonary artery and pulmonary capillary wedge pressure in non-critically ill patients. *Heart Lung* 1976; 5:83
36. Wright J, Gong H: Auto-PEEP: Incidence, magnitude, and contributing factors. *Heart Lung* 1990; 19:532.

Chapter 12

Discontinuation of and Weaning From Mechanical Ventilation

With David Shelledy, Ph.D., R.R.T.

On completion of this chapter the reader will be able to:

1. State the number-one factor to be considered when evaluating a patient for ventilator discontinuation or weaning.
2. Summarize the steps that should be taken to optimize patient condition prior to attempting ventilator discontinuation.
3. List all commonly used weaning parameters and include the range of values for each which are considered favorable for ventilator discontinuation.
4. Summarize the procedure used to achieve classic or conventional ventilator weaning.
5. Summarize the procedure used during weaning when using IMV or SIMV.
6. Compare the rationales for conventional weaning and IMV or SIMV.
7. Explain the rationale for the use of pressure support and mandatory minute volume as adjunctive ventilation techniques to facilitate ventilator discontinuation.
8. List common causes for failure in efforts to achieve ventilator discontinuation and explain each.

DISCONTINUATION AND WEANING OF THE VENTILATED PATIENT

When the need for mechanical ventilation no longer exists, the patient can be removed from support. In the majority of patients this is a simple maneuver. In some patients it requires a more lengthy process. The first we call *discontinuation* or *disconnection;* the second we call *weaning*. Disconnection or discontinuation from mechanical ventilation implies that a patient no longer needs that form of treatment. It is estimated that about 80% of patients requiring temporary mechanical ventilation do not require a weaning process before treatment is discontinued.[110] These patients can be disconnected within a few hours of initial support. Examples of these situations include postoperative ventilatory support for recovery from surgery and anesthesia and the treatment of uncomplicated drug overdose. The rapidity of the process is dependent upon individual patient needs. In a study of 910 ventilated patients, 583 (64%) were discontinued in less than 24 hours. But 327 (36%) required support for longer than 24 hours, some for as long as 23 days and more.[77] In a few rare cases, ventilatory support is continued for the duration of the patient's life.

Weaning implies that the need for support still exists and that the patient is still ventilator-dependent.[100] Weaning is a gradual process that is begun only after there is evidence that the problem leading to the need for ventilation has been corrected. Deciding whether a patient needs to be weaned or discontinued depends greatly on the patient's overall clinical condition and psychological state. These must be evaluated prior to attempting to remove the patient from ventilatory support.

PATIENT EVALUATION

A great deal of interest in recent years has focused on establishing specific criteria which predict the success of weaning patients from mechanical ventilation. To date, no one single measure has been established that is uniformly successful in predicting patient "weanability." Therapists and physicians routinely evaluate such factors as spontaneous volumes and rates, vital capacity, inspiratory force, and blood gases in an attempt to determine when patient weaning is indicated and to predict success. The number-one factor in determining if weaning from mechanical ventilation is appropriate, however, is often overlooked. Has there been improvement or reversal of the disease process or condition which caused the patient to be placed on the ventilation? If the answer to this question is no, then assuming that mechanical ventilation was indicated in the first place, weaning is not likely to succeed. If the answer to that key question, however, is yes, then other factors are assessed. These include the patient's overall medical condition, the results of a physical assessment related to cardiopulmonary reserve and work of breathing, and the patient's psychological readiness.

Evaluation of Clinical Profile

Table 12–1 lists the clinical factors which help in the evaluation of the patient's overall condition. Anything which is not in a normal range may inhibit the patient's ability to breathe spontaneously without mechanical support. It needs to be pointed out that sometimes one or more of these items will be outside the normal range, but the patient may still be able to support his or her

TABLE 12–1.
Clinical Factors in Evaluation of the Weaning Candidate's Overall Condition

Acid-base balance
Anemia or the presence of abnormal hemoglobin
Body temperature
Cardiac arrhythmias
Caloric depletion (malnutrition or protein loss)
Electrolytes
Exercise tolerance (sit up in a chair, etc.)
Fluid balance
Hemodynamic stability (blood pressure, cardiac output)
Hyperglycemia or hypoglycemia
Infection
Pain (minimize without oversedation)
Psychological condition
Renal function
Sleep deprivation (an important and often overlooked problem)
State of consciousness

own ventilation successfully. It is hard to predict when the patient will be successful and when not.

Measurements for Respiratory Assessment

Measurements for evaluation of respiratory physiologic readiness for discontinuation are listed in Table 12–2. Measurements of maximum inspiratory pressure (MIP), vital capacity (VC), maximum voluntary ventilation (MVV), tidal volume (V_T), and minute volume ($\dot{V}_E$) are used to assess respiratory muscle strength in preparing for discontinuation of the ventilator. High airway resistance and stiff lungs (low compliance) may require too much work of breathing (WOB) for the patient to be able to breathe spontaneously.

Mechanical ventilation with positive end-expiratory pressure (PEEP) is sometimes used to reverse hypoxemia. If a ventilated patient requires high fractional concentrations of oxygen in inspired gas (F_{IO_2}) and has low arterial levels, then the underlying disease process has probably not improved enough to allow the patient to breathe on his or her own. That is why we examine the arterial oxygen tension–F_{IO_2} ratio (Pa_{O_2}/F_{IO_2}), the arterial–alveolar oxygen tension ratio ($Pa_{O_2}/P_{A_{O_2}}$), the alveolar-arterial oxygen pressure difference [$P(A-a)_{O_2}$], and shunt ($\dot{Q}s/\dot{Q}t$) before discontinuing ventilation.

Work of Breathing

Work of breathing[112] during mechanical ventilation is an important consideration of weaning from ventilatory support.[39, 79–83, 107, 115, 116] If the WOB becomes too high for the patient, he or she will not be able to continue to breathe without assistance. One of the problems is that a patient may have been on complete ventilatory support for several days to weeks. The respiratory muscles may be too weak from lack of use to breathe unassisted. Another problem is that a patient may be undernourished prior to or during ventilatory support. Like any other muscle, lack of food will weaken it. A third common problem is a high level of work of breathing during mechanical ventilation when using the IMV mode in patients with high spontaneous respiratory rates. The resultant fatigue of ventilatory muscles can be an important part of ventilator dependency.

Two schools of thought exist about when to rest a respiratory muscle and when and how to exercise it. Some believe that the diaphragm is an endurance muscle. Like the muscles of a long-distance runner, it needs long periods of low levels of work and periods of rest in between. Others believe that the diaphragm is more like a strong man's arm. It needs short intense periods of exercise to fatigue with rest in between. Neither side denies that you need to feed the muscle for rebuilding and energy. Nevertheless, much attention has been fo-

TABLE 12–2.

Respiratory Physiologic Values for Evaluating Readiness for Weaning*

Respiratory rate (f)	Preferably <25 breaths/min (normal 12–18 breaths/min)
Tidal volume (V_T)	3–5 mL/lb of body weight or >300 mL; in adults if V_T <300 mL (or >700 mL) there may be difficulty in weaning the patient
Minute volume ($\dot{V}_E$)	<10 L/min is usually acceptable; if >20 L/min, the patient cannot support this spontaneously for long periods
Vital capacity (VC)	Preferably >15–20 mL/kg of ideal body weight; 20 mL/kg or 3 × V_T (predicted) is needed in order for the patients to be able to cough and deep-breathe on their own If <13 mL/kg or 2 × predicted V_T, weaning may be a problem
Maximum inspiratory pressure (MIP)	If > −20 cm H_2O within 20 sec, the patient probably has a VC ≥15 mL/kg; preferably >30 cm H_2O (normal MIP is ≥ −80 cm H_2O within 10 sec.)
Maximum voluntary ventilation (MVV)	At least >2 × $\dot{V}_E$; if the patient is able to double spontaneous $\dot{V}_E$ on command, this is a good sign
Ventilatory pattern	Preferably a synchronous and stable pattern; asynchronous breathing or periods of apnea or irregularity are bad signs
Shunt ($\dot{Q}s/\dot{Q}t$)	<30% maybe, <20% good (<10% normal or near-normal on a ventilator patient)
Oxygen status	Pa_{O_2}/F_{IO_2} > 238 mm Hg Pa_{O_2}/P_{AO_2} > 0.47 mm Hg $P(A - a)_{O_2}$ < 350 mm Hg on F_{IO_2} = 1.0
Dead space–tidal volume ratio (V_D/V_T)	V_D/V_T – <80% may consider attempting <50% probably near-normal on a ventilator patient
Dynamic compliance (Cdyn)	>25 mL/cm H_2O

*Data in part from Stoller JK: *Respir Care* 1991; 36:188.

cused lately on the working of the respiratory muscles—when to rest them and when to exercise them.

A variety of ventilating methods have been tried to allow respiratory muscles to rest while the patient is healing.[1, 15, 47, 75, 76, 80, 83, 115, 116] The initial ventilator setup in acutely ill patients is often designed to provide full or nearly full ventilatory support. This can be accomplished by several different modes of ventilation: control, assist-control, and synchronized intermittent mandatory ventilation (SIMV), used either with or without the addition of pressure support (PS).

Since increased WOB during mechanical ventilation might slow recovery from mechanical support because of muscle fatigue, selecting an appropriate mode is important to the weaning process.[47, 80–83] It is still not known which mode is most effective in decreasing the WOB in the patient who can breathe in spontaneously.[115, 116] It may be helpful to compare these modes in terms of WOB.

Controlled Ventilation.—Controlled ventilation is probably the mode of choice if the WOB is to be eliminated completely.[80, 83] However, this often requires the use of sedatives and neuromuscular blocking agents. These can compromise patient safety in the event of ventilator disconnection or failure. They may also prolong weaning times.[27, 59, 61, 64]

Assist-Control Ventilation.—In the assist-control mode every breath is mechanically supported. Theoretically, this mode provides a lower WOB than intermittent mandatory ventilation (IMV) or SIMV for patients who can still breathe spontaneously. However, it has been found that WOB may increase in some subjects.[81, 82] What appears to happen is that some patients continue to breathe in after triggering the ventilator. Their need for inspiratory gas flow may exceed what is set on the ventilator. When inspiratory muscle activity persists, this may increase WOB.[80–83, 122] The WOB during an assisted breath is also determined by the machine sensitivity. If the ventilator is too insensitive or does not respond rapidly to a patient effort, this can also increase WOB.[81, 82, 107]

IMV Ventilation.—IMV may produce a higher work of breathing than controlled[97, 98] or assist-control ventilation.[108] The differences between assist-control and IMV or SIMV in terms of WOB, however, are not always obvious.[44, 80, 96] IMV may not provide any faster weaning time[87, 109] as was once believed.[22, 68] The demand flow systems used with IMV that are employed on some ventilators may also impose a high WOB.[9, 42, 50]

Some clinicians have started using pressure support with IMV or SIMV since it may reduce the WOB for the "spontaneous breaths and thus overcome the resistance to ventilation imposed by demand valves, patient breathing circuits and artificial airways."[16, 38] This still has not been proved in terms of the oxygen cost of breathing.[58] Although IMV may be better than assist-control in preventing respiratory alkalosis,[55–57] its benefit in relation to increased WOB is uncertain.[23]

TABLE 12–3.
The Physical Signs and Measurements of Increased Work of Breathing (WOB)*

Use of accessory muscles
Asynchronous breathing (chest wall–diaphragm dyssynchrony)
Diaphoresis
Anxiety
Tachypnea
Substernal and intercostal retractions
Patient asynchronous with the ventilator
>1.8 kg/m/min (measured WOB)
15% of total $\dot{V}O_2$ (measured WOB)

*Data from Stoller JK: *Respir Care* 1991; 36:188.

Pressure-Supported Ventilation (PSV).—PSV, used as the sole source of mechanical support, can result in a lower WOB than CPAP[2, 121] or IMV.[62] It may also be as effective in decreasing WOB as controlled ventilation in some patients.[121] But in comparison to assist-control, it may not be much different.[86, 118]

Conclusions.—The choice of mode of mechanical ventilator setup in the spontaneously breathing patient continues to be controversial and may just be a matter of personal preference.[52] It is still essential to evaluate the patient's ability to support his or her own breathing prior to ventilator discontinuation. The physical signs and measurements of increased WOB are listed in Table 12–3.

If the patient is doing a lot of ventilatory work on one particular mode, then there is a good chance he or she will experience muscle fatigue. This makes any attempt to disconnect or wean from ventilation more difficult. It would probably be a good idea to use another mode of ventilation that reduces work. An overview of three newer modes of mechanical ventilation commonly used during weaning from the ventilator follows. They are IMV and SIMV, pressure support, and mandatory minute ventilation (MMV).

ALTERNATIVE METHODS OF VENTILATION FOR WEANING

Intermittent Mandatory Ventilation (IMV)

Prior to the 1970s, weaning from ventilatory support involved a specific routine. The patient was periodically removed from the ventilator and given the opportunity to breathe spontaneously for longer and longer periods of time until ventilatory support was no longer needed. In the early 1970s IMV became popular and provided an alternative mode of weaning and mode of ventilation.

IMV allows spontaneous ventilation to occur between preset mechanical breaths and it provides a way to wean while the patient remains attached to the ventilator. Newer-generation ventilators provide SIMV. SIMV synchronizes the mandatory machine breaths with the patient's effort on a periodic basis between which spontaneous ventilation can occur at ambient pressures.

IMV was originally used as a means of ventilating infants with idiopathic respiratory distress syndrome (IRDS).[67] In 1973, Downs and associates[30] developed a similar system for adults and used it as a method of weaning. Their studies indicated that IMV may shorten weaning time as compared to controlled mechanical ventilation (CMV). Their studies also suggested that IMV lowered the incidence of respiratory alkalosis and changes in oxygen consumption ($\dot{V}O_2$) when compared to CMV. Some of their findings, however, have been criticized for lack of adequate control data.

Most of the literature during the early 1970s recommended that mechanical ventilation be discontinued only after the need for PEEP had ended. It has since been found that some patients do well on CPAP or PEEP with low IMV rates and essentially need no mechanical breathing. Some clinicians wean their patients first from mechanical ventilation, then from PEEP or CPAP, and finally from oxygen therapy.[29] IMV facilitates this type of procedure more than conventional weaning in which the patient is placed directly on a T-tube for a period of time.

Add-on IMV Circuits.—When using an IMV mode some older ventilators may have to be adapted with additional external circuits. Exceptions to this are the IMV Emerson and the newer generation of ventilators which come equipped for SIMV; the BEAR 5, the Puritan Bennett 7200ae, the Siemens Servo 900C and 300, and the Hamiltor Veolar are examples. Some hospitals are still using Puritan Bennett MA-1 ventilators in their units. For these and similar ventilators, if an additional circuit is required, there are two basic types: demand flow IMV and continuous flow IMV. Figure 12–1 shows a demand flow IMV system.[30] This is one of the earliest types of IMV setups. A separate spontaneous breathing circuit is added to the patient ventilator circuit near the patient connector. Demand IMV requires that the patient open a one-way valve. This requires an inspiratory effort of -1 to -2 cm H_2O. Because the WOB is significant in some patients, many clinicians favor the use of continuous flow IMV. Demand flow IMV circuits are now seldom used with the exception of providing expiratory positive airway pressure (spontaneous PEEP, or sPEEP), or for the precise management of expired gases for metabolic measurement or to measure dead space. Such techniques are more difficult with continuous flow IMV.

Figure 12–2 shows a continuous flow IMV system. As before, there is also a separate system added to a volume ventilator. The primary component of the continuous flow breathing circuit is illustrated in Figure 12–3. A blended gas source flows into a reservoir bag which is usually a large (3 L) anesthesia bag. Sometimes the reservoir bag is fitted with an adjustable screw lamp that provides a bleed-off port for excessive gas flow. From this reservoir the circuit is

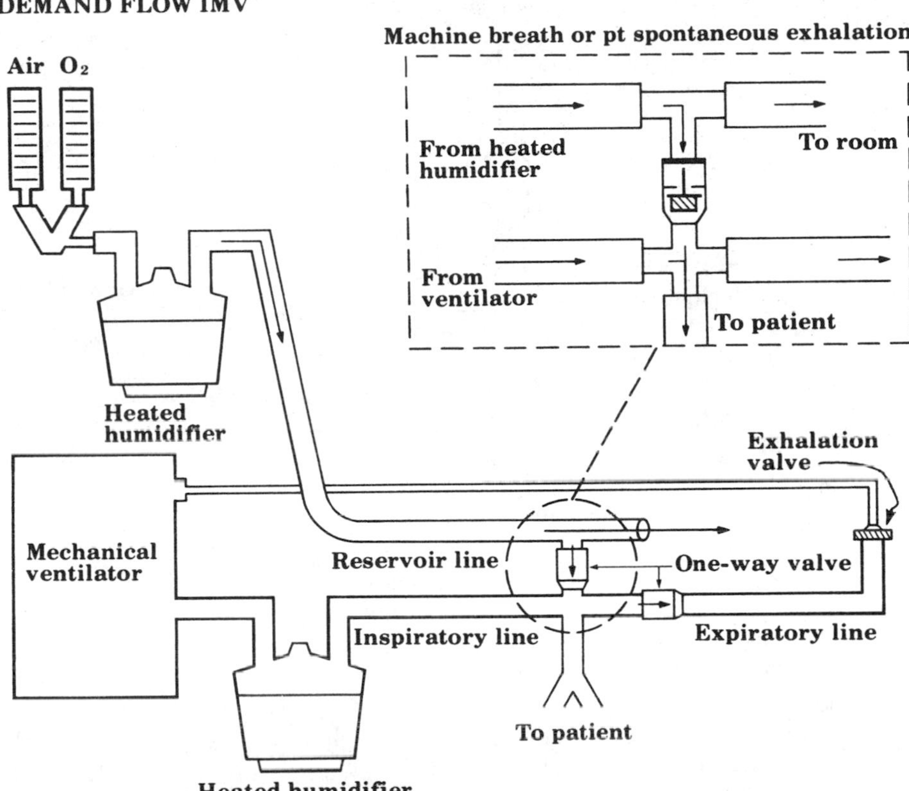

FIG 12–1.
Schematic diagram of a volume ventilator with a demand flow intermittent mandatory ventilation (IMV) circuit added. The ventilator provides one source of oxygen and humidity and the IMV circuit (spontaneously breathing circuit) also has a source of oxygen and humidity. The enlarged portion of the demand IMV circuit shows the connection between the two circuits. During a machine breath the one-way valve and the exhalation valve close and air is forced into the patient's lungs. During spontaneous breathing the patient inspires and opens the one-way valve getting unpressurized air from a humidified source of gas. There is an additional piece of tubing at the end of the spontaneous (IMV) circuit that vents to the room. This allows air from the additional gas source to empty into the room when the patient is exhaling. This piece of tubing also acts as reservoir. When the patient spontaneously inhales, if the inspiratory gas flow rate exceeds what is being provided the IMV circuit, then the patient receives some air from this piece of tubing. This helps to guarantee that the desired, fractional concentration of oxygen in inspired gas (F_{IO_2}) is being delivered. This type of IMV system can also be used to provide expiratory positive airway pressure (EPAP).

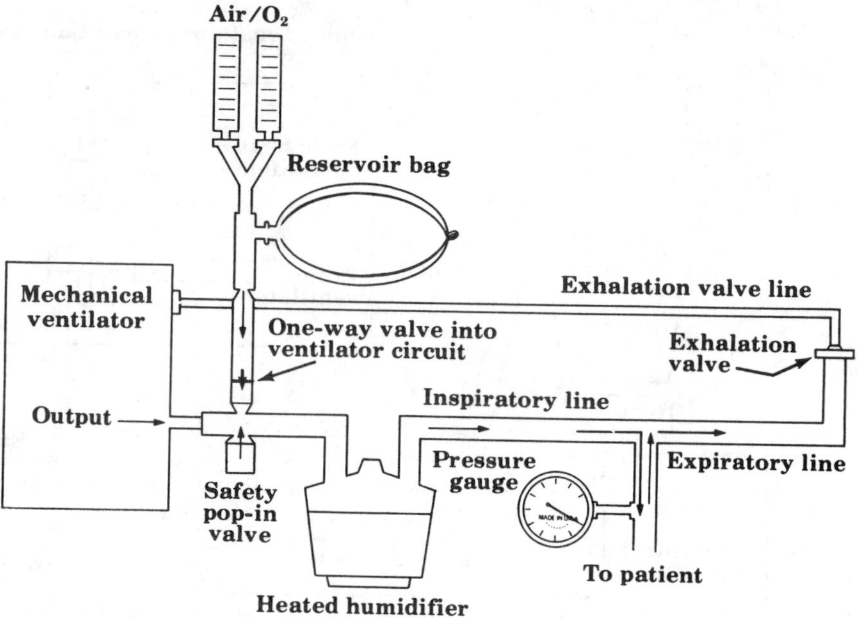

FIG 12–2.
Schematic shows a volume ventilator with the addition of a continuous flow IMV circuit.

connected to the ventilator circuit through a one-way valve. This valve prevents a positive pressure breath generated by the machine from entering the reservoir bag. This gas is then passed through the humidifier. In this way a single humidifier can add humidity to either the reservoir gas or the gas from the ventilator.

With this system there is a continuous flow of gas from the reservoir bag through the humidifier, through the main inspiratory line, and to the patient. Gas then goes to or past the patient, out the main expiratory line, and finally out the exhalation valve into the room. The continuous gas flow keeps the one-way valve slightly open so that the patient does not have to open the valve to receive the desired air. This is only true as long as the flow from the blender or the air and oxygen flowmeters is high enough to keep the reservoir bag from collapsing. In the interest of conserving oxygen, the amount of gas filling the reservoir is usually just enough to keep the reservoir full so that it does not collapse during inspiration. During a positive pressure breath, the high pressure closes the one-way valve preventing machine air from going into the reservoir. Simultaneously, gas continues to flow into the reservoir but this is usually not enough to cause serious overinflation of the bag.

As the continuous gas flow passes through the system between machine breaths, it meets the resistance of the ventilator circuit and the exhalation valve. Because of this resistance and the continuous flow of gas, a slight, but constant, positive pressure is present within the circuit. The manometer connected near the patient's airway will indicate a slight positive pressure. This slight PEEP is not usually clinically significant; however, at the very high flows often required for tachypneic patients, this may cause some resistance to exhalation and should be considered if it appears that the patient has a significantly increased WOB. It may be appropriate in these instances to place the patient on a higher IMV rate or on assisted ventilation. During V_T monitoring on continuous flow IMV, it is easier to measure exhaled gases at the endotracheal (ET) tube than to measure

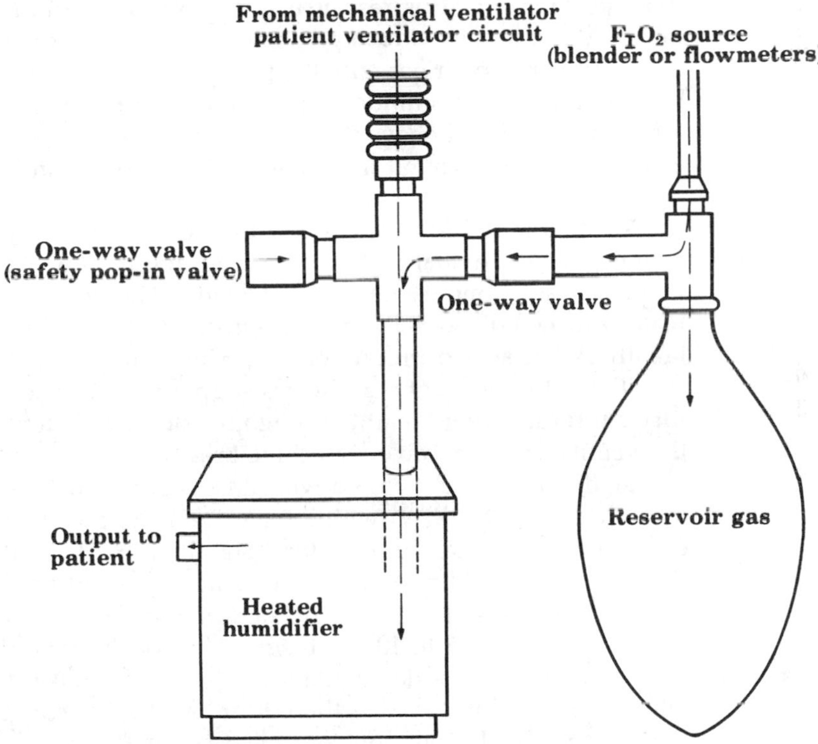

FIG 12–3.
Blended gas fills the reservoir and flows through a one-way valve into the patient ventilator circuit. This gas continues to flow through the humidifier and out to the patient. During a machine breath, positive pressure closes the one-way valve connected to the reservoir and the pressurized air from the machine continues to pass through the humidifier and to the patient.

them at the exhalation port. If a respirometer is placed at the exhalation port with a continuous flow system, the needle of the respirometer will be continuously moving as it measures the constant flow of gas coming from the reservoir. During plateau pressure measurements for the calculation of static compliance (Cs) it is not appropriate to obstruct gas flow out the exhalation valve with a continuous flow IMV system. This will cause the gas coming from the reservoir to build up in both the ventilator circuit and the patient's lungs.

A continuous flow IMV system can also be used to deliver IMV with CPAP by pressuring the reservoir bag to the level of PEEP or CPAP in the main circuit. The desired pressures are maintained during expiration by using a PEEP device at the exhalation port of the ventilator. With continuous flow IMV there is the risk that if the flow of gas to the reservoir is cut off, there is no place where the patient can receive air. The ventilator will not cycle on with patient effort since the sensitivity is usually turned off (control mode) or turned to a very "insensitive" position. For this reason it is important to use a safety pop-in valve or one-way check valve which points into the circuit from the ambient air (see Fig 12–2). If the reservoir gas fails, the patient can then open this one-way valve and breathe room air. Continuous flow IMV circuits can be adapted for ventilators which do not already have this feature built into their system. Figure 12–4 shows a continuous IMV circuit mounted on the inside of an MA-1 ventilator.

Ventilator Adjustments for IMV.—Once the ventilator circuit has been connected to a demand flow or a continuous flow IMV circuit, then certain ventilator adjustments need to be made. The sensitivity of the ventilator is usually turned off so that a patient's inspiratory effort will not trigger a machine breath. As an added precaution some institutions only partially inactivate the sensitivity. In the event that the gas supply fails, a patient with a strong inspiratory effort can either breathe through the one-way safety pop-in valve or trigger the ventilator and receive a machine breath.

Traditionally, the V_T used with IMV is between 10 and 15 mL/kg of patient ideal body weight (IBW) with an average setting of 12 mL/kg. This V_T is large enough to eliminate the need for a sigh breath. The IMV rate is usually at the lowest rate that will provide for the maintenance of normal arterial blood gases and pH and allow the patient to perform part of the WOB. Many institutions start with a rate of 8 to 10 breaths/min.[92] Under these circumstances the patient may be doing very little spontaneous breathing, but for the initial setting this may be appropriate. Even if there is an IMV setup connected to the ventilator, the patient is technically on controlled ventilation if no spontaneous breathing occurs, and the machine does all of the WOB. Initial use of these high IMV rates in ventilating patients who require ventilatory support guarantees a safe $\dot{V}_E$. From this point on the rate can be turned down as appropriate.

If the spontaneous respiratory rate rises above 25 to 30 breaths/min or if the patient's V_T falls to less than his or her anatomic dead space (about 250 mL or

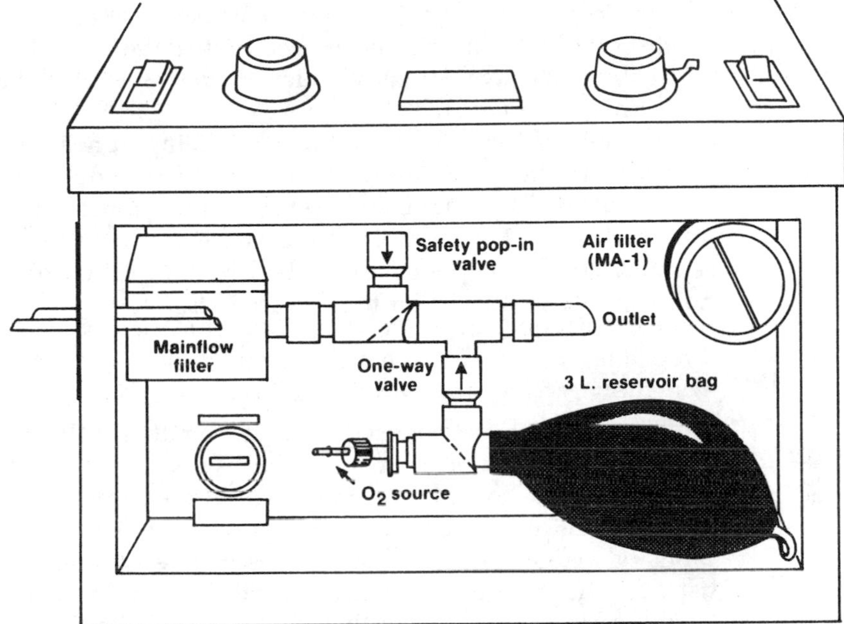

FIG 12–4.
Continuous flow IMV circuit has been added to a Puritan Bennett MA-1 ventilator inside the front panel between the ventilator outlet port and the main flow bacterial filter.

less), then ventilation is becoming ineffective and the IMV rate must either be increased or the patient needs to be placed on assisted ventilation or some other mode that provides more breathing support. The need for additional mechanical breaths may also be required if abnormal patterns of breathing occur, such as Cheyne-Stokes or Biot's respirations, or if the blood gas results indicate respiratory acidosis.

It is important to be sure that the peak pressure limit (pop-off pressure) is set at 10 cm H_2O above the ventilating pressure. During IMV ventilation it is possible for the machine to deliver an inspiratory breath after the patient has just spontaneously inhaled. This is called "breath stacking." Careful setting of the pop-off pressure limit can help to avoid delivery of high airway pressures if breath stacking occurs. It would appear that breath stacking might increase the incidence of barotrauma; however, this has not been clinically proved.[48, 49]

When ventilators are adapted for IMV, the sources of inspired gas for the ventilator and for the IMV circuit are often different. The IMV circuit is usually powered by air and oxygen flowmeters or by an oxygen blender. When this is the case, both the ventilator F_{IO_2} dial and the IMV gas sources must be set at the desired concentration. When changes in the patient's blood gases require a change in the patient's F_{IO_2}, both of these sources must be changed. More sophisticated adaptations and newer ventilators have eliminated the problem. Newer systems have a single blender or "dial" for controlling all of the inspired gas going to the patient.

Because of the risk of a patient becoming apneic on low IMV rates (<4 breaths/min) the use of apnea alarms is needed to detect cessation of breathing by the patient. These are usually set so that the apnea time is less than twice the total cycle time. For example, if the rate is 10 breaths/min, the cycle time is 6 seconds. The apnea period would be less than 12 seconds. An apnea period is normally not set for higher than 20 seconds.

IMV vs. SIMV

Newer ventilators come equipped with either IMV or SIMV built into them so that the addition of separate systems is not necessary (see Chapters 2 and 4). In a comparison of IMV vs. SIMV no difference was found between cardiac index, stroke index, central venous pressure, pulmonary artery or pulmonary capillary wedge pressure, systemic vascular resistance, pulmonary vascular resistance, shunt, arterial blood gas results, or the incidence of barotrauma.[48,49] Further studies have shown that the WOB and the $\dot{V}O_2$ may be increased with demand valve SIMV ventilators compared to IMV systems.[19, 42, 89] This depends on their design and response time. This varies between different brands.

Complications With IMV and SIMV Equipment

The majority of equipment failures associated with IMV and SIMV are due to a disconnection either in the circuit or at the patient connector. For example, the only disconnection or apnea alarm built into the MA-1 system is the spirometer and this spirometer cannot be used with a continuous flow IMV system. Once removed, there is no apnea, disconnection, or low pressure alarm. Compounding this problem is the lack of alarm systems on most add-on IMV systems. That is why it is essential that an apnea or low pressure alarm be added on to this system. Newer ventilators that feature IMV or SIMV have eliminated much of the problem by providing excellent alarm and surveillance systems. Because of the risks involved, it is very important for IMV systems constructed in-house be carefully modified to provide safe ventilation for the patient.

Potential Benefits of IMV

There are several potential benefits of using IMV for weaning as opposed to controlled ventilation with conventional weaning. These benefits are listed in Table 12–4 and a brief discussion of each follows.

TABLE 12–4.
Potential Advantages of Intermittent Mandatory Ventilation (IMV)

Avoidance of sedatives, narcotics, and muscle relaxants
Avoidance of respiratory alkalosis
Maintenance of synchronous breathing
Prevention of muscle weakening or atrophy
Expediting of weaning process
Reduced cardiovascular side effects and risk of barotrauma due to lower mean airway pressures
Fewer staffing problems during weaning process
Reduced tendency for psychological dependency on mechanical ventilation
Maintenance of lung distention independent of mechanical ventilation
More uniform distribution of gas

Avoidance of Sedation and Paralysis.—Prior to the introduction of IMV, most patients were maintained on controlled ventilation with the use of drugs. These drugs reduced the response of the central respiratory centers and kept the patient from breathing asynchronously with the ventilator. With IMV the need for sedatives, narcotics, and muscle relaxants is significantly reduced and often eliminated. Exceptions to this are patients with tetany or seizures where undesirable muscular contractions must be eliminated by the use of paralyzing agents.

Avoidance of Respiratory Alkalosis.—When controlled ventilation is used on sedated or paralyzed patients, respiratory alkalosis is sometimes inadvertently produced. Prolonged respiratory alkalosis can make weaning from ventilatory support more difficult because it reduces the patient's spontaneous breathing efforts. In contrast to controlled machine breaths where the patient's ventilatory drive is suppressed, by using IMV or SIMV the patient can set a breathing pattern and establish his or her arterial carbon dioxide partial pressure ($Paco_2$). This may expedite weaning.

An added risk for patients with COPD is hyperventilation when the patient is initially placed on ventilatory support. Since these patients often have increased bicarbonate levels, inadvertent hyperventilation and iatrogenic respiratory alkalosis can lead to seizures, coma, and death.[123] IMV produces less risk of respiratory alkalosis than controlled ventilation.

As long as the respiratory centers are normal, respiratory alkalosis seldom occurs with assisted mechanical ventilation or IMV. In patients with abnormal respiratory centers, hyperventilation is likely to occur with IMV or assisted ventilation. In these cases, if it is desirable to prevent possible hyperventilation, it may be necessary to sedate the patient and use controlled ventilation.

Maintenance of Synchronous Breathing.—Prolonged periods of controlled mechanical ventilation may result in diaphragmatic-intercostal dyscoordination, which is noted when attempts are made to place these patients on T-piece trials for weaning from ventilation. This lack of synchrony between the motion of the diaphragm and the chest wall muscles does not appear to occur in patients ventilated and weaned with IMV.[36]

Prevention of Muscle Weakening or Atrophy.—Long-term controlled ventilation has been associated with rapid wasting or atrophy of the diaphragm. This does not appear to occur with assisted mechanical ventilation or IMV or SIMV.[125] IMV may act as a form of respiratory muscle exercise and thus help prevent atrophy; however, there is also evidence that IMV may reduce muscle strength through fatigue.[123] This may be caused by attempting to reduce the IMV rate too rapidly or without allowing periods of rest. Short periods of muscle retraining with intermittent periods of rest, as occurs with conventional ventilatory weaning, may be more beneficial than allowing the patient to assume a large portion of the WOB too rapidly.[123]

Expediting Weaning Process.—IMV may help to expedite weaning in some patients who are normally difficult to wean.[30] With IMV weaning can be started almost as soon as mechanical ventilation has begun.[30] The transition from total dependence to complete independence is gradual as the patient assumes increased amounts of work (Figure 12–5); however, weaning time may be rushed when the IMV rate is reduced too rapidly, or it may be slower than is necessary for the patient if the IMV rate is reduced too slowly.

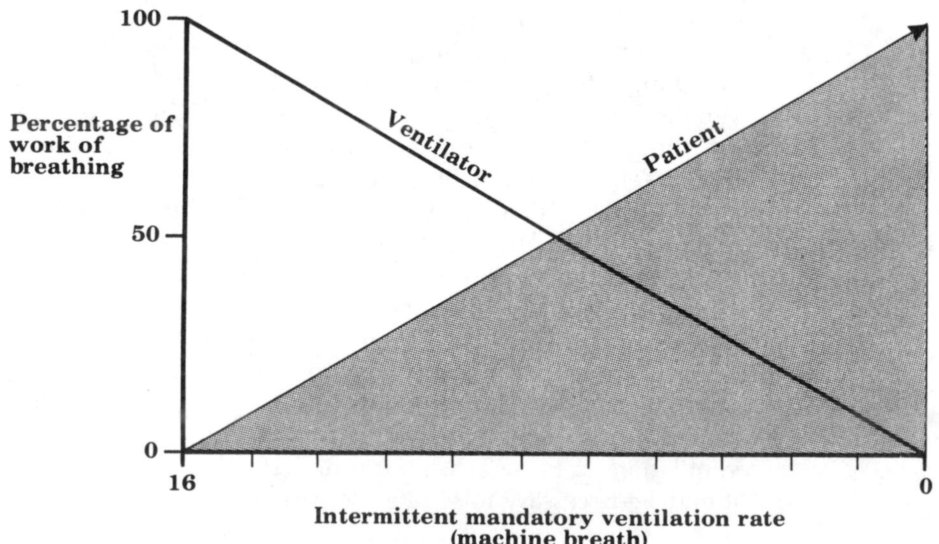

FIG 12–5.
As the IMV rate is decreased, the work performed by the ventilator is reduced and the work of breathing done by the patient increases.

Reducing Cardiovascular Effects and Barotrauma.—Since the major risks of positive pressure ventilation are associated with high mean airway pressures, reduction of high pressures and positive intrapleural pressures by decreasing the machine rate may help to minimize the cardiovascular side effects and the incidence of barotrauma in certain patients.[67, 110, 114] Barotrauma may be better correlated with mean transpulmonary pressures than with peak airway pressures. Studies on the incidence of barotrauma with IMV compared with CMV are not conclusive.[123]

Fewer Staffing Problems.—Staffing limitations is a serious problem in hospitals. Skilled personnel need to be in attendance at all times in the event a problem develops during the weaning process.[36] With IMV, weaning can progress while the patient is still attached to the ventilator and being monitored by a variety of methods. The patient need not be constantly attended to during the gradual IMV weaning procedures. This is cost-effective and still safe for the patient.

Less Psychological Dependency.—Psychological dependency on the ventilator is a problem in some patients. Weaning can be started early with IMV, and users claim that it may help to reduce psychological dependency in patients who must be on ventilatory support for extended periods of time.[30]

Lung Distention Without Mechanical Ventilation.—A very important attribute of IMV is its ability to help to maintain lung distention (PEEP) independent of the need for mechanical ventilation.[36] IMV can be reduced to 1 or 2 breaths/min or less. Once the patient is totally ventilator-independent, the patient can be kept on CPAP through the ventilator until the CPAP is reduced to 0 to 5 cm H_2O, at which time the patient can be extubated.

More Uniform Gas Distribution.—During spontaneous ventilation, inspired gas is preferentially distributed to the dependent parts of the lung because of the diaphragm which displaces caudad. In contrast, gas distribution favors the nondependent portions of the lung during mechanical ventilation in the supine position. This is because the diaphragm is not used and the nondependent lung and chest wall are more compliant than the diaphragm.[123] Theoretically, IMV may improve ventilation-perfusion ($\dot{V}/\dot{Q}$) relations since it allows for spontaneous ventilation.

Potential Problems With IMV

Proponents of IMV support the concept that it is beneficial for a patient to do part of the WOB for reasons cited. Patients in respiratory failure, however, may not be able to breathe effectively on their own. The patient may require complete ventilatory muscle rest which IMV does not provide. The WOB may be increased by the resistance of breathing through ET tubes, ventilator circuits, demand valves, and one-way valves.[123] The results may be discomfort, muscle fatigue, and progressive difficulty in breathing. IMV must be done with careful monitoring so that such a situation does not occur.

The inspiratory flow rates delivered by the IMV setup, both through continuous flow reservoir systems and SIMV demand valve systems, may be slower than the patient's spontaneous efforts. The patient struggles to get a breath, becomes fatigued, and exhibits an increased WOB. This situation can be detected when monitored upper airway pressures decrease by several centimeters of water pressure below the patient's baseline pressure during inspiration. An IMV setup must have a very low resistance and high inspiratory flow rates to avoid this problem.

Inadequate attention by the staff can result in delayed weaning time with IMV resulting in prolonged ET intubation, excessive time on ventilatory support, and perhaps increased time in the intensive care unit (ICU). All of these increase the cost of care to the patient and are avoidable by careful patient monitoring by the staff. Conversely, aggressively reducing the IMV rate when the patient is not ready for weaning or discontinuation can also be a problem.

While IMV has contributed to patient safety and comfort in many institutions, its use must be carefully monitored, as with any mode of ventilation and weaning. IMV is only as effective as the person caring for the patient. It is the clinician and not the technique which is the crucial element.

PRESSURE-SUPPORTED VENTILATION (PSV)

History

Pressure-supported ventilation originally appeared in 1981 in two European-designed ventilators (the Engström Erica and the Siemens Servo 900C). The first reports of this technique appeared in the United States in the mid-1980s.

Definition and Classification

Pressure-supported ventilation is a pressure-triggered (assist mode), pressure-limited, flow-cycled method of mechanical ventilatory support that assists the patient's spontaneous inspiratory efforts. Airway monitoring of pressure-supported breaths usually shows an initial deflection of pressure below baseline caused by the patient's inspiratory effort, followed by a rapid rise in pressure to the set value (Fig 12–6). Inspiration ends when a predetermined percentage or portion of the patient's peak inspiratory flow is detected. Most

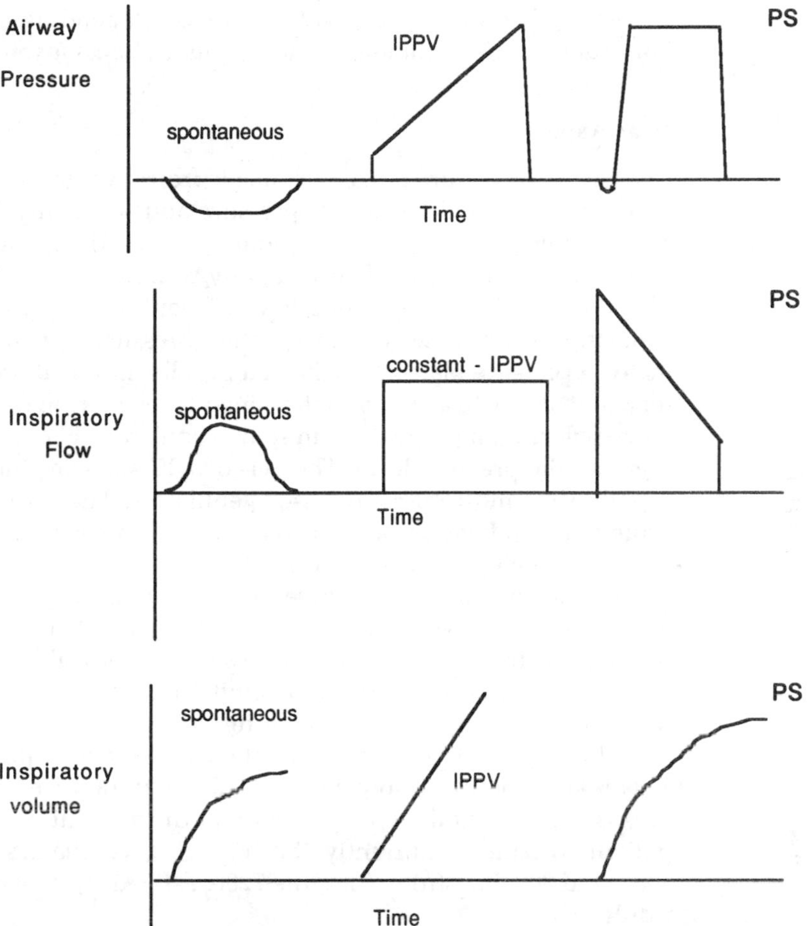

FIG 12–6.
Pressure support compared with a spontaneous and an intermittent positive pressure ventilation *(IPPV)* breath. Airway pressure, inspiratory flow, and inspiratory volume delivery are compared.

commonly this is 25% of peak flow. Other ventilators use a preset flow. The 7200ae uses a measured inspiratory flow of 5 L/min to end-inspiration.

Inspiration can also be limited by pressure or time. If pressure rises about 1 to 3 cm H_2O above the set PS level, inspiration ends. For example, in the 7200ae, if the airway pressure exceeds the PSV plus end-expiratory pressure by 1.5 cm H_2O for 100 ms, inspiration ends. This is to avoid a rise in pressure for whatever reason.

A maximum time consisting of a set number of seconds or a set percentage of total cycle time can also end inspiration depending on the ventilator in use. For example, the Hamilton Veolar ventilator limits inspiratory time to 3 seconds.

Technical Aspects

The PSV pressure range is available from 1 to 100 cm H_2O, depending on the ventilator. The clinician selects pressure and sensitivity. The patient determines rate, inspiratory flow, and inspiratory time. Tidal volume is determined by patient effort, lung compliance, airway resistance, and PSV level.

At the beginning of inspiration sufficient flow of gas enters the circuit as the exhalation valve closes to allow system pressure to reach the preset level. Normally, a pressure plateau is achieved rapidly and held until the patient's inspiratory flow drops to a system-determined level. During inspiration, the exhalation valve will remain partly open in some ventilators, like the Servo 900C. This helps regulate the pressure level. The Servo 900C achieves the PSV level much more rapidly than most microprocessor ventilators. The Bird 6400ST and the 7200ae achieve PS midway through inspiration. The Veolar may not reach preset pressure until the end of inspiration.[59, 61]

Ventilators must be sensitive to the patient's inspiratory effort to trigger the PSV breath. Some ventilators are less responsive than others. The WOB imposed by most of these microprocessor systems is probably not clinically important since even the worst-performing unit that has been evaluated was only one tenth of the normal WOB of the lung.[59, 61]

At the present, only the Irisa offers a flow rate adjustment for the PS mode. This feature will probably soon be added to other microprocessor ventilators. This is because studies have shown that the amount of flow needed varies from patient to patient. Currently the following ventilators provide PS: the Servo 900C and 300, Engström Erica, the 7200ae, BEAR 5, Veolar, Ohmeda Advent, and Adult Star.

Physiologic Benefits of PSV to Normal Breathing

During normal inspiration, pressure at the mouth begins at 0 cm H_2O. Normal intrapleural pressure is about -10 cm H_2O. This results in an intrapulmonary, or alveolar pressure (P_A) of about -5 cm H_2O. The transairway pressure (P_{TA}) between the mouth and the alveoli is about 5 cm H_2O. With a normal Cs of 100 mL/cm H_2O, this results in a V_T of about 500 mL. If the Cs is decreased to 50 mL/cm H_2O, the same inspiratory effort results in a V_T of only 250 mL.

If 5 cm H_2O of PS is applied during inspiration, a pressure gradient of 10 cm H_2O will result at the same level of inspiratory effort (Pawo = +5; P_A = -5). With a Cs of 50 mL/cm H_2O, PS will increase the V_T from 250 to 500 mL. PSV allows patients with a mechanical impairment to breathing the chance to acquire a larger inspiratory V_T at the same level of effort. It also permits a patient to maintain the same V_T at a lower level of work. These benefits apply to patients with reduced lung or thoracic compliance; increased airway resistance due to secretions, mucosal edema, or bronchospasm; reduced ventilatory muscle strength as in neuromuscular disease; and increased resistance to ventilation due to artificial airways, mechanical ventilator circuits, or slow demand flow systems found on some mechanical ventilators.[111]

Imposed Work of Breathing by Artificial Airway

Pressure-supported ventilation has received much attention in relation to imposed WOB (WOBi). This section presents some of the findings of the effects of WOBi and the use of PSV to reduce WOBi.

The pressure gradient needed to keep a constant flow through a fixed resistance (R), such as an ET tube, increases as the flow increases. $R = \Delta P/\text{flow}$. The higher the inspiratory flow demand, the higher the pressure change required to overcome the resistance imposed by the system. As tube size decreases and $\dot{V}_E$ increases, WOB by the lung and imposed by the system increases. For every millimeter of inner diameter decrease in an ET tube, work increases 34% to 154% (depending on flow).[59, 61]

When the manometer pressure drops below baseline as a patient breathes in, this indicates the inability of the system to meet patient inspiratory demands. Sometimes these negative deflections in the manometer are not visible even when the patient is actively breathing in. That is because of where pressure measurement is made in the system. These deflections or signs of active inspiration on a ventilator demand system are usually affected by (1) trigger sensitivity, (2) demand flow capabilities, and (3) the type of humidifier used.[59, 61]

To summarize, demand systems and poorly designed continuous flow systems cause WOBi which may represent a fatiguing workload on the spontaneously breathing patient if (1) the ET tube is small, or (2) ventilatory muscle fatigue, or chronic obstructive pulmonary disease (COPD) or neuromuscular or neurologic disease is present.[59, 61]

Pressure support can overcome the work of breathing imposed by an ET tube at various flows.[59, 61, 102] The amount of PSV required increases as tube size decreases and patient flow increases.[61] In individual patients, the exact level needed depends on the flow pattern, V_T, and the trigger sensitivities of the ventilators.[101, 102] The value is usually between +5 and +10 cm H_2O.

Indications and Contraindications

Pressure-supported ventilation is a fairly new mode of ventilation. Scientific studies have not firmly established when it should be used. Even without this scientific support, it is still widely used in the ICU setting. For this reason, the currently accepted indications and contraindications are reviewed.

Contraindications.—A patient with absent or depressed respiratory drive or a patient with impaired neuromuscular respiratory function who can perform little, if any, spontaneous ventilatory work is not a good candidate for PSV.[75,76] In this patient population controlled ventilation is appropriate.[66]

Indications.—When the need for full ventilatory support has passed, it may be beneficial to switch to PSV or to another mode that provides partial ventilatory support, e.g., SIMV. If not, the prolonged use of controlled ventilation may lead to muscle atrophy. Once the respiratory drive has returned to normal, a switch to PSV or SIMV is appropriate.[75] PS can be used when a patient is ready to begin doing some of the WOB. During PSV the amount of work done depends on how much pressure is given. Patients do no work if the pressure is high enough, except to trigger the valve open. The work and the work pattern will vary as the pressure varies.[74]

Methods of Using PSV

There are three uses of PSV: (1) at low levels to overcome the resistance of the ET tube, ventilator circuit, and demand valve system; (2) at low levels with SIMV. Again, this relieves the work of the spontaneous breath but provides some mechanical support; (3) at high levels as a form of stand-alone ventilation. This is called PSmax, maximum pressure support.[75]

Low-level PSV is used with CPAP or spontaneously breathing patients for airway management purposes. Its function is to reduce or eliminate the resistive work of the ET tube. This is especially important for patients with small ET tubes who may require some ventilatory support, especially if the spontaneous rate is more than 20 breaths/min and spontaneous $\dot{V}_E$ is more than 10 L/min.[59,61]

PSV with SIMV may be indicated in any patient on SIMV who is tachypneic, dyspneic, or asynchronous and these signs are believed to be at least partially due to the spontaneous ventilatory muscle work imposed by the ET tube, the demand valve system, and the circuit. The purpose is to decrease inspiratory work imposed by poorly designed demand valve systems (low flow rate on demand; long response time, highly resistant breathing circuit, and a flow resistor expiratory pressure valve) and ET tube resistance.[66] However, unless PS is set to match only the pressure drop needed to overcome the system resistance, positive pressure ventilation results.[66] SIMV with PSV is an example of partial ventilatory support. One example is a patient with a history of COPD or evidence of ventilatory muscle weakness who requires ventilatory support for 24 to 48 hours and is being maintained on demand system SIMV at rates of 4 breaths/min or less, or on CPAP.[59,61] Weaning from SIMV plus PS in these instances is accomplished by progressive reduction of SIMV breaths.

As the level of PS is increased, a constant amount of ventilatory muscle work results in a progressively larger "spontaneous" V_T. This may allow the clinician to rapidly reduce the frequency of mandatory SIMV breaths provided. Whether one has really achieved anything in terms of weaning by exchanging one form of ventilatory support (i.e., mandatory SIMV breaths) for another (i.e., level of PSV) is highly questionable.

There may be an inherent advantage to PSV which favors improving ventilatory muscle endurance.[72, 73] In healthy volunteers, endurance conditioning of the ventilatory muscles can be achieved by continuous repetition of relatively low levels of ventilatory work. Strength conditioning can be achieved by maximal ventilatory effort for shorter periods of time.[71] PSV theoretically allows the clinician to adjust the ventilatory workload associated with each spontaneous breath, and might be used to facilitate endurance conditioning.[72, 73] It must be pointed out that little is known about respiratory muscle conditioning as it applies to the critically ill patient in ventilatory failure. What is stated is speculative at this time.

PSVmax can only be used as a stand-alone method of support in patients with a reliable ventilatory drive and some stability in ventilatory requirements.[11, 75, 76] This approach to PSV is primarily used in the recovery phase of respiratory failure.[75] Criteria for PSVmax, as established by Fiastro, et al.[38] is a V_T equal to or less than 3 mL/kg of IBW, a respiratory rate of 35 breaths/min or greater, with a $Paco_2$ and pH that are normal for the patient. When PSV is used in this way the need for monitoring $\dot{V}_E$ and V_T and rate is essential. If V_T or rate change, the level of PSV may also need to be changed. Most ventilators do not provide a back-up mode of ventilation if the patient becomes apneic. Of course, if the apnea monitor (low rate, low volume, or low pressure) is working, this will alert the clinician to the problem.

The advantages of PSVmax may include an improvement in subjective comfort for awake and alert patients. PSV allows the patient to control the initiation of inspiration, inspiratory times, flows, and volumes, as well as termination of inspiration.[90] SIMV mandatory breaths allow the patient to initiate inspiration only. Inspiratory times, flows, and volumes are preset by the clinician. PSV may provide a more comfortable and compatible breathing pattern that more closely matches the patient's ventilatory drive. PSV may also reduce the $\dot{V}o_2$ of the ventilatory muscles when compared to SIMV. Until clear scientific evidence becomes available as to the benefits of PSV over conventional ventilation, it cannot be advocated as a primary stand-alone mode of ventilation for routine use.

Initial Settings With PSVmax

When PSVmax is initiated with adults it is set to establish a V_T of 10 to 12 mL/kg.[72–74] This represents full support and zero work for the patient. When PSV is used alone, the clinician must be sure V_T is at least 7 mL/kg. Smaller volumes without sighs may lead to atelectasis, decreased compliance, and progressive respiratory failure.[90] Achieving PSVmax requires support as high as 20 to 30 cm H_2O.[38, 111] PSVmax of more than 50 cm H_2O is rarely needed. Varying levels of PS affect the depth and rate of spontaneous breathing without always changing the overall level of spontaneous $\dot{V}_E$.[41] The need for high pressures indicates an unstable patient who needs back-up controlled ventilation as a safety net. PSVmax is then reduced as tolerated.

With PS, no minimum level of machine support is guaranteed. Back-up low $\dot{V}_E$ alarms may alert one to changes. Back-up modes like mandatory minute ventilation (MMV) may provide needed ventilation in the event of an emergency.

Effect of Flow-Limiting Characteristic on Tidal Volume Delivery with PSV

The common method of cycling of a PSV breath is by a measured flow rate value. This is usually 25% of peak expiratory flow rate. Some ventilators, like the 7200ae, cycle out of a PS breath at a specific flow rate, in this case when the flow falls to 5 L/min.

It has been shown that ventilators with a preset flow rate cycling like the 7200ae can deliver larger volumes in some cases than those that terminate inspiration as a percentage of peak flow.[13] Those with the highest peak flows, and which use cycling out of inspiration based on percentage of peak flow, delivered smaller V_T. Examples are the Servo 900C, BEAR 5, and Veolar.[59, 61]

Complications

Most of the time the descending flow pattern provided by a PS breath is adequate to meet the patient's needs. However, sometimes the flow through the system on PS may not be adequate. Perhaps a better design would allow flow adjustment as well.[74] PSV is a form of mechanical ventilation and patients must not be considered to be breathing spontaneously. A patient with normal Pa_{CO_2} values, a low PS of 5 cm H_2O on a CPAP of 5 cm H_2O may look normal. However, premature extubation can result in dyspnea, tachypnea, and hypercapnia.[66] Again, PSV is *not* to be used with patients with impaired or unstable ventilatory drives.

Several mechanical problems can occur in various ventilator systems when PSV is used. These are presented here to alert the practitioner to these possible complications.

Problems With System Leak.—A system leak can result in application of high flow and no cessation of inspiration during PSV. For example, in the 7200a with a PSV at 20 cm H_2O, if a leak occurs in the circuit and flow does not drop to 5 L/min, flow and pressure persist. The result is an inadvertent CPAP.[66] Fortunately, time and pressure can act as safety limits to inspiration. For example, the Veolar limits inspiratory time to 3 seconds. The 7200a limits pressure to 1.5 cm H_2O PSV plus PEEP.

Problems With High Flow and Too Small ET Tube Size.—The Servo 900C may prematurely end inspiration during ventilation of infants if the working pressure is set too high and results in very high inspiratory flow rates. This high flow, along with small ET tube size, appears to cause the premature cycling. Working pressure needs to be set about 5 to 10 cm H_2O above the PS level.[14, 24, 91, 119]

Problems With In-line Nebulizers.—Use of in-line nebulizers powered by outside gas sources can affect the ventilator function in the PS mode on the Servo 900C. Inserting a continuous flow nebulizer between the patient and the ventilator's sensing device makes it more difficult for the patient to initiate a pressure-supported breath. In some cases the patient may be unable to do so. This will not cause any ventilator alarm systems to be activated. The patients will be underventilated.[7] It is suggested that the practitioner switch to another mode of ventilation such as assist-control or SIMV to deliver an externally added, micronebulizer treatment. This problem has been reported with the Servo 900C, but may occur with other microprocessor ventilators if the manufacturer's directions for giving aerosolized treatments are not followed.

Summary

To summarize, it has been found that PSV may be more comfortable for patients than other forms of ventilation.[38, 72, 73] It helps to overcome the imposed work of the ET tube, ventilator circuits, and the demand valve systems on ventilators, and in SIMV systems.[38, 59, 61, 111] It may be of value in patients with respiratory muscle fatigue.[72, 73, 77, 78, 111, 118] PSV may improve abdominal-to-chest wall synchrony,[35] increase V_T, and reduce respiratory rate[35, 111] and decrease $\dot{V}O_2$.[59, 61] No differences have been seen between PSV and controlled ventilation or SIMV in terms of oxygenation or hemodynamic data.[111]

PSV, as a mode of ventilation, has become widely available on the newer mechanical ventilators. At present, little scientific data are available about the benefits of PSV compared with more established modes of mechanical ventilation. Its use should probably be avoided as the primary mode of ventilation in patients requiring high levels of ventilatory support. PSV can be a useful adjunct to SIMV. With the advent of sophisticated ventilatory monitoring and alarm systems, a nonvolume-orientated ventilatory mode such as PSV can be safe and effective. Once a sound research basis is established, there is little doubt that like IMV and SIMV, PSV will find a permanent place in the repertoire of the respiratory care practitioner.[111]

MANDATORY MINUTE VENTILATION

Mandatory minute volume ventilation (MMV) was introduced in Great Britain in 1977 by Hewlett, Platt, and Terry.[53] In its early forms it was not very successful, mostly because of limited technology. Since that time, MMV has been developed in conjunction with a few newer-generation ventilators as an optional mode of ventilation. MMV is currently available on the Ohmeda CPU-1 and Advent, and the Erica, BEAR 5, Veolar, Irisa, and Dräger EVA.[37, 99]

As initially developed, MMV was considered a new way of solving the problems associated with weaning patients from mechanical ventilation using traditional IMV.[53] Most methods of weaning, such as IMV and PSV, do not guarantee a constant level of ventilation in the presence of minute-to-minute changes in a patient's ability to breathe spontaneously. It was thought that a system which provided a constant level of $\dot{V}_E$ might permit patients whose ventilation was precarious to be safely maintained during the weaning process.[111] The advantage of MMV is that, if the patient's spontaneous ventilation decreases, the system automatically increases the level of mechanical support. Conversely, patients who recover the ability to breathe spontaneously can increase their own $\dot{V}_E$ and the machine automatically lowers mechanical support. This is done without having to change any specific ventilator settings. MMV was originally introduced as a sort of automatic IMV system with the ventilator, as opposed to a human operator, adjusting the frequency of mechanical breaths.[53]

Potential Benefits

The possible advantages of MMV are as follows[53, 111]:

1. MMV may offer greater control over Pa_{CO_2} than IMV.
2. Acute hypoventilation or apnea occurring in patients receiving MMV will not result in a sudden hypercarbia.
3. There is less concern of acute hypoventilation following the administration of sedatives, narcotics, or tranquilizers, because pain, anxiety, and agitation are eliminated in patients receiving MMV.
4. MMV provides a smooth transition from mechanical support to spontaneous ventilation in patients recovering from a drug overdose or anesthesia.

Potential Complications

Depending on the system employed, the ventilator may not respond rapidly enough to quickly correct for a complete apneic episode. This, of course, depends on how the ventilator provides this mode of ventilation. In addition, a rapid shallow respiratory pattern may meet the preset $\dot{V}_E$. But this type of pattern increases dead space ventilation and could lead to hypercapnea. The typical physiologic response to a decreased ability to maintain adequate spontaneous alveolar ventilation is an increase in spontaneous respiratory rate and a decrease in spontaneous V_T.[21] This type of pattern can result from a decrease in compliance from pulmonary congestion, pulmonary edema, pleural effusion, fibrosis, atelectasis, pneumonia, abdominal disorders, etc., or a decrease in ventilatory muscle strength. As spontaneous V_T declines and respiratory frequency increases, physiologic dead space begins to assume a larger proportion of the total $\dot{V}_E$. Spontaneous V_T values of less than 7 mL/kg without an intermittent deep breath may promote progressive collapse of alveoli.[8, 90]

As a protection, the ventilator needs to have a high rate alarm and a low V_T alarm to guard against this possibility. The ventilators which have MMV also have several added safeguards. The CPU-1 incorporates a low spontaneous volume alarm. This alarm can only be adjusted to three eighths or one fourth of the set machine V_T.[12] The Veolar offers a low $\dot{V}_E$ alarm,[45, 46] which must be used with caution since it does not tell if low rate or V_T is the problem. The Erica features a high-frequency alarm which might guard against acute hypoventilation.[34] The BEAR 5 offers a relatively easy-to-program low spontaneous V_T alarm.[5, 6, 111]

At this time, not many studies have been performed to evaluate this mode.[99] The ventilators that do have this mode available are not widely used in the United States at present. For this reason, use of MMV as an independent mode needs to be done with caution.

Like IMV in the 1970s a number of unsubstantiated benefits have been attributed to MMV. These include improved regulation of the patient's Pa_{CO_2}, enhanced patient safety, a smooth transition from mechanical support to spontaneous breathing, and potential improvement in efficiency by reducing manpower requirements without jeopardizing patient safety. As a mode of mechanical ventilation originally designed to maintain a constant level of ventilation in the presence of fluctuations in the level of a patient's spontaneous breathing, MMV has a potentially fatal flaw.

Methods of Application

The current generation of ventilators offer different methods for accomplishing MMV. The CPU-1, the Advent, the Erica, Irisa and BEAR 5 all work in a similar fashion. These ventilators "compare" the level of the patient's spontaneous breathing to the set MMV level and either increase, decrease, or maintain the frequency of mechanical breaths as indicated.[5, 6, 12, 34] The mechanical V_T is preset in each case.[99, 111]

The Veolar takes a different approach to maintaining a constant MMV level. Rather than increasing or decreasing the number of mechanical breaths to achieve a desired MMV, the Veolar uses PSV to achieve the desired $\dot{V}_E$. The

Veolar MMV system used a spontaneous mode in which additional $\dot{V}_E$ is delivered by varying inspiratory PS levels. The ventilator adjusts the pressure support level up or down to ensure that a minimum $\dot{V}_E$ is maintained in the spontaneously breathing patient. If the $\dot{V}_E$ is less than the target $\dot{V}_E$, the PSV is increased in increments of 1 to 2 cm H_2O until the $\dot{V}_E$ is achieved.[99] The Veolar provides for a programmable back-up rate and volume if the patient becomes apneic.[45, 46]

PSV as a method of maintaining a patient's level of ventilation has the advantage that as the level of pressure is increased, the patient receives a larger and larger "spontaneous" breath at the same level of ventilatory work.[72, 73] In theory, the use of stand-alone PSV to accomplish a constant level of MMV has some merit over the original technique. The machine can compensate for a tendency on the part of a patient to take very shallow spontaneous tidal breaths. No machine breaths with a preset V_T are delivered to the patient in the MMV mode using the Veolar.[111]

While MMV is not yet clinically well established, it may prove to be a new adjunct to conventional mechanical ventilation. It has the potential of providing greater control over Pa_{CO_2} than IMV alone in some patients. MMV may decrease the possibility of acute hypoventilation and thus be safer than traditional IMV or PSV. MMV may also provide a smoother transition from the ventilator and has the potential to be more efficient than traditional IMV. Future studies will help determine if MMV is able to live up to expectations.

TECHNIQUES FOR DISCONTINUATION OF OR WEANING FROM VENTILATION

Guidelines

Discontinuation or weaning from ventilation begins when the underlying disease process has been significantly improved or reversed. As discussed earlier, the patient's clinical profile and parameters for respiratory assessment must be evaluated. The patient must be able to breathe spontaneously and needs to be psychologically ready and prepared for the process.

Patients on ventilatory support for short-term ventilation (<2 days) can be discontinued quickly and simply. Following their evaluation, they can simply be connected to a T-piece setup with a warm, humidified oxygen source. If the patient is comfortable and breathing at a low steady respiratory rate, with stable vital signs, for a period of 15 to 30 minutes, then it is likely that he or she is ready for spontaneous ventilation. At this point the blood gases are checked, as needed. The ET tube is removed and the patient placed on an oxygen mask.[57]

If this patient fails this preliminary T-piece trial, he or she is not ready for disconnection. Besides this group, patients who have been on mechanical ventilatory support for long periods of time will require a longer weaning process. Both groups, however, must meet the same criteria and evaluation process.

The clinical and respiratory physiologic values for evaluating and measuring the patient's readiness for weaning are presented in Tables 12–1 and 12–2. In general, the patient needs to be alert, fully orientated, and have a normal drive to breathe. Vital signs must be stable and within normal limits. The arterial blood gases will be within normal limits for the patient at a safe level of inspired oxygen. Ventilatory reserve can be evaluated based on the $\dot{V}_E$, VC, MIP, and respiratory rate. Once all data have been considered the patient is prepared for the process of weaning.

The process must be explained to the patient. Patients should be told that alternative methods are available. In this way, if one method is tried and is unsuccessful, the patient will not feel hopeless or at fault. In addition to the patient, the nursing personnel, respiratory personnel, and all physicians involved in the patient's care need to be informed of the process and procedure. In this way, individual groups won't be at odds about the goal that is sought.

Conventional or Traditional Weaning (Unattached to the Ventilator)

Conventional, or traditional, weaning is the oldest of the available techniques. It consists of removing the ventilator from the patient based on a predetermined time schedule. The weaning process starts when the patient can breathe spontaneously for 5 to 10 minutes without ventilator support, and the criteria for weaning are met.

The patient is prepared for the procedure by an explanation of what will occur. It is important to reassure the patient that ventilator support can be resumed whenever it is desired. The equipment is then prepared. A heated humidifier with a large reservoir is connected to an oxygen flowmeter set at a minimum of 10 L/min in order to provide high humidity gas at the desired F_{IO_2}. This is connected to a T-piece (Briggs adaptor) by large-bore tubing which is then attached to the patient's ET tube. Another piece of large-bore tubing is attached to the exhalation side of the T-piece (volume about 120 mL) to provide a reservoir or "afterburner." If the patient inhales and the gas flow through the tubing from the humidifier is inadequate, some of the patient's inhaled air can come from this reservoir and will contain gas at the desired F_{IO_2}. The F_{IO_2} setting is usually placed at 10% above the F_{IO_2} that was set on the ventilator, except for patients who have COPD, where F_{IO_2} remains low.[17]

The patient is kept on the ventilator until the procedure has been explained, the additional equipment has been prepared, a continuous electrocardiogram (ECG) monitor has been attached, and the patient's airway has been suctioned as needed. Patients are usually sitting or semirecumbent for the procedure. The patient is then disconnected from the ventilator and given a few manual breaths. This helps to augment the initial spontaneous breaths. The patient is then connected to the T-piece and oxygen equipment, and kept disconnected from the ventilator for 5 to 10 minutes while being continuously monitored for signs of dyspnea, fatigue, pain, anxiety, sweating, paleness or cyanosis, drowsiness, restlessness, or the use of accessory muscles. The following indications are also monitored and noted:

1. A rise in the respiratory rate above 25 to 30 breaths/min (increases >10 breaths/min, or drops <8 breaths/min) is a sign of fatigue.
2. A fall in V_T below 250 to 300 mL is undesirable.
3. A significant change in blood pressure (a drop of 20 mm Hg systolic or a rise of 30 mm Hg systolic or a change is diastolic of 10 mm Hg may indicate a problem).
4. A rise in the heart rate of more than 20 beats/min or above 110 beats/min may also signal problems.
5. Frequent PVCs (premature ventricular contractions) (>4–6/min) may indicate cardiac instability.
6. Any clinical signs showing deterioration in the patient's condition may indicate that the patient is not ready to be weaned and must be returned to ventilatory support. Some underlying problem is interfering with the weaning process.

If the patient remains stable without ventilatory support, then an arterial blood gas sample can be obtained. The patient is then returned to ventilatory support for the remainder of the hour. This process is repeated once an hour and gradually the time off the ventilator is increased until the patient is off the ventilator for 30 minutes and on for 30 minutes. The WOB for the patient with traditional weaning is represented graphically in Figure 12–7. When this figure is compared with Figure 12–5, it can be seen how IMV and traditional weaning affect the WOB. The off time is then increased to 1 hour.[100] Once the patient is off the ventilator for 30 to 60 minutes without difficulty, then he or she can be checked every 15 minutes. Weaning time can also progress more rapidly. Attempting to wean the patient through the night may overtax a patient's energy reservoirs. It is best, then, to allow the patient to receive full ventilatory support during the night so he or she can sleep restfully and be ready for weaning the next day.[17, 100] This also allows the respiratory muscles to recover from their bout of exercise.

The rate at which weaning by this method progresses depends entirely on the length of time the patient was on ventilatory support, and on his or her current clinical condition. Most patients require only a few hours before discontinuation of ventilatory support is accomplished. Others may require days or weeks. Sitting up and eating, mobilization while on ventilatory support, and good bronchial hygiene can all facilitate the weaning process in patients who

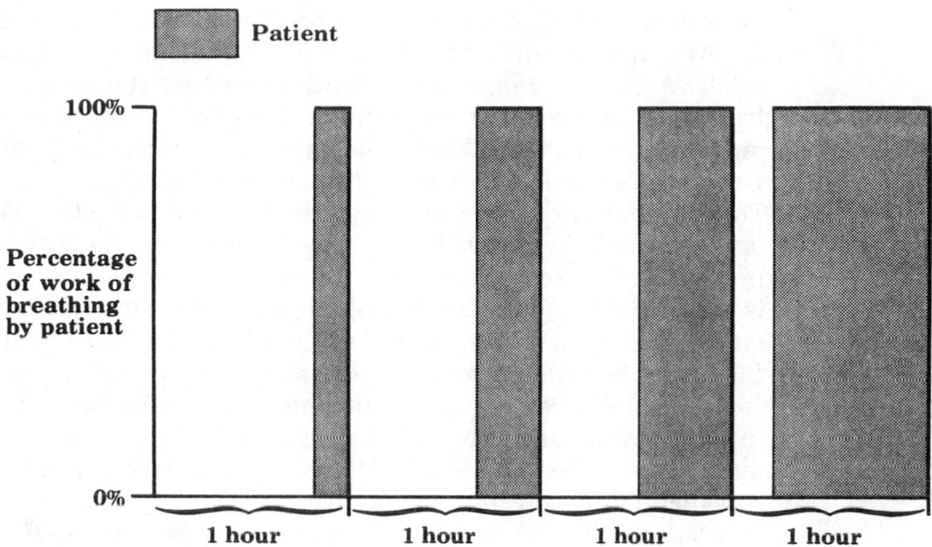

FIG 12–7.
Simple example of the distribution of the work of breathing with conventional weaning. Either the machine or the patient does 100% of the work. The amount of time the patient must do the work is increased progressively as the patient is weaned.

require extended weaning time. Once weaning is complete, the patient can be extubated.

The development of noninvasive monitoring procedures such as capnometry and pulse oximetry have facilitated the weaning procedure by providing close evaluation techniques of the patient's progress. Use of these devices may reduce the necessity of drawing frequent arterial blood samples as long as these parameters and the patient's clinical picture remain stable and optimal.

IMV Weaning Techniques

Before the use of IMV, patients were most often mechanically ventilated because of neuromuscular failure and the inability to eliminate carbon dioxide. Mechanical ventilation was discontinued only when they were able to breathe without support and still maintain a normal $Paco_2$ and pH. Since the 1970s more patients are given mechanical and ventilatory support because of severe hypoxemia and increased WOB. Often these patients do not have a problem with CO_2 elimination, but do have trouble maintaining the WOB with low arterial oxygen levels and low lung compliance. The weaning criteria may not be the same for these patients because CO_2 elimination is not their problem.[29] For these patients, the use of IMV and CPAP or IMV and PEEP may provide the answer. The IMV rate can be just low enough to prevent acidosis. Weaning is achieved by lowering the IMV rates in decrements as long as acidosis and increased WOB do not occur.[29]

IMV weaning progresses in much the same way as traditional weaning. Patients must have their initial problem resolved, must be in stable condition, must be capable of breathing spontaneously, and must meet clinical criteria for weaning. They may, however, still be on some level of end-expiratory pressure. This does not preclude weaning by the IMV method. Once PEEP or CPAP is optimized and the criteria for weaning are met, then the IMV rate is decreased progressively as long as pH is near normal, the F_{IO_2} is at a safe level, and the Pa_{O_2} is 60 to 100 mm Hg. Respiratory rate must stay at a reasonable level (<25 breaths/min in the adult) and $\dot{V}_E$ less than 10 L/min. When the IMV rate is zero, CPAP can be reduced and the patient extubated and weaned from oxygen. Generally, IMV weaning is a continuous reduction in the ventilator rate from 8 to 6 breaths/min, then from 6 to 4 breaths/min, and so on as the patient assumes more of the WOB (Table 12–5). This is gradually reduced to 1 or 2 breaths/min and then finally to zero (same as T-piece). The rate at which the ventilator is reduced depends on how long the patient has been on mechanical ventilation and how stable and strong the patient is. Postoperative ventilator management may last no longer than a few hours, while severely ill patients may take several days to weeks before they are weaned.

A few precautions must be taken while weaning with IMV or SIMV. If the patient's spontaneous respiratory rate rises above 25 breaths/min in the adult or the Pa_{CO_2} rises more than 10 mm Hg with a corresponding fall in pH, then the decrease in the IMV rate is progressing too rapidly. Patients who do not progress well on IMV weaning may do better with some other methods. With continuous flow IMV, the gas flow rate is inadequate if the manometer needle indicating upper airway pressure dips below the patient's baseline pressure by several centimeters of water pressure. A similar situation may occur with SIMV in which the patient must use a great inspiratory effort to receive an adequate flow of gas from the ventilator. These situations increase $\dot{V}_{O_2}$, carbon dioxide production ($\dot{V}_{CO_2}$) and $\dot{V}_E$. In some cases the cost of the WOB on a demand valve

TABLE 12–5.

Example of Reduction of IMV Rate as Part of Weaning Procedure in Patient Who Appears to Be Ready for Discontinuation of Ventilatory Support (pH Normal)

Time	Tidal Volume (mL/kg)	Machine Rate (breaths/min)	Spontaneous Rate (breaths/min)	Pa_{CO_2} (mm Hg)
9:00 A.M.	800	6	6	38
9:30 A.M.	800	4	8	38
10:00 A.M.	800	2	12	38
10:30 A.M.	500*	0	14	38

*Spontaneous tidal volume.

SIMV system is more significant than it is on a continuous flow IMV system. If the patient seems to be using considerable inspiratory effort to breathe on such a system, it may be desirable to use a PSV at low levels (5–10 cm H_2O) and then gradually reduce the SIMV rate.

Weaning With Pressure Support

In patients who fail an initial T-piece trial or in those who have been on mechanical ventilation for a long time, then PSV, like IMV or SIMV, is an alternative. When PSV is used with IMV or SIMV or with CPAP and spontaneous breathing through an ET tube, the pressure is set at a level to prevent a fatiguing workload on the respiratory muscles. Some authors recommend calculation of PS from bedside estimations of total ventilatory system resistance (patient plus circuit).[59,61] This value is calculated during a regular intermittent positive pressure ventilation (IPPV) breath with the use of a constant (rectangular) flow pattern.

$$R = (P_{Peak} - P_{Plateau})/\text{flow}$$

The patient's peak flow is measured or estimated during spontaneous inspiration. The PS level needed will equal the calculated resistance times the patient's inspiratory gas flow rate (PS = R × flow). The value calculated will probably be higher than that required to overcome WOBi, but it is a logical starting point.

Probably the most reasonable method of establishing the PS level for the purpose of overcoming WOBi is to set the PS at a level that establishes a reasonable ventilatory pattern in a given patient.[59,61] This assumes that tachycardia, hypertension, tachypnea, diaphoresis, paradoxical breathing, respiratory alternans, and excessive accessory muscle use signal cardiopulmonary stress and possible muscle fatigue.[78] Set the PS so it does not elicit these responses. In general, levels between 5 and 15 cm H_2O will accomplish these goals in most patients. Trying to reestablish the patient's baseline respiratory rate (15–25 breaths/min) and V_T (300–600 mL) is another sound approach.[59,61] As improvement is noted, the PS level can be reduced to a minimum of 5 cm H_2O, from which the patient is either extubated or put on Briggs' T-piece with continuous flow.

If a traditional weaning method is being used, the use of appropriately set SIMV or assist-control ventilation can be used to rest patients between CPAP or T-tube trials. During SIMV rest periods, PSV at low levels can be used to unload any spontaneous breaths interposed between the SIMV breaths.[59,61] As the patient improves, the number of mandatory breaths is decreased.

When weaning is going too fast, fatigue is shown clinically by tachypnea, abdominal paradoxical movements, and finally CO_2 retention and respiratory arrest.[75,76] A slow rate suggests that the patient is not being overworked. Conversely, if the rate is at or above 30 to 40 breaths/min, work is excessive. If this occurs as SIMV or PSV is reduced, it suggests that loads are not tolerated.

Although PS has not been compared with conventional weaning techniques, it has become a very popular form of both ventilatory support and weaning. The use of PSV for weaning has resulted in patient comfort, and more physiologic workloads on the ventilatory muscles.[78]

Weaning With MMV

Although MMV is a fairly new technology, there are some guidelines for using it as a method of weaning. Again, the patient needs to be evaluated prior to weaning to establish his or her readiness. Setting the $\dot{V}_E$ is the most important decision with this mode. Next in importance is setting the high rate and low V_T alarms. There are not much data to support any particular settings. If MMV is being used to be sure adequate $\dot{V}_E$ is going to the patient it needs to be set like any initial setting (see Chapter 4). Arterial blood gases can then be used to determine its effectiveness.

If the MMV is a method of weaning, then the target $\dot{V}_E$ needs to be at a level that is slightly below what is needed. This results in mild hypoventilation that requires that the patient provide some of the alveolar ventilation. If patients are being weaned from ventilator conditions in which they are not hypocarbic or alkalotic, then using 80% of their previous $\dot{V}_E$ may be appropriate. If they are slightly alkalotic or hypocapneic, then 75% or less may be enough.[99] It seems logical that for patients on IMV or SIMV that they would not need a $\dot{V}_E$ higher than the $\dot{V}_E$ set on their ventilator. This is supported by some research findings. A $\dot{V}_E$ of 90% of the set IMV or SIMV $\dot{V}_E$ appears to be correct.[99] Tidal volumes are set at normal settings (10–15 mL/kg). If PS is used with MMV it is usually set to achieve a V_T of 5 to 7 mL/kg for the spontaneous breaths.

Although MMV appears to have a role in the weaning of mechanically ventilated patients, what the role is is not known at this time. It may be useful in shortening weaning time since it allows patients to establish the rate at which they assume control of the breathing, unlike any other mode.[26] It does not appear to cause hypoventilation even in situations where respiratory depression is caused by drug administration.[33] This finding, however, has not been evaluated with all available MMV systems. There are no studies to date that evaluate whether MMV with changes in rate is different from MMV with changes in PS levels. MMV offers tempting possibilities since it is responsive to a patient's ventilating effort or lack of it.

Summary

Controversy exists over which mode of weaning is the best. Each method offers benefits for selected patients and should be used accordingly. If one procedure does not work well for a patient, then another might. The greatest benefit to weaning is the expertise and care of the administering personnel and the cooperation of the patient.

COMPLETING WEANING PROCESS

Discontinuation of Endotracheal Tube

It is often difficult to predict when a patient will be able to sustain a patent airway on his or her own. Sometimes excessive secretions make it necessary to keep an ET tube in place even after mechanical ventilatory support and CPAP have been discontinued. At other times, a patient is unable to tolerate a T-piece after weaning from ventilation once CPAP or PEEP has been decreased from +5 H_2O to zero. In this patient it is best to remove the ET tube once criteria for weaning are met at +5 cm H_2O of CPAP.

Once extubated, a patient can also develop subglottic edema and require treatment with racemic epinephrine. If the edema is severe and the patient develops inspiratory stridor, respiratory distress, and severe dyspnea that is refractory to treatment, then reintubation may be necessary. It is often the fear of having to reintubate that makes clinicians reluctant to remove an ET tube. If the patient is alert and orientated, and removal of secretions is no longer a problem, then the success of extubation is fairly certain.[105] Table 12–6 outlines a brief procedure for extubation and lists the appropriate equipment to be used.

Tracheostomy Tubes During Weaning

Patients who have been on mechanical ventilatory support for extended periods of time may have tracheostomy tubes in place. By partially or completely blocking a tracheostomy tube after the cuff has been deflated, the patient is obliged to move air around the tube past the deflated cuff and into the upper airway again; however, the tube does obstruct air flow and increases the resistance to breathing. Use of a fenestrated tube can help to wean these patients. This tube has an opening (fenestration) cut into its back border (convex surface) which faces the posterior (dorsal) wall of the trachea. It is also suppled with an inner cannula and a cuff on its outer cannula. When the inner cannula is removed and the cuff is deflated, the patient can move air through the tube itself, around the tube, and out to room air. It also allows the patient to talk and expel secretions more easily. A fenestrated tube must be used with care since both the opening and the inner end of the tracheostomy tube can impinge on tissues in the airway and cause obstruction to breathing. Airway tissue can enter the fenestration when the inner cannula is replaced; this can cause tissue damage.

Removal of a tracheostomy tube is not difficult and can proceed as with extubation. Once the tube is removed, the stoma is covered with one or two

TABLE 12–6.
Extubation Procedure and Equipment

Procedure

1. A monitoring ECG should be in place.
2. The patient should be in semi-Fowler's or high Fowler's position.
3. The procedure should be explained to the patient.
4. Preoxygenate the patient with a manual resuscitation bag.
5. Suction the mouth and pharynx.
6. Squeeze the resuscitation bag while deflating the cuff. This forces secretions into the mouth from above the cuff for suctioning.
7. Repeat this procedure until the airway is clear.
8. Deflate the cuff and loosen the tape supporting the tube.
9. Oxygenate and hyperinflate the patient, withdrawing the ET tube when pressure is built up in the lungs.
10. Have the patient cough while the tube is being removed. (Air in the lungs helps force secretions into the mouth.)
11. Have the patient cough once the tube is removed.
12. Administer the same F_{IO_2} as prior to extubation.
13. Monitor the patient while encouraging coughing and deep breathing. Measure respiratory rate, heart rate, and blood pressure frequently for about 30 minutes.
14. Monitor the patient for changes over the next hour. It may be desirable to obtain an arterial blood gas assessment at this time to be sure the patient is stable.

Equipment

Resuscitation bag, oxygen source, and oxygen mask.
Suctioning equipment.
Equipment and tubes for reintubation, if necessary.
A 5-mL unit dose of normal saline or a 5 mL syringe for irrigation with normal saline during suctioning, if necessary.
A 10-mL syringe for cuff deflation.

gauze pads held in place with tape. The stoma is like an open wound and will heal in a few days in most patients, barring complications. Patients are taught to support the stomal opening when they cough by applying pressure to the gauze bandage with the flat surface of their hand. The secretions, once brought to the mouth, can be expectorated.

If it is necessary for the stoma to remain open because of excessive secretions, or some other reason, then a Kistner tracheostomy tube or Moore button can be used. These short tubes are placed into the stomal opening and held in place by flanges on their inner side. These tubes can be capped in order to occlude the tube opening if it is desired.

Weaning COPD Patients From Mechanical Ventilation

Most patients with COPD and acute or chronic respiratory failure are managed conservatively. Failure of conservative measures are suggested by increasing Pa_{CO_2} with acidosis, and mental obtundation with hypoxemia. Treatment then requires mechanical ventilatory support. Ventilatory support of these patients is difficult. There is a high mortality rate. These patients frequently have fluctuations in blood pressure and electrolyte balance. They often have congestive heart failure and are cachectic. Support with IPPV can result in barotrauma from the rupture of blebs or weakened lung tissues.

Weaning is hampered in the presence of respiratory or metabolic alkalosis, malnutrition, and sedation. The loss of functional lung tissue owing to superimposed pulmonary infections may make weaning impossible. It is generally accepted that the longer this type of patient is on controlled mechanical ventilation, the more dependent he or she becomes. With controlled ventilation the respiratory muscles may weaken or atrophy.

The longer mechanical ventilatory support is necessary, the smaller the patient's chance of survival. Some clinicians believe that patients with COPD should be started on weaning immediately after being placed on mechanical ventilation. They are of the opinion that controlling ventilation and deliberate sedation to allow rest may lead to serious problems in weaning.[29] These clinicians use IMV for ventilation and weaning with COPD patients and avoid sedation and muscle relaxants. They keep F_{IO_2} values low (<30%) and V_T at 10 mL/kg to avoid high peak pressures. Initial IMV rates may be as low as 2 to 3 breaths/min.[28, 31] Their rationale is that this helps to avoid the rapid reduction in Pa_{CO_2} and the development of severe and sudden alkalosis. These patients are treated with appropriate bronchodilators, bronchial toilet, low F_{IO_2} values, and little or no PEEP. The use of PS at low levels can overcome the WOBi of the tubes and patient circuits. When the ventilator rate is at zero, and PS is at +5 cm H_2O, the patient is extubated. If PSV is not used, the patient is extubated as soon as possible to avoid having to breathe through the high resistance of the ET tube.

Other physicians advocate giving this type of patient a 1 or 2-day rest period in order to overcome whatever problem it was that led to the need for mechanical ventilatory support. These patients are given controlled ventilation or assist-control ventilation, and sedation and muscle relaxants. Ventilator support is discontinued by traditional means when it has been determined that the patient meets the weaning criteria. No studies have proved the superiority of one method of ventilation and weaning over another in this patient population.

Nutritional Status and Weaning

Weakening of the respiratory muscles may occur in any patient receiving inadequate nutrition or who is nutritionally depleted on admission; however, overfeeding, particularly with solutions using carbohydrates as the primary calorie source, may result in increased $\dot{V}_{O_2}$, increased $\dot{V}_{CO_2}$, and increased $\dot{V}_E$.

This may interfere with weaning from mechanical ventilation. Feedings need to be carefully monitored and nutritional solutions given which contain emulsified fats. These do not appear to elevate the metabolic rate and ventilatory needs as significantly as high carbohydrate solutions.[94]

Weaning in Patients With Left Ventricular Dysfunction

During abrupt disconnection from mechanical ventilation, as with traditional weaning, there is occasional hemodynamic instability caused by the rapid drop in intrathoracic pressures. In normovolemic patients with good cardiac response this is not a problem. What occurs temporarily is a redistribution of blood volume from the systemic venous system to the central veins. This results in increased cardiac filling pressures. In patients with preexisting heart disease this can result in acute cardiac decompensation.[123] This may contribute to difficulty in weaning.

The IMV methods of weaning and ventilation may compromise cardiac function, particularly in patients with left ventricular dysfunction. One mechanism that may explain the adverse hemodynamic response with IMV is that with a decrease in mean airway pressure, there may be an increase in venous return. In the presence of a poorly functioning left ventricle this may lead to an acute increase in preload and finally cardiac decompensation. Another explanation is that increased right ventricular volume with increased venous return may change the function and shape of the right and left ventricles, and thus worsen the left ventricular dysfunction. The more negative intrapleural pressure with IMV during spontaneous breaths may increase the left ventricular transmural pressure and afterload. This may cause a decreased stroke volume.[123]

Regardless of the causes, the hemodynamic response to weaning with either conventional weaning or with IMV can result in undesirable hemodynamic responses that are not easily predicted and which can result in the failure of a patient to wean from ventilatory support.

Problems in Weaning From Ventilatory Support

In addition to problems with poor nutritional status, psychological dependency, and adverse cardiovascular responses, other factors can hamper the weaning process. These include depressed consciousness and drive to breathe due to sedation or the use of narcotics; excessive secretions; weak respiratory muscles; atelectasis; anxiety; fever; acid-base imbalance; electrolyte imbalance; dehydration; renal failure; shock; sleep deprivation; attempting to wean before the patient is ready; the presence of an illness preventing weaning; and malfunction of the weaning apparatus (Table 12–7). Sometimes, in spite of all efforts on the

TABLE 12–7.
Problems in Weaning

Cardiovascular collapse (shock, heart failure)
Poor muscle strength or atrophy
Increased work of breathing
Excessive secretions
Patient not psychologically or physiologically ready
Primary illness not resolved
Improper weaning procedure or patient cannot be weaned (terminal illness)
Pulmonary complications (e.g., atelectasis, pulmonary infection, bronchospasm)
Poor nutrition
Continued use of sedatives or analgesics
Acid-base imbalance
Electrolyte imbalance
Abdominal distention
Anemia
Fluid overload
Renal failure
Malfunction of equipment

part of the health care team, it is not possible to remove ventilatory support from the patient. Chronic disease or a neuromuscular condition may require continuous long-term ventilator care.

Long-Term Ventilation in Ventilator-Dependent Patients

Following the polio epidemics of the 1950s some patients were sent home with iron lung ventilators to support their breathing. The iron lung was used both on a continuous basis or periodically, such as night use or when patients became fatigued. Some of these patients have survived more than three decades of paralyzing polio and continue to live on home mechanical ventilation. Patients with chronic conditions such as polio, muscular dystrophy, severe chronic lung disease, loss of the central drive to breathe, phrenic nerve damage or paralysis, cervical fracture leading to paralysis, and other neuromuscular or chronic disorders may require mechanical ventilation on a permanent basis. The negative pressure ventilators such as the Emerson iron lung or the chest cuirass are still used for this purpose since they do not require an artifical airway. Small portable positive pressure ventilators are also popular for home use, but are generally used on patients who have permanent tracheostomy tubes in place.

Ventilator dependency is unfortunate, but it is not completely confining and many such patients have found valuable lives for themselves outside of the hospital environment (see Chapter 14).

SUMMARY

Weaning from mechanical ventilation is started as soon as the reason for the initial institution is no longer present and the patient is ready for it. Successful weaning requires careful patient evaluation, and overall clinical stability. Problems encountered in weaning can come from unexpected sources, so all organ systems must receive careful evaluation and attention. The advent of additional methods of weaning with PS and MMV offer new alternatives.

STUDY QUESTIONS

1. Which of the following are reported to be advantages of IMV?
   I. It may help avoid the use of sedation and paralysis.
   II. Correction of carbon dioxide abnormalities may be facilitated.
   III. Cardiac depression may be minimized.
   IV. It allows for use of much lower F_{IO_2} values.
   a. II and IV.
   b. II, III, and IV.
   c. I, II, and IV.
   d. I, II, and III.
   e. I and III.
2. A patient is receiving continuous flow IMV via a Puritan Bennett MA-I ventilator with a 5-L reservoir bag in the system. The mandatory rate is 6 breaths/min and the patient is not receiving PEEP therapy. During the patient's spontaneous respirations, the practitioner notes that the system pressure manometer reads -10 cm H_2O. Based on the above information, the therapist should perform which of the following corrective actions?
   a. Increase the continuous flow rate.
   b. Increase the sensitivity as well as the continuous flow rate.
   c. Decrease the sensitivity.
   d. Use a smaller reservoir bag system.
   e. Decrease the continuous flow rate.
3. Once the patient is stable and the initial goals for mechanical ventilation have been achieved, weaning from mechanical ventilation can begin. Which of the following is used to assess the patient readiness for weaning?
   I. VC of 15 mL/kg body weight.
   II. MIP between -20 and -30 cm H_2O.
   III. Dead space–tidal volume (V_D/V_T) ratio of less than 0.6.
   IV. Spontaneous respiratory rate less than 25 breaths/min.
   V. Patient body weight.
   a. I, II, III, IV, and V.

b. II, III, and IV.
c. I and II only.
d. III and IV only.
e. I, II, III, and IV.

4. All of the following are used when a patient is being weaned from a mechanical ventilator *except*:
   a. IMV or SIMV.
   b. Pressure support.
   c. MMV.
   d. Optimal PEEP.
   e. Trial on T-piece.
5. While weaning a patient using progressively longer trials on a T-piece, the respiratory therapy practitioner would need to do all the following *except*:
   a. Monitor vital signs and blood gases.
   b. Prepare the patient psychologically for weaning.
   c. Return the patient to the ventilator at night to rest (for the first few nights).
   d. Increase the patient's physical activities to strengthen all muscles.
   e. Closely supervise the weaning process.
6. You are called to the ICU to extubate a patient who has been successfully weaned from mechanical ventilation. Which of the following is the most significant problem that is likely to occur following extubation?
   a. Hemorrhage.
   b. Pneumothorax.
   c. Laryngospasm which does not respond to treatment.
   d. Lethal cardiac arrhythmia.
   e. None of the above.
7. Which of the following is a disadvantage of the demand valve IMV method?
   a. Imprecise control of FIO_2.
   b. Imprecise control of humidification.
   c. Requires an increased WOB.
   d. It is more cost-effective.
   e. Inability of measure exhaled V_T.
8. You are asked to evaluate a patient with amyotrophic lateral sclerosis in the ICU for possible implementation of continuous mechnical ventilation due to insufficient muscle strength. Which of the following parameters will provide an index of respiratory muscle strength?
   I. PaO_2.
   II. V_D/V_T.
   III. MIP.
   IV. VC.
   V. Spontaneous V_T and respiratory rate.
      a. I, IV, and V.

b. I, III, and V.
c. II and IV.
d. III, IV, and V.
e. I, II, III, IV, and V.

9. Which of the following indicate that a patient is ready for extubation?
   I. Presence of abundant and purulent secretions.
   II. Respiratory rate of 14 breaths/min, spontaneous.
   III. VC of 26 mL/kg.
   IV. Pressure support less than or equal to 5 cm H_2O.
   V. CPAP of +15 cm H_2O.
   a. II, III, and IV.
   b. I and V.
   c. I and III.
   d. III and IV.
   e. I, II, III, and V.
10. On PSV, spontaneous inspiration by the patient results in a manometer pressure reading of −5 cm H_2O. An appropriate action would be to:
    a. Increase machine sensitivity.
    b. Increase gas flow.
    c. Increase the rate.
    d. Sedate the patient.
    e. Switch to assist-control.
11. MMV is appropriate for which of the following situations?
    I. Weaning from mechanical ventilation.
    II. For the patient who can assume part of the WOB.
    III. During cardiopulmonary resuscitation.
    a. I only.
    b. II only.
    c. III only.
    d. I and II.
    e. I, II, and III.
12. A patient on SIMV has the following arterial blood gases and ventilation settings: V_T = 1,000 mL, respiratory rate = 6 breaths/min, F_{IO_2} = 0.4, pH = 7.30, Pa_{CO_2} = 58 mm Hg, Pa_{O_2} = 75 mm Hg. The most appropriate therapy is to:
    a. Implement PEEP.
    b. Increase V_T.
    c. Increase the respiratory rate.
    d. Increase F_{IO_2}.
    e. Switch to assist-control.
13. Which of the following are reported to be advantages of MMV?
    I. The machine responds to changes in patient $\dot{V}_E$.
    II. Abrupt changes in CO_2 from a drop in ventilation can be avoided.

III. Cardiac depression may be minimized.
IV. It allows for use of a much lower F_{IO_2}.
   a. II and IV.
   b. II, III, and IV.
   c. I, II, and IV.
   d. I and III.
   e. I and II.

14. A patient with absence of a normal ventilatory drive may be placed on pressure support. True or false?
15. A patient is on IMV with a set rate of 5 breaths/min and a V_T of 800 mL (set $\dot{V}_E$ = 4 L/min). The patient is being switched to MMV. What should the $\dot{V}_E$ setting be for the MMV mode?
   a. 3.2 L/min.
   b. 3.6 L/min.
   c. 4.0 L/min.
   d. 3.0 L/min.
   e. 2.0 L/min.

ANSWERS TO STUDY QUESTIONS

1. d.
2. a.
3. e.
4. d.
5. d.
6. c.
7. c.
8. d.
9. a.
10. a.
11. d.
12. c.
13. e.
14. False.
15. b.

REFERENCES

1. Aldrich TK: Respiratory muscle fatigue. *Clin Chest Med* 1988; 9:225–236.
2. Annat GJ, Viale JP, Dereymez CP, et al: Oxygen cost of breathing and diaphragmatic pressure-time index. Measurement in patients with COPD during weaning with pressure support ventilation. *Chest* 1990; 98:411–414.
3. Banner MJ, Kirby RR: Similarities between pressure support ventilation and intermittent positive pressure ventilation (letter). *Crit Care Med* 1985; 13:997.
4. Banner MJ, Kirby RR: Pressure support ventilation (letter). *Crit Care Med* 1986; 14:666–667.
5. *BEAR 5: Ventilator operator's manual.* Riverside, Calif, Bear Medical Systems.
6. "Introducing the Bear 5 Ventilator" (sales brochure). Riverside, Calif, Bear Medical Systems, Inc, 1985.
7. Beaty CD, Ritz RH, Benson MS: Continuous in-line nebulizers complicate pressure support ventilation. *Chest* 1989; 96:1360–1363.
8. Bendixen HH, Egbert LD, Hedley-Whyte J, et al: *Respiratory Care.* St Louis, Mosby–Year Book, Inc, 1965, pp 9–11.

9. Bersten AD, Rutten AJ, Vedig AE, et al: Additional work of breathing imposed by endotracheal tubes, breathing circuits and intensive care ventilators. *Crit Care Med* 1989; 17:671–677.
10. Boysen PG: Weaning from mechanical ventilation: Does technique make a difference? *Respir Care* 1991; 36:407–416.
11. Boysen PG, McGough E: Points of view: Pressure support. *Respir Care* 1989; 34:129–134.
12. BOC Health Care: *The Ohmeda CPU-1: Operation and Maintenance Manual*. Columbia, Mo, Ohmeda, 1985.
13. Branson RD, Campbell RS, Davis K, et al: Comparison of the effects of pressure support ventilation delivered by two ventilators. *Respir Care* 1990; 35:1049–1055.
14. Branson RD, Campbell RS, Davis K, et al: Altering flowrate during maximum pressure support ventilation (PSV_{max}): Effects on cardiorespiratory function. *Respir Care* 1990; 35:1056–1064.
15. Braun NM: Intermittent mechanical ventilation. *Clin Chest Med* 1988; 9:153–162.
16. Brochard L, Pluskwa F, Lemaire F: Improved efficiency of spontaneous breathing with inspiratory pressure support. *Am Rev Respir Dis* 1987; 136:411–415.
17. Burton GC, Gee GN, Hodgkin JE (eds): *Respiratory Care: A Guide to Clinical Practice*. Philadelphia, JB Lippincott Co, 1977.
18. Burton GC, Hodgkin JE (eds): *Respiratory Care: A Guide to Clinical Practice*. Philadelphia, JB Lippincott Co, 1984, p 837.
19. Christopher KL, Good TJ Jr, Bowman JL, et al: Should COPD patients be weaned by T-piece or intermittent mandatory ventilation (IMV)? A comparison of pressure and resistance in different systems. *Chest* 1981; 80:381.
20. Christopher KL, Neff TA, Bowman JL, et al: Demand and continuous flow intermittent mandatory ventilation systems. *Chest* 1985; 87:625–630.
21. Comroe JC, Forster RE, Dubois AB, et al: Mechanics of breathing, in *The Lung*. St Louis, Mosby–Year Book, Inc, 1962, pp 162–203.
22. Cullen P, Modell JH, Kirby RR, et al: Treatment of flail chest. Use of intermittent mandatory ventilation and positive end-expiratory pressure. *Arch Surg* 1975; 110:1099–1103.
23. Culpepper JA, Rinaldo JE, Rodger RM: Effect of mechanical ventilator mode on tendency towards respiratory alkalosis. *Am Rev Respir Dis* 1985; 132:1075–1077.
24. Czervinske MP, Shreve J, Lester KB, et al: Effects of pressure on respiratory pattern and airway pressure during pressure support ventilation (PSV) in infants with chronic lung disease (abstract). *Respir Care* 1988; 33:930.
25. Davies S, Linton D: MMV vs IMV weaning. Presentation to the Seventh Australasian Congress of Anesthesiologists. Hong Kong, September 1986.
26. Davis S, Pogieter PD, Linton DM: Mandatory minute volume weaning in patients with pulmonary pathology. *Anaesth Intensive Care* 1989; 17:170–174.
27. Desautels DA, Blanch PB: Mechanical ventilation, in Burton GC, Hodgkin JE, Ward JJ (eds): *Respiratory Care: A Guide to Clinical Practice,* ed 3. Philadelphia, JB Lippincott Co, 1991, p 520.
28. Downs JB, Block AJ, Vennum KB: Intermittent mandatory ventilation in the treatment of patients with chronic obstructive pulmonary disease. *Anesth Anal* 1974; 53:437–443.

29. Downs JB, Douglas ME: Intermittent mandatory ventilation and weaning, in Kirby RR, Graybar GB (eds): *Intermittent Mandatory Ventilation. International Anesthesiology Clinics.* Boston, Little, Brown Co, 1980, pp 81–85.
30. Downs JB, Klein EF Jr, Desautels D, et al: Intermittent mandatory ventilation: A new approach to weaning patients from mechanical ventilators. *Chest* 1973; 64:331–335.
31. Downs JB, Perkins HM, Modell JH: Intermittent mandatory ventilation: An evaluation, *Arch Surg* 1974; 109:519–523.
32. Dupuis YG: *Ventilators: Theory and Clinical Application.* St Louis, Mosby–Year Book, Inc, 1986, pp 493, 419, 301.
33. East TD, Elkhuizen PH, Pace NL: Pressure support with mandatory minute ventilation supplied by the Ohmeda CPU-1 prevents hypoventilation due to respiratory depression in a canine model. *Respir Care* 1989; 34:795–780.
34. *The Engström Erica: Reference Manual,* Rockville, Md, 1988, Engström Co.
35. Ershowsky P, Krieger B: Changes in breathing pattern during pressure support ventilation. *Respir Care* 1987; 32:1011–1016.
36. Fairley HB: Critique of intermittent mandatory ventilation, in Kirby RP, Graybar GB (eds): *Intermittent Mandatory Ventilation. International Anesthesiology Clinics.* Boston, Little, Brown Co, 1980, pp 143–177.
37. Fevrier MJ, Pilorget A, Lemaire F: *Mandatory Minute Volume (MMV) Ventilation: A Clinical Assessment.* Unpublished manuscript. Cretail France, Service de Réanimation Médical, Hôpital Universitaire Henri Mondor et Université, Paris–Val de Marne, 1986.
38. Fiastro JF, Habib MP, Quan SF: Pressure support compensation for inspiratory muscle work to endotracheal tubes and demand continuous positive airway pressure. *Chest* 1988; 93:499–505.
39. Field S, Kelly SM, Macklem PT: The oxygen cost of breathing in patients with cardiorespiratory disease. *Am Rev Respir Dis* 1982; 126:9–13.
40. Forrette TL, Billson D, Cook EW: Case report: Ventilator weaning of an AIDS patient by EMMV with inspiratory assist. *Respir Manage* 1987; 17:14–18.
41. Forrette TL, Cairo JM: Changes in ventilatory dynamics during mechanical ventilation with pressure support (abstract). *Respir Care* 1988; 33:930.
42. Gibney RTN, Wilson RS, Pontoppidan H: Comparison of work of breathing of high gas flow and demand valve continuous positive airway pressure systems. *Chest* 1982; 82:692–695.
43. Graybar GB, Smith RA: Apparatus and techniques for intermittent mandatory ventilation, in Kirby RR, Graybar GB (eds): *Intermittent Mandatory Ventilation. International Anesthesiology Clinics.* Boston, Little, Brown & Co, 1980, pp 53–77.
44. Groeger JS, Levinson MR, Carlon GC: Assist control versus synchronized intermittent mandatory ventilation during acute respiratory failure. *Crit Care Med* 1989; 17:607–612.
45. Hamilton Medical: *The Respirator for Critical Care From Controlled Ventilation to Spontaneous Breathing.* Hamilton Medical Engineering, Reno, 1985.
46. Hamilton Medical: *Veolar: Operator's Manual.* Reno, 1988.
47. Harpin RP, Baker JP, Downer JP, et al: Correlation of the oxygen cost of breathing and length of weaning from mechanical ventilation. *Crit Care Med* 1987; 15:807–812.

48. Hasten RW, Downs JB, Heenan TJ: A comparison of synchronized and nonsynchronized intermittent mandatory ventilation. *Respir Care* 1980; 25:554–557.
49. Heenan TJ, Downs JB, Douglas ME, et al: Intermittent mandatory ventilation: is synchronization important? *Chest* 1980; 77:598–601.
50. Henry WC, West GA, Wilson RS: A comparison of the oxygen cost of breathing between a continuous flow CPAP system and a demand flow CPAP system. *Respir Care* 1983; 28:1273–1281.
51. Herve P, Simonneau G, Girard P, et al: Total parenteral nutrition induces hypercapnea in mechnically ventilated patients with chronic respiratory insufficiency. *Am Rev Respir Dis* 1983; 127:255.
52. Hess DR, Hodgkin JE, Burton GG: Mechanical ventilation: Initiation, management and weaning, in Burton GG, Hodgkin JE, Ward JJ (eds): *Respiratory Care: A Guide to Clinical Practice*, ed 3. Philadelphia, JB Lippincott Co, 1991, p 602.
53. Hewlett AM, Platt AS, Terry VG: Mandatory minute volume: A new concept in weaning from mechanical ventilation. *Anaesthesia* 1977; 32:163–169.
54. Higgs BD, Bevan JC: Use of mandatory minute volume ventilation in the perioperative management of a patient with myasthenia. *Br J Anaesth* 1979; 51:1181–1183.
55. Hooper LD, Hurlow RS, Craig KC, et al: Does intermittent mandatory ventilation correct respiratory alkalosis in patients receiving assisted mechanical ventilation? *Am Rev Respir Dis* 1985; 132:1071–1074.
56. Hooper RG, Browning M: Acid-base changes and ventilator mode during maintenance ventilation. *Crit Care Med* 1985; 13:44–95.
57. Hudson LH: Weaning techniques, in Kacmarek RM, Stoller JK (eds): *Current Respiratory Care*. Philadelphia, BC Decker, Inc, 1988, pp 195–200.
58. Hurst JM, Branson RD, Davis K, et al: Cardiopulmonary effects of pressure support ventilation. *Arch Surg* 1989; 124:1067–1070.
59. Kacmarek RM: The role of pressure support ventilation in reducing work of breathing. *Respir Care* 1988; 33:99–120.
60. Kacmarek RM: Points of view: Pressure support. *Respir Care* 1989; 34:136–138.
61. Kacmarek RM, McMahon K, Staneck K: Pressure support level required to overcome work of breathing imposed by endotracheal tubes at various peak inspiratory flowrates (abstract). *Respir Care* 1988; 33:933.
62. Kanak R, Fahey PJ, Vanderwarf C: Oxygen cost of breathing: Changes dependent upon mode of mechanical ventilation. *Chest* 1985; 87:126–127.
63. Kirby RR: Weaning from mechanical ventilation. *Curr Rev Respir Ther* 1985; 6:lesson 10.
64. Kirby RR: Modes of mechanical ventilation, in Kacmarek RM, Stoller JK (eds): *Current Respiratory Care*. Toronto, BC Decker Inc, 1988, pp 128–131.
65. Kirby RR: Synchronized intermittent mandatory ventilation versus assist control: Just the facts, ma'am. *Crit Care Med* 1989; 17:706–707.
66. Kirby RR, Banner MJ, Downs JB: *Clinical Applications of Ventilatory Support*, ed 2. New York, Churchill Livingstone Inc, 1990.
67. Kirby R, Robinson E, Schultz J, et al: Continuous flow is an alternative to assisted or controlled ventilation in infants. *Anesth Analg* 1972; 51:871–875.
68. Klein EF: Weaning from mechanical breathing with intermittent mandatory ventilation. *Arch Surg* 1975; 110:354–357.
69. Knak R, Fahey PJ, Vanderward C: Oxygen cost of breathing. Changes dependent upon mode of mechanical ventilation. *Chest* 1985; 87:126–127.

70. Laaban JP, Lemaire F, Baron JF, et al: Influence of caloric intake on the respiratory mode during mandatory minute volume ventilation. *Chest* 1985; 87:67–72.
71. Leith DE, Bradley M: Ventilatory muscle strength and endurance training. *J Appl Physiol* 1976; 41:508–516.
72. MacIntyre NR: Respiratory function during pressure support ventilation. *Chest* 1986; 89:677–683.
73. MacIntyre NR: Pressure support ventilation (editorial). *Respir Care* 1986; 31:189–190.
74. MacIntyre NR: Pressure support ventilation: Effects on ventilatory reflexes and ventilatory-muscle workloads. *Respir Care* 1987; 32:447–457.
75. MacIntyre NR: Weaning from mechanical ventilatory support: Volume-assisting intermittent breaths versus pressure-assisting every breath. *Respir Care* 1988; 33:121–125.
76. MacIntyre NR: Pressure support: Inspiratory assist, in Kacmarek RM, Stoller JK (eds): *Current Respiratory Care*. Philadelphia, BC Decker, Inc, 1988, pp
77. MacIntyre NR, Leatherman NE: Ventilatory muscle loads and the frequency-tidal volume pattern during inspiratory pressure-assisted (pressure-supported) ventilation. *Am Rev Resp Dis* 1990; 141:327–331.
78. MacIntyre NR, Stock MC: Weaning mechanical ventilatory support, in Kirby RR, Banner MJ, Downs JB (eds): *Clinical Applications of Ventilatory Support*, ed 2. New York, Churchill Livingstone Inc, 1990, pp 263–276.
79. Marini JJ: The role of the inspiratory circuit in work of breathing during mechanical ventilation. *Respir Care* 1987; 32:419–427.
80. Marini JJ: Work of breathing, in Kacmarek RM, Stoller JK (eds): *Current Respiratory Care*. Toronto, BC Decker Inc, 1988, pp 188–194.
81. Marini JJ, Capps JS, Culver BH: The inspiratory work of breathing during assisted mechanical ventilation. *Chest* 87 (1987):612–618.
82. Marini JJ, Rodriquez RM, Lamb V: The inspiratory work load of patient-initiated mechanical ventilation. *Am Rev Respir Dis* 1986; 134:902–909.
83. Marini JJ, Smith TC, Lamb VJ: External work output and force generation during synchronized intermittent mechanical ventilation. Effect of machine assistance on breathing effort. *Am Rev Respir Dis* 1988; 138:1160–1179.
84. Mathru M, Rao TL, Venus B: Ventilator-induced barotrauma in controlled mechanical ventilation. *Crit Care Med* 1983; 11:359–361.
85. Martz KV, Joiner J, Shepherd RM: *Management of the Patient-Ventilator System. A Team Approach*. St Louis, Mosby–Year Book, Inc, 1982.
86. McGough EK, Banner MJ, Boysen PG: Pressure support and flow-cycled, assisted mechanical ventilation in acute lung injury. *Chest* 1990; 98:458–462.
87. Muir JF, Aubry P, Levi-Valensi P: Two methods of weaning patients from respirators (with and without IMV). A comparative study in 22 subjects with acute or chronic respiratory failure. *Rev Fr Mal Respir* 1982; 10:131–141.
88. Nunn JF, Lyle JR: Bench testing of the CPU-1 ventilator. *Br J Anaesth* 1986; 58:653–662.
89. Op't Holt TB, Hall MW, Bass JB, et al: Comparison of changes in airway pressure during continuous positive airway pressure (CPAP) between demand valve and continuous flow devices. *Respir Care* 1982; 27:1200–1209.
90. Perel A: Newer ventilatory modes—temptations and pitfalls (editorial). *Crit Care Med* 1987; 15:707–709.

91. Perlman ND, Schena J, Thompson JE, et al: Effects of ET tube size, working pressure and compliance on pressure support ventilation (abstract). *Respir Care* 1988; 33:928.
92. Petty TL: In defense of IMV (editorial). *Respir Care* 1976; 21:121–122.
93. Pilbeam SP: *Mechanical Ventilation.* St Louis, Mosby–Year Book, Inc, 1986, p 293.
94. Pilbeam SP, Head A, Grossman GD, et al: Undernutrition and the respiratory system. *Respiratory Therapy* September/October 1983, pp 65–70; November/December 1983, pp 72–78.
95. Pinilla JC: Acute respiratory failure in severe blunt chest trauma. *J Trauma* 1982;22:221–226.
96. Popovich J: Mechanical ventilation. Physiology, equipment design and management. *Postgrad Med* 1986; 79:217–220.
97. Prakash O, Meij SH: Oxygen consumption and blood gas exchange during controlled and intermittent mandatory ventilation after cardiac surgery. *Clin Care Med* 1985; 13:556–559.
98. Prakash O, Meij S: Cardiopulmonary response to inspiratory pressure support during spontaneous ventilation versus conventional ventilation. *Chest* 1985; 88:403–408.
99. Quan SF, Parides GC, Knoper SR: Mandatory minute ventilation (MMV) ventilation: An overview. *Respir Care* 1990; 35:898–905.
100. Rattenborg CC, Via-Reque E: *Clinical Use of Mechanical Ventilation.* St Louis, Mosby–Year Book Inc, 1981.
101. Ritz R, Bishop M, Robinson C: Guidelines for choosing the appropriate level of pressure support (PS) with a Bear 5 to overcome imposed work of breathing (WOBi) (abstract). *Respir Care* 1988; 33:933.
102. Robinson C, Bishop M, Ritz R: Guidelines for choosing the appropriate level of pressure support with a Servo 900C to overcome imposed work of breathing (WOBi) (abstract). *Respir Care* 1988; 33:933.
103. Rodgriquez J, Weissman C, Askanazi J et al: Metabolic and respiratory effects of glucose infusion (abstract). *Anesthesiology* 1982; 57:A119.
104. Ruppel GL: *Manual of Pulmonary Function Testing*, ed 5. St Louis, Mosby–Year Book, Inc, 1991, p 138.
105. Sahn SA, Lakshminarayan S: Bedside criteria for discontinuation of mechanical ventilation. *Chest* 1973; 68:1002–1005.
106. Saltzman HA, Salzano JV: Effects of carbohydrate metabolism upon respiratory gas exchange in normal men. *J App Physiol* 1971; 30:228–331.
107. Sassoon CS, Mahutte CK, Te TT, et al: Work of breathing and airway occlusion pressure during assist-mode mechanical ventilation. *Chest* 1988; 93:571–576.
108. Savino JA, Dawson JA, Agarwal N, et al: The metabolic cost of breathing in critical surgical patients. *J Trauma* 1985; 25:1126–1133.
109. Schachter EN, Tucker D, Beck GJ: Does intermittent mandatory ventilation accelerate weaning? *JAMA* 1981; 256:1210–1214.
110. Shapiro BA, Harrison RA, Trout CA: *Clinical Application of Respiratory Care.* St Louis, Mosby–Year Book Inc, 1979.
111. Shelledy DC, Mikles SP: Newer modes of mechanical ventilation; part 1: Pressure support. *Respir Manage* 1988; (July/August):14–20.

112. Shelledy DC, Rau J, Thomas L: A comparison of the effects of assist-control, SIMV and SIMV with pressure support on ventilation, oxygen consumption and ventilatory equivalent, in press.
113. Siemans M: *Operating Manual, Servo Ventilator 900C Model.* Schaumberg, Ill, Siemens-Elema Life Support Systems, 1985.
114. Spearman CB, Sheldon RL, Egan DF: *Egan's Fundamentals of Respiratory Therapy.* St Louis, Mosby–Year Book, Inc, 1982.
115. Stoller JK: Establishing clinical unweanability. *Respir Care* 1991; 36:186–198.
116. Stoller JK: Physiologic rationale for resting the ventilatory muscles. *Respir Care* 1991; 36:290–296.
117. Thompson DJ: Computerized control of mechanical ventilation: Closing the loop. *Respir Care* 1987; 32:440–444.
118. Tokioka H, Saito S, Kosaka F: Comparison of pressure support ventilation and assist control ventilation in patients with acute respiratory failure. *Intensive Care Med* 1989; 15:364–367.
119. Trevino MD, Walters PR: The effects of working pressure on tidal volume and inspiratory flow during pressure support ventilation with the Siemens 900C (abstract). *Respir Care* 1988; 33:926.
120. Trunet P, Dreyfuss D, Bonnet JL, et al: Augmentation de la Pa_{CO_2} due à la nutrition entérale au cours de la ventilation artificielle. *Presse Med* 1983; 12:2927–2930.
121. Viale JP, Annat GJ: Oxygen cost of breathing postoperative patients. Pressure support vs continuous positive airway pressure. *Chest* 1988; 93:506–509.
122. Ward ME, Corbeil C, Gibbons W, et al: Optimization of respiratory muscle relaxation during mechanical ventilation. *Anesthesiology* 1988; 69:29–35.
123. Weisman LM, Rinaldo JE, Rogers RM, et al: Intermittent mandatory ventilation. *Am Rev Respir Dis* 1983; 127:641–647.
124. Wissing DR, Romero MD, George RB: Comparing the newer modes of mechanical ventilation. *J Crit Illness* 1987; 2:41–49.
125. Zelt BA, LoSasso AM: Prolonged nasotracheal intubation and mechanical ventilation in the management of asphyxiating thoracic dystrophy: A case report. *Anesth Analg* 1972; 51:342–348.

Chapter 13

Initiating Resuscitation and Respiratory Support in Newborn and Pediatric Patients

Cathleen Patterson, MSN, R.N.
Robert L. Chatburn, R.R.T.

On completion of this chapter the reader will be able to:

1. List and describe the six steps of initial resuscitation following delivery of the newborn.
2. State the cause of respiratory distress syndrome in the premature infant.
3. Name and describe the tool used in assessment of the severity of respiratory distress.
4. Describe the clinical signs and symptoms associated with respiratory distress of the newborn.
5. Establish the ventilation decision that needs to be made following evaluation of respiratory pattern and heart rate.
6. Provide four situations that describe the criteria for endotracheal intubation in the newborn.
7. Describe the condition of respiratory distress in the child.
8. Interpret acid-base balance values.
9. State the ways in which respiratory physiology of the newborn is different from that of the adult.
10. List four indications for mechanical ventilatory support in the newborn.
11. Describe the ideal ventilator.
12. Explain the function of the available controls for adjusting mechanical ventilation in the newborn.
13. Compare the use of pressure-controlled, volume-controlled, and high-frequency ventilation in the neonate.
14. Discuss what ventilator changes can be made to change arterial blood gas findings.
15. Discuss some of the problems encountered in humidification of inspired air in the NICU environment.

NEWBORN ASSESSMENT, RESUSCITATION, AND STABILIZATION

The initial assessment and care of the cardiopulmonary system is critical to the stabilization of the newborn. Health care workers such as physicians, nurses, and respiratory care practitioners (RCPs) evaluate and intervene on a continuous basis during the first moments of life and thereafter as needed. This team works together efficiently to stabilize the newborn.

Initial Evaluation

Assessment begins at birth as soon as the infant is delivered. It is based primarily on evaluation of respirations, heart rate, and color. These help guide the action, evaluation, and decision process during the first moments of life. A commonly used tool in the evaluation of the newborn is Apgar scoring. This procedure provides an objective assessment of the infant's heart rate, respiratory effort, color, muscle tone, and reflex irritability (Fig 13–1). It is normally "scored" at the first and fifth minutes following delivery.

Along with Apgar scoring, the infant is also evaluated as it is cared for during the normal procedure following delivery. This procedure includes the initial steps of neonatal resuscitation (Fig 13–2). During part of this process the baby is checked for response to touch or tactile stimulation and level of breathing (Fig 13–3). If the assessment shows that the infant is not responding as normal, then the process of neonatal resuscitation is begun.

Overview of Neonatal Resuscitation

The American Heart Association (AHA) and the American Academy of Pediatrics (AAP) have developed standards for neonatal resuscitation. This process includes a continuous cycle of action, evaluation, and decision as shown in Figures 13–2 and 13–3. The initial steps of resuscitation include the well-known AHA basic life support (BLS) criteria: the "ABCs of resuscitation": *A,* establish an open airway, *B,* initiate breathing, *C,* maintain circulation.

Once the baby is delivered, the initial steps of resuscitation then follow those outlined in Figure 13–4 and briefly described here.

Prevention of Heat Loss.—Prevent heat loss by placing the infant on a radiant, heated surface, drying the baby, and removal of wet linen. This intervention is performed rapidly with the goal of providing an optimal thermal environment for the neonate and preventing hypothermia. The neonate's skin temperature should be maintained between 36.3 and 36.7° C.

Positioning the Infant.—The infant is positioned with the neck slightly extended to establish an open airway. This can be easily accomplished by

SIGN	0	1	2
HEART RATE	Absent	Slow (< 100)	Fast (> 100)
RESPIRATORY EFFORT	Absent	Weak cry	Strong cry
MUSCLE TONE	Limp	Some flexion of extremities	Well flexed
COLOR	Blue, pale	Body pink Extremities blue	Completely pink
REFLEX RESPONSE			
Response to catheter in nostril (tested after oropharynx is clear)	No response	Grimace	Cough or sneeze
Tangential foot slap	No response	Grimace	Cry and withdrawal of foot

FIG 13–1.
Apgar scoring chart. Each of the five signs is scored individually. Then the overall score is added. (From Apgar V, Holaday DA, James LS, et al: *JAMA* 1958; 168:1985–1988. Used by permission.)

placing a small shoulder roll beneath the shoulders and using the head tilt–chin lift procedure with care not to hyperextend the neck.

Suctioning.—First the oral, and then the nasal passages are suctioned to remove secretions. If meconium is present in the amniotic fluid upon delivery of the neonate's head and prior to delivery of the shoulders, then the upper airway is suctioned. This includes the nasopharynx, oropharynx, hypopharynx, and

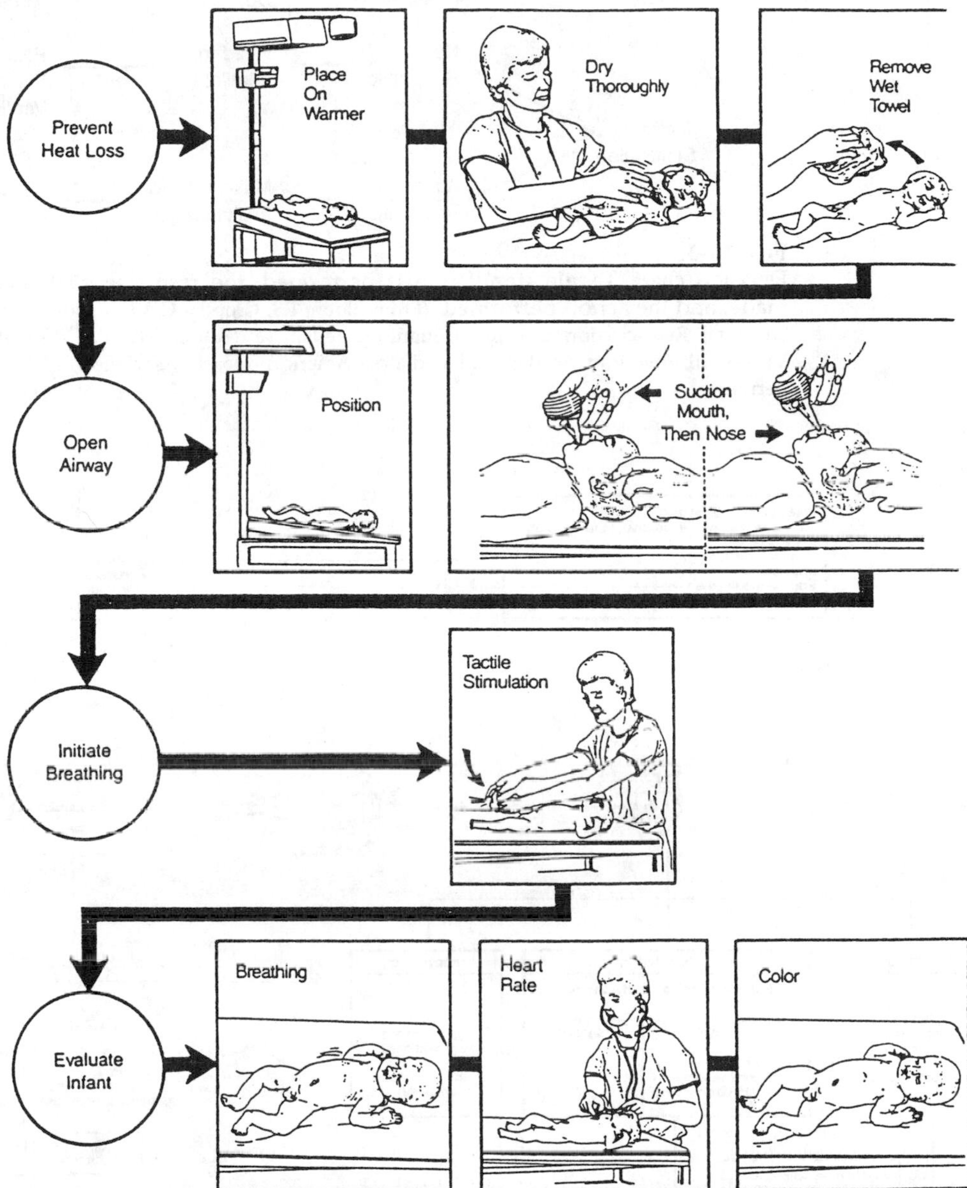

FIG 13–2.
Initial steps of resuscitation. (From Bloom RS, Cropley C, Chameides L, and the AHA/AAP Neonatal Resuscitation Steering Committee (eds): *Textbook of Neonatal Resuscitation.* Elk Grove Village, Ill, American Academy of Pediatrics/American Heart Association, 1990, pp 2–8. Used by permission.)

Action
Evaluation
Decision
Action
No Respirations
Need to Ventilate
Positive-Pressure Ventilation
Tactile Stimulation
Adequate Respirations
Make Additional Evaluation
Check Heart Rate

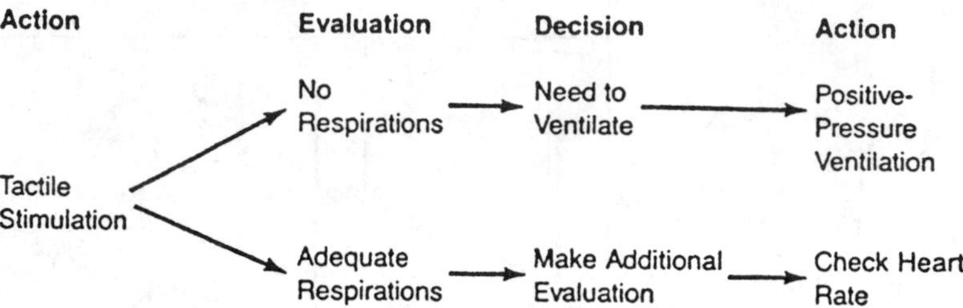

FIG 13–3.
Decision chart. Tactile stimulation is performed, the response evaluated, a decision is made, and the action performed. (From Bloom RS, Cropley C, Chameides L, and the AHA/AAP Neonatal Resuscitation Steering Committee (eds): *Textbook of Neonatal Resuscitation.* Elk Grove Village, Ill, American Academy of Pediatrics/American Heart Association, 1990, pp 1–21. Used by permission.)

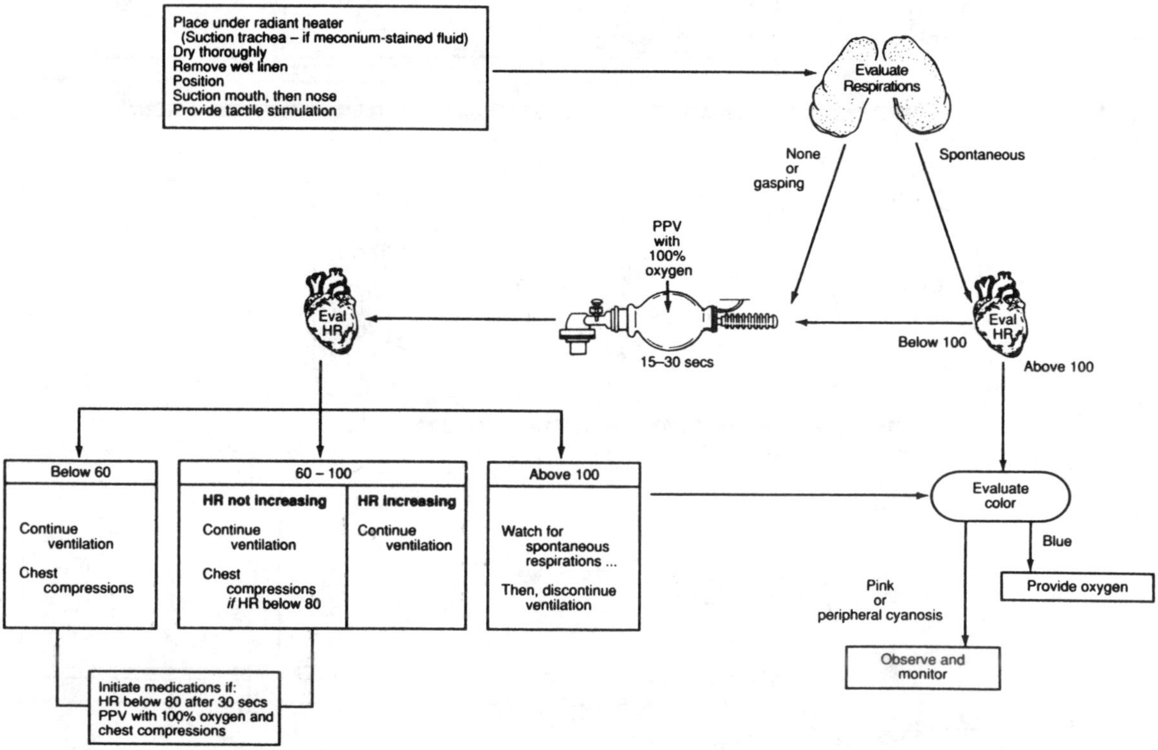

Place under radiant heater
(Suction trachea – if meconium-stained fluid)
Dry thoroughly
Remove wet linen
Position
Suction mouth, then nose
Provide tactile stimulation
Evaluate Respirations
None or gasping
Spontaneous
PPV with 100% oxygen
15–30 secs
Eval HR
Below 100
Above 100
Eval HR
Below 60
Continue ventilation
Chest compressions
60 – 100
HR not increasing
Continue ventilation
Chest compressions if HR below 80
HR increasing
Continue ventilation
Above 100
Watch for spontaneous respirations ...
Then, discontinue ventilation
Evaluate color
Blue
Provide oxygen
Pink or peripheral cyanosis
Observe and monitor
Initiate medications if:
HR below 80 after 30 secs
PPV with 100% oxygen and chest compressions

FIG 13–4.
Overview of resuscitation in the delivery room. (From Bloom RS, Cropley C, Chameides L, and the AHA/AAP Neonatal Resuscitation Steering Committee (eds): *Textbook of Neonatal Resuscitation.* Elk Grove Village, Ill, American Academy of Pediatrics/American Heart Association, 1990, pp 0–5. Used by permission.)

posterior pharynx. These steps are done before the baby's first breath. The infant is then quickly placed on the radiant warmer table. As soon as the infant has been placed on the radiant warmer and before drying, the following two steps are taken: (1) residual meconium in the hypopharynx is removed by suctioning under direct vision, and (2) the trachea is intubated and residual meconium is removed from the lower airway. Whenever meconium is found on the vocal cords when viewing the airway, the infant is generally intubated, irrigated, and suctioned until the secretions come back clear.

The decision may need to be made as to whether the difficulty of intubating a very vigorous and active infant outweighs the advantages of full meconium removal. In addition, the infant with severe asphyxia should be managed by clinical judgment to determine the number of reintubations since it may not be possible to remove all meconium before initiating positive pressure ventilation (PPV).

Once the trachea is suctioned, the stomach is suctioned to prevent aspiration of gastric contents with meconium. If positive pressure ventilation is not required, the suctioning of the gastric contents can be deferred until the infant is 5 minutes old so that the risk of producing a vagal response is minimized.[2]

Assessment of Breathing.—Assessment of breathing is rapidly established. If the infant is apneic, then, tactile stimulation is given for no longer than 2 seconds and a reassessment of respiratory effort is made. If apnea persists, PPV is immediately administered with 100% oxygen via an anesthesia bag or a self-inflating bag. PPV is administered for a cycle of 15 to 20 seconds and the heart rate assessed so that the decision can be made if further action is needed. When neonates are ventilated with a face mask, or bag-and-mask system for more than 2 minutes using PPV, an oral gastric catheter is usually inserted so that the stomach is decompressed and does not inhibit lung expansion. The gastric tube is left to open drainage.

Assessment of Heart Rate.—If spontaneous respirations are present in the initial assessment, then the heart rate is evaluated (see Fig 13–4). Assessment of heart rate is established by listening directly to the apical pulse with a stethoscope for 6 seconds and converting to a 1-minute reading (multiply by 10). A heart rate of above 100 beats/min is considered adequate.

A heart rate of less than 100 beats/min is indicative of inadequate cardiac output, and inadequate O_2 delivery to the tissues. PPV with 100% O_2 needs to be administered when the neonate shows poor respiratory effort and the heart rate is less than 100 beats/min. If the neonate's heart rate is below 60 or remains 60 to 80 beats/min and is not rising despite PPV with 100% O_2 for 30 seconds, then chest compressions are initiated at a rate of 120/min.

Assessment of Color.—The practioner can move on to the assessment of color if the infant's heart rate is above 100. If the infant has regular respirations

	Liter flow: 5 per minute
½"	Approximately 80%
1"	Approximately 60%
2"	Approximately 40%

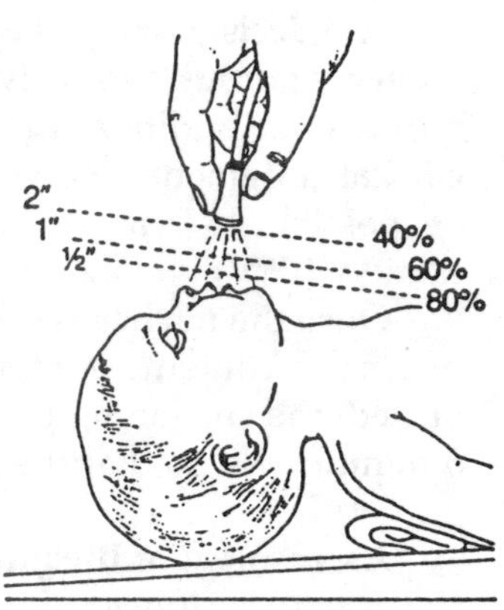

FIG 13–5.
Oxygen administration at various distances (inches) from the nose. The concentrations in the chart apply only if a flow of 5 L/min is used, and the tubing is held steady, aimed at the nares. Waving the end of the tubing back and forth in front of the nose decreases the oxygen concentration considerably. (From Bloom RS, Cropley C, Chameides L, and the AHA/AAP Neonatal Resuscitation Steering Committee (eds): *Textbook of Neonatal Resuscitation.* Elk Grove Village, Ill, American Academy of Pediatrics/American Heart Association, 1990, pp 2–28. Used by permission.)

and central cyanosis, 100% free-flow O_2 is administered to relieve the cyanosis. This can be done by holding O_2 tubing with a flow of 5 L directly over the neonate's nose, and at least ½ in. from the nose. This will deliver at least 80% free-flow O_2 (Fig 13–5).

Once the neonates' color improves and the infant becomes pink, the O_2 can be withdrawn gradually while the practitioner continues to assess the infant. The decision-making cycle is continued until the infant is stabilized.

Oxygen Administration Considerations

When time allows, heated and humidified O_2 can be delivered by way of an O_2 hood. This helps prevent drying of the respiratory tract mucosa and heat loss. But, during an emergency, dry O_2 can be administered briefly.[2]

The temperature of the O_2 hood is maintained between 32 and 35° C with 100% humidity at a flow of 5 to 7 L/min for a small- to medium-sized hood, and 7 to 10 L/min for a large hood. Inspired gas used for continuous positive airway pressure (CPAP) or ventilation is warmed to 35° C and with 90% to 100% humidity.

Summary of Neonatal Resuscitation

During neonatal resuscitation, the heart rate is taken every 15 to 30 seconds so that the need for ongoing treatment can be determined based on the decision-making cycle (see Fig 13–4). Further resuscitation procedures are described in detail in the AAP-AHA *Textbook of Neonatal Resuscitation.*[2]

PREMATURITY AND RESPIRATORY DISTRESS SYNDROME IN THE NEWBORN

At birth, the lungs of a newborn must adapt to extrauterine life by taking the responsibility of oxygenating the circulating blood volume as soon as the placental blood supply is stopped. This is easily assumed in the majority of full-term infants. However, there are infants that will require additional assistance to achieve their optimal respiratory function.

Prematurity

Prematurity accounts for the highest number of admissions to a neonatal intensive care unit (NICU). Most of the neonates who are admitted to the NICU have respiratory problems. Respiratory distress syndrome (RDS) is the leading diagnosis encountered in the NICU. RDS was also formally called hyaline membrane disease (HMD) but this term has become less frequently used since HMD refers to a variety of nonspecific responses of the lungs to various insults, which include mechanical ventilation.

RDS is responsible for more infant deaths than any other disease.[13] The prognosis for infants with RDS has improved dramatically with advances in neonatal care. It is primarily seen in the premature infant, i.e., those born prior to the 37th week of gestation. The full-term or term infant is 38 to 42 weeks' gestation. The postmature or postterm infant has a gestational age of 42 weeks or greater.[2] Lung tissue is not completely developed in the preterm infant. The terminal airways begin to develop at 24 weeks' gestation and surfactant production is established at 22 weeks and continues through the 35th week of gestational age.

RDS presents with clinical symptoms that result from abnormal lung mechanics due to immature lung development and surfactant deficiency. Surfactant is a phospholipid and protein mixture that coats the inner surface of the alveoli. Surfactant decreases the natural tendency of the alveoli to collapse. Insufficient surfactant production results in decreased lung compliance which is caused by an increased surface tension. There is a tendency for alveolar collapse and diffuse atelectasis. These factors increase pulmonary artery pressure and the pulmonary hypertension resulting in extrapulmonary shunting of blood from right to left. An increased ventilation-perfusion ($\dot{V}/\dot{Q}$) mismatch is shown by an increased alveolar-arterial oxygen gradient [$P(A - a)O_2$] and high arterial-alveolar carbon dioxide gradient [$P(a - A)CO_2$].[4]

Prematurity is the most important single factor in the development of RDS. However, the preterm infant is also at the greatest risk for the development of other problems due to the state of immaturity of organs and systems. The determination of neonatal maturity or gestational age helps guide the practioner's plan of patient care.

Identification of Respiratory Complications in the Newborn

Identifying an infant who is having respiratory complications following delivery is very similar to assessment at birth for resuscitation. The newborn is observed and assessed for initial respiratory effort and pattern.

Disorders That Cause Respiratory Distress

Factors that contribute to the evolution of neonatal respiratory distress can be described under two categories. They include: (1) pulmonary disorders and (2) extrapulmonary disorders (Table 13–1). These disorders require a multidisciplinary approach to the clinical management by the health care team in the NICU. Every neonate requires astute assessment and management by the practioner based on the process of the decision cycle. The goal is to provide prompt and immediate assessment and intervention. This helps promote optimal stabilization and oxygenation of the newborn until the infant's problem is corrected.

Clinical Characteristics of RDS

Infants with RDS may develop clinical signs of respiratory distress immediately after birth and within the first 4 hours of life. The clinical course is characterized by a gradual worsening that occurs during the first 2 to 3 days. RDS may be complicated by the presence of a patent ductus arteriosus, pneumothorax, and dislodgement or obstruction of the endotracheal (ET) tube. The presence of fluctuating or persistent pulmonary hypertension caused by arterial constriction will alter blood gases significantly. Recovery is preceded by a spontaneous diuresis. Some seriously ill and preterm neonates may require a prolonged recovery period that can result in the development of bronchopulmonary dysplasia.

TABLE 13–1.
Differential Diagnosis of Respiratory Distress During the First Days of Life*

Pulmonary Disorders		
Common	**Less Common**	**Uncommon**
Respiratory distress syndrome	Pulmonary hemorrhage	Congenital lung cysts, tumors
Transient tachypnea of the newborn	Pulmonary hypoplasia/agenesis	Congenital lobar emphysema
Meconium aspiration	Wilson-Mikity syndrome	Tracheoesophageal fistula
Congenital pneumonia	Upper airway obstruction	Pulmonary lymphangiectasia
Pneumothorax/air leaks	Tracheomalacia	Tracheal lesions
Persistent fetal circulaton	Abdominal distention	Rib cage anomalies
	Pleural effusion/chylothorax	Extrinsic masses
	Diaphragmatic hernia	

Extrapulmonary Disorders		
Cardiovascular	**Metabolic**	**Neurologic/Muscular**
Hypovolemia	Acidosis	Cerebral edema
Anemia	Hypoglycemia	Cerebral hemorrhage
Polycythemia	Hypothermia	Drugs
Persistent fetal circulation	Hyperthermia	Muscle disorders
Cyanotic heart disease		Spinal cord diseases
Congestive heart failure		Phrenic nerve damage

*From Carlo WA, Chatburn RL: Neonatal respiratory care, in Walsh MC, Carlo C, Miller M (eds): *Respiratory Diseases of the Newborn*. St Louis, Mosby–Year Book, Inc, 1988, p 265. Used by permission.

RDS is rarely found in infants of greater than 38 weeks' gestation. Selected perinatal factors may increase the incidence and severity of RDS. These include maternal diabetes, asphyxia, and cesarean section delivery. Males are more likely to develop RDS than females. With the case of multiple births, it is commonly noted that the second-born twin may exhibit a higher degree of RDS than the first-born twin.

Assessment for Severity of RDS

One of the tools used in evaluating for RDS is Silverman's chart (Fig 13–6). The infant's upper chest, lower chest, and nares are observed along with audible assessment for degree and pitch of breath sounds. Characteristics of the breath sounds, such as audible grunting upon expiration with unequal air exchange, are noted. The pattern of retractions and grunting assessed is indexed according to the chart.

The chart illustrates the pattern and configuration of chest movement upon inspiration and expiration. In preterm infants with pulmonary difficulties retractions are a prominent feature owing to the compliant chest wall. The weak

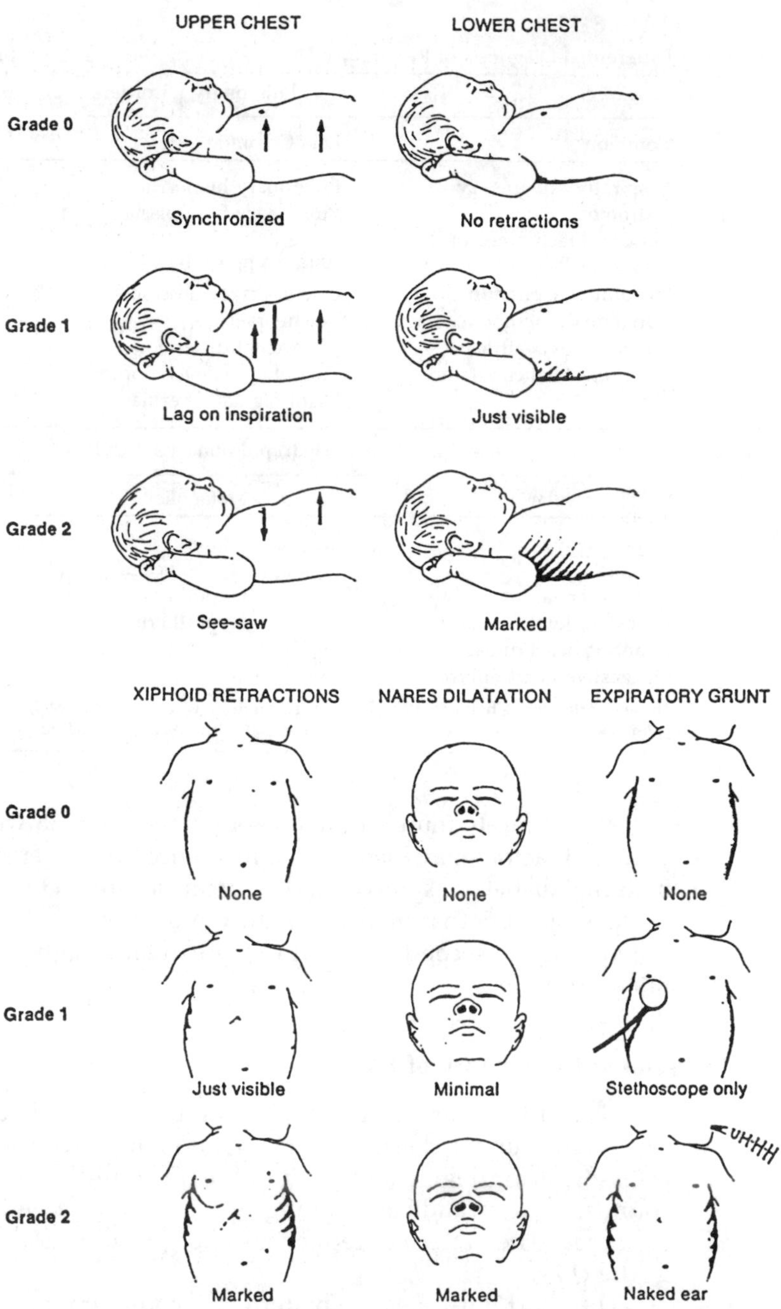

FIG 13–6.
Observation of retractions. (From Silverman WA, Anderson DH: *Pediatrics* 1956; 17:1. Used by permission.)

muscles of the chest wall along with the highly cartilaginous rib structure promotes an extremely elastic rib cage. During the initial period, the neonate attempts to produce higher negative intrathoracic pressure changes to promote alveolar expansion. During this early phase, the infant's color remains satisfactory and breath sounds remain normal with good air entry and exchange. However, the work of breathing is high as the infant produces high negative intrapleural pressures. Respiratory distress becomes more clinically evident when the infant's respiratory rate increases from the normal rate of 40 to 60 breaths/min to a tachypneic rate of 80 to 120 breaths/min. The respiratory pattern becomes increasingly labored with increased retractions and nasal flaring.

Neonates characteristically increase their respiratory rate instead of the depth of their respiratory effort when in respiratory distress. The pronounced substernal retractions are due to the high negative intrapleural pressures. The diaphragm is working hard to inflate collapsed alveolar sacs. At this stage of respiratory distress, breath sounds will reveal fine rales upon inspiration along with a grunt noted during expiration. The expiratory grunt serves as a method of maintaining or increasing the end-expiratory pressure in the lung. This helps keep the alveolar sacs expanded, promoting better alveolar-capillary gas exchange.

Nasal flaring is also an indicator of respiratory distress that accompanies retractions, tachypnea, and grunting. Cyanosis also becomes evident and can usually be relieved by providing 100% O_2 until the neonate's color improves. An appropriate degree of oxygenation and ventilation is demonstrated by blood gas analysis. Transcutaneous partial pressure of oxygen (Po_2) monitoring can assess tissue Po_2. Careful monitoring of arterial oxygen tension (Pao_2) in the neonate is essential in the prevention of hyperoxygenation and retrolental fibroplasia (RLF).

As respiratory distress progresses the newborn becomes markedly more cyanotic, pale, and mottled in appearance despite increased delivery of O_2 concentration. Frequent episodes of apnea, a cessation of breathing for greater than 10 to 15 seconds with a heart rate less than 100/beats/min, along with a decreased state of consciousness, are common. The clinician may also note the presence of decreased muscle tone and flaccidity.

The breath sounds are diminished and the infant will demonstrate late-stage "shocklike" symptoms that include a low arterial blood pressure (late sign) suggesting a decreased cardiac output. Generally, neonates that survive the first 96 hours of life with RDS have a greater chance of recovery. Although results are still under investigation, recent clinical data have demonstrated that the new treatment of surfactant replacement therapy can also enhance the neonate's recovery from RDS related to prematurity.

The major complications of RDS include patent ductus arteriosus, congestive heart failure, intraventricular cerebral hemorrhage, persistent pulmonary hypertension, and necrotizing enterocolitis.

Clinical Management of Respiratory Distress

The management of neonatal respiratory distress is based upon many factors. Infants with respiratory distress due to pulmonary or nonpulmonary causes can develop respiratory insufficiency immediately during the postnatal period or over several hours. Prompt intervention with the provision of airway management, O_2, and ET intubation with the application of PPV are used to stabilize the newborn with respiratory distress.

Oxygenation.—The administration of O_2 can be the single most effective therapeutic intervention in the management of the neonate with respiratory distress. Oxygen must be administered by trained practitioners with careful monitoring so that the potential side effects can be prevented or diminished. Oxygen is carried in the blood by a chemical bond with hemoglobin. Fetal hemoglobin differs slightly in its affinity for O_2 compared to normal adult hemoglobin (Fig 13–7). For example, a Pa_{O_2} of 90 to 100 mm Hg indicates that the blood is almost completely saturated. Cyanosis can be observed at saturations of 75% to 85%. This correlates with the O_2 tension of 32 to 42 mm Hg on the fetal

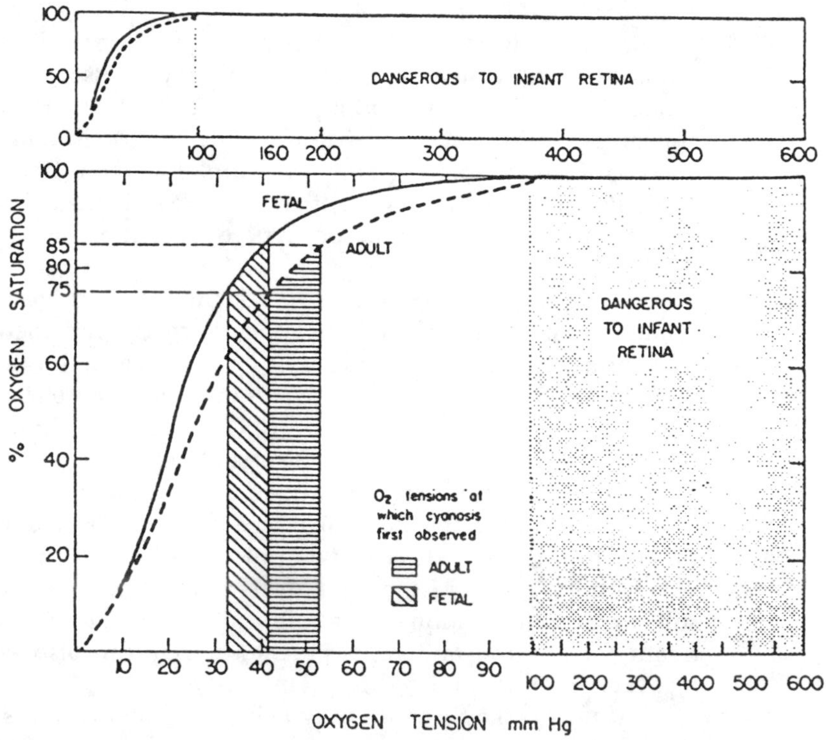

FIG 13–7.
Oxygen dissociation curve. (From Klaus M, Meyer BP: *Pediatr Clin North Am* 1966; 13:731. Used by permission.)

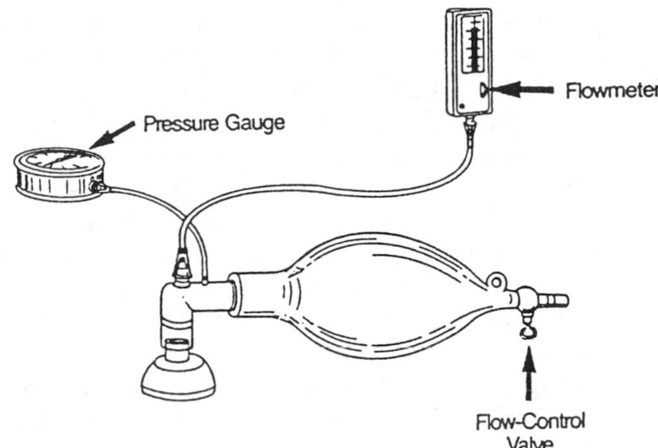

FIG 13–8.
Anesthesia bag assembly which inflates only when gas flow is provided. (From Bloom RS, Cropley C, Chameides L, and the AHA/AAP Neonatal Resuscitation Steering Committee (eds): *Textbook of Neonatal Resuscitation.* Elk Grove Village, Ill, American Academy of Pediatrics/American Heart Association, 1990, pp 3A–14. Used by permission.)

dissociation curve. The Pa_{O_2} is dependent on the lung's ability to transfer O_2 and can be affected by the presence of cardiac and pulmonary problems. Giving 100% O_2 will enhance O_2 saturation in the presence of diffusion abnormalities or inadequate ventilation.

However, in neonates with a fixed right-to-left shunt, such as a true cyanotic cardiac lesion, particularly those with transposition of the great vessels, the Pa_{O_2} will rarely rise above 40 mm Hg, even with continuous exposure to 100% O_2. The newborn with persistent fetal circulation (PFC) may have transient periods with a P_{O_2} greater than 100 mm Hg only when hyperventilation is provided for aproximately 5 to 10 minutes, which decreases the partial pressure of carbon dioxide in arterial blood (Pa_{CO_2}) to ranges of 18 to 25 mm Hg.[4]

Clinical signs of hypoxia in the newborn include tachypnea, tachycardia, pallor, abdominal distention, cyanosis, and fall in temperature. If hypoxia is not corrected, the infant will develop acidosis and a subsequent fall in blood pressure and heart rate. Hypoxia is a complication of respiratory distress and can be corrected by the administration of PPV given by face mask and bag ventilation or by ET tube and bag ventilation.

Ventilation by Bag and Mask.—Ventilation by the bag-and-mask system can be effective in correcting hypoxia. The mask must fit securely over the infant's nose and mouth by creating an adequate seal so that ventilation can be delivered at a rate of 40 to 60 breaths/min. An anesthesia bag or self-inflating bag can be used to ventilate the infant (Figs 13–8 and 13–9).

With an anesthesia bag, the inflation of the bag depends on the seal that is created at the infant's face, and an adequate supply of O_2 from the flowmeter. The flow control or pressure release valve regulates the amount of gas escaping from the bag. This establishes the CPAP level if the bag is not squeezed and the peak inspiratory pressure (PIP) when it is. The pressure gauge or manometer connected to the anesthesia bag monitors the amount of pressure that is being delivered with each breath. Ventilating pressures for infants without lung disease range between 15 and 20 cm H_2O. Infants with RDS need to be ventilated with pressures ranging between 20 and 40 cm H_2O.

A self-inflating bag (Fig 13–9) must have an O_2 reservoir attached so that the bag is capable of delivering 90% to 100% O_2. Self-inflating bags without O_2 reservoirs are totally inadequate for resuscitation of the newborn. The self-inflating bag must be connected to an O_2 flowmeter or a blender set at 100%. Unlike the anesthesia bag, the self-inflating bag is equipped with only a pressure release valve and no pressure gauge. The pressure release valve is designed so that ventilation pressures do not exceed 35 cm H_2O unless the valve is occluded or bypassed. Any self-inflating bag in which the pop-off valve is bypassed should have a pressure gauge attachment.

Ventilation Decisions.—The infant should be ventilated based on three categories of respiratory and heart rate decisions as shown in Figure 13–10. First, if the heart rate is above 100 beats/min and the infant is spontaneously breathing, then O_2 is being circulated through the system and the color should improve. At this point, the practitioner discontinues PPV and provides mild tactile

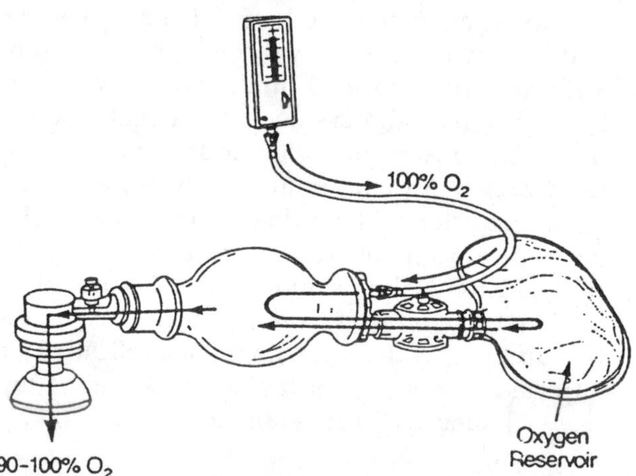

FIG 13–9.
Self-inflating manual resuscitation bag. (From Bloom RS, Cropley C, Chameides L, and the AHA/AAP Neonatal Resuscitation Steering Committee (eds): *Textbook of Neonatal Resuscitation.* Elk Grove Village, Ill, American Academy of Pediatrics/American Heart Association, 1990, pp 3A–23. Used by permission.)

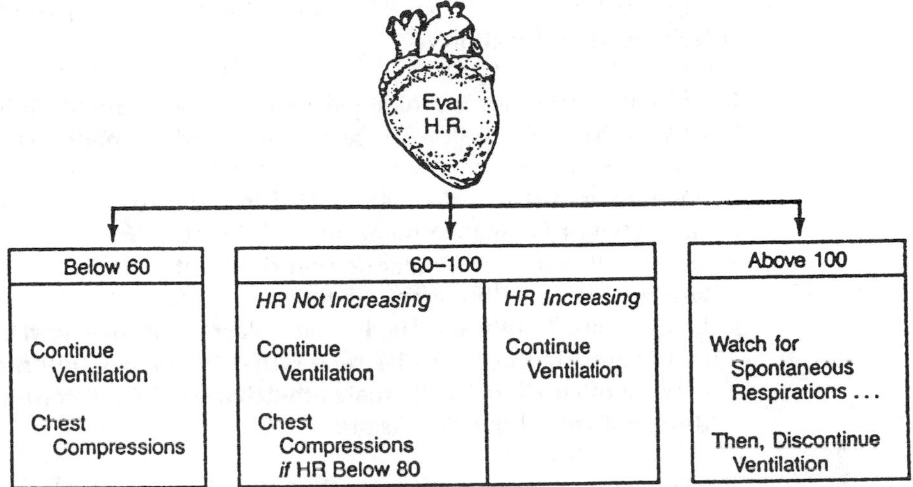

FIG 13–10.
Heart rate decision flow diagram. (From Bloom RS, Cropley C, Chameides L, and the AHA/AAP Neonatal Resuscitation Steering Committee (eds): *Textbook of Neonatal Resuscitation.* Elk Grove Village, Ill, American Academy of Pediatrics/American Heart Association, 1990, pp 3C–14. Used by permission.)

stimulation while monitoring the infant's progress. If the infant does not breathe spontaneously and if the infant becomes cyanotic, then 100% O_2 needs to be provided via assisted ventilation at a rate of 40 to 60 breaths/min.

If the neonate's heart rate is between 60 and 100 and increasing, then assisted ventilation with 100% O_2 is provided for 15 to 30 seconds and the heart rate is rechecked. If the heart rate is 60 to 100 beats/min and not increasing, the practitioner continues ventilation. If the rate is less than 80 beats/min, chest compressions are performed by a second practitioner. On the other hand, if the heart rate is 60 to 100 beats/min and the rate is increasing, then the practitioner checks for adequacy of ventilation by assessing breath sounds and ensures that 100% O_2 is being administered via pressure-monitored positive pressure ventilation (PPV) system.

If the 6-second heart rate assessment is below 60 beats/min, the neonate is in serious trouble and will require the continuation of ventilation with 100% O_2 and chest compressions. Resuscitative medications are administered if the neonate's heart rate remains below 80 beats/min after 30 seconds of PPV with 100% O_2 and chest compressions.

Endotracheal Intubation

Positive pressure ventilation can usually be administered effectively by a mask-and-bag system. Unfortunately, there are circumstances when the PPV must be administered by an ET tube. The following four situations describe the criteria for ET intubation:

1. PPV is required for a prolonged period to ventilate the infant.
2. PPV by bag and mask is ineffective as noted by inadequate response and chest expansion.
3. Suctioning of the trachea is required in order to clear the airway of infants suspected of having aspirated formula or other foreign material. The trachea is intubated and suctioned on those infants who have thick or particulate meconium in the amniotic fluid.
4. If congenital diaphragmatic hernia is suspected, the newborn is immediately ventilated using an ET tube rather than a bag and mask. Ventilation by way of an ET tube eliminates the chance of air entering the bowel and thus inhibiting lung expansion.

The intubation equipment is selected and prepared. The appropriate sizes of laryngoscope blades and ET tubes are selected prior to intubating the infant or child. The supplies and equipment needed are listed in Tables 13–2 and 13–3. The infant or child is positioned supine with the neck slightly extended. Hyperextension of the neck should be avoided, since it occludes the straight alignment of the trachea. Manual ventilation is performed for at least 15 to 20 seconds with 100% O_2. If the intubation attempt extends beyond 20 seconds, the procedure is stopped so that the infant can be ventilated with 100% O_2 again. The practitioner assisting with the intubation is responsible for monitoring the time and assessing the neonate for distress. The heart rate is continuously monitored since

TABLE 13-2.
Equipment Needed for Intubation of the Newborn

Laryngoscope
Blades
Size 1 (full-term infant)
Size 0 (preterm infant)
Endotracheal tubes cut to 13 cm and adaptor-reconnected
Sizes
2.5 mm
3.0 mm
3.5 mm
4.0 mm
Suctioning device
Meconium aspirator
#10F suction catheter
Shoulder roll
½ in. cloth adhesive tape
Scissors
Resuscitation bag and mask connected to 100% oxygen
Stylet or ice for stiffening endotracheal tube (optional)

TABLE 13–3.
Equipment Guidelines According to Age and Weight*

	Age (50th Percentile Weight)					
Equipment	Premature Infant (1.0–2.5 kg)	Neonate (2.5–4.0 kg)	6 mo (7.0 kg)	1–2 yr (10–12 kg)	5 yr (16–18 kg)	8–10 yr (24–30 kg)
Airway—oral	Infant (00)	Infant/small (0)	Small (1)	Small (2)	Medium (3)	Medium/large (4/5)
Breathing						
Self-inflating bag	Infant	Infant	Child	Child	Child	Child/adult
O_2 ventilation mask	Premature	Newborn	Infant/child	Child	Child	Small adult
Endotracheal tube	2.5–3.0 (uncuffed)	3.0–3.5 (uncuffed)	3.5–4.0 (uncuffed)	4.0–4.5 (uncuffed)	5.0–5.5 (uncuffed)	5.5–6.5 (cuffed)
Laryngoscope blade	0 (straight)	1 (straight)	1 (straight)	1–2 (straight)	2 (straight/curved)	2–3 (straight/curved)
Suction/stylet (F)	6–8/6	8/6	8–10/6	10/6	14/14	14/14
Circulation						
BP cuff	Newborn	Newborn	Infant	Child	Child	Child/adult
Venous access						
Angiocatheter	22–24	22–24	22–24	20–22	18–20	16–20
Butterfly needle	25	23–25	23–25	23	20–23	18–21
Intracatheter	—	—	19	19	16	14
Arm board (in.)	6	6	6–8	8	8–15	15
Orogastric tube (f)	5	5–8	8	10	10–12	14–18
Chest tube (f)	10–14	12–18	14–20	14–24	20–32	28–38

*From Chameides L: *Textbook of Pediatric Advanced Life Support.* Dallas, American Heart Association/American Academy of Pediatrics, 1990, p. 105. Used by permission.

mechanical stimulation of the airway can induce reflex bradycardia. If a bradyarrythmia occurs with a heart rate of less than 80 beats/min in the infant and less than 60 beats/min in the child, then the procedure is interrupted and PPV with a mask-bag-valve system and 100% O_2 are provided.

Once the ET tube is placed, proper positioning of the tube must be immediately confirmed. Initially, the chest is observed for symmetric chest rise with ventilation. The practitioner then listens to breath sounds to be sure they are present and equal bilaterally. The area over the stomach can be ausculated to note the absence of breath sounds. The ET tube is inspected for the presence of condensation during exhalation. If the above initial criteria are not met, and gastric distention is noted with ventilation, the ET tube is removed and a second attempt to intubate is carried out after the infant or child is ventilated with 100% O_2 with a bag-valve-mask device for at least 30 seconds.

If breath sounds are noted to be unequal with greater air entry heard over the right side, right mainstem bronchial intubation is suspected and the ET tube needs to be withdrawn 1 to 2 cm. Hopefully, this will position the tube in the midtrachea. The breath sounds are then rechecked for equality. If the ET tube is correctly placed but ventilation or chest expansion is inadequate, several factors

TABLE 13–4.
Complications of the Intubation Procedure*

Complication	Causes
Hypoxia	Taking too long to intubate Incorrect placement of tube
Bradycardia, apnea	Hypoxia Vagal response due to the laryngoscope blade, ET tube, or suction catheter stimulating the posterior pharynx
Pneumothorax	Overventilation of one lung due to placement of tube in a main bronchus (usually the right)
Contusions or lacerations of tongue, gums, pharynx, epiglottis, trachea, vocal cords, or esophagus	Rough handling of laryngoscope or ET tube Laryngoscope blade that is too long or too short
Peforation of esophagus or trachea	Stylet protruding beyond end of tube
Infection	Introduction of organisms via equipment or hands

*From Bloom RS, Cropley C, Chameides L, and the AHA/AAP Neonatal Resuscitation Steering Committee (eds): *Textbook of Neonatal Resuscitation.* Elk Grove Village, Ill, American Academy of Pediatrics/American Heart Association, 1990, pp 5–42. Used by permission.

are considered. A first consideration may be that the tube is too small and that an air leak is present at the glottis. This is corrected by placing a larger tube or, for the child older than 8 years, by inflating the cuff on the ET tube. It is preferable to have a slight audible air leak so that the glottis does not become irritated or traumatized.

Another consideration might be that the infant or child may require a slight increase in ventilation pressure. This is accomplished by adjusting the pressure-release valve on the anesthesia bag and by occluding the pop-off valve on the self-inflating bag. The pressure gauge is carefully monitored, along with clinical signs, if additional ventilatory pressure is indicated.

The presence of loose connections or a leak may inhibit the proper inflation of the anesthesia bag. All tubings and connections are checked for correct attachment and securely adjusted. The bag can be briefly disconnected from the patient and manually checked to ensure that it inflates and functions properly. The manual breaths are assessed for shallowness and adjusted to give a fuller or larger breath as indicated.

Following correct ET tube placement, the centimeter marker is noted at the level of the upper lip and documented. The ET tube is secured to the face by using tape and benzoin or similar materials to prevent dislodgment. The tube must not extend more than 4 cm from the infant's lips to keep mechanical dead space to a minimum. Final confirmation of correct ET tube position is ensured by a chest film. Complications associated with the intubation procedure are listed in Table 13–4.

PEDIATRIC RESUSCITATION AND STABILIZATION

Annually in the United States approximately 40,000 infants under 1 year of age die.[13] Sixteen thousand children die between 1 and 14 years of age.[4] These deaths are caused by cardiac arrest resulting from hypoxemia secondary to a respiratory or circulatory condition. The events that may result in death and that require resuscitation are many. These are grouped into five categories: (1) injuries (44%), including motor vehicle accidents (45% of total), drowning (17% of total), and poisoning, firearms, and burns (21%); (2) suffocation caused by foreign body, i.e., toys, foods, plastic covers, etc.; (3) smoke inhalation; (4) sudden infant death syndrome (SIDS); and (5) infections, especially of the respiratory tract.[4]

In the pediatric age group the incidence of cardiac arrest is often the result of a prolonged period of hypoxemia, secondary to inadequate oxygenation and ventilation. The resulting circulatory shock may be initiated by many predisposing conditions such as the pulmonary and extrapulmonary disorders shown in Table 13–1.

General Principles in Management of Pediatric Respiratory Distress

The management goals for the pediatric patient in respiratory distress are similar to the goals previously described for neonatal resuscitation. The decision-making cycle for the pediatric patient centers on the goal of anticipating and recognizing the many causes of respiratory problems and supporting or supplanting those functions that are absent or compromised so that cardiovascular and neurologic recovery are supported.

Assessment of Respiratory Performance.—Assessment of respiratory performance in the pediatric patient relies on the assessment of clinical features that are characterized by the child's ability to eliminate CO_2 and adequately oxygenate the blood. Normal respiration or ventilation is accomplished with minimal work. With increasing age the normal range for respiratory and heart rates decreases. The normal respiratory rate for newborns ranges between 30 and 80 breaths/min. During late infancy and early childhood the range is 20 through 40. During late childhood and early adulthood (reaching adult level at age 15 years) the respiratory rate ranges between 15 and 25 breaths/min.[4] The normal respiratory rate in infants and children has an extensive range that is more responsive to disease, illness, emotion, and exercise than that of adults. Tidal volume (V_T) or the volume of each breath per kilogram of body weight remains relatively constant throughout life at about 5 to 7 mL/kg. Normal pediatric values for heart rate and temperature are provided in Tables 13–5 and 13–6.

Assessment of Respiratory Failure.—Like the neonate, the pediatric patient will exhibit similar clinical signs of respiratory distress and impending respira-

TABLE 13–5.
Normal Heart Rates for Infants and Children*

Age	Heart Rate (beats/min)		
	Resting (Awake)	Resting (Sleeping)	Exercise (Fever)
Newborn	100–180	80–160	Up to 220
1 wk–3 mo	100–220	80–200	Up to 220
3 mo–2 yr	80–150	70–120	Up to 200
2 yr–10 yr	70–110	60–90	Up to 200
10 yr–adult	55–90	50–90	Up to 200

*From Gillette PC: Dysrhythmias, in Adams FH, Emmanouilides GC (eds): *Moss' Heart Disease in Infants, Children, and Adolescents*, ed 3. Baltimore, Williams & Wilkins Co, 1983, p 729. Used by permission.

TABLE 13–6.
Average Body Temperatures in Well Children Under Basal Conditions*

Age	Temperature	
	°F	°C
3 mo	99.4	37.5
6 mo	99.5	37.5
1 yr	99.7	37.7
3 yr	99.0	37.2
5 yr	98.6	37.0
7 yr	98.3	36.8
9 yr	98.1	36.7
11 yr	98.0	36.7
13 yr	97.8	36.6

*Modified from Lowrey GH: *Growth and Development of Children*, ed. 8. St Louis, Mosby–Year Book.

tory failure. Various diseases of the pulmonary or neuromuscular system along with head injury or trauma can cause acute respiratory failure. Additional causes of respiratory failure can result from the administration of certain pharmacologic agents, such as opiates. The resultant hypercapnia or hypoxemia determines the severity of respiratory failure.

Infants and children with impending respiratory failure can be identified as those with (1) an increased respiratory rate, effort, and diminished or abnormal breath sounds, (2) a decreased level or responsiveness to pain with a diminished level of consciousness, (3) poor musculoskeletal tone, and (4) cyanosis, individually or generally. A thorough assessment of respiratory function includes careful observation of respiratory mechanics. Inspection of the skin and mucous membranes for color will guide the clinician's assessment and decisions in the clinical management of the infant or child in respiratory failure.[4]

The respiratory rate often serves as the first indicator of respiratory distress in infants. Tachypnea without respiratory distress can indicate the presence of nonpulmonary causes such as metabolic acidosis associated with shock, severe dehydration, chronic renal insufficiency, inborn errors of metabolism, salicylate poisoning, and diabetic ketoacidosis. This "quiet tachypnea" is the result of the body's attempt to maintain a normal pH by increasing the minute ventilation ($\dot{V}_E$) which results in a compensatory response.[4] A slow respiratory rate is an ominous sign in the acutely ill infant or child. It may be caused by factors such as fatigue, hypothermia, and depression of the central nervous system (CNS). An infant or child that becomes fatigued in the midst of respiratory distress will need prompt intervention.

The mechanics of respiration that signal impending respiratory failure in the infant or child are similar to those previously described for the newborn. The cause of respiratory distress can be determined by the presenting characteristic symptoms. In children with airway obstruction and alveolar disease, an increased level of work is required to facilitate breathing. Nasal flaring and intercostal, subcostal, and suprasternal inspiratory retractions may be noted. The increased work of breathing requires an increased cardiac output to keep up with the demand of the respiratory muscles. Respiratory acidosis may develop. The respiratory acidosis can become combined with a metabolic acidosis if the continued work to support breathing exceeds the ability to meet the increased demand of the tissues for O_2.

Signs such as stridor, prolonged expiration, grunting, and head bobbing are indicators of additional mechanical work effort. Head bobbing is especially crucial to note in that it indicates impending respiratory failure. Asymmetric chest expansion can be noted in the "seesaw" or rocking respirations that facilitate lung inflation with the chest drawn in on inspiration while the abdomen is thrust out. The presence of stridor, or high-pitch inspiratory sounds, may indicate an upper airway obstruction located between the trachea and the supraglottic space. Conditions such as congenital abnormalities, airway tumor, cyst, or vocal cord paralysis present with the signs of upper airway obstruction. More common causes include infections such as epiglotittis and croup. Foreign body aspiration also is a cause of upper airway obstruction in infants and children. The infant or child with asthma or bronchiolitis presents with prolonged expiration characterized by wheezing. This indicates that the bronchioles are obstructed due to the underlying disease. As described earlier in the section on respiratory distress in the newborn, grunting can be noted in infants and children whose disease results in the need to maintain a physiologic functional residual capacity (FRC). Grunting is noted in infants and children with atelectasis, alveolar collapse, loss of lung volume, pneumonia, pulmonary edema, and adult respiratory distress syndrome (ARDS).

The presence of cyanosis is a late indicator and inconsistent sign of respiratory failure. Cyanosis can best be identified in the mucous membranes of the mouth and nail beds. Peripheral cyanosis, cyanosis of the extremities, is most likely the result of shock or circulatory failure than pulmonary failure. The assessment of the severity of respiratory failure can be determined through the measurement of blood gases in the presence or absence of cyanosis.

The Pediatric Advance Life Support Program developed by the AAP and AHA is similar to the Neonatal Resuscitation Program in that it provides a construct for practitioners and clinicians to complete rapid assessments and provide interventions based on standardized protocols (Table 13–7).

Infant and pediatric cardiopulmonary resuscitation (CPR) interventions are based on the AHA's BLS protocol. The goal of management is to anticipate, identify, and correct compromised ventilatory and circulatory function in the infant and child. An in-depth description of the procedures for pediatric resuscitation can be found in the textbook on pediatric advanced life support developed by the AAP and AHA.[5]

Summary.—The basic approach in the management of the infant or child with respiratory failure is as follows (AHA BLS format): (1) secure an open airway, (2) initiate breathing, and (3) assess the circulation. If, despite the administration of free-flow O_2 concentration, the infant or child's ventilation is inadequate, with poor chest movement and diminished breath sounds, then assisted ventilation is initiated. The administration of gentle positive pressure breaths are given by either a mask-bag-valve device or by an ET tube–bag-valve system. The

TABLE 13–7.
Rapid Cardiopulmonary Assessment*

Respiratory Assessment	Cardiovascular Assessment
Airway patency	Circulation
Breathing	Heart rate
Rate	Blood pressure
Air entry	Peripheral pulses
Chest rise	Present/absent
Breath sounds	Volume
Stridor	Skin perfusion
Wheezing	Capillary refill time
Mechanics	Temperature
Retractions	Color
Grunting	Mottling
Accessory muscle use	CNS perfusion
Nasal flaring	Recognition of parents
Color	Reaction to pain
	Muscle tone
	Pupil size

*From Chameides L: *Textbook of Pediatric Advanced Life Support*. Dallas, American Heart Association/American Academy of Pediatrics, 1990, p 7. Used by permission.

administration of PPV is carefully timed and coordinated with the child's efforts. Positive pressure breaths that are not coordinated may be ineffective and cause retching, coughing, and gastric distention.[5]

Oxygen Delivery Systems for the Spontaneously Breathing Child in Respiratory Distress

Infants or children that are alert and present with signs of respiratory distress are immediately provided with the highest concentration of humidified O_2 available. The humidification is essential so that the child's small airway does not become obstructed with dried secretions. Heated humidification is preferable to cool so that hypothermia is not produced.

However, children with chronic respiratory insufficiency, such as bronchopulmonary dysplasia and advanced cystic fibrosis, should be carefully monitored since they have a characteristic chronically elevated $Paco_2$. The administration of high concentrations of O_2 may diminish the infant or child's respiratory drive and result in respiratory failure.

Alert children in respiratory distress assume a position that promotes airway patency. These children must be allowed to maintain their position of comfort and are not forced to lie supine since this may add to oxygen consumption ($\dot{V}o_2$) and increase their respiratory distress. Young alert children in respiratory distress are often frightened by O_2 masks and can be comforted by the parent holding the child and administering a flow of humidified O_2 by the child's nose and mouth. The infant or child that becomes somnolent or unconscious requires assistance in securing an open airway. The airway is opened by performing the head tilt–jaw thrust maneuver. The insertion of an oral or nasal airway will facilitate the patency of the airway by preventing the tongue from falling against the posterior wall of the pharynx. Suctioning of the mouth and nasal passages for secretions is also an adjunct intervention for achieving a clear airway.

Oxygen delivery systems for the infant and child can be divided into low flow and high flow systems. The systems depend on the $\dot{V}_E$ and can be adjusted to deliver O_2 within the range of 23% to 90%. For low flow systems, the O_2 from the flowmeter does not meet all the inspiratory requirements of the infant or child and room air is entrained. The high flow system provides enough O_2 to meet the inspiratory requirements and can also be adjusted to deliver a low flow O_2 concentration using a blender. The systems are: (1) nasal cannulas, (2) O_2 hoods, (3) O_2 tents, (4) O_2 face tents, and (5) O_2 masks.

Nasal cannula O_2 delivery is appropriate for infants and children that require only a minimal amount of supplemental O_2 (about 22%–42%).[4] The O_2 hood is well tolerated by infants up until 1 year of age. It allows the clinician easy access to the chest, trunk, and extremities. The O_2 hood is a reliable source of controlled O_2 delivery since it can be powered by a blender or similar device.

The O_2 tent is suitable for the large infant or child over 1 year of age. The O_2 tent is capable of maintaining a fractional concentration of oxygen in inspired gas (FIO_2) of 0.5 with high flows, but this is especially difficult since the tent is frequency manipulated and tends to mix with room air. The face tent or face shield provides high flow O_2 that is often well tolerated by children. An O_2 flow rate of 10 to 15 L/min is required. The face tent is large and permits access to the child's face for procedures such as suctioning. Stable O_2 concentrations cannot be guaranteed. It is usually used for an FIO_2 of less than 0.40. Oxygen masks for infants and children are available in various shapes and sizes. A simple O_2 mask will deliver approximately 35% to 60% O_2 with a flow rate of 6 to 10 L/min. A minimum flow of 6 L/min is necessary to prevent rebreathing of exhaled CO_2. A partial rebreathing mask provides a reliable concentration of inspired O_2 at 50% to 60%. Generally a flow of 10 to 12 L/min is required. A nonrebreathing mask has the capability of providing an inspired O_2 concentration of 90% to 100% with an O_2 flow rate of 10 to 12 L/min and a well-secured face seal.[5]

Manual Resuscitation Bags

The infant or child can be ventilated effectively with a face mask or ET tube connected to an anesthesia or self-inflating bag (see Figs 13–8 and 13–9). The size of the ventilation bag varies for the infant and child. The neonate and infant require a small ventilation bag with a capacity between 250 and 500 mL. The small infant and young child require a ventilation bag with a capacity of from 750 to 1,000 mL. The older, larger child can be ventilated with either a 1,000-mL bag or an adult-sized bag. The mask must cover the child's nose and mouth securely.

Positive Pressure Ventilation by Endotracheal Tube–Bag-Valve Device

After initial attempts to provide PPV with a mask bag-valve system, if the child fails to improve or requires prolonged ventilatory assistance, the placement of an ET tube is the next step in respiratory stabilization. The advantages of ET tube placement are: (1) the ET tube isolates the larynx and trachea from the pharynx and this helps to prevent aspiration and gastic distention; (2) the presence of the ET tube allows the clinician to suction the airway for secretions; (3) the ET tube also serves as a mode of delivery for certain resuscitation medications such as epinephrine and atropine; (4) PPV via an ET tube–bag-valve system is used to improve the $\dot{V}/\dot{Q}$ match. The application of positive end-expiratory pressure (PEEP) in conjunction with improving the residual capacity of the lungs can promote oxygenation and ventilation.[5] Steps in pediatric intubation are similar to those for infants.

NEONATAL VENTILATORY SUPPORT

Recognizing Need for Mechanical Ventilation

The neonate, infant, or child that requires continued PPV via manual resuscitator to maintain oxygenation needs to be placed on a system of mechanical ventilation and monitored for ongoing cardiopulmonary status. The RCP is responsible for the decision to initiate mechanical ventilation in collaboration with the physician responsible for the management of the infant or child's plan of care. The nurse works with the RCP to provide ongoing assessment and evaluation of the clinical management provided for the neonate, infant, or child during the postresuscitation and stabilization phase of care in the intensive care unit (ICU).

Goals of Assisted Ventilation

The primary goal of mechanical ventilation for infants and children is to promote gas exchange and to decrease the amount of effort (work) to sustain ventilation.

Neonatal Blood Gas Interpretation

A complete assessment of gas exchange requires knowledge of (1) oxygenation and O_2 transport; (2) ventilation and CO_2 transport; and (3) blood gas interpretation (see Chapter 3). Physical assessment provides additional information for the clinician in determining the quality of gas exchange. Observations of skin and mucous membrane color along with a measurement of capillary refill and tissue perfusion status provide useful physical assessment data.

Neonatal and infant blood gas values have ranges that are different from pediatric and adult values. Table 13–8 shows acceptable ranges for management of the neonate on mechanical ventilation. In general, the accepted pH range for

TABLE 13–8.

Acceptable Blood Gas and pH Values for Management of the Neonate on Mechanical Ventilation*

	Age (hr)	
	≤72	>72
pH	7.25–7.45	7.25–7.45
$Paco_2$ (mm Hg)	35–45	45–55
Pao_2 (mm Hg)	60–90	50–80

*Term infant Pao_2 = 75 mm Hg on room air; $Paco_2$ < 40 mm Hg. Premature infants Pao_2 = 65 mm Hg; $Paco_2$ < 50 mm Hg.

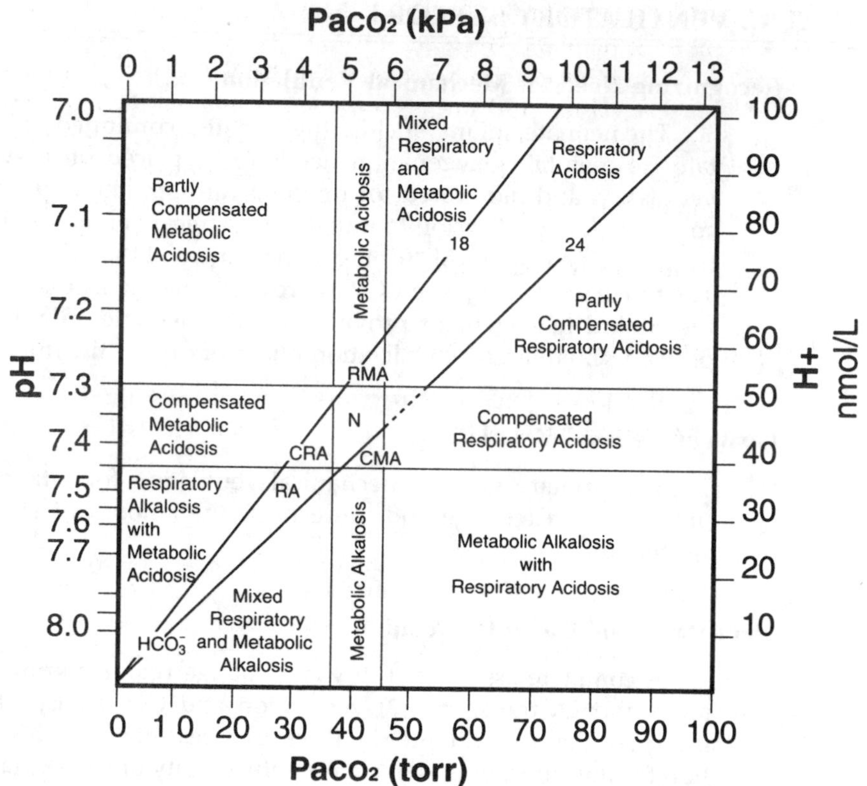

FIG 13–11.

Neonatal acid-base map. *N* = normal acid-base status; *CRA* = compensated respiratory alkalosis; *CMA* = compensated metabolic alkalosis; *RMA* = mixed respiratory and metabolic acidosis; *RA* = respiratory alkalosis. (From Chatburn RL, Carlo WA: Assessment of neonatal gas exchange in Carlo WA, Chatburn RL (eds): *Neonatal Respiratory Care.* St Louis, Mosby–Year Book, Inc, 1988, p 58. Used by permission.)

a sick neonate is from 7.25 to 7.45. The lower pH range is tolerated because of the risk associated with the administration of sodium bicarbonate. There is often concern over increasing alveolar ventilation and the increased risk of pulmonary barotrauma.

The neonatal acid-base map (Fig 13–11) assists with the process of determining the clinical diagnosis based on a respiratory or metabolic process. As an example, a very premature neonate with a high partial pressure of carbon dioxide (P_{CO_2}) along with a high HCO_3^- would most likely have been given too much sodium bicarbonate and also has respiratory acidosis occurring at the same time. The diagnosis of metabolic alkalosis with a component of respiratory acidosis is confirmed by this map. This system is used as a basis for the management of neonatal ventilation.[14]

The interpretation of blood gas disorders, their compensatory mechanisms, normal values, and normal ranges are generally straightforward. Figure 13–12 illustrates the mental decision-making process helpful in interpreting blood gases. This flow chart does not cover every possible combination of blood gas values but serves as a useful instructional and diagnostic algorithm for the practitioner. Table 13–8 gives acceptable limits of blood gas and pH values for infants for use with the algorithm.

Respiratory Physiology in Newborn

The physiologic mechanisms that control ventilation in the newborn are different from those in the adult. The infant has a much higher risk of developing respiratory failure. In fact, it is one of the leading causes of morbidity and mortality in neonates.[12] The occurrence of apneic episodes and periodic breathing is not unusual in newborn infants. They are known to occur most commonly during sleep. These patterns of breathing are even more common in preterm babies. Apneic and periodic breathing are associated with bradycardia and hypoxia. Frequently, premature infants require intervention such as tactile stimulation, oscillating or bumper beds, or medications like theophylline or caffeine to stimulate breathing.

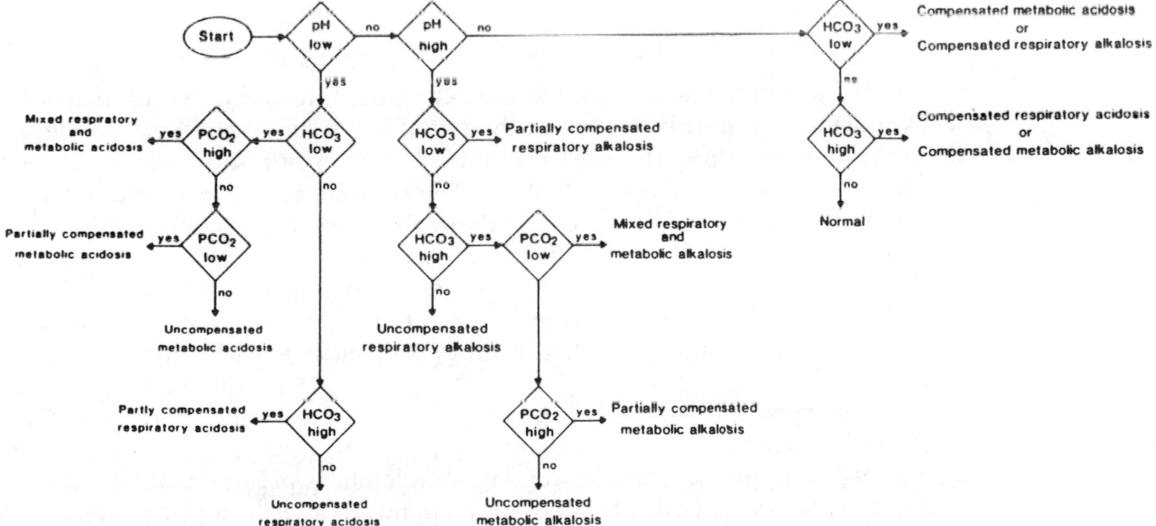

FIG 13–12.
Blood gas flow chart illustrating the mental process by which a set of blood gas values may be interpreted. (From Hess D: *Respir Care* 1984; 29:375. Used by permission.)

In addition to abnormal breathing patterns, the response to arterial CO_2 and O_2 are different in the infant. Premature infants have a reduced response to CO_2 compared to adults. The presence of hypoxia seems to further reduce the CO_2 response. They are also less responsive to hypoxia than adults. Premature infants respond less to low PO_2 than do full-term infants. The latter respond to hypoxia with periods of stimulated breathing followed by apneic episodes.[12] As a result, whenever an infant exhibits periods of apnea, it is important to evaluate arterial blood gases to assess oxygenation. This can be followed, but not replaced, by continuous monitoring with pulse oximetry or transcutaneous monitoring (see Chapter 9). Evaluation of Pa_{O_2} is very important since infants can have a Pa_{O_2} of 40 mm Hg before they become cyanotic (see Fig 13–7).

Besides differences in control of breathing, neonates also differ with respect to lung mechanics. Their chest wall is not as rigid as that of the adult because of the presence of more cartilage in their thoracic skeletal structure. Their very small conductive airways increase resistance to gas flow. The presence of secretions worsens this problem. In addition, they tend to have a lower lung compliance than adults. When lung compliance is further reduced from disorders such as hyaline membrane disease or pneumonia, the condition is more pronounced. When they make a strong inspiratory effort, intrapleural pressures become very negative and the chest wall tends to collapse inward. This causes paradoxical movement of the chest wall and abdomen. As mentioned, the resulting high work of breathing can quickly lead to respiratory muscle fatigue and respiratory failure.

Indications for Ventilatory Support

As in the adult, determining the moment when intervention with mechanical ventilatory support is needed in the infant is not an exact science. A single criterion for establishing the presence of respiratory failure does not exist. The practitioner must rely on several criteria. The decision to use mechanical ventilation is based on the need to decrease the work of breathing, decrease $\dot{V}_{O_2}$, and decrease cardiac work. For small children, the decision is most often made on the basis of arterial blood gas analysis, i.e., respiratory acidosis or severe hypoxemia, along with an increased respiratory rate and use of accessory muscles. Indications for mechanical ventilatory support include the following[9, 10]:

1. Marked hypoxemia—a Pa_{O_2} of less than 50 to 60 mm Hg on an F_{IO_2} greater than 60% to 80%.
2. A rising Pa_{CO_2} greater than 50 mm Hg with a falling pH of less than 7.20.
3. Frequent apneic episodes that do not respond to other forms of therapy (e.g., medications, CPAP).
4. Premature infants weighing less than 1,000 g with accompanying asphyxia or respiratory distress.

Ventilator Selection

Ideally, a neonatal ventilator should have the following characteristics[9]:

1. Small size, low cost, and quiet.
2. Minimal system compliance and resistance to breathing.
3. Visible and audible alarm systems.
4. Sensitive and rapid response time.
5. Availability of intermittent positive pressure ventilation (IPPV), intermittent mandatory ventilation (IMV), and CPAP or PEEP modes.
6. Respiratory rates up to 150 breaths/min.
7. Tidal volume range of 10 to 200 mL.

The clinician must choose between volume control and pressure control modes. This may involve the selection of a particular type of ventilator because all ventilators do not conveniently offer the ability to deliver both modes. Most "infant" ventilators are designed to be used primarily in the pressure control mode, meaning that the clinician can set the parameters that define the airway pressure waveforms (e.g., peak inspiratory pressure, PEEP, inspiratory-expiratory ratio (I/E), and rate). On the other hand, most larger children are ventilated with "adult" ventilators that are designed primarily for use in the volume control mode, meaning that the clinician can set inspiratory flow rate and V_T.

There are no conclusive scientific data suggesting that pressure-controlled ventilation is superior to volume-controlled ventilation. However, pressure-controlled ventilation is often preferred for small children because the ventilators are less expensive and somewhat easier to manage although the gas exchange of the patient is harder to control. The advantages of pressure-controlled ventilation are listed below.[9]

Initial Settings for Mechanical Ventilation

Initial settings for pressure-controlled ventilation of infants are shown in Table 13–9.[6, 9, 10] For volume ventilation, a V_T of 6 to 8 mL/kg is set. Other parameters will parallel those in Table 13–9. Minute ventilation is calculated in terms of body surface area (BSA) since infants and children have such a wide range of sizes. BSA is estimated in square meters by the following equations:

For neonates and infants weighing 2.5 to 20 kg:

$$\text{BSA} = \frac{(3.6)(\text{weight}) + 9}{100}$$

For children with weights ranging between 20.1 and 40 kg:

TABLE 13–9.
Suggested Initial Ventilator Settings for Newborn Infants*

	With Normal Lungs	With Noncompliant (Stiff) Lungs or RDS
PIP	12–18 cm H_2O	20–25 cm H_2O
Respiratory rate	10–20 breaths/min	20–40 breaths/min
PEEP	2–3 cm H_2O	4–5 cm H_2O
Flow rate	4–10 L/min	4–10 L/min
Inspiratory time	0.4–0.8 sec	0.3–0.5 sec
I/E ratio	1:2–1:10	1:1–1:3
F_{IO_2}	To maintain Pa_{O_2} > 50 mm Hg	To maintain Pa_{O_2} > 50 mm Hg

*RDS = respiratory distress syndrome; PIP = peak inspiratory pressure; PEEP = positive end-expiratory pressure; I/E ratio = inspiratory-expiratory ratio; F_{IO_2} = fractional concentration of oxygen in inspired gas; Pa_{O_2} = partial pressure of arterial oxygen.

$$BSA = \frac{(2.5)(\text{weight}) + 33}{100}$$

Figure 13–13 shows the required $\dot{V}_E$ per square meter of BSA required to achieve the desired Pa_{CO_2} for a given dead space–tidal volume ratio (V_D/V_T). The $\dot{V}_E$ required is multiplied by the calculated BSA to get the $\dot{V}_E$ that must be delivered by the ventilator.

Available Controls for Adjusting Mechanical Ventilation in the Newborn

Ventilator adjustments are made on the basis of arterial blood gas analysis and clinical signs and symptoms. Prior to reviewing how to make adjustments based on Pa_{O_2}, Pa_{CO_2}, and pH, we will look at the controls available on most pressure-controlled ventilators.

Peak Inspiratory Pressure.—On a pressure-controlled ventilator, this is a set value. In general, an increase in PIP results in a decrease in Pa_{CO_2}, and an increase in V_T, alveolar ventilation, mean airway pressure ($\overline{P}aw$), and oxygenation. On a volume-controlled ventilator, PIP changes when the V_T is changed, when the inspiratory flow rate is changed, or when lung mechanics change.

The level of PIP needed is based on arterial blood gas values, O_2 saturation, chest expansion, breath sounds, and chest film findings. Low PIP levels (<30 cm H_2O) result in low V_T values which may reduce the risk of pulmonary air leak, barotrauma, and bronchopulmonary dysplasia (BPD). The patient may recover more rapidly because of fewer ventilator-imposed problems. On the other hand, low PIP may not be adequate to ventilate the lungs. Pa_{CO_2} may rise as Pa_{O_2} falls and $\dot{V}/\dot{Q}$ mismatch increases.

High PIP (>30 cm H_2O) may be needed if lung compliance is low. If compliance improves, the PIP must be watched closely to avoid inadvertent increases in VT that would increase the risk of pulmonary air leaks, barotrauma, and BPD.

Respiratory Rate.—Normally, increasing the respiratory rate results in an increase in $\dot{V}$E, a lower PaCO_2, and a higher pH. Very high rates (>75 breaths/min) may increase air trapping (auto-PEEP) and increased FRC because of shorter exhalation time. This may increase PaCO_2 and $\dot{V}$E may decrease. High rates that are achieved without gas trapping can be used to produce respiratory alkalosis which can be used in the treatment of persistent pulmonary hypertension. Alkalosis reduces pulmonary vascular resistance and may increase oxygenation. This can help in the closure of a patent ductus arteriosus.

Inspiratory Time, Expiratory Time, and I/E Ratio.—Inspiratory time is normally set at 0.4 seconds or more to begin. This usually provides time for the pressure delivery to result in an adequate VT. The time needed for complete inspiration or expiration will depend on the overall time constant of the infant's lungs. During pressure-controlled ventilation, about four to five time constants

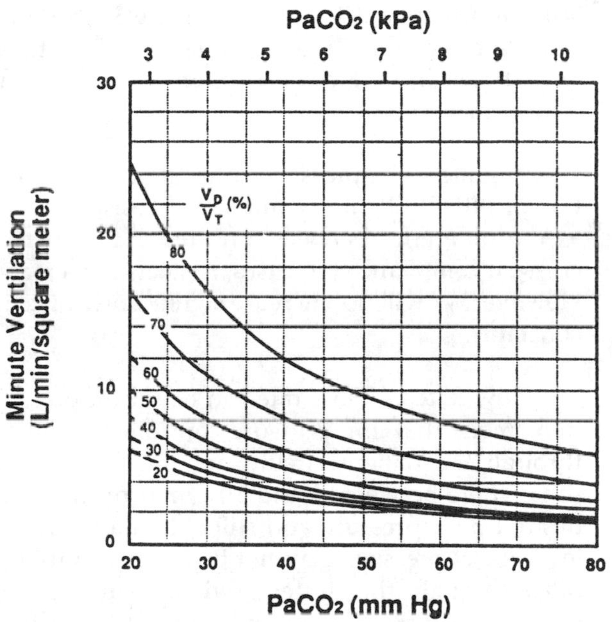

FIG 13–13.
Graph relates minute ventilation ($\dot{V}$E) and arterial carbon dioxide tension (PaCO_2) for different values of physiologic dead space–tidal volume ratio (VD/VT) (assuming atmospheric pressure is 760 mm Hg [101 kPa]), and body temperature is 37° C and carbon dioxide output is 112 mL × min^{-1} m^{-2}). (From Chatburn R: *Respir Care* 1991; 36:571. Used by permission.)

are needed to achieve 98% to 99% inflation or deflation of the lungs. This must be kept in mind when setting inspiratory and expiratory times. Normal lung compliance in the newborn is about 0.003 to 0.006 L/cm H_2O (3–6 mL/cm H_2O). In infants with RDS this may be much lower—0.5 to 1.0 mL/cm H_2O. Normal airway resistance is about 20 to 40 cm H_2O/L/sec. The ET tube can increase airway resistance to 50 to 100 cm H_2O/L/sec.

For example, if compliance were 0.005 L/cm H_2O and resistance 30 cm H_2O/L/sec, the time constant would be 0.005 L/cm H_2O × 30 cm H_2O/L/sec = 0.15 second. An inspiratory (or expiratory) time needed to provide 99% lung volume change would be 5 × 0.15 second = 0.75 second. Using less than five time constants (99%) may result in incomplete delivery of the V_T during inspiration. Using an expiratory time of less than five time constants may result in incomplete exhalation. Five time constants or more will allow expiratory time. Pressure-controlled ventilators usually have inspiratory time controls. You can calculate total cycle time, inspiratory and expiratory times, and I/E, as shown in Chapter 6.

I/E ratios are generally set as follows: for newborn infants with normal lungs, and during weaning, an I/E ratio of 1:2 to 1:10 is set; for newborn infants with noncompliant (stiff) lungs or RDS, an I/E ratio of 1:1 to 1:3 is set. Inverse ratios are occasionally used to increase $\overline{P}aw$ to improve oxygenation. It has the risk of air trapping since expiratory times are usually very short and cardiac output may fall.

Volume.—On pressure-controlled ventilators, volume is not set. It is a function of PIP, PEEP, lung compliance, resistance, and time. In general, V_T increases as the difference between PIP and PEEP increases. Also, volume tends to increase if compliance increases, resistance decreases, or inspiratory time increases. However, V_T will not increase significantly once inspiratory time equals five time constants.

Flow Rates.—Flow rate can be set on pressure-controlled infant ventilators. Remember that for pressure-controlled ventilation, the set flow is the flow through the patient circuit, not the flow into the lungs. Initially flow is set somewhere between 4 and 10 L/min or at a value high enough to deliver the desired peak pressure and still obtain a pressure plateau. If the flow rate is too low, preset pressure may not be reached until the very end of inspiration. Flow rates through the system, whether for machine-delivered or spontaneous breaths, must be high enough to meet the patient's inspiratory demand.

While volume ventilators sometimes have a variety of waveforms available for delivering flow, such as constant (rectangular) and ascending ramp, infant pressure-controlled ventilators do not. With pressure controllers, changing flow rate can alter the pressure waveform. At low flow rates, a curved waveform is seen. This is sometimes described as an exponential waveform (Fig 13–14). This has the advantage of a smoother rise to PIP and a lower $\overline{P}$aw. At higher flow rates, the waveform is nearly rectangular. This has the advantage of increasing $\overline{P}$aw which helps improve oxygenation.

Mean Airway Pressure.—The $\overline{P}$aw is not set on the ventilator, but it is a very important part of infant ventilation. To review, $\overline{P}$aw is the average pressure during one total respiratory cycle (see Chapter 7). In infants, it has long been known that oxygenation is strongly affected by $\overline{P}$aw. This value is often reported on the control panel of the ventilator as one of the many monitored parameters. Increases in $\overline{P}$aw tend to improve oxygenation. However, increases can also reduce venous return and cardiac output.

Factors that increase $\overline{P}$aw include: increase in PIP, PEEP, I/E ratio (long inspiratory times), and waveform (the longer the pressure plateau, as occurs with high flow rates, the higher the $\overline{P}$aw). An optimal $\overline{P}$aw is somewhere in the neighborhood of 10 to 15 cm H_2O. On the other hand, with acute phases of RDS the $\overline{P}$aw may need to be increased to maintain oxygenation. Once severe disease states have resolved and lungs return to normal, the $\overline{P}$aw can be reduced.

Inspired Oxygen Tension (F_{IO_2}).—In addition to $\overline{P}$aw as a means to improve oxygenation, the traditional methods of F_{IO_2} and PEEP offer the normal alternatives. Inspired O_2 concentration must be regulated to maintain Pa_{O_2}, while minimizing the risk of O_2 toxicity. For premature infants, Pa_{O_2} in general should be maintained between 50 and 88 mm Hg, and should not exceed 100 mm Hg to minimize the risk of RLF. Once an F_{IO_2} of greater than 0.6 is reached, most clinicians look to PEEP as an alternative method to improve oxygenation, hoping to avoid O_2-related problems such as RLF and O_2 toxicity. When lung

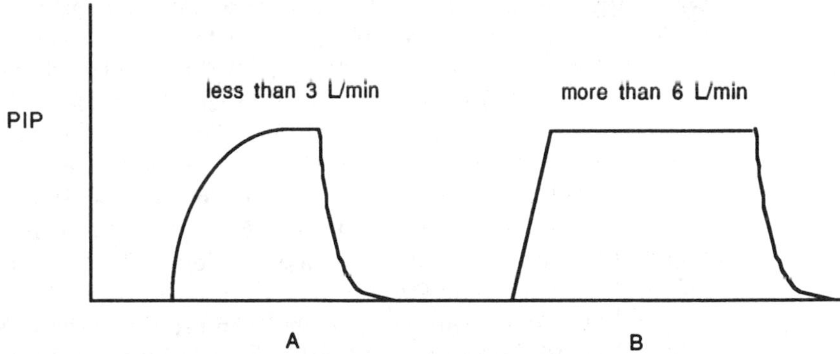

FIG 13–14.
Changes in waveform patterns on pressure-controlled ventilators used in infants. At a low flow rate, a rounded waveform is seen. At high flow rates, the pattern is nearly rectangular (constant). *PIP* = peak inspiratory pressure.

condition improves and F_{IO_2} can be lowered, it is usually done in increments of 1% to 2% while maintaining Pa_{O_2} above 50 mm Hg.

PEEP.—Whereas in adults PEEP is used to recruit atelectatic areas of lung tissue, in infants it is more often used to help maintain alveolar inflation and prevent collapse during exhalation. The use of PEEP may help improve $\dot{V}/\dot{Q}$ mismatch, reduce shunt, improve lung compliance, and improve oxygenation. Problems associated with PEEP in the neonate, as in the adult, are related to the transmission of positive pressure to the intrapleural space. This can increase pulmonary vascular resistance, and reduce venous return and cardiac output. This will compromise O_2 delivery to the tissues. It can also lead to increased dead space. Hyperinflation may occur with PEEP greater than 10 cm H_2O, leading to CO_2 retention. PEEP is indicated when Pa_{O_2} is less than 50 mm Hg on an F_{IO_2} of greater than 0.6. It is generally used in all newborns at levels of 2 to 5 cm H_2O (see Table 13–9). PEEP and F_{IO_2} are titrated to maintain a Pa_{O_2} of 50 to 70 mm Hg.

When PEEP is used with a time-cycled, pressure control mode, its use narrows the pressure amplitude (PIP − PEEP). This could reduce volume delivery to the lungs and thus reduce ventilation. On pressure-controlled ventilation when PEEP is increased, PIP may need to be increased to maintain the same ventilating pressure (PIP − PEEP = ΔP). If it is not increased, the pressure gradient used to establish the V_T will decrease and Pa_{CO_2} may increase.

Management of Variables During Pressure-Controlled Ventilation

When using pressure-controlled ventilation, the V_T is not set on the ventilator, is usually not measured, and thus is unknown. Therefore, the clinician must have at least a general understanding of how ventilator settings interact with lung mechanics to achieve gas exchange. Figure 13–15 illustrates these interactions. In this figure, the time constant is calculated by multiplying compliance times resistance (see Chapter 2). The relationship of V_T, flow, rate, I/E ratio, and inspiratory and expiratory times is discussed in Chapter 6. The pressure gradient is the difference between PIP and the end-expiratory pressure. Values affecting $\overline{P}aw$, such as I/E ratio, flow rate, and pattern, and PEEP are evaluated in Chapter 7. Within reasonable limits, as $\overline{P}aw$ increases, mean lung volume increases, which usually results in less shunt and better oxygenation. Unfortunately, the risk of cardiovascular depression and pulmonary barotrauma also increase.

Basically, the compliance of the respiratory system determines how much volume will be delivered by the pressure gradient generated by the ventilator. If compliance decreases, as it does when RDS worsens, the delivered V_T will decrease even though the set pressure gradient stays the same. Respiratory system resistance affects the time it takes to deliver the V_T. If resistance changes,

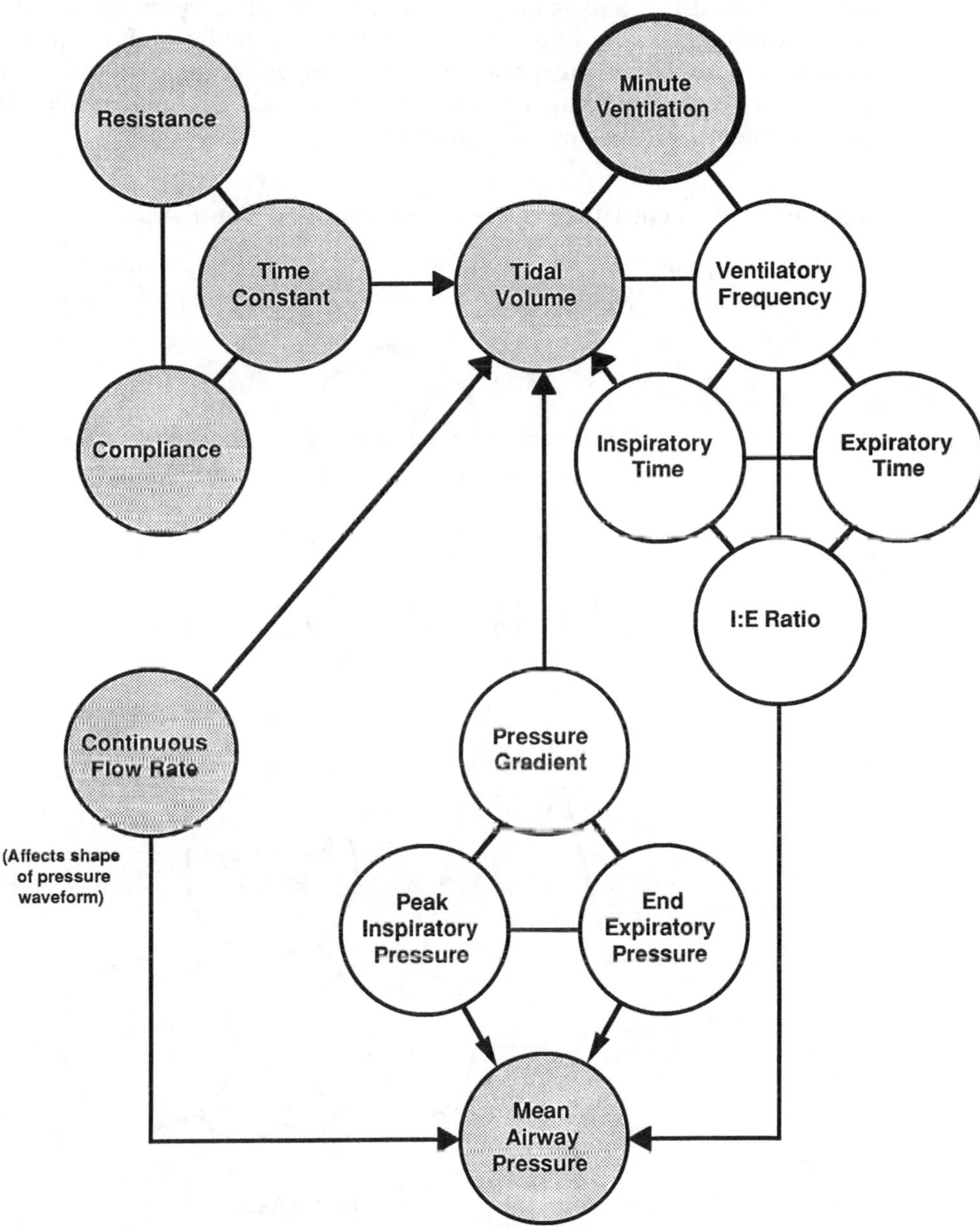

FIG 13–15.
Factors affecting pressure-controlled ventilation.

for example, due to secretions in the ET tube, it will take longer to deliver an adequate VT. If this time is longer than the set inspiratory time, the patient will be hypoventilated. Use of a volume monitor may be helpful. Frequent assessments of gas exchange must also be made using either invasive procedures, like arterial blood gas sampling, or noninvasive methods, such as pulse oximetry or transcutaneous monitoring (see Chapter 9).

Volume-Controlled Ventilation vs Pressure-Controlled Ventilation

In our opinion, patients who initially can be oxygenated and ventilated easily by manual ventilation and who do not have significant lung disease

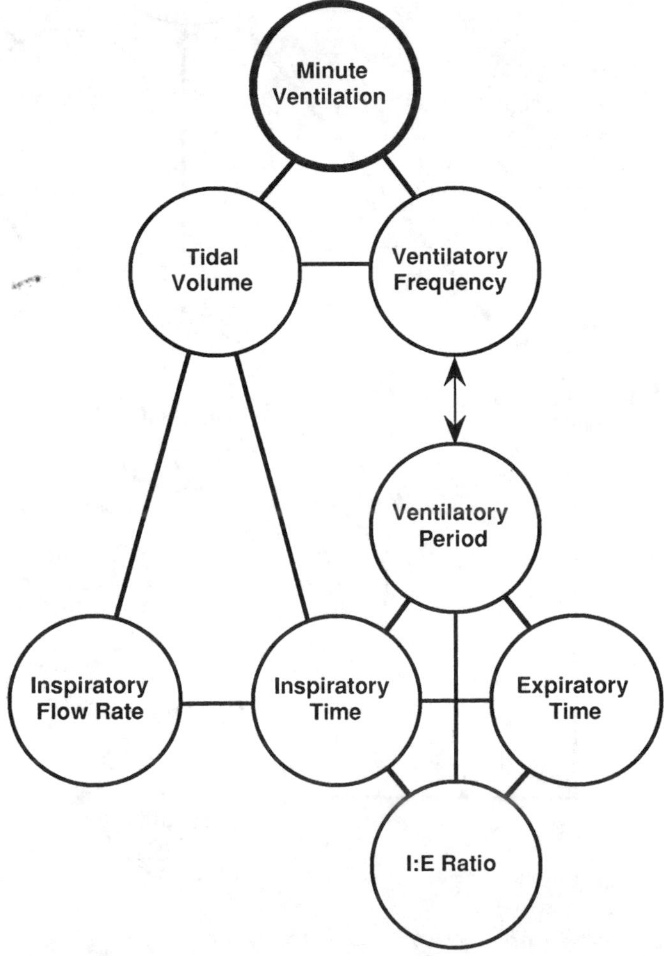

FIG 13–16.
Factors affecting volume-controlled ventilation.

should be ventilated with a volume control mode with VT in the range of 5 to 6 mL/kg, and minimal PEEP (e.g., 2–3 cm H_2O) and no inspiratory hold. Theoretical data suggest that for a given VT, an ascending ramp inspiratory flow waveform (if available) minimizes the work of distending the lungs. This may minimize the risk of barotrauma and minimize mean intrapleural pressure. The latter reduces the risk of hemodynamic compromise. Figure 13–16 illustrates the interaction of variables that takes place during volume-controlled ventilation (see Chapter 6). On the other hand, these same patients may also be candidates for pressure-supported ventilation. It may be that for patients with normal lungs, the mode of ventilation has no clinically important effect on gas exchange.

Patients who have surfactant-deficient lungs (e.g., both RDS and ARDS), or who are difficult to oxygenate with volume-controlled ventilation, need to be managed with pressure-controlled ventilation, specifically with a time-cycled, pressure-limited mode, and which, preferably, provides VT monitoring. One might consider switching from volume-controlled to pressure-controlled ventilation when the PaO_2/FIO_2 ratio is below 100, peak airway pressure (with I/E = 1:1) is higher than 35 cm H_2O, and PEEP exceeds 8 cm H_2O. The pressure gradient is set to deliver a VT of about 5 to 7 mL/kg. Frequency is set no higher than that required to maintain the desired $PaCO_2$, and PEEP is adjusted to maintain oxygenation at the lowest FIO_2. Inspiratory time is set just long enough to deliver the desired VT, and expiratory time just long enough to allow complete expiration of that VT.

Indications for High-Frequency Ventilation

If the patient has life-threatening barotrauma in the form of pulmonary interstitial emphysema or bronchopleural fistula, a high $PaCO_2$ despite all efforts to optimize ventilation, or if the $\overline{P}aw$ is unusually high, then a trial of high-frequency ventilation (HFV) is warranted. The idea here is to carry the small VT–high PEEP approach to the extreme. This can be accomplished with a HFV rather than trying to increase the rate on a conventional ventilator. Conventional ventilator control mechanisms and delivery circuits make HFV inefficient.

One possible index of the need for HFV is the pressure cost of oxygenation. This can be calculated by dividing the $\overline{P}aw$ by the $P(A - a)O_2$ gradient. When this is equal to about 100 cm H_2O, then HFV is indicated. We have been successful with high-frequency jet ventilation at frequencies of 100 to 250 cpm, and the I/E fixed at about 1:3. Adolescents and large children need lower frequencies than do premature infants to prevent gas trapping. Gas trapping is suspected if a ventilator parameter change seems to cause an increase in both PaO_2 and $PaCO_2$. The pressure gradient or amplitude (PIP − PEEP) is adjusted to obtain the desired $PaCO_2$ while $\overline{P}aw$ is adjusted (via PEEP) to control oxygenation. The ventilatory frequency is usually not changed once an optimal rate is found, as small changes (e.g., 10 cpm) have negligible effect on gas exchange.

The underlying philosophy for either conventional ventilation or HFV is to maintain open alveoli throughout the ventilatory cycle by using $\overline{P}aw$ as an index of mean lung volume and then to use either a small-to-normal V_T for compliant lungs or a very small V_T for noncompliant lungs at high risk for overdistention.

Making Parameter Changes

Once the method of ventilation is selected and ventilation has begun, an arterial blood gas sample is obtained to determine the level of ventilation and oxygenation. The results are compared with monitored pulse oximetry or transcutaneous monitor readings to establish a baseline. If arterial blood gas results are outside of acceptable limits, then a change in some variable needs to be made. In the newborn, any change is done in small increments and is followed by another blood gas analysis. Table 13–10 shows the incremental changes in some common variables.[9, 10]

Increasing Oxygenation.—In general, to improve Pa_{O_2}, F_{IO_2} is increased to about 0.6, and PEEP is increased, if it has not already been done, to greater than 5 cm H_2O. Changes in Pa_{CO_2} need to be evaluated at this point to be sure PEEP has not increased dead space. Then, PIP is increased up to 25 cm H_2O in steps of 1 to 2 cm H_2O at a time. Next, the rate may be increased up to about 45 breaths/min in appropriate steps. The rate adjustment may require inspiratory time to be shortened to less than expiratory time so that air trapping is avoided. If the Pa_{O_2} is still unacceptable after these changes, then PIP and F_{IO_2} are increased further in careful steps. If oxygenation continues to be a problem, a trial of longer inspiratory times and possible reversed I/E ratios (usually after sedating the patient) can be used. It may take as long as 24 hours for significant improvement to occur. The general philosophy is to use small V_T values and high PEEP rather than large V_T values and low PEEP.[1] Once the desired Pa_{O_2} is achieved, it is maintained and monitored closely in case the infant's lung condition changes.

Changing Pa_{CO_2} Through Changes in Ventilation.—If Pa_{CO_2} is high and the pH acidotic (respiratory acidosis), ventilation needs to be increased to achieve a Pa_{CO_2} of less than 50 mm Hg and a pH range of 7.25 to 7.45. The first step is to

TABLE 13–10.
A Guideline for Changing Variables During Ventilation of the Neonate*

Parameter	Increase	Decrease
F_{IO_2}	5%–10%	1%–2%
PIP	1–2 cm H_2O	1–2 cm H_2O
PEEP	1 cm H_2O	1 cm H_2O
Rate	2–3 breaths/min	1–2 breaths/min

*Data from references 9, 10.

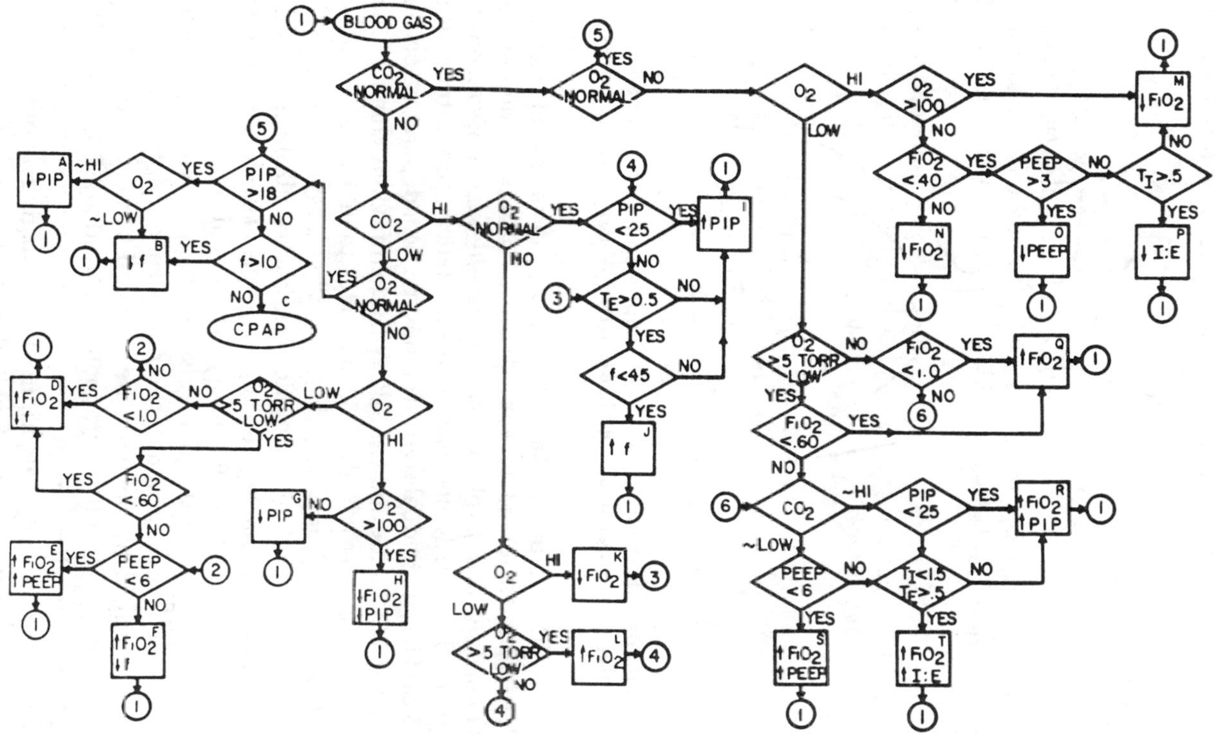

FIG 13–17.

Algorithm for management of RDS with an infant ventilator. F_{IO_2} = fractional concentration of oxygen in inspired gas; *PIP* = peak inspiratory pressure; T_I = inspiratory time; f = respiratory rate; *PEEP* = positive end-expiratory pressure; *I:E* = inspiratory-expiratory ratio; T_E = expiratory time; *CPAP* = continuous positive-airway pressure. (From Chatburn RL, Carlo WA, Lough MD: *Resp Care* 1983; 28:1579. Used by permission.)

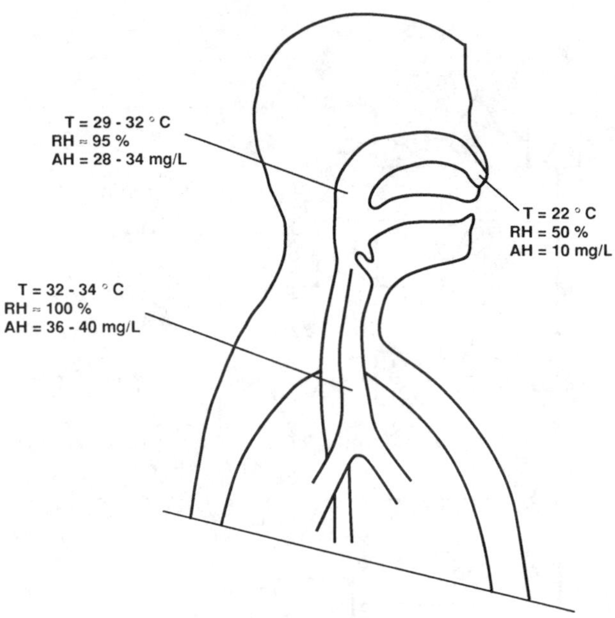

FIG 13–18.
Heat and humidification guidelines. *T* = temperature; *RH* = relative humidity; *AH* = absolute humidity. (From Chatburn RL: *J Pediatr* 1989; 114:417. Used by permission.)

increase the PIP in steps (see Table 13–10) until PIP is 25 cm H_2O. If $Paco_2$ is still high, the rate is increased in appropriate steps up to the upper limit of 45 breaths/min, if needed. Expiratory time is usually kept at greater than 0.5 second at this point. If there is no change in ventilation status, the PIP is increased above 25 cm H_2O in gradual steps. The next option, depending on the expiratory time, is to adjust the rate and the PIP. With the previous changes, the Pao_2 needs to be checked. If it is less than 50 mm Hg, then Fio_2 or PEEP, or both, are increased.

If $Paco_2$ is low and pH alkalotic (respiratory alkalosis), ventilation needs to be decreased to achieve the desired levels. The first step is to check the Pao_2 and make sure it is satisfactory. Then reduce the PIP if it is above 25 cm H_2O by 1 to 2 cm H_2O. If PIP is less than 25 cm H_2O, then reduce the rate first by 1 to 2 breaths/min. If the rate is changed, the inspiratory time may need to be changed to maintain the proper I/E ratio. If the $Paco_2$ is still less than 35 mm Hg, then PIP is gradually reduced by 1 to 2 cm H_2O until the correct $Paco_2$ is reached.

Figure 13–17 gives an algorithm for managing a pressure-limited, time-cycled infant ventilator for an infant with RDS. This was developed by Chatburn and associates.[7] The preceding section describes some of the steps of this algorithm. While it may, at first glance, seem complicated and difficult to follow, it

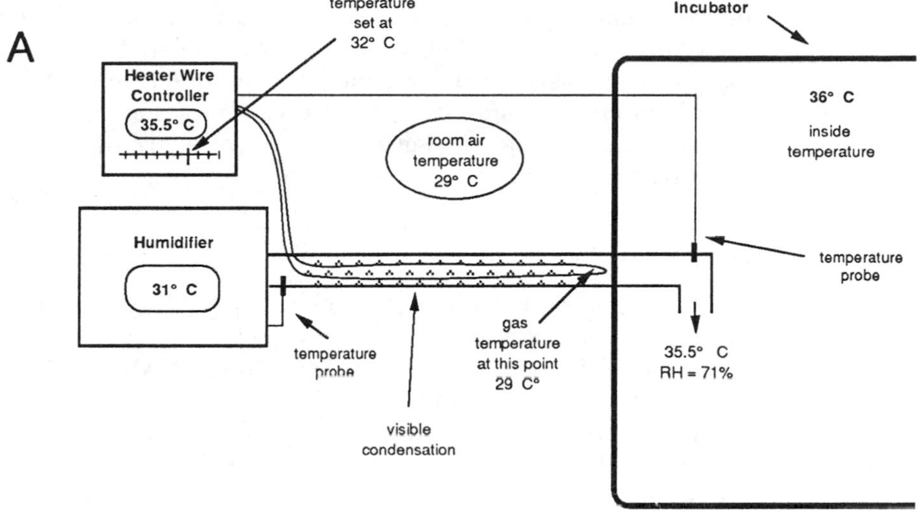

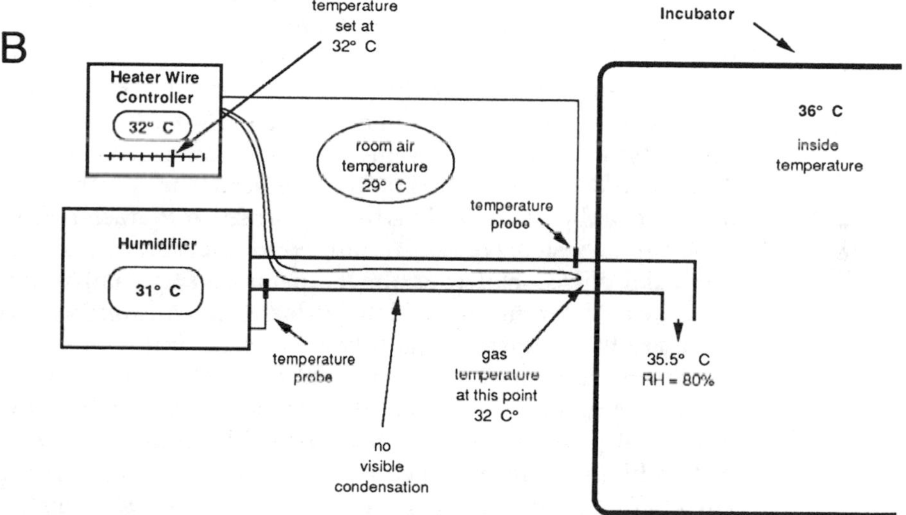

FIG 13–19.
Illustration of a problem encountered during the use of a patient circuit with a heated wire inside an incubator. **A,** when the temperature probe is placed inside an incubator whose temperature is set higher than the output temperature of the humidifier, the temperature of the inspired gas increases, the temperature probe sends a signal to shut off the heating wires, condensation forms in the circuit, and the relative humidity *(RH)* of inspired gas drops. **B,** when the probe is placed just outside the incubator, the heating wires function properly and the RH of the inspired gas is increased. (From Chatburn RL: *Respir Care* 1991; 36:585. Used by permission.)

offers an important advantage. Staff using an algorithm will always follow the same procedure. It also helps prevent the errors that can occur when ventilator management is switched from one practitioner to the next during shift change. Ventilator changes are made more consistently and staff know what rationale others are following. Similar algorithms are being discovered to be useful in adult management as well.

Humidification

An important but often overlooked aspect of mechanical ventilation is the problem of humidification of inspired gas. There are actually two main problems, one having to do with physiology and one with methodology (i.e., design principles and clinical application). The first is how inspired gas should be conditioned to mimic normal physiology. The upper airway physiology suggests that inspired gas delivered to the trachea be heated to 32 to 34° C and that the humidified water vapor content be 36 to 40 mg/L (Fig 13–18). But there are other physiologic concerns such as the maintenance of body temperature in premature neonates and the relationship between humidification and clinical outcome. These issues have just begun to be recognized in the pediatric literature.

A look at the designs of humidifiers and the complex clinical environments in which they are used leads to interesting problems. Heated humidifiers designed for use on intubated patients are intended to supply gas saturated with water vapor over a wide range of temperatures. The temperature and relative humidity of the gas leaving the device are affected by many factors, including: (1) the surface area of the liquid-gas interface inside the humidifier, (2) the gas flow rate and pattern, and (3) the performance characteristics of the temperature controller. These factors are accounted for and controlled to a large extent by the particular device. However, the temperature and relative humidity of the gas at the airway opening is affected by many uncontrollable factors. Chief among these are the temperature and flow patterns of the air surrounding the patient circuit and the amount of incidental thermal radiation, such as from a radiant warmer. Ambient air temperature can be above or below the desired temperature of inspired gas. This can change the performance of the humidification system by the transfer of heat or cold across the walls of the patient circuit.

Heating wires placed within the circuit to replace heat lost to room air can be effective in preventing pooled condensation, but this can cause other problems. Figure 13–19 illustrates one extreme situation that occurs when a patient circuit with heated wires passes through two distinct environments: room air at 29° C and incubator air at 36° C.

We mention these issues to call attention to the fact that humidification of inspired gas, particularly during neonatal ventilation, is more complicated than it appears. There is some evidence that links improper conditioning of inspired gas to an increased incidence of pneumothorax and severity of chronic lung disease in low-birth-weight infants. Just as there is currently no "ideal" ventilator, so too there is no ideal humidification system, nor is there any real consensus about how to use either.

SUMMARY

In this chapter, basic neonatal assessment and resuscitation are reviewed so that a practitioner might be able to perform evaluation of an infant or child and respond to an emergency. Neonatal and pediatric ventilation are very complex subjects and have only been briefly covered here. Our intention has been to provide information about indications, goals, initial settings, and basic ventilator changes. In this way, the general practitioner might have enough information to at least stabilize an infant or child on ventilation until a neonatal or pediatric intensive care specialist is available to assist.

STUDY QUESTIONS

1. What are the six steps involved in the initial resuscitation of the premature newborn?
2. What is the usual cause of RDS in the premature newborn?
3. Name the tool used in assessment of the severity of respiratory distress and list the factors given on this tool.
4. Describe the clinical signs and symptoms associated with respiratory distress of the newborn.
5. A ventilation decision needs to be made in the following situation: the heart rate is greater than 100 beats/min., the infant is currently breathing spontaneously, and oxygen has improved the infant's color. What is the next appropriate action?
6. What four situations describe the criteria for intubation in the newborn?
7. Describe the condition of respiratory distress in the child.
8. Interpret the following acid-base balance values: pH = 7.20, Pa_{CO_2} = 64 mm Hg.
9. State the ways in which respiratory physiology of the newborn is different from that of the adult.
10. List four indications for mechanical ventilatory support in the newborn.
11. Describe seven characteristics of the ideal infant ventilator.
12. Explain the function of the flow rate control for adjusting mechanical ventilation in the newborn.
13. What measured parameter has significant effect on oxygenation in the newborn?

14. If a neonatal patient had a condition of respiratory acidosis, what would be the first step in improving ventilation?

ANSWERS TO STUDY QUESTIONS

1. Prevention of heat loss, positioning the infant, suctioning, assessment of breathing, assessment of heart rate, and assessment of color.
2. The cause of RDS in the premature infant is a result of abnormal lung mechanics due to immature lung development and surfactant deficiency.
3. Silverman's chart. The infant's upper chest, lower chest, and nares are observed along with audible assessment for degree and pitch of breath sounds. Characteristics of the breath sounds, such as audible grunting upon expiration with unequal air exchange, are noted. The pattern of retractions and grunting assessed are indexed according to Silverman's chart.
4. Infants in respiratory distress exhibit tachypnea (80–120 breaths/min), substernal retractions, fine inspiratory rales on auscultation, expiratory grunting, nasal flaring, and cyanosis. This can become progressively worse with cyanosis and a mottled appearance that does not improve with oxygenation, periods of apnea, a drop in heart rate, a reduced state of consciousness, and decreased muscle tone and flaccidity.
5. The practitioner discontinues any assisted positive pressure ventilation and provides tactile stimulation while monitoring the infant's progress. If the infant does not breathe spontaneously and becomes cyanotic, then 100% O_2 needs to be provided via assisted ventilation at a rate of 40 to 60 breaths/min.
6. The following four situations describe the criteria for endotracheal intubation: (a) PPV is required for a prolonged period to ventilate the infant. (b) PPV by bag and mask is ineffective as noted by inadequate response and chest expansion. (c) Suctioning of the trachea is required in order to clear the airway in infants suspected of having aspirated formula or other foreign material. The trachea is intubated and suctioned on those infants who have thick or particulate meconium in the amniotic fluid. (d) If congenital diaphragmatic hernia is suspected, then the newborn is immediately ventilated using an ET tube rather than a bag and mask. Ventilation by way of an ET tube eliminates the chance of air entering the bowel and thus inhibiting lung expansion.
7. The infant or child with respiratory failure shows increased work of breathing (increased rate, nasal flaring, and retractions in the intercostal, subcostal, and suprasternal spaces) and possibly stridor, prolonged expiration, grunting, and head bobbing. Asymmetric chest and abdominal movement may also be present, as well as cyanosis.

8. Respiratory acidosis.
9. They may have periods of apnea and periodic breathing. They have a reduced response to CO_2 and hypoxia seems to further reduce this response to CO_2. They are less responsive to hypoxia. Their chest wall is not as rigid, their lungs less compliant, and their airways more resistant to ventilation.
10. (a) Marked hypoxemia—a PaO_2 of less than 50 to 60 mm Hg on an FIO_2 greater than 60% to 80%; (b) a rising $PaCO_2$ greater than 50 mm Hg with a falling pH of less than 7.20; (c) frequent apneic episodes that do not respond to other forms of therapy (e.g., medications, CPAP); and (d) premature infants weighing less than 1,000 g with accompanying asphyxia or respiratory distress.
11. The ideal ventilator for infants would have the following characteristics: (1) small size, low cost, and quiet; (2) minimal system compliance and resistance to breathing; (3) visible and audible alarm systems; (4) sensitive and rapid response time; (5) IPPV, IMV, and CPAP or PEEP available as modes; (6) respiratory rates up to 150 breaths/min; (7) V_T range of 10 to 200 mL.
12. Flow rate is usually set at four times $\dot{V}_E$. If it is too low, the preset pressure may not be reached until the end of inspiration on a pressure-controlled machine. This produces a rounded curve. When set high, the waveform is nearly rectangular.
13. Mean airway pressure. PEEP and FIO_2, of course, also affect oxygenation.
14. Increase the PIP first until it is 25 cm H_2O.

REFERENCES

1. Bates B: *A Guide to Physical Examination.* Philadelphia, JB Lippincott Co, 1974.
2. Bloom RS, Cropley C, Chameides L, and the AHA/AAP Neonatal Resuscitation Steering Committee (eds): *Textbook of Neonatal Resuscitation.* Elk Grove Village, Ill, American Academy of Pediatrics/American Heart Association, 1990.
3. Burton GG, Hodgkin JE, Ward JJ (eds): *Respiratory Care: A Guide to Clinical Practice,* ed 3. Philadelphia, JB Lippincott Co, 1991.
4. Carlo WA, Chatburn RL (eds): *Neonatal Respiratory Care.* St Louis, Mosby–Year Book, Inc, 1988.
5. Chameides L: *Textbook of Pediatric Advanced Life Support.* Dallas, American Heart Association/American Academy of Pediatrics, 1990.
6. Chatburn RL: Principles and practice of neonatal and pediatric mechanical ventilation. *Respir Care* 1991; 36:569–595.
7. Chatburn RL, Lough MD: Mechanical ventilation, in Lough MD, Doerchuk D, Stern R: *Pediatric Respiratory Therapy,* ed 3. St Louis, Mosby–Year Book, Inc, 1985, pp 148–191.
8. Fanaroff AA, Martin RJ (eds): *Neonatal-Perinatal Medicine: Diseases of the Fetus and Infant.* St Louis, Mosby–Year Book, Inc, 1987.

9. Harwood R: *Perinatal/Pediatric Respiratory Care: A Comprehensive Manual.* Atlanta, Georgia State University, College of Health Sciences, Dept of Cardiopulmonary Care Sciences, 1991.
10. Kacmarek RM, Mack CW, Dimas S: *The Essentials of Respiratory Therapy,* ed 3. St Louis, Mosby–Year Book, Inc, 1991.
11. Nicks J, Schrum M, Schumacher R: Continuous end tidal CO_2 monitoring reflects disease severity in newborn RDS. *Pediatr Res* 1987; 21–461A.
12. Null D, Berman LS, Clark R: Neonatal and pediatric ventilatory support, in Kirby RR, Banner MJ, Downs JB: *Clinical Applications of Ventilatory Support,* ed 2. New York, Churchill Livingstone, Inc, 1990, pp 199–238.
13. Statistical Resources Branch, Division of Vital Statistics: *Final Mortality Statistics 1981.* and *Monthly Vital Statistics Report* 32: 16. Hyattsville, Md, National Center for Health Statistics, 1984.
14. Whaley LF, Wong DL: *Nursing Care of Infants and Children.* St Louis, Mosby–Year Book, Inc, 1987.

Chapter **14**

Home Mechanical Ventilation

Theresa Gramlich, M.S., RRT

On completion of this chapter, the reader will be able to:

1. List the goals of home mechanical ventilation.
2. Discuss the patient and family characteristics and financial factors that must be considered in patient selection for home mechanical ventilation.
3. Identify the most important operational features that a home mechanical ventilator should possess.
4. Describe the different types of negative pressure ventilatory support devices that may be used in the home.

5. Describe the basic operational features of positive pressure ventilators that can be used in the home.
6. List ancillary equipment that is needed in the home for ventilator-dependent patients.
7. Explain the cleaning and disinfecting procedure for home mechanical ventilation equipment.
8. Discuss the roles of the health care team in preparing the patient for home mechanical ventilation.
9. Describe several important tasks that are involved in the comprehensive discharge plan.
10. Explain the importance of the follow-up and evaluation of ventilator-assisted patients in the home.
11. Identify the indications for nasal mask CPAP and NIPPV.
12. List the advantages of NIPPV over conventional methods of mechanical ventilation.
13. Describe the general function of nasal mask CPAP and NIPPV systems.
14. List the potential complications of nasal mask CPAP and NIPPV therapy.
15. Discuss the preparation for home care for patients utilizing nasal mask CPAP or NIPPV therapy.

HOME MECHANICAL VENTILATION

Care of the ventilator-dependent patient at home is not a new concept. The 1950s gave birth to this home care concept as a result of the polio epidemic. Faced with high costs and high readmission rates of ventilator-dependent polio victims, many patients were discharged to home or other alternative sites where they received general care and rehabilitation. After the polio epidemic subsided, interest in home mechanical ventilation decreased. Continued advances in pulmonary medicine and technology contributed to increased survival rates among critically ill adults and children. However, this was largely confined to acute care hospitals.

Care of the ventilator-dependent patient has now come full circle as seen in the past decade by an upsurge in home mechanical ventilation. The development of medical equipment which makes home care a less costly alternative to prolonged hospitalization, and the psychosocial benefits for many patients and their families, have made the renewed concept of home mechanical ventilation a reality.

GOALS OF HOME MECHANICAL VENTILATION

The overall goal of long-term mechanical ventilation in the home or other alternative care site is to improve the patient's quality of life. While different patients will require different levels of care, it is hoped that each patient will progress to the point of maximum activity and take an active role in his or her own care. If this is accomplished, then the psychosocial well-being of the patient will also improve. Other goals include reducing the amount of hospitalizations, extending life, and reducing the costs as compared to hospitalization. Table 14–1 lists five goals of home mechanical ventilation developed by the American College of Chest Physicians.[13]

TABLE 14–1.
Goals for Home Mechanical Ventilation: American College of Chest Physicians Guidelines*

1. Extend life
2. Enhance the quality of life: continue progress in development and social growth
3. Reduce morbidity: decrease hospitalizations; reduce episodes of medical complications
4. Improve the physical, psychological, and social function of the individual
5. Cost-effectiveness: home care should be less costly than care in an institution

*Data from Make B: *AARC Times* 1987; 11:56–58.

PATIENT SELECTION

Patient selection is the key to success for any home care ventilation program. Although many factors must be considered in this selection, they can be broadly grouped into three areas: (1) disease process and clinical stability, (2) psychological evaluation of the patient and family, and (3) financial considerations.

Disease Process and Clinical Stability

Previous studies have shown that some disorders causing ventilator dependency may be more successfully managed than others. From these studies, a system has been devised which separates ventilator-dependent patients into three categories:

1. Patients who are unable to maintain adequate spontaneous ventilation over long periods of time, either daytime or nighttime.

2. Patients who require continuous ventilatory support in order to survive.
3. Patients who have been diagnosed as terminally ill and have little prognosis for long-term survival.

Table 14–2 lists the disorders grouped in each category.

Neuromuscular conditions, skeletal disorders, central hypoventilation syndromes, and stable chronic lung disease are more compatible with long-term success than disorders causing failure of gas exchange. Severe disease affecting organ systems other than the pulmonary system offer a high risk of complications and are not suitable for long-term ventilation outside the hospital.

Patients who are considered candidates for home mechanical ventilation must be clinically and physiologically stable to the degree that they are free from any medical complications for at least 2 weeks prior to discharge. This includes cardiopulmonary stability, acceptable arterial blood gas (ABG) values, freedom from acute respiratory infections and fever, no large fluctuations in fractional concentration of oxygen in inspired gas (F_{IO_2}), and preferably, no positive end-expiratory pressure (PEEP). Other considerations include the ability to clear secretions (either spontaneously or by suctioning), and the presence of a tracheostomy tube, if using positive pressure ventilation. In addition, major diagnostic studies or therapeutic interventions should not be anticipated for at least 1 month after discharge.

Psychosocial Factors

In addition to the assessment of the patient's disease process and clinical stability, certain psychosocial aspects of care must be addressed. The psychological stability of the patient and family are most important since the family, in most cases, will become the primary caregivers. The family must be made aware of the patient's prognosis and the advantages and disadvantages of long-term

TABLE 14–2.
Patient Groups Requiring Mechanical Ventilation at Home

Group	Description	Diseases
1	Patients with diseases that allow some spontaneous ventilation for extended periods of time. Ventilatory support is used mainly at night.	Severe kyphoscoliosis Amyotrophic lateral sclerosis Diaphragmatic paralysis Central hypoventilation syndrome
2	Patients who require continuous ventilatory support	Chronic obstructive lung disease (COPD) High spinal cord injuries Muscular dystrophy (late stage)
3	Patients whose care is primarily supportive. The patient is usually terminal.	Terminal cancer End-stage COPD

mechanical evaluation. In some cases a detailed psychological evaluation is necessary to determine the ability of the patient and family members to cope with stress.[20] If the requirements for the patient's care exceed the family's capabilities, then outside help is sought. The availability of other support services such as support groups, home health agencies, and psychological consultants is often critical to the success or failure of home care candidates.

Financial Considerations

The financial obligations of home care mechanical ventilation are also considered in patient selection since the family is almost always responsible for some expenses, even if insured. The cost of home mechanical ventilation will vary depending on the need for home care personnel, the type of ventilator selected, accessory supplies, and the resources available to the patient. Studies have shown that the major factor affecting the cost of home care is the need for professional caregivers. This cost is dependent on the availability of family members, patient independence and self-care abilities, and the number of hours and level of care required from others.[16] As much as possible, an estimate of the actual cost to the patient is determined and presented to the patient and family during the selection process.

EQUIPMENT SELECTION

Ventilator Selection

Many types and models of ventilators are available for home use. Some of these are quite sophisticated, offering an array of modes, alarms systems, and other complex ventilatory techniques. Although occasionally these machines may be necessary for medical stability outside the hospital, the goal of ventilator selection is geared toward simple technology as much as possible.[16]

Many factors are considered in choosing a ventilator for home use. The most important of these are the following:

1. **Reliability:** the ventilator must be mechanically dependable and trouble-free for extended periods of time without breakdown or need for costly maintenance.
2. **Safety:** the ventilator must be safe to operate in oxygen-enriched environments and have an adequate alarm system to warn of low ventilation pressure, high ventilating pressure, machine disconnection, and mechanical failure.
3. **Versatility:** the mechanical ventilator needs to be portable from room to room or adjusted for travel outside the home. This necessitates the use of a reliable internal or external battery source.

4. **User-friendly:** the ventilator controls must be easy to understand and manipulate. The circuit must be simple and easy to change.
5. **Easy patient cycling:** the ventilator must be easy to cycle in the assist-control mode. For those patients with some spontaneous effort, the ventilator should incorporate the intermittent (IMV) or synchronized intermittent mandatory ventilation (SIMV) mode.

For all home ventilator patients, back-up ventilatory support must be available in case of electrical failure or malfunction. All ventilator-assisted patients require a self-inflating manual resuscitator. If a patient can tolerate extended periods of being off the ventilator, a manual resuscitator as back-up may be all that is necessary. For those patients who are totally dependent on ventilatory support, or for those patients who live a significant distance from medical support, a second mechanical ventilator as back-up is often necessary. In addition, for those patients who require supplemental oxygen, a concentrator and E-cylinder back-up are also needed.

Evaluation of the electrical adequacy of the patient's home is important and is done before the ventilator is selected. This includes a complete assessment of the circuit on which the home ventilator will be installed. Table 14–3 provides instructions for mapping electrical circuits in the home. For medical equipment, grounded outlets are required. If electrical support is not sufficient to provide safe operation, additional electrical support must be added. Arrangements are made with local utility companies and fire departments of the patient's location and condition. In the event of a power outage or other interruption of services, the home ventilator patient is usually given priority for restoration of service.

Negative Pressure Ventilators

For patients who require limited ventilatory support, the negative pressure ventilator has proved to be very useful. Its simplicity of operation and the lack of

TABLE 14–3.
Mapping Electrical Circuits in the Home*

1. Place a number by each of the circuit breakers or fuses in the main electrical panel.
2. Using a piece of paper for each room in the home, draw a square representing the room and mark each receptacle or light in the room.
3. Make sure each receptacle has a small appliance or light plugged into it. Turn on all the lights and small appliances you have plugged in.
4. Turn off the number one circuit and note the appliances affected (they will be off). Mark the circuit number by the receptacles and lights in that room on the drawing for that room.
5. Turn that circuit back on and turn off the next circuit in the numbering sequence.
6. Continue until all appliances or lights in all rooms have been assigned to a circuit.

*From May D: *Rehabilitation and Continuity of Care in Pulmonary Disease.* St Louis, Mosby–Year Book, Inc. 1990, p 117. Used by permission.

necessity for tracheostomy has made it a preferential ventilator for patients with such disorders as neuromuscular disease, spinal cord injuries, or central hypoventilation syndromes. Some patients, however, will not benefit from negative pressure ventilation if there are excessive airway secretions, decreased pulmonary compliance, increased airway resistance, or patients at risk for aspiration.

A description of negative pressure ventilation has already been given in Chapters 1 and 6. Table 14–4 is a brief summary of those ventilators and ventilatory assists used in home care mechanical ventilation.

Positive Pressure Ventilators

The most commonly used equipment for providing ventilatory support for the home care patient is the positive pressure ventilator. Unlike the large and sophisticated positive pressure ventilators used in the intensive care unit, these easy-to-operate ventilators for use in home care have an array of advantages, most notably their compact size, light weight, and portability. Most of these units are designed to utilize three different power sources: normal ac current, internal dc battery, and external dc battery.[8] The last-named power source makes these ventilators relatively easy to be mounted on a wheelchair or placed in a motor vehicle. This enhances a patient's chance of greater mobility and

TABLE 14–4.
Negative Pressure Ventilators and Ventilatory Assists

Full body chamber (iron lung by J.H. Emerson): Rate and pressure are adjustable; I/E ratio is fixed at 1:1.
  Advantages: simple to use; noninvasive.
  Disadvantages: lack of access to patient; lack of mobility; may cause upper airway obstruction.

Chest cuirass: Half-body chamber; ideally should be made from a cast of patient's chest.
  Advantages: more mobility; better tolerated.
  Disadvantages: leaks around chest if not custom-fitted; may cause upper airway obstruction.

Raincoat (wrap): A poncho-type device that surrounds the chest and is secured at the hips.
  Advantages: inexpensive; patient can get into and out of it with ease.
  Disadvantages: leaks at arms, legs, and hips.

Pneumosuit: A complete body suit with a shell-like grid around the chest.
  Advantages: best system other than iron lung.
  Disadvantages: must be custom made which makes it expensive.

Pneumobelts: Used only for ventilatory assistance. Belt is attached around the abdomen and then a hose is attached to a positive pressure ventilator. Inflation of the belt compresses the abdomen allowing the diaphragm to rise. Deflation allows the diaphragm to fall. Works best in the sitting position.

Rocking bed: Gas movement is due to the rocking motion of the bed. The motion shifts the abdominal contents which then alters intrathoracic and intrapulmonary pressures. Best for patients with accessory muscle use. Motions of the bed help mobilize secretions.

participation in other activities. In the past 10 to 20 years, many home care positive pressure ventilators have been developed. While this text cannot completely describe all of the available features of each home care ventilator, a comprehensive description of their basic features follows.

General Information.—Current portable positive pressure ventilators used for home care are primarily volume-cycled, piston-driven machines which produce either a sine wave or descending ramp waveform pattern. Tidal volume (V_T) capabilities range from 0 to 3,000 mL, and mandatory rates average from 4 to 35 breaths/min with either a fixed (1:1 or 1:2.5) or variable inspiratory-expiratory (I/E) ratio.

Modes.—All of the volume-cycled positive pressure portable ventilators currently on the market will function in the control mode (time-triggered) and most will offer the assist-control mode as well (pressure/time-triggered). Until recently, these were the only two modes available because it was believed that most patients are more easily managed in these modes of ventilation. On some of the earlier models, e.g., Life Products LP-3, and Lifecare PVV, IMV modes were possible only with the addition of an external IMV system. This increased the cost and complexity of ventilator support. The newer microprocessor ventilators designed for home care, such as Life Products LP-4, LP-5, LP-6, and Lifecare PVL-100, offer IMV or SIMV without the addition of an external system.

Alarms.—Standard alarm controls incorporated in the home care ventilator include low battery or power loss alarms and low pressure alarms. Many newer models offer additional alarms such as high pressure, I/E ratio, inspiratory flow, and apnea. If such alarms are not incorporated into the ventilator unit and are necessary for the patient, separate alarms can be purchased or rented.

Oxygen.—Only about half of the current portable positive pressure ventilators have a reservoir for the addition of oxygen. This may be due to the fact that most home care candidates are weaned to room air before discharge. In the ventilators where oxygen is added, the patient's F_{IO_2} requirements usually remain under 0.4. The need for an F_{IO_2} greater than 0.4 indicates clinical instability which requires more respiratory care than is available in the home.

PEEP.—Very few of the portable positive pressure ventilators have PEEP capabilities. PEEP is more difficult to provide, usually requiring more complex equipment and technology. It is also difficult to monitor in the home. Its use indicates clinical instability, particularly when it is necessary to maintain adequate arterial oxygenation.[16]

Ancillary Equipment

In addition to the mechanical ventilator, the patient requires other supplies for daily general care. These include supplies for airway care, humidification, supplemental oxygen, disposable circuits, and an emergency back-up ventilator. Table 14–5 lists the equipment and supplies which are suggested for home care of the ventilator-assisted patient.[8]

TABLE 14–5.
Equipment List for Home Mechanical Ventilation

- Ventilator equipment
  - Primary ventilator
  - Back-up ventilator
  - Manual resuscitator
  - External 12-V battery
  - Connecting cable
  - Disposable or nondisposable circuits
  - Humidifiers and heater (or heat moisture exchanger)
  - Replacement ventilator filters
  - Patient monitor and alarms (if not incorporated in ventilator)
- Airway management equipment
  - Suction machine (preferably portable)
  - Suction container
  - Appropriate-size catheters
  - Connecting tubing
  - Latex gloves
  - Spare tracheostomy tubes
  - Tracheostomy care kits
  - Hydrogen peroxide
  - Sterile saline or sterile water solution
  - Water-soluble lubricant
  - Syringes
  - Antibiotic ointment
- Oxygen equipment
  - Concentrator
  - E-cylinder back-up
  - Oxygen tubing
  - Tracheostomy collar or T-tube adaptor
  - Large-bore tubing
- Miscellaneous
  - Air compressor for aerosolized medications
  - Wheelchair
  - Hospital bed
  - Bedside commode
  - Equipment disinfectant solution

Disinfection Procedures

The presence of an artificial airway in a compromised ventilator-assisted patient makes the potential for infection from contaminated equipment a risk in the home setting as it is in the hospital setting. For this reason, infection control and decontamination procedures are taught to all persons involved in the care of the patient in the home.

Infection control measures emphasize the avoidance of contamination from person to person, and from objects to person. Family members and other caregivers are encouraged in the practice of thorough handwashing before and after touching the patient or equipment. The use of gloves (nonsterile) is encouraged when performing such tasks as suctioning or tracheostomy care.

In 1988, the American Respiratory Care Foundation (ARCF) developed guidelines for the disinfection of respiratory care equipment used in the home.[3] The committee recommended that all ventilatory equipment be cleaned and disinfected every 24 hours if possible. Equipment is disassembled, rinsed first with cool water, washed in warm soapy water, drained, and soaked in an effective disinfectant solution. Then it is thoroughly rinsed and air-dried and placed in a plastic bag. Ideally, a patient would have at least three circuits so that one can be in use while the other is being disinfected.

Previous information has endorsed the use of quaternary ammonium compounds, or 2% white vinegar and distilled water as an adequate disinfectant solution. There are now conflicting data on the efficacy of these solutions as disinfectants. The ARCF has recommended the use of activated gluteraldehyde

TABLE 14–6.

American Respiratory Care Foundation Guidelines for Disinfecting Home Ventilator Equipment*

Preparation:

1. Choose a clean dry area.
2. Have all supplies ready for use.
3. Wash hands (gloves may be worn).

Procedure

1. Disassemble circuit completely. Wipe small tubes with clean, damp cloth.
2. Rinse large-bore tubings, connectors, humidifier, and exhalation valve with cold water.
3. Soak equipment in warm soapy water for several minutes.
4. Scrub equipment with a small brush to remove dirt and organic material.
5. Rinse thoroughly to remove any soap residue and drain off excess water.
6. Place equipment parts in disinfectant solution. Be sure all parts are submerged.
7. After 15 minutes, rinse equipment thoroughly.
8. Drain off excess water, hang tubes to dry, place small parts on a clean surface to dry.
9. When equipment parts are dry, reassemble circuit and store in a clean plastic bag.
10. Repeat procedure every 24 hours.

*Data from American Respiratory Care Foundation: *Respir Care* 1988; 33:801–808.

for home use. Although this may be the disinfectant solution of choice, its cost and availability may be a limiting factor in its use. Other studies in infection control in the home setting have shown that a wide range of effective disinfection procedures for home equipment are being used. Whatever method is used, the processing of equipment needs to be done in a clean, dry space separated from food preparation areas.

The ARCF also recommended that water to be used as diluents or in humidifiers be boiled for 30 minutes and stored in a sterile container in the refrigerator. After 24 hours, the water is then discarded. Table 14–6 is a summary of the ARCF guidelines for the cleaning and disinfection of equipment.[1, 3]

PREPARATION FOR DISCHARGE

The preparation for discharge to a home of a ventilator-assisted patient begins almost simultaneously with patient selection and includes the process of equipment selection. Together with the coordinated efforts of the multidisciplinary health care team, a comprehensive discharge prescription, and an educational program for home care management is developed.

The health care team consists primarily of the patient's primary physician, a pulmonary physician, a nurse, a respiratory care practitioner, and a social worker. Depending on the patient's level of care, other disciplines included might be physical therapist, psychologist, occupational therapist, and a clinical dietician. The medical equipment supplier will also be a crucial member of this team once equipment has been selected. Finally, the team must include the patient and family.

Each member of the team is responsible for educating the caregivers in the management of the ventilator-dependent patient. The education component includes detailed instructions in cardiopulmonary resuscitation, use of manual resuscitators, aseptic suctioning technique, tracheostomy care, methods of disinfecting equipment, and bronchial hygiene therapies such as chest physiotherapy and aerosolized medication administration. The family is also taught to recognize the early signs and symptoms of a respiratory infection and what action must be taken if such a situation arises. A written protocol with directions for respiratory treatments and other aspects of care also needs to be given to the family (Fig 14–1).

As part of the discharge plan, the medical supplier or respiratory care practitioner looks over the patient's home environment for proper electrical outlets and available space (Fig 14–2). Detailed instructions regarding the function of the mechanical ventilator, and its settings and alarm functions are provided for each caregiver. Daily ventilator flow sheets can be provided to the family for monitoring the patient (Fig 14–3).

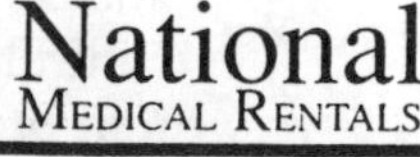

CERTIFICATE OF MEDICAL NECESSITY

Prescription for Home Ventilator Equipment

Here When You Need Us.

PATIENT INFORMATION

Patient's Name

Address

Telephone

Discharge Date

Diagnosis that requires home ventilator | Prognosis

Arterial Blood Gas Results	PaO_2	$PaCO_2$	pH
	HCO_3	SaO_2	FIO_2

Duration of Medical Necessity ________ months "Lifetime" and "Indefinite" are not accepted by all insurances

P 2 3 **INSURANCE INFORMATION (for office use only)**

Medicare #

Medipak #

Medicaid #

Carrier

Policy #

Address

City, State Zip

Employer

Telephone

Subscriber

PRESCRIBED PROCEDURES

Previous Forms of Treatment Attempted

Home ventilator is still required Yes No | Oxygen is still required Yes No

Home Ventilator	Type		Tidal Volume	ml.	FIO_2	%
Mode/Rate	Control	BPM	Assist	BPM	IMV	BPM
	Flow Rate	LPM	PEEP	cm H_2O	Sigh Volume	ml.
	Ventilation Hours	per day				

Other Instructions or Information

Supplemental O_2 | Liquid System ☐ | Concentrator ☐ | Cylinders ☐

If you choose a supplemental *liquid system*, choose the one, if any, of lines A, B, C and D that best describes your patient. Check all boxes in the chosen line that apply.

A. ☐ Patient is fully ambulatory | is able to work outside the home ☐ | is able to ambulate outside the home with little or no restriction ☐

B. ☐ Patient has limited ambulation | is to perform prescribed exercise program in or out of home ☐ | is able to do occasional shopping or visit doctor ☐

C. ☐ Patient is homebound | is to perform prescribed exercise program inside the home ☐

D. ☐ Patient is bedfast with some ability to ambulate, and a portable oxygen system is required in order to ambulate beyond the limitations of the stationary oxygen system

Suction Unit

Suction unit is appropriate for home use without technical or professional supervision Yes No

Stationary Yes No | Suction as needed to clear secretions Yes No | Hyperinflation prior to and following suctioning Yes No

Portable Yes No | Manual Resuscitator Yes No | Sterile Saline for instillation Yes No | Suction Catheter Size FR

Tracheostomy Care By

Tube Type | Tube Size | Change Stoma Dressing and tracheostomy ties as needed to keep them clean and dry Yes No

Remove, clean and replace inner cannula Yes No | ____ times per day | Tracheostomy tube change every ________ weeks

Due to the above diagnosis, a home ventilator is mandatory for this patient to be safely discharged from the hospital. I, the undersigned, certify that the above prescribed equipment and procedures are reasonable and necessary according to accepted standards of medical practice in the treatment of this condition.

PHYSICIAN CERTIFICATION INFORMATION

Signature | Date

Printed Name

Address

Telephone

FIG 14–1.

Prescription for home ventilatory equipment. (Courtesy of National Medical Rentals, Little Rock, Ark.)

Prior to discharge, the patient is placed on the home ventilator for several days to allow patient and family members to become familiar and comfortable with its operation. All family members involved in the patient's care need to demonstrate adequate hands-on performance in all aspects of patient care before patient discharge.

The primary physician makes arrangements with the local physician, and nursing service if the patient lives far away. A local hospital emergency room

CHECKLIST FOR HOME VENTILATOR INSTALLATION

Patient Name: ____________ Physician: ____________

Address: ____________ Phone: ____________

Phone: ____________ Prescription: ____________

Examine each of the following items listed and note your findings. Make comments in the space provided.

HOME/CAREGIVER	COMMENTS
___ Accessibility to home - roads	
___ Number of entrances/exits to the home	
___ Proper electrical grounding - circuit capacity	
___ Availability of telephone	
___ Location & size of patient's bed	
___ Location & size of patient's bedroom	
___ Accessibility of respiratory equipment	
___ Location of back-up systems for equipment	
___ Location & type of heaters	
___ Storage space for supplies	
___ Distance in the home to be walked from bedroom	
___ Availability of EMS/Rescue Squad	
___ Local utility company	
___ Availability of other caregivers	
VENTILATOR SET-UP	
___ Mini-instructions given	
___ Operating manual given	
___ Flowsheets given and explained	
___ Operation of equipment checked	
___ Explanation of alternate power source	
___ Alarm functions explained	
___ Decontamination procedures explained	

GENERAL COMMENTS: ____________

Installation performed by: ____________

Date: ____________

FIG 14–2.
Checklist for home ventilator installation.

HOME VENTILATOR FLOW SHEET

DATE:

Time													
Mode													
Oxygen %													
Volume													
Rate (mach./pt.)													
Pressure													
Flow rate													
ALARMS													
High pressure setting													
Low pressure setting													
Apnea setting													
OTHER													
Humidifier setting													
Sputum characteristics													
Aerosol therapy													
Tube care done													
Circuit changed													

COMMENTS: ______________________________

____

FIG 14–3.
Flow sheet for home ventilation.

needs to be designated for emergency care, and emergency plans must be clearly outlined. The local power company is notified in writing of the patient's condition and need for priority status for electricity in case of power failure. Figure 14–4 provides an example of a discharge plan from a community hospital.

FOLLOW-UP AND EVALUATION

Before the patient is discharged, equipment and supplies are set up in the patient's home and checked for proper placement and function. The medical supplier and other members of the health care team are often present when the patient arrives home to assure both patient and family and relieve any apprehensions. Initially, the patient may require frequent home visits or daily calls

T.J. SAMSOM COMMUNITY HOSPITAL
HOME HEALTH AGENCY
CARE GIVER INSTRUCTION LIST

I have been given adequate instructions, including demonstrations and return demonstration on the following procedures:

RESPIRATORY THERAPY SKILLS	Inst. Begun	Inst. Comp.	Return Demon.	NA
Suctioning Procedures				
- Hyperinflation/hyperoxygenation with manual resuscitator				
- Tracheal and nasopharyngeal suctioning				
- Aseptic technique				
- Instillation of normal saline solution				
Ventilator Operation				
- Circuit change				
- Equipment cleaning/disinfection				
- Checking alarm system				
- Safety precautions				
- Checking and charging electrical back-up				
- Troubleshooting				
Safety Precautions				
- Adequate grounding				
- Response to alarms				
- Response to power/machine failure				
- Recognition of early signs of respiratory distress				
- Response to airway occlusion				
- Prevention of infection				
- Prevention of barotrauma				

I feel comfortable assuming the care of ______________________ without supervision.
(Patient name)

Signed: ______________________
(Caregiver)

____
(Date)

We the undersigned have instructed ______________________ in the
(Caregiver)

procedures as indicated and feel that he/she can care for ______________________ with competency.
(Patient name)

Signed: ______________________ ____________
(Instructor) (Date)

______________________ ____________
(Instructor) (Date)

FIG 14–4.
An example of a caregiver instruction list. (Courtesy of T. J. Sampson Community Hospital, Home Health Agency, Glasgow, Ky.)

PATIENT EVALUATION/FOLLOW-UP REPORT

Date ____________
Time____________

Name ____ Phone ______________

Address____

City ____________________ State ____________ Zip Code ________

Diagnosis ____

Physician ________________________________ Phone ______________

Prescribed Equipment and Procedures : ___________________________
____

ASSESSMENT

Vital Signs Temp. __________ Pulse __________ Resp. Rate ______ BP ______

Ōximetry: ______________ % Saturation on ______________

Breath Sounds: ____

Dyspnea: ____

Cough: ____

Sputum:____

Difficulty Sleeping: _______________________________________

Appetite: ____

Level of Consciousness: ____________________________________

Skin/Edema: ____

Medications: 1. ____________ 2. ____________ 3. ____________
4. ____________ 5. ____________ 6. ____________

Psychosocial: ____

Environmental: ____

Comprehension of Equipment and Procedures: ____________________

Compliance w/Therapeutic Plan: _____________________________

Functioning of Equipment: __________________________________

Plan: ____

____
N.M.R. Representative

FIG 14–5.
A patient evaluation and follow-up report. (Courtesy of National Medical Rentals, Little Rock, Ark.)

until he or she is stable and adjusted to a routine of care. Once this routine is established, only formal monthly visits are necessary to evaluate the patient and report on progress.

Evaluation by home visit may include arterial blood gas studies, pulse oximetry, bedside pulmonary function studies, and vital signs. It may also include observation of the home environment, equipment assessment, and any other problems the patient or family members may have. A written report is completed after the monthly visit and copies sent to the patient's physician, home care agency, and other members of the health care team (Fig 14–5).

The task of caring for ventilator-dependent patients may create increasing frustration and anxiety for family members who are the primary caregivers. If problems are noticed during home visits, the patient's physician is notified. It may be necessary to provide psychological counseling to family members or contact alternative means of care (e.g., respite care) to allow a rest for family members.

ALTERNATIVES TO CONVENTIONAL MECHANICAL VENTILATION AT HOME: CPAP AND NIPPV

Many patients with chronic respiratory disorders have only moderate impairment of respiratory function during waking hours, but develop severe respiratory failure during sleep. For these patients, some system of nocturnal ventilation needs to be supplied. For years, the negative pressure ventilator or positive pressure ventilator via tracheostomy tube had been the only nocturnal ventilation system available for these people. Since the early 1980s, alternatives to conventional methods of mechanical ventilation have been steadily increasing. The effectiveness of nocturnal intermittent positive pressure ventilation (NIPPV) through a nasal mask or CPAP through a nasal mask has been examined in several studies for patients with neuromuscular disorders, chest wall defects, obstructive and restrictive intrinsic lung diseases, and obstructive sleep apnea.[4, 6, 7, 9, 10] In all of these previous studies, patients exhibited varying degrees of hypoventilation, and hypoxemia during sleep requiring some periods of assisted ventilation. The results of all of these studies have shown that NIPPV or CPAP through a nasal mask prevented episodes of severe hypoxemia and hypercapnia. The nasally applied positive pressure actually stabilized the oropharyngeal airway structures and prevented any episodes of upper airway obstruction. In addition, daytime partial pressures of arterial oxygen (Pa_{O_2}) and carbon dioxide (Pa_{CO_2}) improved in all patients in all studies. There was also reported improvement in respiratory muscle strength and stabilization of lung volumes.[11] Patients also reported subjective improvement in symptoms of headaches, daytime somnolence, and an increase in their ability to perform activities of daily living. There is now sufficient evidence to support the effectiveness of noninvasive ventilatory assistance in the home care setting.

Indications

The decision to use nocturnal CPAP or NIPPV depends on the degree of upper airway obstruction the patient experiences and his or her respiratory muscle strength. For those patients who have adequate muscle strength and require no mechanical ventilation but who become hypercapnic and hypoxemic during sleep, nasal CPAP may be all that is necessary to alleviate hypoxemia and alveolar collapse. This is especially true for the patient who suffers from obstructive sleep apnea (OSA). CPAP levels can be titrated to increase expired lung volumes during sleep and reduce inspiratory and expiratory resistance. This will result in improvement of the Pao_2, decrease respiratory rate, and prevent air trapping.

NIPPV may be needed when respiratory muscle strength is inadequate to support effective ventilation during sleep. Such patients as those with progressive neuromuscular disease or chest wall deformities often experience severe hypoxemia and hypocapnia during sleep. For these patients, NIPPV can be an alternative to intermittent positive pressure ventilation (IPPV) via intubation or tracheostomy tube provided that:

1. Oropharyngeal muscle strength is adequate for swallowing, speaking, and clearing oral secretions.
2. The patient is alert and cooperative.
3. There is no acute pulmonary disease or intrinsic lung disease requiring oxygen therapy or extensive airway management.
4. The patient is free of seizures.
5. There are no orthopaedic problems such as facial fractures that would interfere with the use of a nasal mask.[4]

The advantages of nasal mask NIPPV over more conventional methods of mechanical ventilation have been well documented.[9] In addition to the physiologic improvements associated with all forms of nocturnal mechanical ventilation, nasal mask ventilation:

1. Is less cumbersome than the tank, curaiss, or poncho negative pressure ventilators, allowing better patient mobility.
2. Is simple to apply by the patient or caregiver.
3. Allows the patient to coordinate his or her breathing effort.
4. Mechanically dilates the upper airway, preventing upper airway obstruction.
5. Removes or postpones the need for tracheostomy.
6. Is more cost-effective since it eliminates the expenses associated with tracheostomy care, such as suction equipment and supplies.

CPAP Systems

A nasal CPAP system for home care consists of two main elements: an air blower unit and the nasal mask system. The blower incorporates an electrically powered motor, fan assembly, and a mechanism for setting and controlling the pressure that is delivered to the circuit. A continuous flow of air from the blower, ranging from 15 to 30 L/min, is delivered to the nasal mask through a lightweight 22-mm-diameter corrugated plastic hose attached to a one-way valve or whisper swivel valve (Respironics). These valves prevent the flow of expired gas into the inspiratory limb.

The nasal mask system usually consists of a soft translucent mask made of medical-grade silicone. These masks come in a variety of sizes designed to custom-fit faces (Figs 14–6 and 14–7). An alternative to the nasal mask is the nasal pillow (Fig 14–8: Puritan Bennett ADAM). The nasal pillows are short silicone tubes that fit securely in a plastic shell device and seal the patient's nares securely to virtually eliminate leaks. A small opening on the surface of the plastic

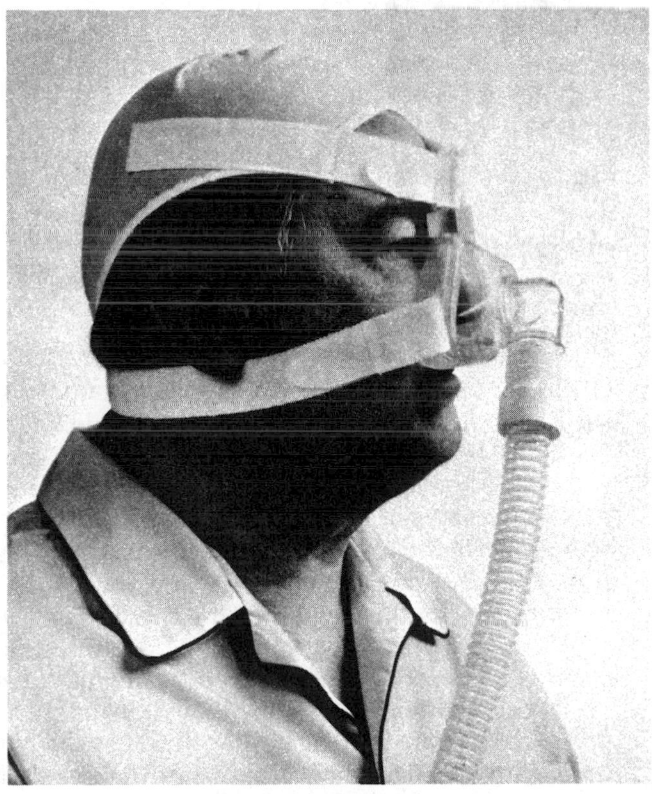

FIG 14–6.
CPAP nasal mask and tubing (Softcap). (Courtesy of Respironics Inc., Murrysville, Pa.)

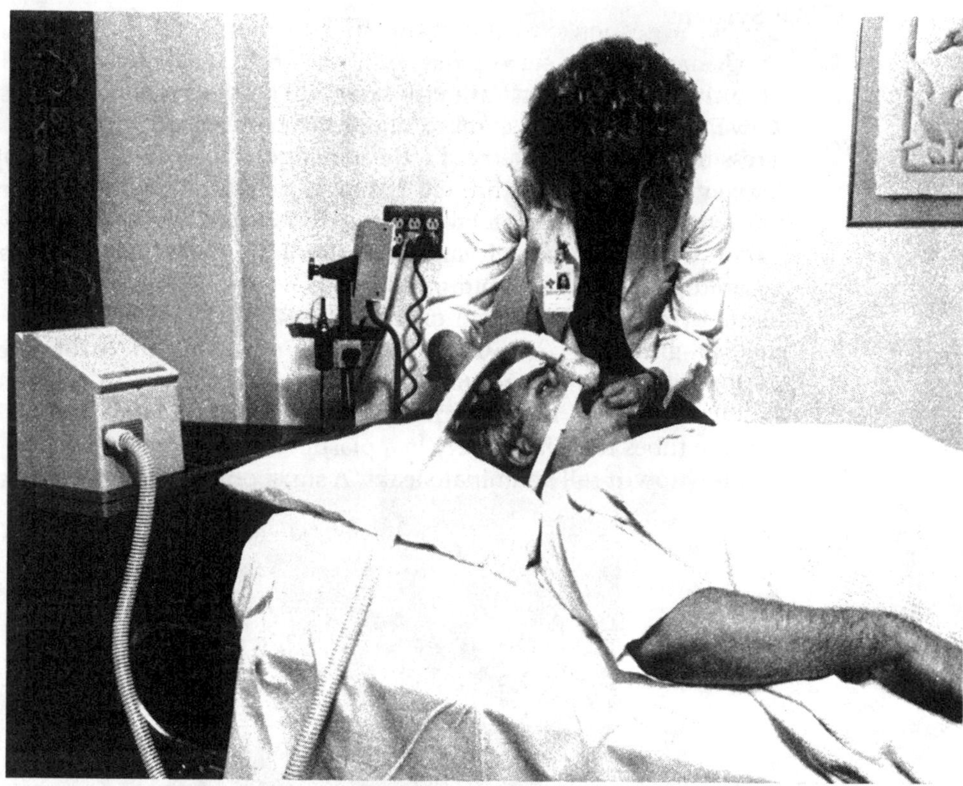

FIG 14–7.
A nasal CPAP mask attached to the CPAP generator. (Courtesy of Healthdyne Technologies, Marietta, Ga.)

shell allows for exhalation of gases. Both the nasal masks and nasal pillows are secured to the face by lightweight adjustable headgear.

CPAP levels ranging from 2.5 to 20 cm H_2O are available on most home care units. These levels are achieved in one of two ways. The older units utilize various fixed-level spring-loaded valves (e.g., 5, 7.5, 10, 15 cm H_2O) that are screwed in-line with the CPAP circuitry. The pressure is developed by tension from curved springs applied to a disc valve. Gas flow rates are then adjusted until the level of threshold pressure is achieved. The newer units used for home CPAP therapy incorporate electronic pressure transducers that sense pressure changes in the circuit and regulate the amount of airflow into the circuit. Figure 14–9 illustrates that as the patient inhales and the circuit pressure decreases, the pressure transducers increase the blower speed allowing more air to move into the circuit. As the patient begins to exhale and circuit pressure increases, the amount of air flowing into the circuit decreases. This increase and decrease of airflow in response to circuit pressure changes allows the patient to inhale and exhale against the same pressure.

Although constant flow is maintained through the system, these newer CPAP units do not incorporate any mechanisms for measuring the amount of flow moving through the circuit. The pressure level is held constant and the patient must maintain full effort of breathing.

Operation of these CPAP units by the patient or family involves turning the on/off switch to the on position. The level of CPAP pressure is set by the practitioner or medical supplier when the unit is installed in the home. This is done by adjusting a screw or control knob in the control panel located on the rear of the units. Once the controls are set to the prescribed levels, the panel locks and conceals the controls. The patient turns the power switch on to activate the unit.

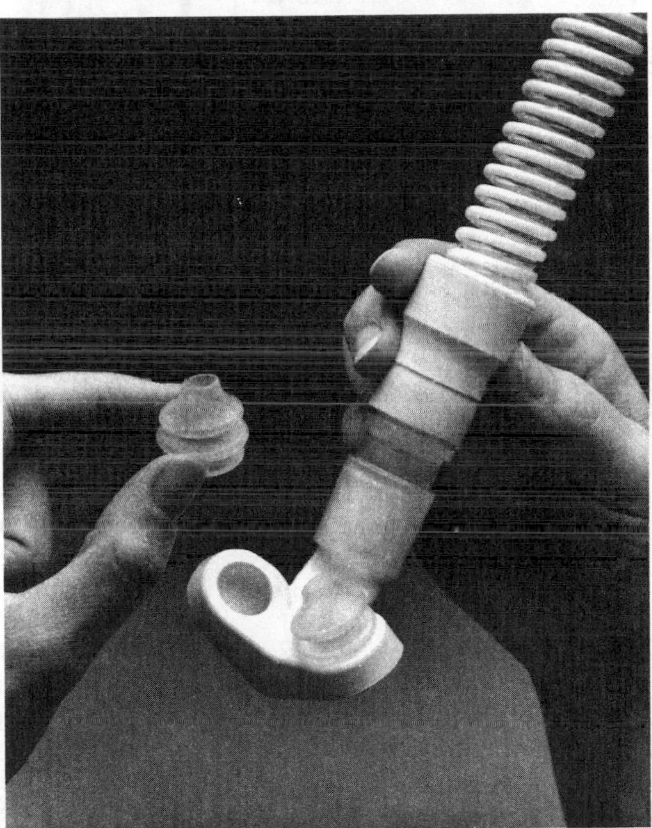

FIG 14–8.
ADAM nasal pillows for providing nasal CPAP. (Courtesy of Puritan/Bennett, Puritan Group, Lenexa, Kan.)

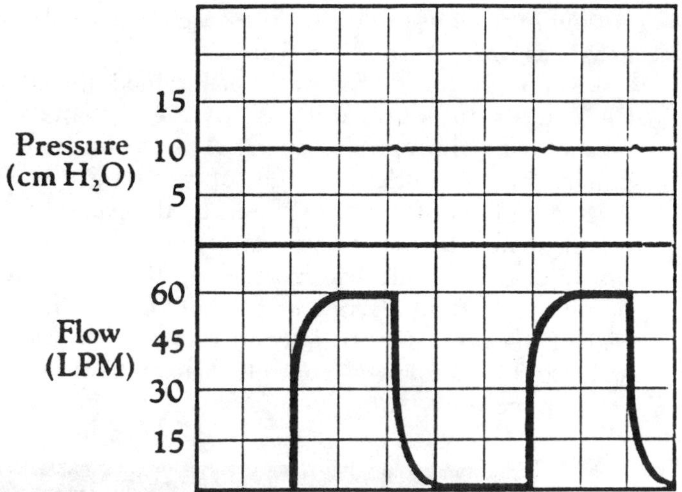

FIG 14–9.
The pressure changes *(top)* compared to flow changes *(bottom)* during CPAP ventilation using the Tranquility Plus CPAP unit. *LPM* = liters per minute. (Courtesy of Healthdyne Technologies, Marietta, Ga.)

NIPPV SYSTEMS

The NIPPV system for home care consists of the nasal mask system and either a portable volume ventilator designed for home care such as Life Products-LP6, Lifecare-PVL 100, or a small pressure-supported ventilator (PSV) like Respironic's BiPAP S/T. The nasal mask system for IPPV is similar in design to those used for the administration of nasal CPAP. A standard ventilator circuit using an inspiratory and an expiratory limb can be attached to the mask. With the use of nasal pillows (see Fig 14–8), a circuit design similar to that used with intermittent positive pressure breathing (IPPB) machines is used. A single lightweight 22-mm corrugated hose with an exhalation valve is attached to the nasal shell.

When using a volume ventilator, a V_T and inspiratory time, or rate, is set. The machine can be set in the assist mode to simply augment each patient respiratory effort, or in the assist-control mode to guarantee a minimum respiratory rate from the machine. Since ventilation is nasal ventilation, mouth air leaks can occur, especially at end-inspiration.[10] If air leaks are large, NIPPV becomes inefficient. To compensate for mouth leaks, the V_T or rate, or both, can be increased until the patient adapts to the system. Since these volume ventilators were originally designed for continuous positive pressure ventilation, they will contain the standard alarms: high pressure, low pressure, apnea, and ventilator inoperative. If excessive mouth leaks occur, low pressure alarms may need to be readjusted.

PSV is an alternative to standard volume ventilation in nasal mask IPPV. With pressure support, the patient has complete control over the respiratory pattern. Each breath is supported by positive pressure allowing the patient to take a larger breath than he or she is able to take alone. This helps reduce the work of breathing.

Most of the newer models like the Respironics BiPAP S/T (Fig 14–10) and S/T-D used for PSV have two pressure settings which, when combined with the patient's respiratory effort, help determine the delivered V_T. The control settings are the inspiratory positive airway pressure (IPAP) control setting and the expiratory positive airway pressure (EPAP) control setting.

The calibrated pressure ranges for both the EPAP and IPAP controls is 4 to 20 cm H_2O. The IPAP and EPAP pressures are maintained by electronic pressure transducers that sense pressure changes and then increase or decrease the amount of airflow from the blower unit. A continuous flow of air through the circuit, ranging from 15 to 30 L/min, is present at all times, making it easier for the patient to breathe. When the patient begins to take a breath, the pressure transducer senses a decrease in the level of circuit flow. The system then cycles to the IPAP level and increases the amount of airflow in the circuit. This additional flow supports the patient's own effort and allows a larger tidal breath.

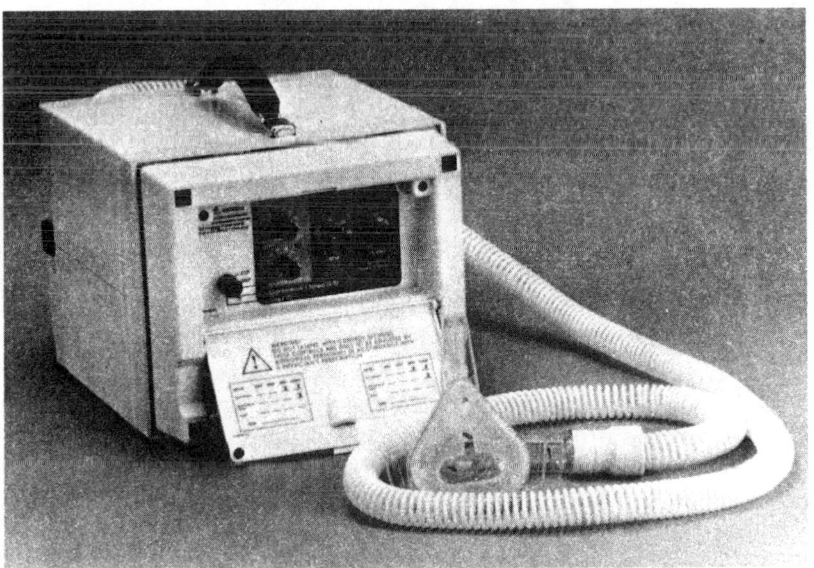

FIG 14–10.
The Respironics BIPAP S/T ventilatory support system used to deliver controlled levels of IPAP and EPAP. (Courtesy of Respironics, Inc., Murrysville, Pa.)

The change in flow detected by this device is called the "spontaneous trigger threshold." The unit is flow-triggered into inspiration. A minimum inspiratory effort of only 40 mL/sec is required to initiate machine support.

The system will also respond to changes in circuit flow at end-inspiration. As the inspiratory flow decreases, the pressure in the circuit will quickly drop to the baseline level allowing the patient to exhale. The EPAP level allows the patient's airways to be supported during exhalation, preventing upper airway collapse.

The unit also responds to changes in circuit flow caused by leaks in the breathing circuit. Leaks into the system cause a decrease in circuit airflow whereas leaks out of the system cause an increase in circuit airflow. In this way, both IPAP and EPAP pressures are maintained and the machine functions reliably to support patient breathing.

There are three options for providing PSV with the Respironics BiPAP S/T: spontaneous, spontaneous-times, and timed modes. In the spontaneous mode, cycling to the IPAP and EPAP levels occurs in response to the patient's own respiratory effort. In the spontaneous-timed mode, all respiratory efforts initiated by the patient are supported to the IPAP level as in the spontaneous mode, but a minimum breathing rate may also be set. In this way, if the patient fails to make an inspiratory effort within a set interval of time, the machine will cycle to the pressure-supported IPAP level (time-triggered). This acts much in the same manner as the assist-control mode on conventional mechanical ventilators.

The timed mode will deliver pressure-supported breaths based on control settings and not patient effort. The amount of IPAP and EPAP levels, the number of breaths per minute, and the inspiratory time are determined by the clinician after the appropriate testing and monitoring of physiologic values. The levels are then adjusted on the machine so that the patient's ventilatory needs are fully met.

These pressure support home units do not include any integrated alarms or monitors since their primary use is to intermittently augment or assist ventilation. Patients who require continuous ventilatory support need these volume ventilators equipped with appropriate alarms and monitors. A separate airway pressure monitor can be interfaced with these home units. These monitors give an audible and visual indication of such conditions as low pressure, high pressure, and apnea.

The newer home CPAP and PSV units require very little maintenance. Both of the units contain an air inlet filter located on the front or back surface of the machine. These filters are replaced monthly. The circuit and accessory equipment are cleaned and disinfected in the same manner as conventional mechanical ventilation equipment.

Potential Complications

All forms of positive pressure ventilation may cause pulmonary problems such as barotrauma. Although this remains a potential problem with both nasal mask CPAP and nasal mask NIPPV, the risk of such problems occurring is greatly reduced. An important complication associated with the delivery of positive pressure by mask is aerophagia and gastric distention. Encouraging the patient to use a lateral sleeping position or using an abdominal strap may alleviate this problem. With continued use, the incidence of gastric distention decreases.

Another potential complication is hypoventilation due to air leaks through the mouth. This is especially true for patients who have low lung compliance. In some cases of NIPPV, V_T may need to be increased and supplemental oxygen applied to compensate for these problems. When using nasal mask CPAP, the CPAP level can be increased to compensate for leaks. A more common complaint from patients utilizing nasal mask CPAP or NIPPV is nasal dryness or congestion due to high airflows through the nasal mask. Increasing the humidification or irrigating the nasal passages with saline has proved helpful.

Finally, eye irritation often occurs from mask leaks. Commercially produced nasal masks can often be adjusted for patient comfort and to reduce air leaks. If this does not alleviate the problem, it helps for the patient to have a custom-made nasal mask. This is usually fabricated by modeling a mixture of silicone paste and catalyst on the patient's face. Two holes are then drilled into the mask opposite the patient's nostril imprints, and cannulas are pushed into the holes. Tubing is then connected via an adaptor to the two cannulas (Fig 14–11). The custom-made mask contoured to the patient's face is more comfortable and reduces air leaks.

Air leaks may also be alleviated by use of the nasal pillows (Puritan Bennett ADAM). The soft silicone tubes fit comfortably into the patient's nares and are

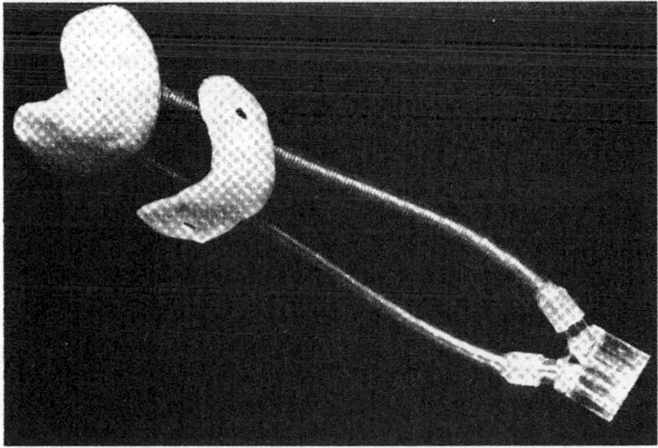

FIG 14–11.
The complete nasal mask with head strap and tubing. (From Leger P, Jennequin J, Gerard M, et al: *Respir Care* 1989; 34:75. Used by permission.)

TABLE 14–7.
Complications Associated with Mask CPAP or NIPPV Therapy*

Patient discomfort from head straps
Aerophagia – gastric distention
Hypoventilation
Nasal dryness, congestion
Eye irritation

*CPAP = continuous positive airway pressure; NIPPV = negative intermittent positive pressure ventilation.

held in place by a plastic shell attached to adjustable headgear. Table 14–7 has a summary of potential complications.

Preparation for Home Care

Before initiating nasal CPAP therapy or nasal mask NIPPV in the home, the patient is monitored over a period of several nights in the hospital setting. This allows close observation of sleep patterns and any periods of oxyhemoglobin desaturation. Under the direction of a physician, CPAP, pressure support levels, or V_T and rate can then be prescribed for normalization of ABG values. The nasal mask system can then be applied and adjusted for comfort. As with conventional home mechanical ventilation, the patient and caregiver must learn to apply the mask correctly and manage the ventilator or continuous gas flow unit. The family is further educated about potential complications and how these problems can be minimized or alleviated. The same procedure for discharge and home preparation of the patient on continuous home mechanical ventilation is followed here.

Although these two methods of noninvasive assisted ventilation are safe, close monitoring and supervision are necessary. As disease progression continues or setbacks due to respiratory infections occur, it may be necessary to temporarily or permanently switch to more conventional methods of mechanical ventilation.

CASE STUDIES

Case 1

A 50-year-old man with the diagnosis of spinal muscular atrophy had been using a chest cuirass negative pressure ventilator at night only for the past 8 months. The patient had been complaining of increasing daytime somnolence and headaches. On the request of his physician, the patient was admitted to the hospital for a routine diagnostic workup and also to see if he would benefit from nasal mask NIPPV.

On the first day of his admission, baseline ABG analysis, bedside pulmonary function tests, and continuous pulse oximetry were performed with the patient breathing spontaneously in Fowler's position. The results showed that his spontaneous vital capacity (VC) was only 34% of predicted, negative inspiratory force (NIF) was -21 cm H_2O, Pa_{O_2} was 58 mm Hg, and oxygen saturation by pulse oximetry was at 89%.

That evening, the patient was placed in the chest cuirass ventilator during a sleep study. Continuous pulse oximetry and electrocardiogram (ECG) monitoring were also performed during the sleep study. Throughout the night, it was noted that the patient had three episodes of hypoxemia lasting several minutes in duration. These hypoxemic episodes occurred during rapid eye movement (REM) sleep indicating possible upper airway obstruction.

The following night, the patient was fitted with a nasal mask utilizing lightweight adjustable headgear. A portable home volume ventilator (Lifecare LP3) and disposable circuit were then attached to the mask. Tidal volume was set at 700 mL with an assist-control rate of 10 breaths/min and an F_{IO_2} of 0.21. Continuous pulse oximetry during ventilation showed saturations above 90% for the entire duration of sleep. The following morning, the patient complained only of slight dryness of the nose and mouth. A pass-over humidifier was added to the circuit for the remaining nights and no other complaints were voiced. It was noticed that on the third night exhaled V_T and peak inspiratory pressure had decreased due to air leaks through the mouth. To correct this problem, the patient's sleeping position was changed and the V_T increased to 800 mL. No other problems were encountered during the hospital stay.

Three days before discharge, the patient's wife and two other family members were given detailed instructions on the operation of the volume ventilator and applying the nasal mask system to the patient. Further education included appropriate actions to take in response to ventilator alarms, an emergency plan in case of power failure, and detailed instructions for the cleaning and disinfecting of equipment. Having already been on a negative pressure ventilator in the home, the medical supply company knew the location and size of the patient's bedroom and the physical outlay of his home. The change to the positive pressure volume ventilator was completed without problems.

Follow-up visits by the medical supply company and home health care agency continued once weekly for the first month. A routine pulse oximetry check revealed a daytime spontaneous oxygen saturation of 92%. The patient and family appeared to be adjusting well to the new method of ventilation. In fact, the patient stated that his headaches had disappeared and he felt he had more physical endurance to perform more activities.

Case 2

A 62-year-old woman with a history of chronic obstructive pulmonary disease (COPD) had been hospitalized on a volume ventilator for 5 weeks following an acute exacerbation of her condition. Although her ABG results, ECG, and electrolytes were stable, numerous attempts to wean her from mechanical ventilation had proved unsuccessful. Mechanical ventilator settings were: V_T, 600 mL; SIMV rate of 8 and a total rate of 14 breaths/min; and F_{IO_2} of 0.3. Her spontaneous VC was 25% of predicted and her maximum inspiratory pressure was −20 cm H_2O.

After 3 weeks on mechanical ventilation, a tracheostomy tube was inserted. There was no evidence of any acute infectious process. The patient was alert and cooperative and has a very supportive husband and son. The physician elected to discharge this patient to the home on a portable volume ventilator and asked the other members of the health care team to prepare the patient for discharge in 1 week.

A medical equipment supply company was contacted to come to the hospital and talk to the patient and family about home mechanical ventilation. The medical equipment supplier interviewed the patient and family before making an assessment of the patient's home environment. Upon arrival at the patient's home, the medical equipment supplier made note of the access roads, the number of entrances to the home, the location of heaters, and the adequacy of electricity available in the patient's room. He determined that the patient's room was quite small, but would accommodate a small portable volume ventilator, hospital bed, and portable suction machine. A small cart was used to store circuits and suction catheters. A concentrator was also needed for supplemental oxygen. The local utility company was then contacted and the patient's name was placed on a priority list in case of power failure.

The following day, a small portable volume ventilator was brought to the patient's room. A respiratory care practitioner began the process of educating the patient's spouse and son in the operation of the unit. Each day for the next week, the spouse and son were taught to perform ventilator checks, to change circuits, to suction the patient, to manually ventilate the patient, and to recognize signs and symptoms of respiratory failure. Together with the medical supplier, physician, and a local nursing service, an emergency plan was formulated and a local hospital designated for emergency care. The patient and family received additional education from nurses and dieticians regarding proper medications and diet. One week after the education program began, the patient was discharged home.

Upon arrival at the home, the medical equipment supplier and a nurse from the local home health agency were there to meet the patient and ensure proper setup and function of the ventilator system. The family was left with a list of important telephone numbers and instructed to call if there were any problems or questions. Routine weekly visits continued for the next 4 weeks at which the patient and family were evaluated.

After 1 month of home mechanical ventilation, the evaluation report revealed that the family was very cooperative and capable of caring for the patient, but were physically and emotionally tired. The patient expressed an interest in becoming more involved in her own care, and had learned to suction and manually ventilate herself with a manual resuscitator. Pulse oximetry and routine vital signs were within normal limits. It was recommended that the family hire a part-time nurses' aide from the local home health agency to allow them periodic time away from home.

STUDY QUESTIONS

1. All of the following are realistic goals of home mechanical ventilation *except:*
   a. Life extension.
   b. Improved physical, psychological, and social function.
   c. Minimization of patient activity.
   d. Lessening the number of hospitalizations.
2. According to the criteria for patient selection, which of the following conditions would be most suitable for successful home care ventilation?
   a. A patient with fibrotic lung disease on continuous ventilatory support with a high F_{IO_2} and PEEP.
   b. A patient with progressive muscular dystrophy.
   c. A patient with severe COPD, cor pulmonale, and recurrent respiratory tract infections.
   d. A patient with terminal lung cancer who is post pneumonectomy.
3. Which of the following factors must be considered when selecting a ventilator for home care ventilation?
   I. Electrical adequacy of the patient's home.
   II. The versatility of the ventilator to accommodate the patient in all areas of the home.
   III. A sophisticated and elaborate alarm system.
   IV. The ease with which the ventilator can be operated by caregivers.
   a. I and II only.
   b. I, II, and III.
   c. II and IV only.
   d. I, II, and IV.
   e. III and IV only.
4. Which of the following negative pressure ventilators can be used *only* for ventilatory assistance and not ventilatory support?
   a. Pneumobelt.
   b. Chest cuirass.
   c. Full body chamber.
   d. Pneumosuit.
   e. Raincoat.
5. A patient with stable COPD has been selected for home care ventilation. His ABGs are stable while on a volume ventilator with the following settings: V_T = 700 mL, rate = 10 breaths/min, SIMV, F_{IO_2} = 0.3. What operational features will need to be considered when selecting this patient's home mechanical ventilator?
   a. Available modes of operation.
   b. Reservoir capabilities for the addition of oxygen.

c. Low pressure and high pressure alarms.
d. Power loss alarm.
e. All of the above.

6. A patient with a high spinal cord injury has been selected for home mechanical ventilation. The patient has a tracheostomy and is on a volume ventilator with room air administration. In addition to this patient's home care ventilator, what other equipment will be needed in the home?
   I. A back-up ventilator.
   II. Tracheostomy care kits.
   III. Concentrator.
   IV. Portable suction unit.
   V. Manual resuscitator.
   a. I, II, and IV.
   b. I, II, III, and V.
   c. I, II, IV, and V.
   d. I, II, III, IV, and V.
   e. I and IV only.
7. While preparing the patient for discharge home, the respiratory care practitioner should instruct the patient and family to:
   a. Wash and dry the ventilator equipment once daily.
   b. Soak the equipment in warm soapy water, rinse, and towel-dry twice daily.
   c. Soak the equipment in warm soapy water, scrub to remove organic material, rinse, and place in disinfectant solution once daily.
   d. Soak the equipment in disinfectant solution once weekly.
   e. Boil the equipment in water for 10 minutes, then allow to air-dry before packaging.
8. A patient with a progressive neuromuscular disorder has been selected for home mechanical ventilation. As part of the discharge plan, the health care team should:
   a. Instruct the family or caregivers in aseptic suction procedures.
   b. Give detailed instructions in cardiopulmonary resuscitation.
   c. Provide a written protocol with directions for respiratory treatment and other aspects of care.
   d. Assess the home environment for proper electrical safety.
   e. All of the above.
9. All of the following should be considered in preparing a patient for home mechanical ventilation *except:*
   a. The family's critical care experience.
   b. The family's willingness to learn and participate in the patient's care.
   c. The geographical location of the patient's home.
   d. The electrical safety and available space in the patient's home.
   e. The family's ability to adequately operate the ventilator.

10. A written report should be completed monthly during the follow-up and evaluation of patients on home mechanical ventilation. Which of the following conditions should this monthly report include?
    I. Pulse oximetry data.
    II. Patient and family apprehensions.
    III. Proper functioning of the equipment.
    IV. Compliance with the therapeutic plan.
    a. I, III, and IV.
    b. I and III only.
    c. I, II, and IV.
    d. I, II, III, and IV.
    e. II and III only.
11. Which of the following patients would benefit from NIPPV?
    I. A patient with progressive neuromuscular disease who requires the use of a chest cuirass at night only.
    II. A patient diagnosed with obstructive sleep apnea but who has good respiratory muscle strength.
    III. A patient with stable COPD who requires nocturnal ventilation.
    IV. A patient with kyphoscoliosis who experiences episodes of hypercapnia and hypoxemia at night.
    a. I only.
    b. II and IV.
    c. III only.
    d. I, III, and IV.
    e. III and IV.
12. All of the following are considered advantages of NIPPV over conventional methods of mechanical ventilation *except:*
    a. It requires the use of a tracheostomy tube.
    b. It is less cumbersome and allows for better patient mobility.
    c. It decreases the risk of infection.
    d. It is cost-effective.
    e. It allows better coordination of the patient's breathing effort.
13. A patient on nasal mask IPPV experiences mouth leaks during sleep. Which of the following procedures would minimize this problem?
    a. Decrease the IPAP pressure level.
    b. Increase the IPAP pressure level.
    c. Decrease the flow rate through the circuitry.
    d. Decrease the inspiratory time.
    e. Decrease the EPAP pressure level.
14. A patient on nasal mask CPAP complains of dried, irritated nasal passages and eyes. All of the following would be beneficial in solving this problem *except:*
    a. Readjusting the nasal mask for better fit.

b. Periodic irrigation of the nasal passages with normal saline.
c. A nasal mask custom-made to fit the patient's face.
d. Addition of a humidifier to the circuit.
e. A heated nebulizer placed in-line with the circuitry.

15. A potential complication of nasal CPAP or NIPPV therapy is:
    a. Reduced cough reflex.
    b. Hypoventilation.
    c. Upper airway obstruction.
    d. Tracheomalacia.
    e. Increased cardiac output.
16. Which of the following statements regarding the indications for nasal mask ventilation is (are) true?
    I. It can be used for continuous ventilatory support.
    II. The patient must have intact cough reflexes.
    III. The patient must have adequate muscle strength.
    IV. The patient must not require extensive airway management.
    a. I, II, and IV.
    b. II and III.
    c. I, II, III, and IV.
    d. II and IV.
    e. I, III, and IV.
17. Which of the following procedures should be followed in the preparation of a patient for home care NIPPV by nasal mask?
    a. Allow the patient several days in the hospital to adjust to the nasal mask system of ventilation.
    b. Instruct the family on the operation and maintenance of the ventilator unit.
    c. Obtain baseline ABGs and pulse oximetry data before setting the desired pressure levels.
    d. Formulate an emergency plan for the family to follow should it be needed.
    e. All of the above.

ANSWERS TO STUDY QUESTIONS

1. c.
2. b.
3. d.
4. a.
5. e.
6. c.
7. c.
8. e.
9. a.
10. d.
11. d.
12. a.
13. b.
14. e.
15. b.
16. c.
17. e.

REFERENCES

1. AARC Home Care Consensus Report: Part 2: Product standards and infection control. *AARC Times* 1990; 57–60.
2. American Thoracic Society: Home mechanical ventilation of 1990; pediatric patients. *Am Rev Respir Dis* 1990; 141:258–259.
3. American Respiratory Care Foundation: Guidelines for disinfection of respiratory care equipment used in the home. *Respir Care* 1988; 33:801–808.
4. Bach JR, Augusta SA: Management of chronic alveolar hyperventilation by nasal ventilation. *Chest* 1990; 97:52–57.
5. Clark K: Psychosocial aspects of prolonged ventilator dependency. *Respir Care* 1986; 31:329–333.
6. Ellis ER, Bye P, Bruderer JW, et al: Treatment of respiratory failure during sleep in patients with neuromuscular disease. *Am Rev Respir Dis* 1987; 35:148–152.
7. Ellis ER, Grunstein RR, Chan S, et al: Noninvasive ventilatory support during sleep improves respiratory failure in kyphoscoliosis. *Chest* 1988; 94:811–815.
8. Kacmarek R, Spearman C: Equipment used for ventilatory support in the home. *Respir Care* 1986; 31:311–328.
9. Kirby G, Mayer L, Pingleton S: Nocturnal positive pressure ventilation via nasal mask. *Am Rev Respir Dis* 1987; 135:738–740.
10. Leger P, Jennequin J, Gerard M, et al: Home positive pressure ventilation via nasal mask for patients with neuromuscular weakness or restrictive lung or chest-wall disease. *Respir Care* 1989; 34:73–78.
11. Linder K, Lotz P, Ahnefeld F: CPAP effect on FRC, VC and its subdivisions. *Chest* 1987; 92:66–70.
12. Lucas J, Golish J, Sleeper G, et al: *Home Respiratory Care.* Norwalk, Conn, Appleton & Lange, 1988.
13. Make B: ACCP guidelines for mechanical ventilation in the home setting. *AARC Times* 1987; 11:56–58.
14. Make BJ: Long-term management of ventilator-assisted individuals: The Boston University experience. *Respir Care* 1986; 31:303–310.
15. O'Donohue WJ, Giovannoni RM, Keens TG, et al: Long-term mechanical ventilation: Guidelines for management in the home and at alternate community sites. *Chest* 1986; 90(suppl):1s–35s.
16. Pierson DJ, George PB: Mechanical ventilation in the home: Possibilities and prerequisites. *Respir Care* 1986; 31:286–270.
17. Scanlan C, Spearman C, Sheldon R: *Egan's Fundamentals of Respiratory Care,* ed 5. St Louis, Mosby–Year Book, Inc, 1990.
18. Schwartz O: Current concepts of ventilation for the home care patient. *AARC Times* 1987; 11:52–54.
19. Sivak ED, Cordasco EM, Gipson TW, et al: Home care ventilation: The Cleveland experience from 1977 to 1985. *Respir Care* 1986; 33:294–302.
20. Splaingard MC, Frates RC, Harrison GM, et al: Home positive-pressure ventilation: Twenty years' experience. *Chest* 1983; 84:376–382.

Appendixes

APPENDIX A. Calculation of Alveolar Ventilation

Per breath: tidal volume (V_T) minus dead space (V_D), which is usually considered to equal anatomic dead space. $V_A = V_T - V_D$
Per minutes: $(V_T - V_D) \times f = \dot{V}_A$ where f is the respiratory rate.
Also, $\dot{V}_E - \dot{V}_D = \dot{V}_A$ where $\dot{V}_E$ is the minute ventilation ($V_T \times$ respiratory rate, f) and $\dot{V}_D$ is the dead space ventilation per minute ($V_D \times f$).

APPENDIX B. Alveolar Air Equation

$$P_AO_2 = (F_IO_2) \times (P_B - 47) - (Pa_{CO_2}) \times \left[(F_{IO_2}) + \left(\frac{1 - F_{IO_2}}{R}\right)\right]$$

where P_AO_2 = alveolar partial pressure of oxygen (mm Hg)
F_{IO_2} = fractional inspired oxygen concentration
P_B = barometric pressure (mm Hg)
47 = partial pressure of water vapor at body temperature (37°C) in mm Hg
Pa_{CO_2} = partial pressure of carbon dioxide in the arteries (mm Hg)
R = respiratory exchange ratio ($\dot{V}_{CO_2}/\dot{V}_{O_2}$)

Modified Alveolar Air Equation

$P_{A}O_2 = P_{IO_2} - Pa_{CO_2}/0.8$

$P_{I}O_2 = F_{IO_2} \times (P_B - 47)$

0.8 = normal respiratory exchange ratio

Alveolar-Arterial Oxygen Gradient $[P(A-a)O_2]$

$P(A - a)O_2 = P_{A}O_2 - Pa_{O_2}$

Normal value is 5 mm Hg at 20 years of age, breathing room air, and increases each decade after 20 by 4 mm Hg

APPENDIX C. Equipment for Tracheal Intubation

- Endotracheal tubes and tracheostomy tubes of varying sizes.
- Laryngoscope with varying blade types and sizes (check light for working condition).
- Stylet.
- Adhesive tape for securing tube; umbilical tape for tracheostomies; scissors.
- Syringes for cuff inflation.
- Endotracheal tube connectors and adaptors.
- Oropharyngeal airways of various sizes. These may be used for bite-blocks when necessary.
- Anesthetic agents: Spray for upper airway and gel (water-soluble) for tube lubrication. Example: 2% xylocaine. A nonanesthetic, lubricating water-soluble gel can also be used.
- Oxygen source, flowmeter, regulator, and oxygen connecting tube for a resuscitation bag with mask. An oxygen mask is also useful.
- Suction source and suction catheters.
- Muscle relaxants and sedatives.
- Access to a well-stocked resuscitation cart.
- A tracheostomy tray.
- Magill forceps and rubber-tipped hemostats.

APPENDIX D. Endotracheal Tubes, Tracheostomy Tubes and Laryngoscope Blades (Tube Thickness May Vary With Manufacturer)

	Endotracheal Tubes*		
Approximate Age or Weight	Internal Diameter (in mm)	External Diameter (in mm)	Length (cm) (avg OD)
Premature infants (2–5 lb)	2.0–3.0	3.7–4.5	8
Newborn infants (5.0–5.5 lb)	3.0	4.5	9
Newborn infants to 3 mo (5.5–11 lb)	3.5–4.0	5.0–5.5	9
3–10 mo (11–18 lb)	4.3	5.7	10
10–12 mo (19–20 lb)	4.5	6.0	11
13–24 mo (20–25 lb)	5.0	6.5	12
2–3 yr (25–33 lb)	5.5	7.0	13
4–5 yr (33–44 lb)	6.0	8.0	14
6–7 yr (44–55 lb)	6.5	8.5	15
8–9 yr (55–70 lb)	7.0	9.0	16
9–10 yr (55–70 lb)	7.0	9.0	16
10–12 yr (70–85 lb)	7.5	9.5	17
12–16 yr (85–130 lb)	7.5	9.5	22.5
Adult females	8.0–9.0	10.0–12.0	19–24
Adult males	8.5–10.0	11.5–13.0	20–28

*Conversion to French scale: 4 × ID or 3 × ED.

	Tracheostomy Tubes	
Age	Jackson Tube Size	OD
Premature to newborn	00	4.5
Newborn to 3 mo	0	5.0
Up to 1 yr	1	5.5
1–3 yr	2	6.0
3–6 yr	3	7.0
6–12 yr	4	8.0
12 yr to adult	5–9	9.0–13.0

Age	Laryngoscope Blades (Type and Size)
Premature	Miller (0)
Infant to 3 mo	Miller (1)
3–12 mo	Miller or MacIntosh (1½)
3–9 yr	MacIntosh (2)
9 yr to adult	MacIntosh (3)

APPENDIX E. Specifications for Some Commercially Available Positive Pressure Ventilators*

Advanced Pulmonary Technologies

APT 100 HFJV

Power source: pneumatic
Control circuit: microprocessor
Cycling control variable: time, pressure
Inspiratory waveform: constant (rectangular) flow
Drive pressure: 15–50 cm H_2O
Frequency: 1–10 H (60–600 breaths/min)
Inspiratory time: 15%–50%
F_{IO_2}: 0.21–1.00

Other features: alarms for airway pressure (operator set), oxygen percentage, valve function, high and low mean airway pressure, battery inoperative and ventilator inoperative. Cathode ray tube (CRT) screen monitor; built-in battery

Bird Ventilators

IMV Bird

Power source: pneumatic
Control circuit: pneumatic
Cycling control variable: time
Inspiratory waveform: nonconstant flow generator
Pressure limit: 20–110 cm H_2O
Tidal volume: 100–2,500 mL
Flow range: 10–66 L/min
Frequency: 1–30 breaths/min
Inspiratory time: 1.0–4.5 seconds
Expiratory time: 0.9–180 seconds
PEEP: 0–35 cm H_2O
F_{IO_2}: 0.21–1.00

* Compiled with Tony Rogers, Respiratory Therapy Program, Greenville Technical College, Greenville, S.C.

Other features: operates on IMV mode and control; has NEEP and expiratory retard available

Bird Mark 7

Power source: pneumatic
Control circuit: pneumatic system regulated by pneumatic clutch and peak flow needle valve
Cycling control variable: pressure or time (expiration)
Inspiratory waveform: constant flow (square wave) on 100% setting; decelerating flow on air-mix mode
Pressure limit: 0–60 cm H_2O
Flow range: 0–50 L/min on 100%; 0–80 L/min on air-mix
Frequency: 0–80 breaths/min
Expiratory time: 0.5–15 seconds
F_{IO_2}: 0.21, 0.4–1.0 (depending on rate, volume, and inspiratory cycle)

Other features: single circuit, low internal resistance; no alarms; sensitivity 0 to −5 cm H_2O

Bird 6400 ST

Power source: pneumatic
Control circuit: microprocessor and stepper motor
Cycling control variable: volume, time, or pressure
Inspiratory waveform: constant or decreasing flow waveform
Pressure limit: 1 140 cm H_2O
Tidal volume: 50–2,000 mL
Flow range: 10–120 L/min
Frequency: 0–80 breaths/min
PEEP or CPAP: 0–30 cm H_2O
F_{IO_2}: 0.21–1.00

Other features: SIMV and CPAP available; alarms for high and low pressure, low PEEP or CPAP, low tidal volume, apnea, low O_2 and air pressure, ventilator inoperative

Bird 8400

Power source: pneumatic
Control circuit: microprocessor and stepper motor
Cycling control variable: volume, time, or pressure
Inspiratory waveform: constant or decreasing flow waveform

Pressure limit: 1–140 cm H_2O
Tidal volume: 50–2,000 mL
Flow range: 10–120 L/min
Frequency: 0–80 breaths/min (assist to 150 breaths/min)
PEEP or CPAP: 0–30 cm H_2O
F_{IO_2}: 0.21–1.00

Other features: SIMV and CPAP available; alarms for high and low pressure, low PEEP or CPAP, low tidal volume, apnea, low O_2 and air pressure, ventilator inoperative; volume monitoring, adjustable apnea with back-up rate, low minute volume alarm, high frequency alarm, graphic monitoring available

V.I.P. Bird (Ventilator for Infant and Pediatrics)

Power source: pneumatic
Control circuit: microprocessor with stepper motor
Cycling control variable: time, volume, pressure
Inspiratory waveform: constant flow or decreasing
Pressure limit: 3–80 cm H_2O (time cycled); 3–100 cm H_2O (volume-cycled)
Tidal volume: 20–760 mL
Flow range: 3–40 L/min (time-cycled); 3–120 L/min (volume-cycled)
Frequency: 4–150 breaths/min
Inspiratory time: 0.1–3.0 seconds
PEEP: 0–24 cm H_2O
F_{IO_2}: 0.21–1.00

Other features: alarms for oxygen failure and air failure; operates IMV or SIMV, PS, PC, A-C; exhaled tidal volume monitor, alarms for high rate, low minute volume, apnea, circuit fault and ventilator inoperative

Bear (Bourns Electronic Adult Respirator) Ventilators

BEAR 1

Power source: electric or compressed gas
Control circuit: electronic solenoids and regulators control pneumatic system
Cycling control variable: volume, time, or pressure
Inspiratory waveform: constant or nonconstant flow generator (square with tapered flow)

Pressure limit: 0–100 cm H_2O
Tidal volume: 100–2,000 mL
Flow range: 20–120 L/min
Frequency: 0.5–60 breaths/min
Inspiratory time: 0.5–10.0 seconds
Expiratory time: 0.95–120 seconds
CPAP or PEEP: 0–30 cm H_2O
F_{IO_2}: 0.21–1.00

Other features: sensitivity setting −1.0 to −5 cm H_2O; inflation hold 0–2 seconds; compliance value 3.0 mL/cm H_2O; SIMV available; alarms for high and low pressure, low volume, loss of power, O_2 failure, ratio, low PEEP or CPAP and ventilator inoperative, sigh mode; single circuit

BEAR 2

Power source: electric or compressed gas
Control circuit: electronic
Cycling control variable: volume, time, or pressure
Inspiratory waveform: constant or nonconstant flow generator
Pressure limit: 0–120 cm H_2O
Tidal volume: 100–2,000 mL
Flow range: 10–120 L/min
Frequency: 0.5–60 breaths/min
Inspiratory time: 0.5–10.0 seconds
Expiratory time: 0.95–120 seconds
CPAP or PEEP: 0–50 cm H_2O
F_{IO_2}: 0.21–1.00

Other features: sigh and SIMV modes available; sensitivity setting from −1 to −5 cm H_2O; alarms for high and low pressure, O_2 failure, low volume, ratio, low PEEP or CPAP, loss of power, high temperature, high rate, and ventilator inoperative

BEAR 3

Power source: electric or compressed gas
Control circuit: electronic
Cycling control variable: volume, time, or pressure
Inspiratory waveform: constant or nonconstant flow generator
Pressure limit: 0–120 cm H_2O
Tidal volume: 100–2,000 mL

Flow range: 10–120 L/min
Frequency: 0.5–60 breaths/min
CPAP or PEEP: 0–50 cm H_2O
FIO_2: 0.21–1.0

Other features: sigh, SIMV, SIMV with pressure support, and pressure support modes; sensitivity setting from −1 to −5 cm H_2O; inflation hold 0–2 seconds; alarms for high and low pressure, oxygen failure, low volume, ratio, low PEEP or CPAP, loss of power, high temperature, high rate, and ventilator inoperative

BEAR 5

Power source: pneumatic
Control circuit: microprocessor-controlled stepper motor
Cycling control variable: volume, time, or pressure
Inspiratory waveform: rectangular, ascending, descending, sine wave
Pressure limit: 0–150 cm H_2O
Tidal volume: 50–2,000 mL
Flow range: 5–150 L/min
Frequency: 0.5–150 breaths/min
Inspiratory time: 0.10–3.0 seconds
PEEP or CPAP: 0–50 cm H_2O
Pressure support: 0–72 cm H_2O
Minimum minute volume: 0.5–40 L/min (called augmented minute volume)
Continuous flow: 5–40 L/min
O_2 concentration: 21%–100%

Other features: IMV or SIMV, time-cycled or pressure-limited IMV, CPAP, and AMV modes available; CRT able to display monitoring, alarms, mechanics, or graphs; alarms for high and low pressure, low tidal volume, high and low minute volume, high and low rate, high and low mean airway pressure, high and low PEEP or CPAP, ratio, low O_2 and air source, and ventilator inoperative (often used)

BP-200 from BEAR

Power source: pneumatic
Control circuit: electronically controlled solenoid and regulators govern pneumatic system
Cycling control variable: time
Inspiratory waveform: constant flow or constant pressure generator
Pressure limit: 10–80 cm H_2O
Flow range: 0–20 L/min

Frequency: 1–150 breaths/min
Inspiratory time: 0.2–5.0 seconds
PEEP: 0–20 cm H_2O
F_{IO_2}: 0.21–1.00

Other features: oxygen or air failure alarm, loss of power alarm; inverse I/E ratios (I/E from 4:1–1:10); IMV mode; single circuit; high internal resistance; CPAP mode

BEAR Cub

Power source: pneumatic
Control circuit: electronic
Cycling control variable: time
Inspiratory waveform: constant flow or nonconstant pressure
Pressure limit: 0–72 cm H_2O
Flow range: 3–30 L/min
Frequency: 1–150 breaths/min
Inspiratory time: 0.1–3.0 seconds
PEEP: 0–20 cm H_2O
F_{IO_2}: 0.21–1.00

Other features: IMV mode; alarms for low pressure, prolonged pressure, low PEEP or CPAP, ratio, air or O_2 failure, loss of power, and ventilator inoperative; add-on monitor available

LS 104-50 Infant Ventilator

Power source: electric
Control circuit: electronic control or linear drive piston
Cycling control variable: volume, time, or pressure
Inspiratory waveform: constant flow
Tidal volume: 5–150 breaths/min
Flow range: 3–12 L/min
Pressure limit: 0–100 cm H_2O
Frequency: 5–80 breaths/min
PEEP: 0–18 cm H_2O
F_{IO_2}: 0.21–1.00 with blender

Other features: sensitivity −0.05 to −1.0 cm H_2O, response time 35 ms; sigh mode, CPAP and IMV, high and low pressure alarm, apnea alarm; single circuit; high internal resistance; inflation hold available

Puritan-Bennett Ventilators

Puritan-Bennett PR-2

Power source: pneumatic
Control circuit: pneumatic system regulated by Bennett valve
Cycling control variable: time, pressure, or flow
Inspiratory waveform: decelerating flow
Pressure limit: 0–50 cm H_2O
F_{IO_2}: air-mix 0.40–0.70, or 1.00 setting

Other features: compliance value 2.5 cm H_2O, flow or 1 L/min ends inspiration, terminal flow for leaks of 1 L/min, fixed I/E ratio (1:1.5); single circuit; low internal resistance, no alarms

Puritan-Bennett MA-1

Power source: electric
Control circuit: electronically powered compressor drives a bellows system
Cycling control variable: volume, time, or pressure
Inspiratory waveform: constant pressure generator with moderate generating pressure (square wave or tapered square wave)
Pressure limit: 10–80 cm H_2O
Tidal volume: 100–2,200 mL
Flow range: 15–100 L/min
Frequency: 6–60 breaths/min
Inspiratory time: 0.4–5.0 seconds
Expiratory time: 0.6–5.0 seconds
PEEP: 0–15 cm H_2O
F_{IO_2}: 0.21–1.00

Other features: compliance value 3 mL/cm H_2O sigh mode, sensitivity -0.1 to -10 cm H_2O, expiratory retard 26–200 L/min, high pressure alarm, low pressure alarm, ratio alarm, O_2 failure alarm, NEEP option, IMV option, circuit, moderate internal resistance

Puritan-Bennett MA-2

Power source: electric or pneumatic
Control circuit: electronic
Cycling control variable: volume, time, or pressure
Inspiratory waveform: constant flow generator
Pressure limit: 10–120 cm H_2O

Tidal volume: 200–2,200 mL
Flow range: 15–100 L/min
Frequency: 0.4–60 breaths/min
PEEP: 0–45 cm H_2O
F_{IO_2}: 0.21–1.00

Other features: compliance value 3 mL/cm H_2O; IMV; demand modes; low circuit and high pressure alarms, low volume alarm, failure-to-cycle alarm, I/E ratio, low PEEP or CPAP alarm, high temperature alarm, oxygen failure; sigh mode available

Puritan-Bennett 7200a Series

Power source: pneumatic
Control circuit: microprocessor
Cycling control variable: volume, time, pressure, or flow
Pressure limit: 10–120 cm H_2O
Tidal volume: 0.1–2.5 L
Flow range: 10–180 L/min
Frequency: 0.5–70 breaths/min
PEEP: 0–50 cm H_2O
F_{IO_2}: 0.21–1.00

Other features: SIMV, CPAP, PS (0–70 cm H_2O) and PC (with SIMV 0–100 cm H_2O) and sigh modes; 100% O_2 delivery for 2 minutes to suction; alarms for high and low pressure, apnea, I/E ratio, power loss, exhalation valve leak, low volume, ventilator inoperative, O_2 failure, low rate, low CPAP or PEEP, low battery; has a self-test mode; sensitivity −0.5 to −20 cm H_2O, inflation hold; 7200 has capability to add on software options such as flow-by (2–10 L/min), respiratory mechanics, pulse oximeter, and plasma screen display

Bio-Med Ventilators

Bio-Med IC2

Power source: pneumatic
Control circuit: fluidic
Cycling control variable: time
Inspiratory waveform: constant (rectangular)
Pressure limit: 10–80 cm H_2O
Tidal volume: 100–2,000 mL
Flow range: 20–75 L/min

Frequency: 1–60 breaths/min
Inspiratory time: 0.4–2.0 seconds
Expiratory time: 0.5–4.0 seconds
PEEP: 0–15 cm H_2O
F_{IO_2}: 0.21–1.00

Other features: SIMV and demand modes available; CPAP

Bio-Med IC-2A (Adult or pediatric use)

Power source: pneumatic
Control circuit: pneumatic
Cycling control variable: time, pressure (volume limit)
Inspiratory waveform: square
Pressure limit:0–100 cm H_2O
Tidal volume: 0–3,000 mL
Flow range: 0–75 L/min
Frequency: 1.33–66 breaths/min
Inspiratory time: 0.4–3.0 seconds
Expiratory time: 0.5–4.0 seconds
PEEP or CPAP: 0–25 cm H_2O
Sensitivity: −20 to +100 cm H_2O
F_{IO_2}: blender

Other features: SIMV and demand modes, CPAP, compatible for MRI

Bio-Med MVP-10 (Neonates to pediatric use)

Power source: pneumatic
Control circuit: pneumatic
Cycling control variable: time, pressure
Inspiratory waveform: rectangular (constant)
Pressure limit: 0–80 cm H_2O
Tidal volume: 0–400 mL
Flow range: 0–20 L/min
Frequency: 1–120 breaths/min
Inspiratory time: 0.2–2.0 seconds
Expiratory time: 0.25–30 seconds
PEEP or CPAP: 0–18 cm H_2O
F_{IO_2}: 0.21–1.00

Other features: IMV mode; alarm module add-on available; compatible for MRI use

Bio-Med IC-5

Power source: pneumatic
Cycling control variable: time, pressure, volume
Pressure limit: 0–120 cm H_2O
Tidal volume: 50–3,000 mL
Flow range: 5–120 L/min
Frequency: 5–150 breaths/min
PEEP or CPAP: 0–35 cm H_2O
F_{IO_2}: 0.21–1.00

Other features: SIMV; plateau 0%–33% of inspiration; sigh mode; alarms for high pressure, temperature, O_2 concentration, exhaled volume, mean airway pressure

Bunnell Ventilator

LifePulse HFJV

Power source: pneumatic
Control circuit: microprocessor (pinch valve or jet valve)
Cycling control variable: time
Inspiratory waveform: ascending ramp
Peak inspiratory pressure (PIP): 8–50 cm H_2O, internal pressure limit: +5 cm H_2O above PIP
Servo pressure: 0–20 psig
Frequency: 0.2–22 breaths/min
Inspiratory time: 0.2–0.34 second
I/E ratio: 1:1.6–1:12

Other features: PEEP; servo control for PIP; monitors for servo pressure (driving pressure, working pressure), mean airway pressure, and ΔP (PEEP − PIP); pressure measured at distal tip of catheter (near carina); alarms: PIP loss, high PIP, cannot meet PIP, low gas supply, vent. fault, and jet valve fault; built-in humidifier with servo-controlled temperature and water level and high/low temperature alarm, and high/low water level

Emerson Ventilators

Emerson IMV

Power source: electric
Control circuit: electronic driven rotary piston

Cycling control variable: time
Inspiratory waveform: sinusoidal
Pressure limit: 50–100 cm H_2O
Tidal volume: 200–2,200 cm H_2O
Flow range: 5.5–60 L/min
Frequency: 0.2–22 breaths/min
Inspiratory time: 1 or 5 seconds
Expiratory time: 2.3–300 seconds
PEEP: 0–25 cm H_2O
F_{IO_2}: 0.21–1.00

Other features: compliance value 4.2 mL/cm H_2O; high and low pressure alarms available; IMV; single circuit; high internal resistance

Emerson 3-PV

Power source: electric
Control circuit: electronic
Cycling control variable: time
Inspiratory waveform: sinusoidal nonconstant flow generator
Pressure limit: 40–160 cm H_2O
Tidal volume: 0–2,000 mL
Flow range: 1.2–260 L/min
Frequency: 10–50 breaths/min
Inspiratory time: 0.4–3.0 seconds
Expiratory time: 0.4–3.0 seconds
PEEP: 0–15 cm H_2O
F_{IO_2}: 0.21–1.00

Other features: compliance value 4.2 mL/cm H_2O; high and low pressure alarms available

Engström Ventilators

Engström 300

Power source: electric
Control circuit: electronic
Cycling control variable: time
Inspiratory waveform: accelerating flow or modified sine wave (nonconstant flow generator)

Pressure limit: 30–90 cm H_2O
Minute volume: 0–50 L/min
Flow range: 1–264 L/min variable
Frequency: 12–35 breaths/min
Inspiratory time: 0.5–1.7 seconds
Expiratory time: 1.2–4.3 seconds
PEEP: 0–20 cm H_2O
F_{IO_2}: 0.21–1.00

Other features: inspiratory hold 0–0.8 second, I/E fixed at 1:2; NEEP available; IMV option; power loss alarm; compliance factor 4.5 mL/cm H_2O; double circuit; high internal resistance

Engström Erica

Power source: pneumatic
Control circuit: electronic
Cycling control variable: flow, time, or pressure
Inspiratory waveform: constant or nonconstant flow generator
Pressure limit: 0–120 cm H_2O
Tidal volume: 100–2,000 ml
Frequency: 0.4–40 breaths/min
PEEP: 0–30 cm H_2O
F_{IO_2}: 0.21–1.00

Other features: SIMV and demand modes; inverse I/E ratios (I/E range 3:1–1:3); sensitivity 0.1 L/sec; sigh mode; alarm for high and low pressure, high and low volume, apnea, power loss, and air or O_2 failure; pressure support mode

Hamilton Ventilators

Hamilton Veolar

Power source: pneumatic
Control circuit: microprocessor
Cycling control variable: flow, time, or pressure
Inspiratory waveform: seven patterns, user-selectable
Pressure limit: 10–110 cm H_2O
Tidal volume: 20–2,000 mL
Flow range: 0–180 L/min
Frequency: 0.5–60 breaths/min

PEEP or CPAP: 0–50 cm H_2O
Pressure support: 0–50 cm H_2O above PEEP up to an actual pressure of 50 cm H_2O
Minimum minute volume: 1–25 L/min
O_2 concentrations: 21%–100%

Other features: SIMV, CPAP, pressure support, pressure control, and MMV modes; alarms for high pressure, high rate, high and low minute volume, high and low O_2 percent, low O_2 and air pressure, apnea, fail to cycle, and power failure

Hamilton Amadeus

Power source: pneumatic
Control circuit: microprocessor
Cycling control variable: volume, time, or pressure
Inspiratory waveform: two patterns user-selectable
Pressure limit: 10–110 cm H_2O
Tidal volume: 20–2,000 mL
Flow range: 0–180 L/min
Frequency: 5–120 breaths/min (SIMV 0.5–60 breaths/min)
I/E ratio: 1:9–4:1
Pause: 0–8 seconds
PEEP or CPAP: 0–50 cm H_2O
Pressure support: 0–100 cm H_2O
Minimum minute volume: 1–25 L/min
O_2 concentrations: 21%–100%

Other features: A-C, SIMV, CPAP; alarms for high pressure, high rate, high and low minute volume, high and low O_2 percent, low source pressure, apnea, disconnection, and power failure

Infrasonics Ventilators

Adult Star

Power source: pneumatic
Control circuit: microprocessor
Cycled into inspiratory: time, flow, pressure
Inspiratory waveform: constant or nonconstant pressure generator
Tidal volume: 100–2,500 mL
Frequency: 0.5–80 breaths/min

Peak flow rate: 10–150 L/min
PEEP or CPAP: 0–30 cm H_2O
Pressure support: 0–70 cm H_2O
FIO_2: 0.21–1.0

Other features: SIMV, SIMV with pressure support, CPAP with pressure support available; sigh; internal nebulizer; all settings via single knob; information and parameter via CRT; 20-minute battery back-up; alarms for high and low pressure, low mechanical volume, low spontaneous volume, low minute volume, low PEEP or CPAP, high rate, apnea, low oxygen and air pressure, low internal battery, loss of power; patient monitoring for exhaled tidal volume, minute volume, spontaneous minute volume, peak pressure, mean airway pressure, PEEP or CPAP, plateau pressure, rate, I/E ratio, inspiratory time

Star Infant

Power source: pneumatic
Control circuit: microprocessor-controlled solenoids
Cycling control variable: time
Inspiratory waveform: constant or demand flow, or constant pressure generator
Pressure limit: 8–90 cm H_2O
Flow range: 4–40 L/min
Frequency: 1–150 breaths/min
Inspiratory time: 0.1–3.0 seconds
PEEP or CPAP: 0–24 cm H_2O
FIO_2: 0.21–1.00

Other features: IMV with continuous or demand flow, CPAP with continuous or demand flow; internal battery system; alarms for low inspiratory pressure, low PEEP or CPAP, obstructed tube, insufficient expiratory time, low O_2 or air pressure, loss of power, battery in use, ventilator inoperative

Lifecare Ventilator

PLV-102 Ventilator

Power source: electric
Control circuit: microprocessor
Cycling control variable: time, volume, pressure
Inspiratory waveform: sine wave
Pressure limit: 5–100 cm H_2O

Tidal volume: 50–3000 mL
Flow range: 10–120 L/min
Frequency: 2–40 breaths/min
PEEP or CPAP: 0–20 cm H_2O with PEEP valve
F_{IO_2}: 0.21–1.00

Other features: SIMV, A-C, sigh, available O_2 analyzer, alarms for high and low pressure, apnea, inverse I/E ratio, increased inspiratory flow, internal and external battery, disconnection, power source change, power failure, and unit malfunction

Monaghan Ventilator

Monaghan 225/SIMV

Power source: pneumatic
Control circuit: fluidic mechanism driven bellows system
Cycling control variable: volume, time, or pressure
Inspiratory waveform: constant flow generator (square wave)
Pressure limit: 10–100 cm H_2O
Tidal volume: 100–3,300 mL
Flow range: 0–100 L/min
Frequency: 0.3–60 breaths/min
PEEP: 0–20 cm H_2O
F_{IO_2}: 0.21–100

Other features: sensitivity −0.5–−10 cm H_2O, SIMV mode, high pressure indicator, apnea alarm, I/E ratio 1:1–1:4, two versions: one with a nonferrous body for MRI use and one with a standard body

Newport Ventilators

Newport E 100i (neonates to pediatric use)

Power source: pneumatic
Control circuit: electronic
Cycling control variable: volume, time, or pressure
Inspiratory waveform: rectangular (constant) and modified ascending ramp
Pressure limit: 0–100 cm H_2O
Tidal volume: 10–2,000 mL

Inspiratory time: 0.1–3.0 seconds
Flow range: 0–100 L/min (continuous flow mixed output 0–55 L/min)
Frequency: 1–120 breaths/min
PEEP or CPAP: 0–25 cm H_2O
F_{IO_2}: 0.21–1.00

Other features: SIMV or IMV and CPAP; nebulizer; alarms for high and low pressure, low O_2 and air source pressure, long inspiratory time, and electrical power failure

Newport Breeze

Power source: pneumatic
Control circuit: microprocessor
Cycling control variable: volume, time, or pressure
PIP: 0–60 cm H_2O
Pressure limit: 10–120 cm H_2O
Tidal volume: 30–2,000 mL
Inspiratory time: 0.1–3.0 seconds
Flow range: 3–120 L/min (spontaneous flow 0–50 L/min)
Frequency: 1–150 breaths/min
PEEP or CPAP: 0–60 cm H_2O
F_{IO_2}: 0.21–1.00

Other features: SIMV, A-C, and CPAP; nebulizer; alarms for high and low pressure, apnea, low CPAP, low battery, gas supply failure, and power failure

Newport Model E 200 (Wave)

Power source: pneumatic
Control circuit: microprocessor
Cycling control: volume, time, flow, or pressure
Flow waveform: rectangular (constant) and descending ramp
PIP: 0–75 cm H_2O
Pressure limit: 10–120 cm H_2O
Tidal volume: 30–2,000 mL
Inspiratory time: 0.1–3.0 seconds (inverse ratio limit 3:1)
Flow range: 1–100 L/min (spontaneous flow 1–160 L/min)
Frequency: 1–100 breaths/min
PEEP or CPAP: 0–45 cm H_2O
Pressure support: 0–60 cm H_2O
Sensitivity: 0 to −5 cm H_2O

Bias flow: 0–30 L/min
F_{IO_2}: 0.21–1.00

Other features: SIMV, A-C, sigh, and CPAP; nebulizer; alarms for high and low pressure, high and low minute volume, inspiratory time too long, system failure, gas supply failure, and power failure; monitors tidal volume (VT) inspired, VT set, inspired minute volume, PIP, mean airway pressure, baseline pressure, and peak flow

Sechrist Ventilators

Sechrist IV-100

Power source: pneumatic
Control circuit: electronically and fluidically
Cycling control variable: time
Inspiratory waveform: constant flow
Pressure limit: 5–75 cm H_2O
Flow range: 0–30 L/min
Frequency: 1–150 breaths/min
Inspiratory time: 0.1–2.9 seconds
Expiratory time: 0.3–60 seconds
PEEP: −2 to +20 cm H_2O
F_{IO_2}: 0.21–1.00

Other features: IMV, I/E range of 10:1–1:300; alarms for low and high pressure, power loss, air or O_2 source failure, and failure to cycle; mean airway pressure display; CRT screen monitor for pressure and flow waveform.

Sechrist 2200B (adult or pediatric use)

Power source: pneumatic (built-in compressor optional)
Control circuit: microprocessor
Cycling control variable: time, pressure, volume
Inspiratory waveform: constant (rectangular), descending ramp
Pressure limit: 10–115 cm H_2O
Flow range: 2–120 L/min
Frequency: 0.5–60 breaths/min
Inspiratory time: 0.2–3.0 seconds
PEEP or CPAP: 0 to +30 cm H_2O
F_{IO_2}: 0.21–1.00

Other features: SIMV, A-C, sigh mode, PSV, PCV, MMV; alarms for low and high pressure, apnea, high and low tidal volume, high and low minute volume, high and low rate, source gas failure, and power failure; nebulizer

Siemens Ventilators

Servo 900B

Power source: pneumatic
Control circuit: electronic servo control of pneumatic system
Cycling control variable: volume, time, or pressure
Inspiratory waveform: constant (rectangular)
Pressure limit: 0–120 cm H_2O
Minute volume: 0.5–25 L/min
Flow range: up to 120 L/min measured against 40 cm H_2O back pressure
Frequency: 6–60 breaths/min on A-C or 6–60 divided by 2, 5, or 10 on IMV
Inspiratory time: 15%–50% of cycle time
PEEP: 0–50 cm H_2O
F_{IO_2}: 0.21–1.00

Other features: pause time 0%–30% of cycle time, sensitivity −25 to +45 cm H_2O, sigh mode; alarms for high and low minute volume, high pressure, and disconnection; SIMV mode, single circuit, high internal resistance

Servo 900C

Power source: pneumatic
Control circuit: electronic
Cycling control variable: flow, time, or pressure
Inspiratory waveform: rectangular, and descending and ascending ramp
Pressure limit: 0–120 cm H_2O
Minute volume: 0.4–40 L/min
Flow range: up to 120 L/min measured against 40 cm H_2O back pressure
Frequency: 6–120 breaths/min
Inspiratory time: 20%–80% of cycle time
PEEP: 0–50 cm H_2O
F_{IO_2}: 0.21–1.00

Other features: SIMV, pressure support (0–100 cm H_2O), pressure control (0–100 cm H_2O), sensitivity 0 to −20 cm H_2O, sigh mode; alarms for high pressure, apnea, high and low minute volume, low source gas, high and low O_2 concentration, and loss of power; additional options: inspiratory and expiratory pause buttons, gas change button

Servo 300

Power source: pneumatic
Control circuit: electronic, and microprocessor-controlled
Cycling control variable: volume, time, flow, or pressure
Inspiratory waveform: rectangular, descending ramp, exponential
Pressure limit: 0–120 cm H_2O
Flow range: 6 mL/min–180 L/min;
SIMV: 0.5–40 L/min
Frequency: 5–150 breaths/min
Inspiratory time: 10%–80% of cycle time
Pause time: 0%–30%
PEEP or CPAP: 0–50 cm H_2O
F_{IO_2}: 0.21–1.00

Other features: volume support, SIMV, volume control plus PS, SIMV, PCV plus PS, pressure support, pressure control, pressure-regulated volume control, PS plus CPAP; inspiratory flow rise time percentage, sigh mode; alarms for high pressure, apnea, high and low minute volume, low source gas, high and low O_2 concentration, technical alarm and loss of power; additional options: inspiratory and expiratory pause buttons, gas change button

Sensormedics Corp.

3100A Oscillatory Ventilator

Power: electric
Control: electronic
Cycling control variable: time
Waveform: modified sine
Inspiratory time: 30%–50%
Frequency: 3–15 Hz (180–900 breaths/min)
Pressure limit: 0–95 cm H_2O
Mean airway pressure: 10–45 cm H_2O
External blender
External humidifier
Bias flow: flush gas (adjustable)

Alarms: above or below mean airway pressure, low battery, auto-dump greater than 50 cm H_2O, ventilator overheat, ventilator stopped, gas supply low.

APPENDIX F. Endotracheal Tube Complications and Complications Associated With Tracheostomy

Endotracheal Tube Complications

A. Damage to the nasal passages and lips
   1. During insertion: facial trauma, damage to the nasal structures, or lips during insertion
   2. While in place: lip ulceration, pressure necrosis to the soft tissues, erosion of nasal septum, increased airway resistance from a small tube lumen
   3. During and after extubation: nasal stricture

B. Damage to the oropharynx
   1. During insertion: traumatic damage to the oropharyngeal soft tissues, dental accidents, retropharyngeal or hypopharyngeal perforation
   2. While in place: grooving of the hard palate from chronic pressure, dental deformities from constant pressure

C. Damage to the larynx and trachea
   1. During insertion: soft tissue damage (bleeding and swelling), laryngeal trauma, laryngospasm
   2. While in place: laryngeal injury (ulceration, edema, bleeding), laryngeal muscle dysfunction, subglottic edema, necrosis over the arytenoid cartilages and the vocal cords, in infants trauma to mucosa covering the cricoid cartilage, necrosis of tissue leading to the innominate artery and uncontrolled bleeding, tracheal injury (ulceration, edema, bleeding, tracheomalacia, cartilage and mucosal necrosis), laryngotracheal web formation, laryngotracheal granuloma, tracheal dilation, irritation of the carina, tracheoesophageal fistula, spontaneous dislocation of the tube (into the right mainstem, too high in trachea, extubation), squamous metaplasia of respiratory epithelium
   3. During and after extubation: laryngospasm, laryngeal edema, glottic injury, laryngotracheal granuloma, laryngeal stenosis (glottic, subglottic), laryngeal motor dysfunction (vocal cord paralysis), cricoarytenoid ankylosis, tracheomalacia, tracheal dilation, tracheal stenosis, perichondritis, laryngeal chondritis, laryngotracheal web

D. Patient problems associated with artificial airways
   1. During intubation: intubation of the right mainstem bronchus, bronchospasm, pulmonary aspiration, barotrauma, cardiopulmonary arrest, hypoxemia, cardiac arrhythmias, cervical and spinal cord injuries, patient discomfort
   2. While in place: patient discomfort, difficulty in communicating, pain, retching, salivation, malnutrition, sinusitis, otitis media, atelectasis, pneumonia, pulmonary aspiration, decreased mucociliary transport, ineffective cough, contamination of the airway from suctioning and invasion of the normal lung defenses, bronchial mucosal damage from suctioning
   3. During and after extubation: hoarseness, sore throat, dysphagia, bronchospasm, aspiration, cardiac arrest

E. Mechanical problems with tubes
   Disconnection, kinking, obstruction from secretions, patient biting on the tube, displacement of the tube tip into the tracheal endothelial layer or against the side of the trachea or carina

F. Mechanical problems associated with the cuff
   Herniation of the cuff over the tube tip, compression of the tube by the cuff, excessive pressure (>25 mm Hg) from overinflation leading to tracheal necrosis, leaking or rupturing of the cuff causing inadequate ventilation, laceration of the cuff during insertion, leaking around the cuff preventing adequate ventilation, damage to the pilot balloon or connection preventing cuff inflation

Complications Associated With Tracheostomy

A. During the surgical procedure: bleeding, thyroid injury, inappropriate incision position (too high or too low), injury to the recurrent laryngeal nerve, pneumothorax, tracheoesophageal fistula, subcutaneous emphysema, mediastinal emphysema, placement of the tube into the pretracheal space, cuff laceration during insertion, cardiac arrest, hypoxia
B. While in place: patient discomfort, infection of the wound or trachea, bleeding (skin vessel, tracheoarterial fistula), tracheal injury (inflammation, bleeding, ulceration, necrosis), tracheal dilation, web formation, perforation of trachea, granuloma formation, pseudomembrane formation, irritation of the carina, tracheoesophageal fistula, sepsis, mediastinitis, atelectasis, pneumonia, aspiration, subcutaneous emphysema, mediastinal emphysema, pneumothorax, decannulation, reduced mucociliary transport, ineffective cough, mechanical problems with the tube or cuff (see endotracheal tube), squamous metaplasia of respiratory epithelium
C. During and after decannulation: tight stoma making decannulation diffi-

cult, patient discomfort, scarring, keloid formation, persistent open stoma, dysphagia, tracheal stenosis, tracheomalacia, tracheal granuloma, tracheal web formation, or tracheal dilation

APPENDIX G. Suctioning of the Airway and Tracheostomy Tube Care

Suctioning

Technique

1. Use sterile procedure and universal precautions (gloves, mask, goggles).
2. Preoxygenate and hyperinflate patient with 100% oxygen and resuscitation bag.
3. Select suction catheter, vacuum source, vacuum regulator and bottle, and wye connector. Suction catheter outer diameter should not exceed one-half the inner diameter of the endotracheal tube. Its length should be sufficient to pass the distal tip of the tube.
4. Insert catheter without applying suction.
5. Apply suction (−80 to −120 mm Hg in adults) intermittently while rotating and withdrawing catheter. Never exceed −150 mm Hg.
6. Never exceed 15 seconds of suctioning.
7. Hyperoxygenate and hyperinflate between suctioning maneuver and after the final suctioning.
8. With thick secretions, instill 1 to 2 mL of sterile normal saline into the airway, and hyperinflate for two to four breaths and repeat suction procedure
9. Rinse the catheter and suction out the upper airway.
10. Deflate cuff while hyperinflating the airway and repeat oropharyngeal suctioning.
11. Reinflate the cuff and discard equipment.
12. Reevaluate patient's breath sounds.
13. Record findings.

Complications

1. Hypoxemia
2. Cardiac dysrhythmias:
   Bradycardia—vagal stimulation or hypoxemia
   Tachycardia—hypoxemia or sympathetic excitation (stress and anxiety to patient)
3. Mucosal damage

4. Hypotension
5. Lung collapse – decreased FRC
6. Aspiration
7. Cross-infection

Tracheostomy and Tracheostomy Tube Cleaning

1. Perform as needed or about every 4 to 8 hours.
2. Tracheostomy stoma care:
   Use aseptic technique.
   Clean stoma site with 3% hydrogen peroxide after removing old dressings.
   Rinse with sterile water and place a sterile dry gauze dressing around site.
   Change fabric ties to tracheostomy tube.
3. Inner cannula cleaning
   Remove inner cannula.
   Insert a sterile tracheostomy adaptor and reconnect patient to ventilator.
   Place inner cannula into basin of 3% hydrogen peroxide and sterile water and scrub clean.
   Rinse inner cannula with sterile water.
   Reinsert cannula and reconnect patient to ventilator.

APPENDIX H. Calculation of Oxygen Content: Comparison of Normal and Anemic Patients

Combined O_2 (attached to hemoglobin) in vol % = Hb × 1.34 × Sao_2
where Hb is hemoglobin in g/dL and Sao_2 is oxygen saturation

Dissolved O_2 (in the plasma) in vol % = Pao_2 × 0.003

Add dissolved O_2 and combined O_2 to obtain total O_2 content in vol %.

Example with normal patients:
Hb = 15 g/dL
Pao_2 = 100 mm Hg
Sao_2 = 100% = 1.00 (as a fraction)
15 × 1.34 × 1.00 = 20.10 vol %
100 × 0.003 = 0.03 vol %
Total = 20.40 vol %

Example with anemic patients:
Hb = 10 g/dL

Pa_{O_2} = 100 mm Hg
Sa_{O_2} = 100% = 1.00 (as a fraction)
10 × 1.34 × 1.00 = 13.4 vol %
100 × 0.003 = 0.39 vol %
Total = 13.79 vol %

APPENDIX I. Dead Space–Tidal Volume (V_D/V_T) Measurements on Mechanical Ventilator Patients

1. Collect and assemble appropriate equipment as pictured in Figure 9–17 for expired gas collection.
2. Collect the exhaled gas in a 100-L Douglas bag with a three-way stopcock or a 9-L anesthesia bag with an Ambu E valve connected to the exhalation valve assembly.
3. Suction the collection bag until it is empty.
4. Collect gas for 3 to 4 minutes; re-empty the bag and then collect again for 3 to 4 minutes.
5. Draw an arterial blood gas sample.
6. If the expired air is collected at the normal exhalation valve, measure the volume lost due to tubing compliance before making the calculations.
7. Check the patient's V_T (delivered).
8. Analyze the samples for Pa_{CO_2} and $P\bar{E}_{CO_2}$.
9. Remove the unnecessary equipment and calculate the results.

APPENDIX J. Calculation of the Clinical Shunt Fraction Given Arterial and Venous Blood Values

Barometric pressure (P_B) = 747 mm Hg
Hemoglobin (Hb) = 10 g
FI_{O_2} = 1.0
Pa_{O_2} = 85 mm Hg
Pa_{CO_2} = 40 mm Hg
pH = 7.36
Sa_{O_2} = 94%
$P\bar{v}_{O_2}$ = 39 mm Hg
$S\bar{v}_{O_2}$ = 70%
R = 0.8

$$\dot{Q}s/\dot{Q}t = \frac{P(A - a)O_2 \times 0.003}{C(a - \bar{v})O_2 + P(A - a)O_2 \times 0.003}$$

Step 1: Calculate PAO_2

$PAO_2 = FIO_2\ (PB - 47) - PacO_2\ [FIO_2 + (1 - FIO_2/R)]$

$PAO_2 = 1.0\ (747 - 47) - 40\ [1.0 + (1 - 1.0/0.8)]$

$PAO_2 = 700 - 40 = 660$ mm Hg

Step 2: Calculate $P(A - a)O_2 \times 0.003$

$PAO_2 = 660$

$PaO_2 = 85$

$PAO_2 - PaO_2 = 660 - 85 = 575$

$P(A - a)O_2 \times 0.003 = 1.73$ vol %

Step 3: Calculate $C(a - \bar{v})O_2$

$CaO_2 = (PaO_2 \times 0.003) + (SaO_2 \times 1.34 \times Hb)$

$CaO_2 = (85 \times 0.003) + (94\% \times 1.34 \times 10)$

$CAO_2 = 0.255 + [.94$ (as a fraction) $\times 1.34 \times 10]$

$CAO_2 = 0.26 + 12.6 = 12.86$ vol%

$C\bar{v}O_2 = (P\bar{v}O_2 \times 0.003) + (S\bar{v}O_2 \times 1.34 \times Hb)$

$C\bar{v}O_2 = (39 \times 0.003) + [0.70$ (as a fraction) $\times 1.34 \times 10]$

$C\bar{v}O_2 = 0.117 + 9.38 = 9.5$ vol %

$C(a - \bar{v})O_2 = 12.86 - 9.5 = 3.36$ vol %

Step 4: Solve for shunt fraction

$$\dot{Q}s/\dot{Q}t = \frac{P(A - a)O_2 \times 0.003}{C(a - \bar{v})O_2 + P(A - a)O_2 \times 0.003}$$

$\dot{Q}s/\dot{Q}t = 1.73$ vol %/(3.36 vol % + 1.73 vol %)

$\dot{Q}s/\dot{Q}t = 0.339$ or 34% shunt

APPENDIX K. Calculation of Tidal Volume and Static Compliance During PEEP

The table below shows how to calculate actual tidal volume delivery and static compliance during mechanical ventilation with PEEP when the exhaled tidal volumes are measured at the exhalation valve and not at the endotracheal tube.*

Static compliance (Cs) estimates lung compliance and chest wall compliance together:

Cs = actual tidal volume (VT) exhaled/(plateau pressure minus positive end-expiratory pressure)

Cs = VT/(PPlateau − PEEP); PEEP must include auto-PEEP

Measured tidal volume (Meas VT) is measured at the exhalation valve using a respirometer. Tubing compliance (see Chapter 8) is 3 mL/cm H_2O for this example. Actual VT (Act. VT) is the measured VT minus volume lost to tubing compliance (tubing V) which is the tubing compliance factor (3 mL/cm H_2O) times the plateau pressure. (Static compliance calculation and determination of actual VT uses the plateau pressure reading and not the peak pressure.)

$$\text{Actual tidal volume (Act. V}_T) = \text{measured V}_T - (\text{P}_{Peak} \times 3 \text{ mL/cm H}_2\text{O})$$
$$= \text{measured V}_T - \text{tubing V}$$

Time	Plateau pressure	PEEP	Meas. VT	Act. VT	$Cs = \frac{\text{Act. V}_T}{\text{P}_{Plateau} - \text{PEEP}}$
1	30	0	1000	1000 − [3 × (30−0)] = 1000 − 90 = 910	$Cs = \frac{910}{30 - 0}$ Cs = 30.33 mL/cm H_2O
2	33	5	1000	1000 − [3 × (33 − 5)] = 1000 − 84 = 916	$Cs = \frac{916}{33 - 5}$ Cs − 32.7 mL/cm H_2O
3	38	10	1000	1000 − [3 × (38 − 10)] = 916	$Cs = \frac{916}{38 - 10}$ Cs = 32.7 mL/cm H_2O
4	42	15	1000	1000 − [3 × (42 − 15)] 1000 − 81 = 918	$Cs = \frac{918}{42 - 15}$ Cs = 34 mL/cm H_2O

*See Demers RR, Pratter MR, Irwin RS: *Respir Care* 1981; 26:644–648, for further details.

APPENDIX L. Fluid Volume Challenge for Augmenting Blood Volume and Cardiac Output With PEEP Increases

1. Assess patient's clinical condition and baseline cardiopulmonary data.
2. Administer between 50 and 200 mL of an appropriate solution over a 10-minute period. The volume may be a colloid such as blood, plasma, albumin, or dextran, or it may be a crystalloid such as saline, Ringer's lactate, or 5% D/W depending on the clinician's choice.
3. Observe the clinical condition of the patient and the changes in clinical data such as blood pressure, peripheral perfusion, and urinary output.
4. Measure the PCWP for change:
   a. If PCWP changes less than 3 mm Hg, repeat the challenge until systemic circulation improves or until adverse physical findings occur, such as the presence of crackles (rales) when listening to the breath sounds.
   b. If PCWP rises more than 7 mm Hg, then it is unlikely that more volume will benefit the patient in most clinical situations.

c. If the change in PCWP is between 3 and 7 mm Hg, wait 10 minutes and repeat the PCWP measurement. If the change is less than 3 mm Hg, go to step a (above). If the change is more than 7 mm Hg, go to step b (above). If the change is still between 3 and 7 mm Hg, repeat the fluid challenge, but use less volume.

APPENDIX M. Estimating Transmural PCWP (PCWPtm) With PEEP

1. PCWPtm with spontaneous breathing normal intrapleural pressure = −5 cm H_2O (−3 mm Hg)
   Recall: 1 mm Hg = 1.36 cm H_2O
   Normal PCWP = 10 mm Hg
   PCWPtm = PCWP − intrapleural pressure
   PCWPtm = 10 mm Hg − (−3 mm Hg)
   PCWPtm = 13 mm Hg
2. PCWPtm with PEEP
   Approximately one third to one half of the PEEP will be transmitted to the intrapleural space in a patient with stiff lungs. We use one third for this example.
   If PEEP = 20 cm H_2O (15 mm Hg) the intrapleural pressure ≈ [1/3 × 15 mm Hg − (normal intrapleural pressure)]
   Intrapleural pressure = 5
   PCWPtm = PCWP − (intrapleural pressure)
   PCWP = 15 mm Hg − (5 mm Hg) = 10 mm Hg
   (PCWP will be higher than normal with PEEP in most cases. PCWPtm is near normal.)
   Note: PCWP should be measured during exhalation; estimates of intrapleural pressure are only estimates since variations in compliance between patients will affect the amount of pressure transmitted to the intrapleural space. PEEP should not be removed to measure PCWP if at all possible.

Index

B

C

I

N

O

P

R

S

W